SPORTS AND ATHLETICS PREPARATION, PERFORMANCE, AND PSYCHOLOGY SERIES

ENCYCLOPEDIA OF SPORTS AND ATHLETICS

SPORTS AND ATHLETICS PREPARATION, PERFORMANCE, AND PSYCHOLOGY SERIES

Is Sports Nutrition for Sale?
Ethical Issues and Professional Concerns for Exercise Physiologists
William T. Boone
2005. ISBN: 1-59454-422-0

Doping in Sports
Christopher N. Burns (Editor)
2006. ISBN: 1-59454-683-5

Literature Reviews in Sport Psychology
Sheldon Hanton and Stephen Mellalieu (Editors)
2006. ISBN: 1-59454-904-4

Hot Topics in Sports and Athletics
Samuel R. Bakere (Editor)
2008. ISBN: 978-1-60456-077-0

Sports Injuries and Their Effects on Health
Robert R. Salerno (Editor)
2009. ISBN: 978-1-60741-507-7

A Competitive Anxiety Review: Recent Directions in Sport Psychology Research
Stephen D. Mellalieu, Sheldon Hanton and David Fletcher
2009. ISBN: 978-1-60692-248-4

A Competitive Anxiety Review: Recent Directions in Sport Psychology Research
Stephen D. Mellalieu, Sheldon Hanton and David Fletcher
2009. ISBN: 978-1-60876-405-1 (Online book)

Former NFL Players: Disabilities, Benefits, and Related Issues
Thomas P. Wasser (Editor)
2009. ISBN: 978-1-60692-346-7

Thoroughbred Horseracing and the Welfare of the Thoroughbred
Cameron L. Stratton (Editor)
2009. ISBN: 978-1-60692-724-3

Advances in Strength and Conditioning Research
Michael Duncan and Mark Lyons (Editors)
2009. ISBN: 978-1-60692-909-4

Advances in Strength and Conditioning Research
Michael Duncan and Mark Lyons (Editors)
2009. ISBN: 978-1-60876-661-1 (Online book)

Contemporary Sport Psychology
Robert Schinke (Editor)
2009. ISBN: 978-1-60876-150-0

Handbook of Sports Psychology
Calvin H. Chang (Editor)
2009. ISBN: 978-1-60741-256-4

Aerobic Exercise and Athletic Performance: Types, Duration and Health Benefits
David C. Lieberman (Editor)
2010. ISBN: 978-1-60876-217-0

Strength Training: Types and Principles, Benefits and Concerns
James T. Kai (Editor)
2010. ISBN: 978-1-60876-221-7

Advancements in the Scientific Study of Combative Sports
Jason E. Warnick and W. Daniel Martin (Editors)
2010. ISBN: 978-1-60876-733-5

Aerobic Exercise in Special Populations
Carlos Ayan Perez , Jose Maria Cancela Carral, and Silvia Varela Martinez
2010. ISBN: 978-1-60876-697-0

Sport-Specific Strength Training: Background, Rationale, and Program
Del P. Wong, Michael A. Tse, June Lee-chuen Chin and Christopher Carling
2010. ISBN: 978-1-61668-259-0

Sport-Specific Strength Training: Background, Rationale, and Program
Del P. Wong, Michael A. Tse, June Lee-chuen Chin and Christopher Carling
2010. ISBN: 978-1-61668-600-0 (Online book)

SPORTS AND ATHLETICS PREPARATION, PERFORMANCE, AND PSYCHOLOGY SERIES

ENCYCLOPEDIA OF SPORTS AND ATHLETICS

JACK L. MURRAY
AND
EMILY O. WATSON
EDITORS

Nova Science Publishers, Inc.
New York

Library of Congress Cataloging-in-Publication Data

Encyclopedia of sports and athletics / editors, Jack L. Murray and Emily O.
Watson.
p. cm.
Includes index.
ISBN 978-1-61209-959-0 (hardcover)
1. Sports sciences--Encyclopedias. 2. Athletics--Encyclopedias. 3.
Sports--Physiological aspects--Encyclopedias. 4. Sports--Psychological
aspects--Encyclopedias. I. Murray, Jack L. II. Watson, Emily O.
GV558.E525 2011
613.7'1--dc22

2011005293

Published by Nova Science Publishers, Inc. ✝ New York

Contents

Preface

This new book presents and discusses current research in the study of sports and athletics. Topics discussed include the anti-inflammatory effects of exercise; the role of physical exercise in Parkinson's disease; the health benefits of aerobic activity and physical fitness in young people; physiological evaluation of athletic performance in cyclic sports; social and environmental influences on athlete motivation in sports; self-talk in sports; mental toughness; the role of physical activity in the treatment and prevention of anxiety and depression in children and being superstitious in sports

Chapter I - "Currently, modern chronic diseases are the leading killers in Westernized society and are increasing rampantly in developing nations. Considerable knowledge has accumulated in recent decades showing that physical exercise can be a very effective non-pharmacological strategy in the treatment of these pathologies, and as a result, several types of physical exercise are recommended in this matter. Aerobic exercise has been recognized as a safe and beneficial physical training modality for a number of chronic conditions, yet physicians do not know how to prescribe it. This chapter aims to discuss the effects of aerobic exercise in the treatment of metabolic syndrome-related disorders (diabetes, hypertension and obesity), heart and pulmonary diseases (coronary heart disease, chronic obstructive pulmonary disease and asthma), locomotive apparatus disorders (rheumatoid arthritis, osteoporosis systemic lupus erythematosus and fibromyalgia), neurological diseases (multiple sclerosis), and gastrointestinal disorders (Crohns Disease). The suggested potential mechanisms for the beneficial effects of aerobic exercise are discussed and some basic guidelines for exercise prescription in this kind of populations are given."

Chapter II - Public health physical activity recommendations state that moderate-intensity aerobic physical activity for a minimum of 30 min on at least five days each week confers substantial protection against chronic diseases such as cardiovascular disease, atherosclerosis, type 2 diabetes, insulin resistance, colon cancer and breast cancer. The mechanisms responsible for the protective effects of exercise are not completely clear. Nowadays it is well-known that these diseases are associated with chronic low-grade systemic inflammation. Thus, it has been suggested that the modification of the levels of the inflammation markers may have therapeutic potential.

In general, the plasma cytokines found following acute bouts of exercise suggest that exercise induces a strong anti-inflammatory effect. This finding may provide, in part, a mechanism as to why physical exercise either reduces the susceptibility to, or improves the symptoms of diseases associated with low-grade inflammation. In fact, muscle contraction induced factors with anti-inflammatory actions, which are released to the circulation during exercise, may be involved in mediating the health beneficial effects of exercise and play important roles in the protection against these diseases associated with low-grade inflammation. Furthermore, cross-sectional studies demonstrate an association between physical inactivity and low-grade systemic inflammation in healthy subjects, in elderly people, as well as in patients with intermittent claudication. However, it is not clear how chronic moderate exercise could perform its anti-inflammatory effects. It has been hypothesized that the long-term healthy effect of exercise may to some extend be ascribed to the anti-inflammatory response elicited by acute bouts of moderate exercise. In addition, it has been suggested that following acute exercise, there is a transient increase in circulating levels of anti-inflammatory factors, whereas chronic exercise reduces basal levels of pro-inflammatory cytokines. Recent studies have suggested that continuous an additional subtle changes resulting in reductions in fat and body mass or in improved lipid and glycemic profiles could induce the anti-inflammatory effect of regular moderate-intensity exercise.

The aim of this review is to examine the anti-inflammatory effects of aerobic exercise and to discuss to what extend the exercise induced anti-inflammatory response may play a therapeutic role in chronic diseases associated with low-grade inflammation.

Chapter III - Parkinson's disease is the second most common neurodegenerative disorder, following Alzheimer's disease, affecting approximately 1% of the population older than 50 years. Since the incidence of the disease increases with age (the most important risk factor), it is likely that the number of people suffering from Parkinson's disease will rise as improved health care lengthens the average life span. Classically, Parkinson's disease is considered to be a motor system disease and its diagnosis is based on the presence of a set of cardinal motor signs (e.g. rigidity, bradykinesia, rest tremor and postural reflex disturbance). These symptoms of Parkinson's disease mainly result from the progressive degeneration of dopamine neurons of the *substantia nigra pars compacta* (SNpc) that project predominantly to the striatum. Nowadays there is considerable evidence showing that deficits in olfactory and cognitive functions precede the classical motor symptoms seen in Parkinson's disease. The beneficial effects of the drugs currently available for the treatment of Parkinson's disease (such as levodopa) on improving the cognitive function affected in this disease is controversial. Thus, the management of non-motor symptoms of Parkinson's disease remains a challenge. Over the last decade, regular physical exercise has been implicated to an increased plasticity in the adult brain (such as increase in neurogenesis and cognitive processes and neurotrophic factors production). Research is now emerging on a possible influence of physical exercise in the neurodegenerative process associated to Parkinson's disease. The present chapter attempts to review results reported in different clinical studies and animal models to provide a comprehensive picture of the role of physical exercise in Parkinson's disease. Although many of the training programs investigated were accompanied by some degree of oxidative stress, which should be taken into account in physical training programs for this population, it is important to emphasize that this response did not promote any negative impact on the rehabilitation aspects of Parkinson's disease patients. Taken together, the current literature suggests that regular physical exercise can present beneficial effects in Parkinson's disease patients evaluated through different tests. It might also afford protection against dopaminergic neurons death and motor dysfunction elicited in experimental models. Finally, this chapter shows recent findings from our laboratory indicating that moderate physical exercise plays an important role into improvement cognitive deficits in an experimental model of Parkinson's disease, reinforcing the potential of physical exercise in the management of non-motor symptoms of Parkinson's disease.

Chapter IV – Introduction: The Transalp Challenge (TAC) is one of the most difficult mountainbike (MTB) stage races in the world. Professional and amateur cyclists are required to cope with an altitude difference of 22500 m and a distance of 662 km within eight successive stages. Therefore, the purpose of this study was to determine the nutrient intake during the TAC.

Method: The subject was a female vegan MTBer (age: 30 years, height: 1.61 m, body mass: 49 ± 1 kg) finishing the TAC 2004 (41 hours 59 minutes 45 seconds, final ranking of 16th place). The athlete has been successfully following a vegan lifestyle for five years. Dietary intake was completely recorded over the full period of competition. Fluid intake (FI) and energy intake (EI) were calculated and subdivided into macronutrients carbohydrate (CHO), protein and fat.

Results: The exercise intensity of 88 ± 2 % of HR_{MAX} determined in the field was maintained over eight days. EI was found to be 24.61 MJ/day. Total calories contribute to 83.3 % from CHO, 7.5 % from protein and 9.2 % from fat. The female ingested 17.4 % pre–race, 35.2 % while racing and 47.4 % post–race.

Discussion: This was the first study showing a well planned vegan diet to adequately meet the nutritional demands of severe MTB stage racing. The dietary requirements of a TAC are challenging for several reasons. Opportunities and time available for FI and EI are restricted by a great diversity of terrains and traits (difficult nature of course profile) simultaneously with aggressive riding tactics. After many years of research, mainly focused on health aspects, the effects of a plant–based diet on athletic performance are still unclear. However, any athlete, regardless of whether omnivore or vegan, should plan his/her diet carefully to avoid the risk of nutritional deficiencies and adverse effects on performance. It is broadly accepted that athletes involved in heavy endurance exercise should ingest a higher amount of energy from CHO to maximize muscle glycogen synthesis. The main advantages of vegetarian diets are the higher amount of CHO, lower fat and adequate protein. Especially vegans consume the majority of their energy from CHO. Therefore, endurance athletes may adopt vegetarian diets as an optimum strategy. Generally, endurance training and competition tend to reduce iron stores. However, iron deficiency occurs in 20 % of the world population, reflecting a similar incidence among vegetarians or vegans compared to omnivores.

Chapter V - Over the last decade, there has been growing interest in the health benefits of exercise for the prevention and treatment of metabolic syndrome disorders.

Currently, the effectiveness of exercise to prevent fat mass gain or to improve the health status of obese people has mainly been assessed through the capacity of exercise to elicit the highest rate of whole body fat oxidation. Hence, low to moderate intensity exercise of duration between 30 to 45 minutes is widely recommended. However, numerous factors affect the mechanisms which control substrate mobilization and utilization. For example, maturation induces changes in substrate metabolism as children tend to oxidize more fat at the same relative submaximal intensity than do adults. Also, studies involving women participants have shown a larger contribution of lipids to energy expenditure. These differences are explained by the effects of ovarian hormones on lipids mobilization, muscle free fat and glucose uptake and oxidation. Acute carbohydrate (CHO) ingestion during exercise has been shown to promote increased CHO oxidation. Similarly, long term, diets rich in CHO and fat promote increased oxidation rates. Furthermore, metabolic alterations such as insulin resistance, abdominal obesity or decreased cardiorespiratory fitness are factors associated with alteration of the mobilization and oxidation of lipids in fat depots. If exercise is to be used as a therapy, all these factors must be taken when establishing the intensity, duration and mode of exercise in children and adults.

However, other modes of aerobic exercise could be just as potent in the treatment of diseases associated with obesity. Indeed, results from a smaller number of investigations in trained individuals indicate that higher exercise intensities elicit a higher utilization of intramuscular triglycerides. Furthermore, it has been shown from the work of Essen in the 1970s that high intensity intermittent exercises, which also improve maximal aerobic capacity, can elicit rates of fat oxidation similar to those observed during moderate intensity continuous exercise. Therefore, it remains to be determined if this type of exercise is as effective as low intensity exercises in the treatment of metabolic diseases and to evaluate the relative importance of the fat oxidation rate as the best single criterion outcome.

This review will discuss the relationships between the substrates mobilization and utilization during aerobic exercise and the metabolic health benefits.

Chapter VI - This chapter present the effects of aerobic training on the adaptation of the cardiovascular system to exercise in prepubertal boys and girls. The major results of the scientific literature showed that the training program led to a rise in maximal O_2 uptake (VO_{2max}), brought about however only by an increase in SVmax in both sexes. Moreover, boys increased their VO_{2max} to a greater extent than girls only because of a higher SVmax improvement. No alterations were noticed in the SV pattern from rest to maximal exercise, indicating that the increase in SVrest was a key factor in the improvement of SVmax and thus VO_{2max}. Regarding resting echocardiographic data, an increase in left ventricular end-diastolic diameter, concomitant with an improvement in diastolic function, were observed after training and constituted an essential element in the rise in VO_{2max} after training in these children. Also, during maximal exercise, a decrease in systemic vascular resistances, probably indicating peripheral cardiovascular alterations, could have also play an important role in the increase in VO_{2max}.

Chapter VII - Results from studies involving adult participants have definitively established that physical activity and cardiorespiratory fitness are inversely correlated to morbidity and mortality. The evidence of the health benefits for physically active and fit adults is well known. There is a wealth of data which has shown that physically active and fit adults can help attenuate the effects of hypertension, insulin resistance, hyperlipidemia, obesity and cancer. However, the relationship between activity, fitness and the health benefits during childhood are less well established. Although it is intuitive to propose that an active child will become an active adult, the research evidence is weak. Similarly, the extent to which children's fitness and activity must decrease to seriously compromise their current or future health is also unknown. There is however growing concern for the future health status of children due to the increased levels of overweight and obese children and increased reporting of cardiovascular risk factors. Prospective data is needed to elucidate the complexity of these relationships. This complexity is partially due to problems related to 1) methodology i.e. how do we measure activity and health outcomes precisely; 2) biology i.e. children are growing and maturing at different rates and 3) sociology i.e. the effects of the environment. These problems therefore pose real challenges for policy makers as to whether they should concentrate resources on those child individuals who are deemed 'at risk' i.e. low fitness and low physical activity patterns or to focus across the whole child population. This review will explore the relationships between physical fitness, activity and health in young people as well as describing the evidence for health benefits in this age group. The review will also discuss the implications for strategies of health related physical activity promotion at local and national levels.

Chapter VIII - Physical activity is vital for overall health maintenance, particularly cardiovascular health. Additionally, physical activity is important for decreasing the risk of cancer and osteoporosis in women. Physical fitness, a benefit of physical activity, is important during pregnancy and postpartum periods for both women and their babies. As women became more aware of this issue, their participation in physical activity increased. Upon becoming pregnant, many women posed their Ob/Gyn physicians with the question, "is physical activity during pregnancy safe?" Initially, little was known about the effects physical activity had on the expectant mother or fetal development. Research has led to a better understanding of maternal and fetal physiology and findings highlight the importance of physical activity during this time. This chapter provides an overview, which examines aspects of physical activity in regard to pregnant and lactating women. Based on the available literature, physicians have shifted their focus from assuring patients that physical activity during gestation is safe to encouraging physical activity during pregnancy because of the potential benefits to both the fetus and mother. Ultimately, these benefits are realized at labor and delivery and during the mother's recovery period. Current research into the fetal and neonatal benefits of maternal physical activity is explored. Lactation represents a continuation of the pregnancy, as the mother continues to supply nourishment for her infant. The effects of physical activity during lactation are viewed from the maternal and infant perspective. As research advances, American College of Obstetricians and Gynecologists (ACOG) guidelines continue to reflect these gains in information. An overview of the current ACOG guidelines is considered. Lastly, the chapter expresses what has been done, and what is currently being done to encourage women to stay physically active during their pregnancy.

Chapter IX - The pioneer studies on the biomechanics of martial arts were published in the nineteen sixties and seventies. After these articles were published, several other biomechanical studies have been conducted about martial arts and other related punching sports using a variety of different measures and methods, especially in the last decade. In general, these studies were concerned with the enhancement of performance and extending the understanding of injury risk. This paper presents a comprehensive review on this subject. It is divided in two major topics: the first topic covers articles about the kinetics, kinematics and electromyography of specific hand strikes, kicks, throws and fall techniques; the second topic focus on some aspects of motor behaviors and perceptual abilities fundamental for efficient and successful performances in martial arts and combative sports (i.e. repeatability of movement, reaction times).

Chapter X - Training control and evaluation of athletes is, nowadays, seen as a fundamental tool to increase the efficiency of the training process. Thus, coaches and their collaborators often implement a set of tasks that allow evaluating the level of development of the athletes' performance determinant factors as well as the result and adequacy of the training exercises and programs.

Sport modalities like running, swimming, cycling and rowing, due to their characteristics (individual, cyclic, closed and combined modalities) are more easily measurable. From the several determinants of the specific performance of these athletes, the bioenergetical and biomechanical factors seem to be the most important and, consequently, the most studied.

The purpose of the present chapter is to present recent data obtained in protocols implemented in cyclic sports, giving more emphasis in running and swimming. The bioenergetical studies presented focus on the characterization of the capacity and power of the two larger body energy systems (the aerobic and the anaerobic ones) through the assessment of well-known physiological parameters like the anaerobic threshold, the maximal oxygen uptake (and the corresponding velocities) and the maximal blood lactate concentrations. Complementarily, recently proposed tests are also presented (e.g. critical velocity).

The authors hope that the presented protocols could be well accepted and applied by athletes, coaches and scientists in their training control programs, helping them to increase the training efficiency and even contributing to predict performance.

Chapter XI - The present chapter was designed to investigate the performance and fatigue in an incremental 6 x 1000 m running test. Well-trained endurance athletes performed eight non-fatigued sprints from 5 m $\cdot$ s^{-1} to maximal velocity and the 6 x 1000 m running test on a 200-m indoor track. In order to investigate the fatigue induced changes in force production during running, non-fatigued ground reaction forces and ground contact times were compared to the values measured at the end of the last 1000-m run. The performance in the last 1000 m (V_{1000m}) correlated significantly with VO_{2peak} ($r = 0.68$; $P = 0.001$), velocity at 4 mM blood lactate level ($r = 0.76$; $P = 0.000$), running economy ($r = -0.47$; $P = 0.042$), maximal sprint running velocity ($r = 0.52$; $P = 0.023$) and anaerobic energy production ($r = 0.63$; $P = 0.004$). V_{1000m} was also related to the fatigue at the end of the 6 x 1000 m ($r = -0.63$; $P = 0.004$). When fatigued and non-fatigued running were compared at the same velocity, it was observed that ground contact times increased ($P = 0.001$) and vertical ground reaction forces ($P = 0.000$) decreased in fatigue. The results showed that the performance in the incremental 6 x 1000 m test on a track is not only related to the traditional endurance performance characteristics, but neuromuscular and anaerobic performance characteristics and fatigue resistance are also important determinants of the incremental running test.

Chapter XII – Purpose: To describe the aerobic exercise capacity and its relationship with muscle strength and motor competence in fifteen preterm born school-aged children (9 boys; gestational age (GA) 29.7 ± 1.71 weeks; birth weight (BW) 1313 ± 356 gram; age of assessment 7.99 ± 0.35 years).

Methods: Weight, height and skinfolds were measured in a standardized manner. Muscle strength was assessed with a hand-held dynamometer, pulmonary function using a spirometer, aerobic exercise capacity using a graded treadmill exercise test, and motor competence with the Movement Assessment Battery for Children. In addition, a 3-day physical activity record was filled out.

Results: Aerobic exercise capacity, lower extremity muscle strength and pulmonary function were significantly reduced compared to reference values. Aerobic exercise capacity was associated with pulmonary function and BW.

Conclusion: In the authors pilot study of preterm born children the authors found a reduced aerobic exercise capacity and lower extremity muscle strength in our group. Encouragement of active participation in physical activities from early childhood onwards might be important indicated in preterm born children.

Chapter XIII - This study examined differences in physique and skeletal dimensions between 1146 elite Caucasian athletes classified into endurance, strength, speed, upper body or combined sports categories and controls, to test the hypothesis that athletes of certain types of sport would exhibit a distinct morphology commensurate with their task. Participants were measured by experienced anthropometrists using an internationally-recognised protocol to describe physique. This involved calculating the anthropometric somatotype in terms of fatness, musculoskeletal robustness and linearity. Further skeletal measures were acquired sufficient to describe an array of morphological indices: crural index (tibial height / femur length), skelic index (leg length / sitting height), androgyny index (biacromial breadth / bicristal breadth) and brachial index (forearm length / upper arm length). Significant inter-group differences in indices prevailed after adjustment for age. Endurance athletes had a high crural index and low brachial index, relative to controls. A low skelic index appears characteristic of female strength athletes while a low brachial index is typical of female endurance and strength athletes. Bayesian cluster analysis has shown the crural index in particular is a discriminant in phenotypic categorisation, in addition to the primary somatotype components of endomorphy, mesomorphy and ectomorphy. These findings are congruent with biomechanical imperatives to maximise force and/or minimise energy expenditure offering sports-specific advantage. Because the skeletal relationships do not respond to the conditioning stimulus in the same way adipose and muscle tissue do, the observed inter-group differences suggest a self-selection of athletes into sports in which they are likely to excel.

Chapter XIV - Patients with chronic kidney disease (CKD) have increased cardiovascular morbidity and mortality. They are frequently deconditioned as a result of inactivity, malnutrition, and abnormal muscle function In advanced CKD, hyperparathyroidism, acidosis, and severe catabolism/malnutrition contribute to debility. Patients with CKD often have cardiovascular risk factors such as inadequate blood pressure control, impaired fasting glucose (or overt diabetes), impaired insulin secretion and/or insulin resistance, abnormal lipid profiles, decreased testosterone and/or estrogen levels, and poor quality of life. Other non-traditional risk factors, such as sympathoactivation, inflammation, oxidative stress, and endothelial dysfunction, are also thought to increase cardiovascular morbidity and mortality. In addition to physical disease, CKD is associated with abnormal mental health, including depression, anxiety, and a feeling of helplessness and lack of well-being.

Aerobic exercise has been proposed to have beneficial effects in CKD. This chapter seeks to define the mechanisms whereby aerobic exercise may benefit such patients. The type, duration, and recommended intensity of exercise will be discussed. While aerobic exercise is relatively safe for most CKD patients, the potential pitfalls of aerobic exercise and concerns about its safety will be addressed. The effects of exercise in the adult non-dialysis CKD population and end-stage renal disease (ESRD) population on dialysis will be clarified. Home exercise, and interdialytic versus intradialytic aerobic exercise will be discussed. Children with CKD are also susceptible to muscle weakness, low aerobic capacity, and abnormal fat composition; the impact of aerobic exercise in the pediatric CKD population will also be discussed. The effect of aerobic exercise on muscle weakness, weight loss, graft loss, and mortality in CKD patients post-transplantation will be illuminated. Finally, emphasis will be placed on areas novel to aerobic exercise and CKD requiring further research.

Chapter XV - The aims of the present study were: a) to identify the effects of plyometric training on explosive strength [squat jump (SJ), countermovement jump (CMJ), mechanical power (MP)], agility (AG), and 20-m sprint speed (20 m) variables in young basketball players; and b) to understand the effects of short-term specific detraining and reduced plyometric training on the previously achieved gains.

The sample consisted of nineteen male basketball players (13-14 years old; weight, 61.26.74 kg; height, 175.46.77 cm). The adopted structure was based upon two fundamental phases. First, subjects were submitted to an 8-week plyometric training program (standing jumps, multiple jumps, box drills, depth jumps, jumps with extra-loads), three times a week. At the end of this period, the subjects showed statistically significant increases in all the assessed variables ($p< 0.05$).

Subsequent to the plyometric training application, subjects were randomly assigned to one of two groups: a reduced training group (RT, n=9) and a specific detraining group (SDT, n=10). During the following four weeks, the former performed a single plyometric training session and the latter ceased plyometric activity. Both groups kept on regular basketball practice. In this period, RT group significantly increased ($p< 0.05$) SJ, CMJ, and S20 values, while SDT group showed statistically significant enhances ($p< 0.05$) on 20 m and AG test. The RT and SDT groups maintained the values of the remaining variables. At the end of this period, no statistically significant differences were observed between RT and DTR groups in all the evaluated variables. In conclusion, a) the outcomes highlight the efficacy of the plyometric training design; b) the reduced training program and the specific detraining indistinctly contribute to the explosive strength levels maintenance; and c) basketball training has an obvious power in the maintenance and sustainability of motor performance at least taking into account the applied training program.

Chapter XVI - The home-field advantage is a topic of much debate in the research literature. This experiment attempted to assess whether there was an advantage for boxers performing in a home country in championship bouts due to judging bias. Official records of all championship bouts in 2006 were analyzed to see if the number of judges that shared the champion's home country was associated with a bout's outcome. It was found that the increased number of judges from a champion's home country produced a disadvantage for the champion when the bout occurred in the United States. These findings are discussed in the context of psychological reactivity.

Chapter XVII - According to a recent World Health Organization report, children and adolescents worldwide are physically inactive during 50% of a normal week (http://www.euro.who.int/Document/e82923.pdf) and the low physical activity level tracks into adult life, with one-third of the disease burden in adulthood being related to such youth behaviour as physical inactivity (http://www.who.int/features/factfiles). Current public health policy lacks routine management of asthmatic child patients; therefore, public health promotion for the future referral of paediatric and adolescent asthmatic patients to chest clinics with standardized equipment available for aerobic capacity testing is urgently recommended.

Milgrom & Taussig affirmed that all asthmatic children should be questioned about their "exercise habits and exercise tolerance," and those with a concerning history should have an exercise test. Such recommendations address populations of asthmatic youth in the global community.

Numerous scores of physical activity exist. One was validated recently and originates from a questionnaire concerned with the frequency and extent of vigorous physical recreational and sports activity after school.

Early detection of physical inactivity and low aerobic capacity addressed by relevant public health policy implementations can be expected to reduce individual and public health care costs by preventing morbidity, disability, and mortality from such chronic respiratory diseases as paediatric asthma.

Chapter XVIII- This chapter is intended to provide a comprehensive review of the various theories of social and environmental factors that influence athletes' motivation in sport. In order to achieve this, a short historical review is conducted of the various ways in which motivation has been studied over the past 100 years, culminating in the 'social-cognitive' approach that undergirds several of the current theories of motivation in sport. As an outcome of this brief review, the conceptualisation and measurement of motivation are discussed, with a focus on the manner in which motivation may be influenced by key social agents in sport, such as coaches, parents and peers. This discussion leads to a review of Deci & Ryan's (2000) self-determination theory (SDT), which specifies that environments and contexts which support basic psychological needs (competence, relatedness and autonomy) will produce higher quality motivation than environments which frustrate of exacerbate these needs. The research establishing the ways in which key social agents can support these basic needs is then reviewed, and the review depicts a situation wherein SDT has precipitated a way of studying the socio-environmental influences on motivation that has become quite piecemeal and fragmented. Following this, the motivational climate approach specified in achievement-goals theory is also reviewed. This section reveals a body of research which is highly consistent in its methodology and findings. The following two sections reflect recent debates regarding the nature of achievement goals and the way they are conceptualised (e.g., approach-avoidance goals and social goals), and the implications of this for motivational climate research are discussed. This leads to a section reviewing the current issues and concerns in the study of social and environmental influences on athlete motivation. Finally, future research directions and ideas are proposed to facilitate, precipitate and guide further research into the social and environmental influences on athlete motivation in sport. Recent studies that have attempted to address these issues are reviewed and their contribution is assessed.

Chapter XIX- Superstition can be defined as a person's unrealistic perception of control over behavioral outcomes in different situations. Although it is assumed that superstitious beliefs may help athletes prepare for a competition, they represent a rather unexplored area in sport psychology. The aim of the present study was to investigate the influence of superstitious beliefs on several performance-related dispositions, such as achievement goals, locus of control, self-handicapping and trait anxiety, and then examine the moderating role of athletes' age and years of competitive experience. The sample of the study consisted of 297 male basketball athletes ($M = 23.86$, $SD = 4.63$) participating in Greek professional leagues. The athletes completed a questionnaire regarding measures of positive and negative superstitious beliefs, self-handicapping strategies, internal and external locus of control and luck, achievement goals and trait anxiety. The results of the regression analyses indicated that positive superstitious beliefs significantly predicted self-handicapping and external locus of control. Negative superstitious beliefs were significant predictors of somatic anxiety, worry, and performance avoidance goals. Moderation regression analysis further indicated that the effect of superstitious beliefs on worry was stronger among athletes with less sports experience. The present study provides valuable information regarding the role of superstitious beliefs in better understanding athletes' cognitive and affective responses, and sets the basis for future research in this rather unexplored area.

Paranormal beliefs reflect a person's belief in phenomena that contradict the basic principles of scientific thinking. Those beliefs include superstition (i.e., black cats and breaking mirrors cause bad luck), precognition (i.e., psychics and astrologers can predict the future), extra sensory perception and a range of similar phenomena (i.e., some people can move objects with the power of their mind). In other words, superstitious beliefs reflect people's tendency to make causal inferences and offer explanations for several phenomena without necessarily taking into account, or even sometimes by contradicting, scientific evidence pointing to alternative and more scientifically-grounded explanations.

Past research has shown that superstitious beliefs are associated with adverse psychological outcomes, such as low self-efficacy, high trait anxiety and dissociative experiences , irrational beliefs and external locus of control. On the other hand, Dudley found that higher scores in superstitious beliefs can help improve performance in solving puzzles during instances of uncontrollability because they may prevent this lack of control. The evidenced effect of superstitious beliefs on task performance may have implications for the study of athletes' performance in sports.

Nevertheless, research in this area is scarce. An early study by Neil, Anderson, and Sheppard showed that highly competitive ice hockey athletes were keen on adopting superstitious behaviours, such as rituals. In another study, Buhrmann and Zaugg suggested that higher scores in religiosity led to stronger superstitious beliefs among basketball players. Van Raalte, Brewer, Nemeroff, and Linder further indicated that people who believed they could control chance events through their actions were more likely to adopt superstitious behaviors. Ciborowski suggested that athletes tend to adopt superstitious behaviors as a way to improve their performance, without necessarily admitting a direct connection between the adopted behavior and their actual sports performance. More interestingly, he reported that if an individual believed that a particular behavior could improve performance, that behavior should not be considered superstitious. Furthermore, Bleak and Frederick reported that the use of superstitious rituals varied across sports, and that the most frequently used superstitious behaviors were not necessarily the ones that were rated by the athletes to be most effective in improving sport performance. Finally, a more recent study indicated that superstitious beliefs significantly affected performance in free-throw shot in basketball.

Uncertainty and lack of control have been proliferated as important determinants of superstitious beliefs, similar to the experience of anxiety, In fact, superstitious beliefs may increase during periods of ambiguity, uncertainty, or uncontrollability, and soothe people by providing an illusory sense of control, or at least an explanation of why events are uncontrollable. In simple words, in the face of uncertainty, individuals attempt to achieve control by investing in irrelevant objects or actions, resting on the assumption that there exists a causal link between those objects or actions and particular results.

Despite anecdotal reports published in newspapers and magazines on the influence of superstitious beliefs on sport performance, there is only limited scientific evidence about sport-related superstitions. For instance, Ciborowski and Schippers and Van Lange found that elite athletes are more likely to employ superstitious rituals in high uncertainty and anxiety-provoking situations, as well as in important competitions. Additionally, anxiety was also associated with the use of rituals. Athletes' skill level and task difficulty were also found to influence superstitious beliefs. Specifically, low skill athletes in an easy condition and high skill athletes in difficult condition had the higher scores in superstitious behavior to this evidence, Bleak and Frederick reported that the use of rituals was not associated with anxiety or perceived importance of success in collegiate athletes.

Chapter XX- Developmental risk researchers has made it possible to identify youth who are significantly more likely than their peers to succumb to at-risk and high risk behaviors often leading to emotional or social disturbances. Two forms of risk are recognized by these researchers. The first involves youth with demographic risk are those with multiple environmental at risk experiences that increase the likelihood of disturbance, including poverty, exposure to violence, or familial disruptions. The second focuses on youth with what is commonly referred to as “functional risk.’ Functional risk experiences are those who do not meet recognized criteria for a clinical or psychiatric disorder but do offer evidence of early dysfunctional behaviors that may represent the early stages of such disorders. Both functional and demographic risk has become the basis for selected preventive interventions. This chapter addresses an approach for intervention specialists that offer a case illustration involving student athletes and their use of over the counter pain medications.

Available research suggests that at risk youth are predisposed to drug abuse. Prior to the turn of the century, the NIDA Resiliency and Risk Workgroup convened a group of experienced clinical researchers with expertise in areas of drug abuse and related research to determine how the further application of available research based data can advance prevention effectiveness beyond current levels. Dr. Alan Leshner, Director of the National Institute on Drug Abuse is a psychologist and behavioral scientist and provided the leadership for this team. The research team generated several key recommendations that should be a model for prevention science research. The major recommendations of the group included advocated the development of prevention interventions which target: youth within the family setting and encouraged family functioning and communication as critical buffer against problematic personality characteristics and at risk behaviors among youth.

Chapter XXI- Objective

Characteristics of social relationships such as friendship quality have important motivational implications within the context of sport. The purpose of this study was to examine the utility of Basic Psychological Needs Theory as a framework for understanding friendship quality amongst athletes competing in adapted sport.

Methods

Participants (N = 51; 55.80% male) drawn from cohorts reporting either a congenital or acquired disability completed a self-report instrument on a single occasion assessing perceived competence, autonomy and relatedness experienced when engaged in adapted sport. The instrument also contained the Sport Friendship Quality Scale to assess perceived friendship quality in sport.

Results: Bivariate correlations revealed a pattern of moderate-to-strong correlations between the five SFQS dimensions and a weak-to-moderate pattern of associations between indices of psychological need satisfaction. Simultaneous multiple regression models indicated that perceptions of psychological need satisfaction accounted for small-to-moderate amounts of the variance in the five SFQS constructs. Perceived relatedness was the dominant predictor of sport friendship quality irrespective of the SFSQ dimension investigated with the strongest association evident with SFSQ-Companionship and Pleasant Play and the weakest with SFSQ-Conflict.

Conclusion

Overall, this study offers initial support for the role of BPNT's psychological needs within the realm of adapted sport as a vehicle for understanding sport friendships. It appears that perceived relatedness with fellow athletes in adapted sport contexts is a plausible route for developing secure friendships within the realm of adapted sport. The extent to which perceptions of autonomy and competence matter in relation to friendship experiences within adapted sport contexts beyond perceived relatedness warrants further inquiry.

Chapter XXII- Mental toughness is a term frequently used in the sporting community by athletes, coaches and psychologists alike to differentiate the "good" from the "great" in their pursuit for sporting excellence. When physical, technical and tactical skills are evenly matched, which so often is the case at the highest levels of competition, it is often the 'mentally toughest' of the two that is thought to prevail. In recent years, momentum has gathered and significant developments in the mental toughness literature have been made which has led to growing understanding of the construct. Nevertheless, concurrence concerning its conceptualisation, definition and how it is developed is yet to be established. The aim of this review is to present the current emerging definitions and conceptualisations of mental toughness, to examine the developments in measuring mental toughness and explore recent findings in the literature. Future research directions will then be discussed.

Chapter XXIII- Self-talk (similar terms: inner speech, private speech, egocentric speech, internal dialogue, internal monologue, verbal rehearsal and self-statements) includes all intentional and automatic self-focused thoughts that run through an individual's mind. The notion of automatic self-talk implies individuals are not always aware they are engaging in private inner speech; yet, self-talk is a robust phenomenon that is one of the most frequent cognitive activities in human life. Almost every minute of our waking life we talk to ourselves. According to Morin the frequency, duration and intensity of self-talk increases when conflicting perspectives within the self or between the self and others occurs.

A workable definition of self-talk is still evolving as no universal definition has been agreed upon with the extant literature. To date, different definitions have been posited that vary in the emphasis they place on both the behavioural and cognitive aspects of self-talk.

Chapter XXIV- Previous research found that highly identified fans report a willingness to engage in a variety of behaviors designed to assist their team, including instrumental aggression, illegal/unethical acts, and superstitious behaviors. The current investigation extended past research by investigating a willingness to engage in acts of desperation (e.g., giving up all drinks except water) if doing so would guarantee a championship. It was hypothesized that higher levels of team identification and rooting for a team that had failed to win a recent championship would predict willingness to consider the acts of desperation. Participants (n = 655) completed a questionnaire packet assessing demographics, team identification with one's favorite Major League Baseball team, and willingness to consider 22 acts of desperation. Regression analysis confirmed both hypotheses and also indicated that men were more likely than women to consider the acts of desperation.

Chapter XXV- Engagement in physical activity and sports, either actively as an athlete or in a passive way as a spectator is of great importance in many people's lives across countries and throughout history. Many studies have dealt with the outcomes of active engagement in sports and there has also been research on the impact of sport events on spectators, i.e. individuals who witness a sports event in person or via the media. Attending sports events or watching them on television can impact individual functioning on many levels, including interpersonal behaviour (e.g., violence) and physical and mental health. Sports-related violence usually refers to aggression and riots by sports fans, and includes soccer hooliganism, but watching sports events might also increase the risk of domestic violence against women by legitimizing and reinforcing violent behaviour. Some major sports events, such as international championships and Olympic Games have been found to change patterns of mortality from coronary heart disease and stroke and to have an impact on the number of presentations to Accident and Emergency Departments. However, this relationship cannot be generalised to all sports events and all groups of spectators.

In regards to mental health and wellbeing, watching games might increase a sense of belonging, allow for release of tension, induce positive mood and reduce the number of psychiatric presentations. However, the defeat of the favoured team may lead to high psychological distress, in some cases reaching clinically significant levels similar to the impact of traumatic events, such as physical threats and natural disasters. Being involved in sports as a spectator might also have an impact on suicidal behaviour, either increasing the risk or being a protective factor, and this chapter reviews the existing evidence regarding this relationship.

Chapter XXVI- This study investigated predictors of collective efficacy in elite female athletes using Hierarchical Linear Modeling (HLM). HLM analyses both individual and team level effects simultaneously and addresses a perennial issues in collective efficacy research, namely the unit of analysis and the cross-level effects. The participants were 318 elite female netball players from 31 teams. Participants completed a questionnaire within 24 hours of the start of either of two national level competitions. The questionnaire included a demographic section and questions relating to team functioning as well as four measures (i.e., Perceptions of Success (POS), Sources of Sport Confidence (SSCQ), Group Environment Questionnaire (GEQ), and a Collective Efficacy measure developed for the present study). Using the procedure suggested by Bryk and Raudenbush, the results suggest that the team level predictors accounted for approximately 73 % of the variance in collective efficacy at the team level. Overall, mastery orientations of the POS (at the player level), length of time spent in team meetings and team cohesion (Group Integration-Task subscale of the GEQ) (at the team level) were found to be significant predictors of collective efficacy. The results do not support those of Spink who noted social aspects of team cohesion to be related to collective efficacy. Results concur with previous research by Paskevich, Brawley, Dorsch and Widmeyer who noted task related aspects of team cohesion to be related to collective efficacy.

Chapter XXVII- Social physique anxiety (SPA) is the anxiety experienced in response to others' real or perceived evaluations of one's physique. In physical activity contexts, SPA can exacerbate performance anxiety concerns and diminish self-efficacy. In the present experiment, we examined the effects of positive and neutral performance feedback on self-presentational efficacy and whether SPA moderates those effects. Forty women (M_{age} = 20.93±2.77) were randomly assigned to receive either positive or neutral performance feedback after performing a strength and endurance task. They then completed a measure of self-presentational efficacy and the Social Physique Anxiety Scale. The performance feedback manipulation did not have a main effect on self-presentational efficacy. However, results of a hierarchical multiple regression analysis revealed that SPA did indeed moderate the effects of feedback on self-presentational efficacy. Women with higher SPA had lower self-presentational efficacy after receiving positive feedback than after receiving neutral feedback. Among women with lower SPA, there were no differential effects of feedback condition on self-presentational efficacy. These results are interpreted taken as indication that

SPA can influence how women interpret feedback regarding their performance on physical tasks. In particular, for women with high SPA, it cannot be assumed that positive feedback will always have positive effects on self-presentational efficacy.

Chapter XXVIII- Anxiety and depression were the major mental health disease in worldwide. The prevalence of anxiety and depression in children and adolescents were accelerating at an alarming rate. Previous studies reported that 5.7% to 17.7% children were suffering from anxiety and 2% to 5% of them with diagnosed depression. Anxiety might lead to serious impairment to individual daily lives and depressed individuals were more likely to suffer from other chronic disease (i.e. diabetes, cardiovascular disease), health risk behaviors (i.e. drug abuse and alcoholism) and committed suicide.

Growing body of research indicated that physical activity (PA) was a protective factor of anxiety and depression and adopted it as a non-pharmaceutical for treating anxiety and depression in adults. However, issue in respect to the effectiveness, mechanism and the application of PA in the treatment and prevention of childhood anxiety and depression is still equivocal. Therefore, this chapter provided an overview on 1) the effect of PA in the treatment and prevention of anxiety and depression in children; 2) the mechanism of PA on anxiety and depression, and 3) PA recommendation for treating and preventing anxiety and depression treatment and prevention in children.

Chapter XXIX- Group cohesion is a ubiquitous, multi-dimensional construct investigated within the military, organizational and industrial settings, sports teams and exercise classes. According to Carron, Brawley and Widmeyer (1998), cohesion is "a dynamic process that is reflected in the tendency for a group to stick together and remain united in the pursuit of its instrumental objectives and/or for the satisfaction of member affective needs". This theory-driven definition was posited by Carron, Widmeyer & Brawley and has become the universally accepted definition within the field of sport psychology. Cohesion has been cited as the most important small group variable and has been shown to have a profound impact on group processes, with links to various factors such as collective efficacy, mood, performance and adherence. In addition, intervention studies have demonstrated efficacy, enhancing cohesion through goal-setting and physical exercise programs developed for cancer patients which concurrently improved mental health, performance levels, as well as emotional and social functioning.

Due to its profound impact on group dynamics, cohesion will continue to be a salient research topic investigated well into the 21st century across both the social and psychological sciences; yet important challenges persist, as key questions remain unanswered. Hence, the current paper aims to critically review recent findings, address limitations and provide suggestions for future research.

Chapter XXX- Previous research has focused on the positive effects of the experience of flow in sports, such as peak performance and well-being. In the present research we assumed that, due to some flow characteristics, the consequences of flow are not always beneficial. For example, the dissociative nature of flow and its association with a loss of self-reflection should lead to an underestimation of one's personnel risk. We tested our hypothesis in a field study with 63 male and female kayakers. Right after kayaking (one easy and one demanding route) they rated their flow experience and their perceived risk. Underestimation of risk was operationalized as the difference between participants' subjective rating of risks (e.g. risk of capsizing) and an objective expert's rating of those risks. As expected, the experience of flow was associated with an underestimation of risks in kayaking. This result remained stable even when controlled for fear, which was highly negatively associated with risk perception, and even when controlled for the conceptually related concept of sensation seeking. The positive and negative consequences of flow in sports are discussed critically in terms of practical implications.

Flow experience is defined as a state “in which people are so involved in an activity that nothing else seems to matter; the experience itself is so enjoyable that people will do it even at great cost, for the sheer sake of doing it”. At first sight this state of optimal experience seems highly desirable and previous research has confirmed this view by showing positive consequences of flow experience such as positive affect and high performance. However, on closer inspection the above definition of flow also suggests a potential disadvantage of flow in that individuals are prepared to accept great costs. These costs can be time costs, for example spending night after night writing computer programs, or financial costs, performing an expensive hobby (diving in the South Seas; restoring vintage cars), or costs that result through neglecting other domains of one’s life (e.g., neglecting one’s family and friends). At worst, the cost may be to one’s physical integrity, for example when endangering one’s health or even one’s life in risky sports. In the present paper we will compile theoretical considerations and facts about how flow is associated with risk behavior and we will present a study involving kayakers showing that flow does indeed lead to an underestimation of risk. However, first the phenomenon of flow will be described in detail.

In: Encyclopedia of Sports and Athletics
Editors: Jack L. Murray and Emily O. Watson

ISBN: 978-1-61209-959-0

Chapter I

Aerobic Exercise in Special Populations

Carlos Ayán Pérez, José María Cancela Carral and Silvia Varela Martínez
University of Vigo, Faculty of Education and Sport Sciences, Vigo, Galicia, Spain

Abstract

"Currently, modern chronic diseases are the leading killers in Westernized society and are increasing rampantly in developing nations. Considerable knowledge has accumulated in recent decades showing that physical exercise can be a very effective non-pharmacological strategy in the treatment of these pathologies, and as a result, several types of physical exercise are recommended in this matter. Aerobic exercise has been recognized as a safe and beneficial physical training modality for a number of chronic conditions, yet physicians do not know how to prescribe it. This chapter aims to discuss the effects of aerobic exercise in the treatment of metabolic syndrome-related disorders (diabetes, hypertension and obesity), heart and pulmonary diseases (coronary heart disease, chronic obstructive pulmonary disease and asthma), locomotive apparatus disorders (rheumatoid arthritis, osteoporosis systemic lupus erythematosus and fibromyalgia), neurological diseases (multiple sclerosis), and gastrointestinal disorders (Crohns Disease). The suggested potential mechanisms for the beneficial effects of aerobic exercise are discussed and some basic guidelines for exercise prescription in this kind of populations are given."

1. Osteoporosis

1.1 Disease Characteristics

Osteoporosis is a systemic illness characterized by bone mass loss (osteopenia) and micro-architectural deterioration which increases fracture risk (Compston, 1992). It is an disease which can affect any person. Progressive bone mineral loss starts generally around 25 years of age both in men and women. With the passing of time all people experience a reduction in bone mass, although osteoporosis is especially frequent from 70 years of age on. Postmenopausal women (Alastair, 1998) are a group especially affected by this disease. However,there exist some risk factors which predispose its development.

(A) Genetic factors: Race (Higher predisposition in white race), sex (women, especially after menopause), genetic diseases (Marfan disease, Imperfect Osteogenesis, etc), factors depending on certain hormones and metabolism (hipertiroidism, diabetes, estrogen defficiency, etc) and people with family antecedents.
(B) Enviromental factors: Some illnesses (Rheumathoid arthritis, hyperparatiroidism, chronic hepatic diseases, defficient intestinal absorpiton etc), postmenopausal women, elderly people, inadequate diet and defficiency of calcium, protein and vitamin D. Certain kinds of medication such as cortisone, antiepileptics or thyroid hormones, excess of alcohol, tobacco, coffee or drugs (glucocorticoids, tiroxine, caffeine, anticonvulsants etc)

Although we are inclined to think of osteoporosis as a modern disease, particularly in view of its apparently greater prevalence in the more prosperous societies of the world, the contribution of bone fragility to fractures in the elderly has been known for at least 200 years. It is difficult to say when the term "osteoporosis" was first used in the modern sense, but it was certainly employed by pathologists in the mid-nineteenth century and was clearly distinguished from osteomalacia by Pommer almost exactly 100 years ago. At the clinical level the crush fracture syndrome was still being confused with osteomalacia in the 1930's, but by the end of that decade Albright had definitively identified it with osteoporosis, which he defined as "too little calcified bone," and his teaching has been amply confirmed (Nordin, 2009).

Osteoporosis is a major public health threat for an estimated 44 million Americans or 55 percent of the people 50 years of age and older. In the U.S. today, 10 million individuals are estimated to already have the disease and almost 34 million more are estimated to have low bone mass, placing them at increased risk for osteoporosis. While osteoporosis is often thought of as an older person's disease, it can strike at any age. Of the 10 million Americans estimated to have osteoporosis, eighty percent of those affected by osteoporosis are women. Osteoporosis and osteoporotic fractures are more frequent in white people, followed by the asiatic. Black and hispanic people are the ones who present a lower incidence.

We can state that there are four kinds of osteoporosis:

(A) **Hormonal osteoporosis:** In some patients with osteoporosis the underlying cause is a hormonal imbalance caused by an increase in the secretion of antianabolic hormones (Crannney, 2006).
(B) **Osteoporosis caused by inactivity.** When the body becomes atrophied for lack of exercise bones are no exception (except skull bones). This can happen at any age (Cancela & Ayán, 2007; Karlsson, et al. 2008).
(C) **Postmenopausal and senile Osteoporosis.** These two kinds of generalized osteoporosis are studied in combination because they share many characteristics. The difference between them is somehow arbitrary since, when women develop osteoporosis between menopause and 65 years of age, osteoporosis is called postmenopausal, whereas when men and women develop the same process from 65

years of age on it is called senile (Cooper et al. 1992; Hui et al. 1990; Ahlborg et al. 2003).

(D) ***Reflex*** **Sympathetic Dystrophy (RSD) (Sudek's Atrophy)** It is a localized post-traumatic or subsequent to inmovilization osteoporosis accompanied with pain and edema in the affected zone and hypercalciura. This injury is reversible and it is evident the influence of a negative sympathetic nervous factor (Van der Laan & Goris, 1997).

In order to deal with osteoporosis prevention is the best policy. It is especially important during the first stages of life, that is, during the person's growing process and developement, childhood and adolescence (Del Rio & Roig, 2001). Exercising is an indispensable factor, among others, to reach the maximum peak of bone mass before loss starts at more advanced ages. Aerobic exercise during old age must be performed cautiously because it is during this stage of life when complications are more likely to appear due to the pathology's onset itself and the decrease in neuromotor abilities.

1.2 Aerobic Exercise and Osteoporosis

Aerobic exercise has a direct effect on bone tissue through the tensions provoked by the bones during the performance of the activity. This load provokes a reorentation of the trabecules to adapt their mass and their architecture to de main direction of the load (Del Rio & Roig, 2001). When load is absent the bone becomes atrophied (Bellver & Pujol, 1997), that is, a decrease or lack of load can be the cause for trabecule loss (Henderson, White, Eisman, 1998), whereas an increase of load provokes bone hypertrophy (Bellver & Pujol, 1997). Various techniques and physical agents can offer important benefits to osteoporosis patients but especially physical exercise, because it has an osteogenic effect which is higher the youger the exerciser is (Honda et al. 2001; Robling et al. 2002). Consequently, it has a preventive effect both by providing a greater bone mass peak during youth and by preventing mineral mass loss later in life. Numerous clinical essays and reviews related directly and positively the effect of exercise with bone mass at any age. (Bailey et al. 1999).

Matsumoto et al., (1997) studied total bone mass density (BMD) and different metabolic markers in three groups of sports people in the modality of judo, athletics (long distance runners) and swimming. They did not find differences in total bone mass density of the body between long distance runners and swimmers, however they found that total bone mass density of the body for both sexes was greater in judokas than in the other two groups. They concluded that these differences were caused by the demands of the specific sport and they were reflected in the rest of metabolic indexes.

Bellver & Pujol (1997) found that the highest percentage of frequency of decreased bone mass was observed in swimmers, artistic gymnasts and athletes.

Courteix et al., (1998) compared female swimmers and gymnasts of a control group, all of them in prepuberal age. BMD between swimmers and control group did not present any difference, however, gymnasts presented higher bone mass density than swimmers and control group. They concluded that physical activity is positive only if the practised sport produces enough bone tension in a medium to long term program, like gymnastics and unlike swimming.

According to this evidence we can conclude that aerobic exercise influences bone tissue and it is indirectly related with less falls and fractures which are the most dramatic result of this illness. Consequently, constant aerobic activity adequated to every patient's capability must be an inexcusable part of osteoporosis treatment (Whalen et al. 1988), however, not every kind of aerobic exercise has the same effect on bone tissue loss because, as many studies indicate, aerobic exercise in a non-gravity environment does not produce the desired effects on the bone.

1.3 Mechanism of Action

There exist evidence of beneficial effects of aerobic exercise on osteoporosis patients. Krall et al. (1994) indicate that postmenopausal women who walked more than a mile daily lost less bone density than those who walked shorter distances, which shows how positive aerobic exercise can be in the treatment and prevention of osteoporosis. Lewis & Modlesky (1998), point out that performing repetitive exercise with a light load (walking, cycling) can have a possitive effect on bone mass if intensity is high. Xhardez, (1995) highlights the preventive function of aerobic exercises (cycling, swimming, etc) as a basic kinesiotherapic treatmet of primitive osteoporosis. Apart from the aforementioned benefits, physical exercise provokes an improvement in blood circulation, new coronary vessels stimulation, muscular tissue reaffirmation and tone and increased tension on the bone. Calcification and calcium absorption are increased. Bones are strengthend and risk of fracture is reduced. Circulating adrenalin levels (stress hormone) decrease and endorfin and other cerebral susbtances increase. Emotional tension is reduced and mood is improved, resulting in a greater emotional and social well-being sensation. Therefore, we recommend antigravitatory aerobic exercises (which involve moving the body weight against gravity) as an effective therapy to prevent osteoporosis and fractures (Birge & Daisky, 1989), especially for elderly people and postmenopausal women (Santora, 1987; Prince et al, 1991; Agre et al 1988), because it helps to keep bones and muscles active and avoid the weakness typical of the ageing process.

1.4 Physical Exercise Prescription in Osteoporosis

The best kind of aerobic exercise to strengthen bones is resistance training (Dupple et al, 1997), that is, exercise which forces the patient to work against gravity, such as walking, climbing up slopes, running, climbing stairs, play tennis, dancing etc. The optimal situation is performing 30-60 minutes of exercise four times a week. Before starting any regular exercise program is convenient to consult a doctor, especially if the patient is over 40 or has got any associate pathology. Professionals then will prescribe the aerobic exercise program which best adapts to the patient's requirements in order to enable him/her to strengthen his/her muscles safely and correct bad posture habits. Exercise prescription must be oriented to the patient's needs and state of health. If the aim is to prevent osteoporosis, aerobic exercise programs must include weight-bearing activities such as walking, running or jogging (Lewis & Modlesky, 1998). It is recommendable to combine these activities with weight-lifting exercises, because this activity is related with higher increases of bone mass density (Barbado, 2001). If the patient has a high risk of osteoporosis or fractures, weight-bearing activities are contraindicated. In these cases we recommend swimming, hydrogymnastics and static bicycle (Xhardez, 1995). Physical exercise for osteoporosis patients must always be progressive and adapted to the cardiovascular state of the patient, never surpassing an established threshold (Andreoli et al., 2001).

2. Rheumatoid Arthritis

2.1 Disease Characteristics

Rheumatoid arthritis (RA) is a systemic autoimmune disorder characterized by a chronic inflammation of the joints which produces progressive destruction and different degrees of deformity and functional disability often progressing to destroy cartilage, bones, tendons and ligaments of the joints (Harris, et al. 2005; Smolen, et al. 2007).

The first convincing description of rheumatoid arthritis is found in French medical literature in 1800, in a document written by doctor Landré, who reports the illness indicating its higher frequency in the female sex and its characteristics, and describing it as primitive asthenic gout (Landre, 2001). However it is probable that the disease is much older than this (Short, 1974; Aceves-Avila et al. 2001). The term rheumatoid arthritis was first used in 1859 by Sir Alfred Garrod, who distinguished the disease from gout. However, this term also included polyarticular osteoarthritis and, up until relatively recently, a number of seronegative arthritides, such as psoriatic arthritis. It was Sir Archibald Garrod, Sir Alfred's son, who distinguished rheumatoid arthritis from osteoarthritis in 1907.

Arthritis and other rheumatic diseases are leading causes of disability in the US and are predicted to affect 60 million people by 2020 (CDC, 1994), RA is present in 0.5–1% of the general population, twice as often in women, and the disease's age of onset is mainly between 45 and 65 years. The American College of Rheumatology (formerly American Rheumatism Association [ARA]) has suggested diagnostic criteria for RA (Arnett et al. 1988). The disease course varies and prediction of the prognosis is difficult in any particular case. In the long run, a reduced function, difficulties in activities of daily living (ADL), and a negative psychosocial impact are often seen.

The treatment of RA focuses on decreasing inflammatory activity and symptoms, limiting joint destruction and disability, and improving health related quality of life. It includes a rich variety of medication, surgery, and rehabilitation. Despite earlier fear of aggravation of symptoms, increased disease activity, and joint destruction, there is now scientific support that various forms of exercise are both safe and beneficial (Minor, 1996). Exercise has become an important part of rehabilitation during the last decades. A number of studies of various quality have been carried out to investigate the effects of aerobic exercise in RA, reflecting the benefits of it on this group of patients.

2.2 Aerobic Exercise and Rheumatoid Arthritis

The RA patients' fear of aggravating their illnes, get injured or feel more pain usually disencourages them to practise any kind of physical exercise even aerobic exercise. Recent studies (Stenstrom & Minor, 2003) have proved that the aim of aerobic exercise in this group of patients must be to complement pharmacologic therapy in order to control the disease evolution and reduce inactivity. Sedentarism provokes muscle atrophy, flexibility reduction and important aerobic capacity loss. These factors can be controlled and modified through specific exercise programs (Pool & Axford, 2001), therefore, exercise can be part of the RA patients' daily life. Minor et al., (1989) carried out a piece of research with a group of 120 patients with rheumatoid arthritis or osteoarthritis who volunteered to be subjects for this study of aerobic versus non-aerobic exercise. The aerobic exercise program consisted of walking (Experimental group 1), aerobic aquatics (Experimental group 2), whereas non-aerobic exercise program was based on range of motion (Control group). The obtained results showed that subjects tolerated adequately all the different kinds of aerobic exercise. The aquatics and walking exercise groups showed significant improvement over the control group in aerobic capacity, 50-foot walking time, depression, anxiety, and physical activity after the 12-week exercise program.

Van de Ende et al. (1998) carried out a systematic review to determine the effectiveness of dynamic exercise therapy in improving joint mobility, muscle strength, aerobic capacity and daily functioning in patients with rheumatoid arthritis (RA). They checked the Cochrane Controlled trials Register, MEDLINE, EMBASE and SCISEARCH databases up to May 1997 in order to study controlled trials on the effect of exercise therapy. The results suggest that dynamic exercise therapy is effective at increasing aerobic capacity and muscle strength. No detrimental effects on disease activity and pain were observed.

Westby et al. (2000) assessed the effects of a 12 month, weight bearing, aerobic exercise program on disease activity, physical function, and bone mineral density (BMD) in women with rheumatoid arthritis (RA) taking low dose prednisone. The results showed that subjects in the exercise group had a small but non-significant decrease in disease activity and statistically significant improvements in physical function ($p = 0.05$) and activity levels ($p = 0.05$). The authors concluded that women with RA taking low dose steroid therapy can safely participate in a dynamic, weight bearing exercise programs with positive effects on their physical function, activity and fitness levels, and BMD with no exacerbation of disease activity.

Gaudin et al. (2008) developed a review of the literature from 1964 to 2005 in order to analyze and determine the optimal program, frequency, target population and the best assessment tools for monitoring clinical, functional, and structural parameters during dynamic exercise therapy in patients with RA. The obtained results show that dynamic exercise programs improve aerobic capacity and muscle strength in patients with RA. Their effects on functional capacity are unclear, since many sources of bias influenced the study results.

These studies corroborate the hypothesis that aerobic exercise, by itself or combined, provokes an improvement in the RA patients' functional capability and enables them to perform daily life activities without experiencing any pain increase, disease advance or joint injuries. Nevertheless, future research must try to establish the guidelines and the most adequate kind of aerobic exercise depending on the illness evolution.

2.3 Mechanism of Action

It is widely known that Rheumatoid Arthritis induces in the patient several combined processes. Swelling, pain, reduction in the range of joint mobility and joint deformation provoke disability and impairment of a great number of daily functions which compromise to a higher or lower degree the patient's independence. On the other hand, when the first symptoms appear, the person starts a psychological assimilation of this new health deterioration state which causes him/her continuous stress due to the constant process of adaptation and superation he/she must face every day (Lindroth, 1994). Medical and scientific results (Stenstrom, 2003; Ekdahl & Broman, 1992; Harkcom et al, 1985) obtained during the last decades have shown that exercise in general and aerobic exercise in particular is one of the best forms to minimize pain and limitation caused by RA, and to alleviate other associated pathologies such as bone mass loss, joint damage, depression, anxiety or sleep disorders. Therefore, aerobic exercise programs prescribed by health and exercise professionals must be systematically included in RA treatment.

2.4 Physical Exercise Prescription in Rheumatoid Arthritis

Starting an aerobic exercise program may be a great challenge for the patients. Understanding the benefits of exercise for RA for these people will help health professionals to prescribe adequate and safe training programs especially designed to meet the patient's requirements and recommentations about how to handle the body's response to exercise and how to modify the exercise routine if it is necessary.

Current recommendations include aerobic exercise understood as a programmed activity which involves the rhythmic and repetitive movement of major muscle groups in the body for 45-60 minutes (Westby, et al. 2000) at a moderate intensity 3-5 times a week. The recommended time can be accumulated in 10-minute periods during the day or the week in order to obtain similar health benefits to those obtained of a continuous training session. This offers greater exercise planning flexibility and allows people who experience pain or fatigue to perform shorter sessions within their own personal tolerance range. Moderate intensity (60%-80%) is the safest and most efficacious effort level in aerobic exercise (Minor, et al, 1989). This means that the person who is exercising can talk normally (Speech test) does not become breathless or hot and is able continue the activity for a long time without feeling any discomfort. Any fluctuation in the disease symptoms must be taken into account, such as longer periods of joint stiffness or pain. In these periods, the patient may need more rest and less exercise. (Stenstrom & Minor MA, 2003).

Prior to any aerobic exercise program the patient must take into account the following (Acsm, 1990):

1. Long term and short term real targets should be fixed in order to become motivated when these targets are reached.
2. Exercise should be performed in company (friends, family).
3. A record of exercises and progression must be kept daily.
4. Problems and impediments which stand in the way of exercising should be identified and avoided.
5. The chosen activities must be convenient, motivating and entertaining.

Safe aerobic exercise activities include walking, aquatic exercising, cycling or exercising in static bycicles, treadmills or elliptical walking machines. Daily activities such as mowing the lawn, raking leaves, playing golf or walking the dog are also aerobic exercises if they are performed at normal intensity (Finckh, 2003).

3. Systemic Lupus Erythematosus

3.1 Disease Characteristics

Systemic lupus erythematosus (SLE or lupus) is an often-severe autoimmune rheumatic disease of unclear aetiology and most commonly diagnosed in women in their childbearing years. Although it was first described in the XIIIth century by physician Rogerius (who thought that facial lesions caused by the disease looked like wolf bites), the systemic form was firmly established by doctors Osler and Jadassohn, respectively in the XXth century (Mallavarapu, 2007). Lupus is known as an autoimmune disease because a person's immune system attacks the body's own tissues. In lupus, the signs and symptoms of the disease can be attributed to damage caused directly by autoantibodies, the deposition of immune complexes (the combination of antigen and autoantibody), or cell-mediated immune mechanisms. The course of the disease is unpredictable, with periods of illness (called flares) alternating with remissions. Common initial and chronic complaints are fever, malaise, joint pains, myalgias, fatigue and photosensitivity among others, but the most common symptom are dermatological manifestations such as red scaly patches on the skin or the presence of the classic malar rash (or butterfly rash). Although a gold standard or single conceptual paradigm does not exist for the diagnosis of SLE, the American College of Rheumatology established eleven criteria, which, despite being originally meant to "facilitate formal communication" have become de facto diagnostic criteria. Based on these criteria it has been estimated that SLE affects 241 in 100.000 people in the United States (Ward, 2004). Current treatment includes nonsteroidal anti-inflammatory drugs, although mild or remittent disease can sometimes be safely left untreated.

Despite the fact that SLE patients can present various clinical conditions such as fatigue, pulmonary disease, heart disease, and peripheral neuropathy, they may benefit from exercise, as observed in other populations, suffering from similar chronic pathologies. Because of that, the prescription of aerobic exercise in SLE can be part of their multidisciplinary rehabilitation treatment.

3.2 Aerobic Exercise and Lupus

Reduced exercise capacity is common in SLE patients, which has been attributed to cardiac, pulmonary, parenchymal and vascular lesions. In fact, recent studies have found that SLE patients show some clear signs of reduced exercise capacity (see Table 1), such as a lower anaerobic threshold, maximum minute ventilation and maximum heart rate, reduced resting lung function measures, especially forced vital capacity, and a generally diminished aerobic capacity (VO2max). In this regard, it is important to note that aerobic exercise has been successfully prescribed as a component of therapy for SLE' as the follow-up studies show (Ayán, 2007). One study compared the effects of an 8-week home-based aerobic cycling programme in 16 patients with a non-aerobic stretching programme in a control group, and reported no differences in SLE activity, hematocrit, hours of sleep or depression measures. On the other hand, aerobic capacity improved by 19% and there was a significant difference in fatigue in the treated group, whose members indicated that they had more energy and an improved sense of well-being after the exercise programme. A similar 12-week programme where 37 patients were randomly assigned to stationary cycling or to a control group, showed that exercisers improved fatigue and depression measures, as well as exercise tolerance, but not significantly. Because of that, it was concluded that although it is safe, unsupervised home exercise programmes may benefit few patients. This safety of exercising and the variability of its effects were confirmed afterwards in a pilot study, where five patients participated in an aerobic programme and received an individual exercise prescription based on their initial level of fitness. They were instructed to exercise to 70-80% of their maximum heart rate, and met for 50 minutes, three times per week for 2 months. After that, patients continued to exercise in the supervised setting for one month and then unsupervised at home for 6 months, combining aerobic exercise with muscular resistance training. Another 5 patients underwent an exercise programme limited to arm and leg movement. They met in the same way as the other group, but after 2 months, muscle strengthening was added. At the end of the program the patients showed some improvement in fatigue, functional status, exercise capacity and muscle strength, while the adherence standard was met by 80% of the patients. However, once the intervention ended only 2 of them continued to exercise after a year. This finding shows that although exercise must be beneficial and improve the quality of life, it also needs to include motivating factors to maintain patients' participation. In this regard, it is important to note that home-based programmes are not always as efficient as supervised ones, as the study carried out by Tench et al., (2003) shows. Thirty-three patients were asked to exercise at home at least three times a week for between 30 and 50 minutes for 12 weeks, the main exercise being walking, with cycling and swimming also available. 32 control patients were asked to listen to a relaxation audiotape. After the training programme, 49% of the exercise patients and 28% of the relaxation patients rated themselves as "much" or "very much" better, and there was a trend for the subsidiary outcome of fatigue to improve, while there was a significant increase in exercise duration (18%), and a decrease in pain. On the other hand, patients abandoned both groups, although there was no flare in disease activity or serious adverse events. Aerobic capacity did not improve, owing perhaps to the mild exercise intensity (only 90 minutes of exercise per week at a maximum 60% of VO2max) or poor compliance with therapy. After three months' follow-up, fatigue improvements were not maintained, possibly because only 8 patients continued to exercise.

Finally, Carvalho *et al., (2005)* designed a 12 week aerobic training programme, where the patients met for 60 minutes 3 times a week. The main exercise was walking at a heart rate corresponding to their ventilatory anaerobic threshold. Among the 50 patients assigned to the training group, 41 completed the cardiovascular training programme, and showed a significant improvement in aerobic capacity, exercise tolerance, O_2 pulse, and pulmonary ventilatory capacity, which proves that physical condition can be trained in SLE patients. Moreover, functional capacity, fatigue, depression and quality of life also improved. Thus, cardiovascular training is well tolerated and its effects on physical condition can be transferred to the activities of the patients' daily life.

In spite of all this, it must be taken into account that all the studies that have been mentioned here have included patients with low to moderate disease activity, so the safety of exercise for patients with high disease activity and its effects need to be addressed in future investigations.

3.3 Mechanism of Action

There are a number of reasons for explaining the beneficial effects of aerobic exercise in SLE patients. For instance, it is widely known that the oxygen uptake needed for the instrumental activities of daily living ranges from 10.5 to 17.5 ml/kg/min. The lowest VO_{2max} value reported in SLE patients is 18.1 ml/kg/min, which is very close to this interval. This finding suggests that in patients with mild SLE, the magnitude of aerobic insufficiency may limit the capacity to engage in occupational and recreational tasks and even affect the ability to sustain normal daily activities for more than minimal periods of time. Because of that, it can be stated that if aerobic training improves exercise capacity, SLE patients will obtain a better quality of life. Furthermore, there are a number of related symptoms, such as obesity, depression, sleep disturbances or osteoporosis which affect the patients' well-being and that can be ameliorated by means of exercising too. To this, it must be added that maintaining a good baseline level of physical fitness can help SLE patients to minimize loss of function when lupus flares, to decrease stress on inflamed joints, and to lessen fatigue levels. Lastly, aerobic exercise can reduce the impact of heart and lung problems in lupus as well as limit the risk of injury, such as those due to falls resulting from weakness.

According to Clarke-Jenssen et al.,(2005) walking at an intensity of 70% of the SLE patient's maximum heart rate, three times a week, starting from 25 minutes per session during the first week to 40 minutes from third week onwards, can be an easy way to achieve some improvements in aerobic capacity and fatigue, with no aggravation of the health state. Other activities, such as swimming or stationary cycling at intensity between 70–80% of the maximum heart rate, for 30–50 minutes, three times a week, can be just as effective.

Table 1. Mean VO2max values in SLE patients

Researchers	*Number of patients*	*(VO2max)*ml/kg/minute
Carvalho et al.	**50**	**24.64**
Keyser et al.	**18**	**19.2**
Forte et al.	**13**	**1098**
Tench et al.	**31**	**21.5**
Tench et al.	**93**	**23.2**
Sakauchi et al.	**21**	**810.7**

3.4 Physical Exercise Prescription in Sle

However, it is important to note that sustained physical training effects depend on the patient's determination to continue exercising once the formal supervised programme is over.

Because of that, motivation towards exercising must be the key to a successful aerobic training intervention.

Lastly, it must be pointed out that, although they are usually safe, exercise programmes can have some risks. Some studies have shown significant differences between SLE patients and controls in heart rate at rest, and in blood pressure response to standing. Lower adrenaline and plasma noradrenaline levels have also been found. These parameters must be taken into account, because SLE patients may have difficulties making maximal efforts, such as maximum repetitions, or with prolonged aerobic exercise. In order to avoid risks while exercising, all patients should receive an individual exercise prescription based on their initial level of fitness, and control their own pace.

4. Fibromyalgia

4.1 Disease Characteristics

Fibromyalgia (FM), is the second most common soft tissue disorder in the United States, afflicting approximately 4 to 6 million Americans, mainly women (Katz et al., 2006). The term fibrositis was the most widely used to refer to this pathology until Hench used the term fibromyalgia for the first time in 1975. Although its origin is uncertain, FM is now recognized as one of the "central" pain syndromes, since it includes the phenomenon of allodynia, in which a normally unpainful stimulus is perceived as painful, and hyperalgesia, in which a normally painful stimulus is perceived of as more painful than it really is. Environmental and genetic factors play a role in the pathogenesis of FM, and it has been suggested that trauma and stress as well as infections, may trigger its development (Ablin et al., 2008). Patiens with FM often report diffuse, chronic, widesprain pain, aching and fatigue, often accompanied by stiffness, sleep disturbances and stress.

The diagnosis of the illness is controversial, although it is generally determined by the location of 18 trigger points in the patient's body and the existence of tenderness in at least one of them. A soft and progressive palpation with the thumb helps to identify these points. The lack of an efficacious pharmacologic treatment has brought about abundant research on the effects of disparate alternative therapies such as dietetic modifications, hypnosis and physiotherapy, obtaining contradictory results (Sueiro et al., 2008). Today, it is considered that one of the most efficacious options is to follow a multidisciplinarian rehabilitation treatment which combines strategies for the self-control of the illness (cognitive educational therapy), exercising and different relaxation techniques to reduce the stress.

4.2 Fibromyalgia and Aerobic Exercise

There is a large amount of research these days on the effects of physical exercise applied to FM patients which aims at reducing the intensity of some symptoms and the recovery of the patient's physical condition. According to the excellent review carried out by Mannerkorpi (2003) exercise programs for FM patients can be divided in three main groups:

Walking: The different existing studies which have proposed walking as a physical rehabilitation therapy have obtained disparate, but mainly positive results. Some of them have achieved an increase in the aerobic capacity, a reduction in the number of tender points and a greater feeling of well-being. Others, despite not achieving the first point, have been able to show an improvement in the patient's quality of life, which is reflected in a greater autonomy, efficacy and personal satisfaction. It must be pointed out the fact that combining an educational cognitive therapy with the walking program has given better results than the walking program alone.

Pedaling: The first studies on the effects of aerobic exercise on FM were developed using cycloergometers, where the patients pedaled following an established protocol. This kind of exercise has generally been reported as positive when used as a rehabilitation therapy. It reduces the number of tender points, raises the pain threshold, improves the patients' well-being and increases their aerobic capacity. However, it must be taken into account that the existence of trigger points in the gluteal region could prevent pedaling at an adequate intensity. It has been confirmed that when two exercise programs only differ in intensity, those patients who follow the most intense one get a greater improvement in their physical condition than those who pedal at a lower intensity. However, they showed more post-exercise discomfort, which in some cases forced them to abandon the program. This is the reason why low to medium intensity aerobic exercise is preferable in this case, since it will produce virtually the same effects than high intensity work allowing patients to adhere to the exercise program more easily.

Water exercise: Although water exercise is one of the best ways for FM patients to develop their physical condition, it is not usually proposed as an aerobic training method. Several studies indicate that water temperature should be around 34ºC in order to reduce pain and muscular strain, enable the patients to relax and become aware of their own body. In addition to this, a shallow swimming pool is indispensable to carry out training programs which include aqua-fitness or aqua-aerobic exercises adapted to the patients' characteristics, and it is especially necessary for those people who cannot swim in order to be able to take advantage of the benefits of water. The expected effects will be, apart from an improvement in physical condition, a reduction of important symptoms such as pain, fatigue or anxiety, and a greater feeling of well-being. In this regard, a safe modalito of aerobic conditioning in water has been proposed: deep water running, where the patient performs a running movement in the pool while wearing a floating belt. This modality of aerobic training has been shown to be as effective as land based exercises (Assis et al., 2006).

Since FM can cause slighter degrees of disability, some of patients are able to perform more demanding aerobic activities such as "Aerobic". In this respect, Schachter and col. (2003) compared the effects of 1 long exercise bout versus 2 short exercise bouts per training day (fractionation) on physical function, signs and symptoms of fibromyalgia, and exercise adherence. Both groups progressed in total daily training duration from 10 to 30 minutes, 3 to 5 times a week, for 16 weeks. The main training segment music tempo was progressed from 126 bpm for the first third of the training segment to 132 bpm for the middle third of the training segment and then to 144 bpm for the final third of the training segment. At the end of the program, no differences were seen between both training groups. Thus, fractionation of "Aerobic" training sessions provided no advantage in terms of exercise adherence, improvements in fibromyalgia symptoms or physical function. Although FM patients experienced some improvement in their fitness level, the high attrition rates and the adherence problems observed in the study proves that “Aerobic” might not be the most advisable aerobic training modality for people suffering from FM.

4.3 Mechanism of Action

The reasons why aerobic exercise may be beneficial for people who suffer from FM are many. First, it has been proved that different training programs have reduced the magnitude of the pain which is characteristic of this syndrome. This is probably due to the fact that when exercise is moderately intense and well tolerated by the patient, the aforementioned secretions may cause a state of hypoalgesia as well as a stimulation of the opioid system which induces a feeling of euphoria and well-being. In addition to this, it is known that physical exercise has an effect on the short wave of sleep, decreasing its latency and therefore positively influencing the feeling of well-being. Some authors point out that the benefits of exercise on FM are mainly based on the fact that local muscular circulation is increased and susceptibility to microtrauma is lowered, inducing a reduction in pain and an improvement in glucose metabolism (which is presumably upset in this kind of patients). This means an improvement in muscle relaxation due to the increase of ATP levels and it would explain why those disciplines which involve the lower limbs (cycling, walking) have proved to reduce muscular pain in the gluteal region. On top of this, we must add that this kind of patients not only obtain physical benefits, but also feel emotionally rewarded when health professionals who are aware of the impact of this illness in their lives try to prescribe them some kind of physical therapy to ease their situation, making them feel emotionally and psychologically better. (Valencia et al., 2008).

4.4 Aerobic Exercise Prescription for FM

One of the recommended aerobic exercises for FM is pedaling, especially with modern static bicycles which allow a complete control of the training sessions. An advisable protocol of action for this kind of exercise includes a pedaling session at 25% of maximum HR for 12 minutes approximately 2-3 times a week. Every week HR level can be increased in 5% and the duration of the exercise can be extended to 14 minutes. After a month and a half approximately, HR can reach 60% and maintain that level until the patient is able to perform a total of 25-30 minutes of aerobic exercise. From that point on, it is not advisable to increase the volume of work or combine different exercises, since a high intensity effort could bring about the negative effects already mentioned. In the case of unfit and seriously affected patients two weekly sessions are recommended including two blocks of 6-minute pedaling exercises. If the training frequency is high, it will be possible to perform two 25-minute blocks after three months. The intensity of the exercise must allow the patients to talk comfortably while they are exercising or slightly sweating. This instructions could equally be applied to walking.

An example of a training schedule is shown in Table 1.

Bicycle protocols used in different studies involving people affected by FM.

When establishing an aerobic training protocol, it must be taken into account that most research on fybromialgia and physical exercise has reported a sometimes excessively high percentage of patients who abandon the program (Busch et al., 2007). This indicates that not every patient tolerates physical exercise in the same way and that most of them give up due to fatigue and pain. Researchers speculate that programming low intensity exercise in order to avoid fatigue leads to an insufficient stimulation and production of adrenocoricotropic hormones, beta-endorphines, prolactin and serotonin, therefore, the hypoalgesic effect of exercise does not occur. In order to avoid this kind of problems the best course of action is to individualize as much as possible the training program and encourage group sessions where the patients can openly express all those positive and negative sensations that, in their opinion, may be related to aerobic exercise.

VOLUME	INTENSITY	FREQUENCY	OBSERVATIONS
25 minutes	50% VO_2 Max	2-3 Days /Week	Similar intensity to 65% of Max H.R
30-60 minutes	150 beats/minute	3 Days/Week	Good initial physical condition.

5. Obesity

5.1 Characteristics of the Illness

Obesity is a rapidly growing epidemic worldwide which increases the risk of morbidity and mortality (Thompson et al. 2007). It is estimated that between 60% to 65% of adults in the United States are overweight (Jakicic, 2003).

Obesity is a symptom of overfeeding that may have some underlying emotional causes. It can be the consequence of a metabolic disorder as well. Genetic factors are also important, so obese parents have 80% of possibilities of having obese children. It is defined as an abnormal increase in the fat proportion in the body. Most of the excess of food, either if it is fats, carbohydrates or proteins is accumulated in the subcutaneous tissue and around the internal organs. Obesity is a risk factor in several deadly illnesses, including various types of cancer, diabetes and heart disease (Thibodeau & Patton, 2000).

A method used to diagnose obesity is the Body Mass Index (BMI).There are more precise methods to calculate body fat percentage, but they are too complex to be employed in primary health care.

$$BMI= weight\ (in\ Kg) / height^2\ (in\ m)$$

This method, accepted by the World Health Organization has proved to show a good correlation with body mass especially in truly obese or highly overweight people.

The aim is to reduce fat mass and increase lean body mass, therefore, prescribing exercise for obese people will reduce risk factors of many chronic conditions including diabetes, hypertension, hypercholesterolemia, stroke, heart disease, certain cancers, and arthritis. Of these conditions, diabetes may be most closely linked to obesity, and its prevalence appears to have increased as the prevalence of obesity increased" (Harris et al. 1998).

Classification	BMI (kg/m2)
Insufficient weight	< 18,5
Normoweight	18,5-24,9
Overweight type I	25-26,9
Overweight type II	27-29,9
Obesity type I	30-34,9
Obesity type II	35-39,9
Obesity type III (morbid)	40-49,9
Obesity type IV (extreme)	> 50

5.2 Aerobic Exercise and Obesity

Physical exercise is highly recommendable as a complement to diet for obese people, however, there is no clear consensus about the suitable duration and intensity of exercise to obtain positive benefits from physical activity. The center of Disease Control and Prevention and the American College of Sport Medicine recommend a minimum of 30 minutes of moderate intensity activity on most days of the week (150 min/week), however, the Institute of Medicine recommends a minimum of 60 min/day of exercise on most days of the week to control body weight. Jakicic et al. (2003) studied weight loss and cardiorespiratory fitness during 12 months (in women) with groups which worked at different intensities and durations. At the end of the study results showed that weight loss occurred both in the longer duration and higher intensity group and in the moderate intensity and moderate duration group. In addition to this, there was an improvement of cardiorespiratory fitness in all groups. According to the study results, the author advises to follow the ACSM recommendation of 150 min/week, especially at the beginning of the training program, and to increase gradually to the Institute of Medicine recommendation of 60min/day, according to the patients level progress.

Church et al. (2007) worked in a similar way (also with women) although they focused on the effect of different doses of exercise on cardiorespiratory fitness. They took as a starting point the ACSM recommendations of 150 min/ week to establish work groups. One group worked as control group, another at 50% (4 kcal/kg per week)of the ACSM recommended time, another one following the ACSM guidelines (8 kcal/kg per week) and one last group worked at 150%(12 kcal/kg per week) of those guidelines. Work intensity was maintained for all groups at 50% Vo2 max, and the program was carried out during 6 months. One of the most salient findings was that the group with a smaller aerobic load showed an improvement in fitness compared to the control group. Besides, the 12 kcal group obtained a higher improvement in fitness than the 8 kcal group. This study did not report weight loss in any of the groups, although waist circumference decreased in all, which is important because excessive abdominal fat is related to an increase in insulin resistance risk, diabetes and metabolic syndrom.

Besides the lack of consensus as far as exercise recommendation is concerned, we must take into account the high incidence of obesity in children. As Goran et al.(1999) show in their work: "Although energy intake depends solely on dietary consumption, energy expenditure is dependent on several components, with the major modifiable aspect being physical activity. Thus, both dietary and physical activity patterns have been emphasized as appropriate interventions for the prevention of obesity. However, among children, a reduction in energy intake may compromise growth and essential energy acquisition. In addition, attempts to modify the eating patterns of children may exacerbate the risk of introducing eating disorders. Although it is clear that physical activity has beneficial effects on health, the optimal intensities, volumes and modalities are unclear, especially in children".

5.3 Mechanism of Action

Exercise is an important component in interventions in overweight and obese people because it achieves an improvement in body weight in a short time, combined with an adequate diet, and is one of the best predictors for long term weight loss.

Although many variables play an important role in it, weight is mainly determined by caloric balance. This means the difference between consumed calories (energy equivalent that food intake provides) and energy expenditure (the energy equivalent of resting metabolic index, the thermic effect of food and the performed physical activity).

The effect of exercise, increasing energy expenditure, results more effective if it is accompanied by a balanced diet, if the aim is to reduce body weight (Jakicic & Otto, 2005). One kilogram of fat equals 7.700 kcal of energy approximately. Long duration and moderate intensity exercises (aerobic exercise) encourages fat burning. When caloric balance is negative induced by exercise, weight loss is mainly fat.

Several studies have researched if physical exercise is able to increase appetite, provoking a higher energy intake. It seems that in obese patients practising exercise can induce higher food intake, thus consuming more calories, although this larger amount of energy does not jeopardize weight loss in most cases because it is not larger than the amount of energy consumed during exercise. Therefore, the global effect is positive (Woo & Sunyer, 1982).

It must be taken into account the fact that physical activity means a reduction in energy consumption derived from other activities when prescribing aerobic exercise to elderly people or to people who are very unfit.

A greater amount of induced fat loss was observed in men than in women (Westerterp & Goram, 1997), especially abdominal fat, both cutaneous and perivisceral, possibly due to the faster lipolithic response of fat in this locations and the higher release of catecholamines derived from exercise. It is important to note that abdominal fat, especially perivisceral fat is closely related to arteriosclerosis and cardiovascular disease (Irwin et al. 2003). Apart from the effect of physical exercise on weight loss, positive effects on the rest of obesity related pathologies must be taken into account as well (Fenster et al., 2002).

5.4 Physical Exercise Prescription in Obesity

The optimal program for weight loss involves a combination of moderate caloric restrictions with regular aerobic exercise, always avoiding any kind of nutritional deficiency.

When designing a weight loss training program, a balance between intensity and duration of the exercise must be kept in order to provoke a hight total caloric expenditure (300-500 kcal per session and 1000-2000 kcal per week, in adults). Obese people have a higher risk of suffering orthopedic injuries, that is the reason why intensity should be kept under the recommended intensity for aerobic capacity improvement.

Having in mind the points mentioned above, we have followed the review carried out by Kelly et al. (2005) who include 11 studies where aerobic exercise programs have been employed. The following guidelines are based on the values used by said studies:

Frequency	:	3-5 times a week
Intensity	:	45-75% Vo2max
Duration	:	20 -60 minutes per session.

6. Hypertension

6.1 Disease Characteristics

The World Health Organization (WHO) defines high blood pressure as "a chronic rise in the systolic pressure, the diastolic pressure or both over the established normal limit for every age group or sex." Hypertension is the most common human disease (ACSM, 2000) and it affects over 50 million Americans (Bacon et al., 2004). It is regarded as an important health problem since it represents one of the main risk factors for cardiovascular disease in the developed countries (Hagberg et al., 2000).

Hypertension is classified into two groups: primary or essential hypertension and secondary hypertension. 95% of hypertension cases belong to the first group whose main cause is unknown, although populations who risk suffering from it are obese people, people with a high concentration of sodium in plasma or people with hypercholesterolemia. Secondary hypertension is related to several renal, pulmonary, endocrine and vascular diseases.

It was in 1983 when the WHO recommended a non-pharmacologic approach to treat hypertension. Since then there has been plenty of evidence that physical exercise plays an important role in the disease treatment (Wallance, 2003). According to this organization, hypertension is associated to a systolic pressure over 140 and a diastolic pressure over 90. The values corresponding to pre-hypertension are found in people who are at risk of suffering the illness and must be controlled in order to normalize their blood pressure.

People who suffer from light to moderate hypertension may feel no symptom whatsoever, therefore their daily activities will not be impaired, but the physical limitations will show up when target organs are affected by the disease increasing the risk of suffering cardiovascular pathologies (coronary disease, ictus, heart failure, etc).

Therefore, the aim of hypertension treatment is to minimize the possible repercussion of the illness on target organs. We must take into account here that hypertension involves a wide range of different problems due to the several variables that may have an effect on it (sex, weight, sodium intake, stress level, alcohol consumption, tobacco, etc)

Classification of hypertension		
	SBP (mmHg)	DBP (mmHg)
Normal	<120	<80
Prehypertension	120-139	80-89
Stage 1 hypertension	140-159	90-99
Stage 2 hypertension	≥160	≥100

Source: WHO 2009.

6.2 Aerobic Exercise and Hypertension

The modification of the patient's lifestyle is the first action in hypertension treatment (Baster & Baster-Brooks, 2005), including regular physical activity which not only has a beneficial effect on hypertension but also reduces the risk of suffering any cardiovascular event.

Aerobic exercise has proved to be an effective non-pharmacologic method to reduce blood pressure, both by itself alone and combined with other courses of action (Manfredini et al., 2008). There is concluding evidence that this kind of exercise reduces resting blood pressure (Sharman & Stowasser, 2009) even at a low intensity (50% VO2max). Halbert et al. (1997) reflects in his meta-analysis that aerobic activities such as walking, jogging or cycling produce an average reduction of 10.7 and 7.6 mmHG in the values of resting blood pressure for both Systolic Blood Pressure and Diastolic Blood Pressure in patients with mild to sever hypertension. It is assumed that all aerobic activities provide the patients with the same healthy effects regardless of the type of activity: jogging, walking, cycling and swimming, which is frequently recommended. Cox (2006) studied two groups of women aged 50-70.One group walked and the other swam and after a 6-month training period the group that had been walking reduced their blood pressure, whereas the group that had been swimming experienced an increase in it. The reasons for this rise are unknown but facial immersion, hydrostatic pressure, breath holding or water temperature may be playing a role in it. Thus, adaptation to the medium seems necessary. More research is needed in order to establish more accurate recommendations.

Another aspect that must be taken into account is that exercise produces a different effect on people depending on their age, sex and race. Therefore, middle-aged people reduce their systolic blood pressure to a higher degree than the young or the elderly (The number of people of every group of age in the sample is also an important aspect to have in mind) (Hagberg et al., 2000). It must be noted that elderly people with mild hypertension may experience an intensification of the effects of hypertensive medication (as well as a reduction in blood pressure) due to endurance training.

Regarding sex differences, according to Hagberg et al. (2000) hypertension is equally frequent in men than in women and regular exercise benefits both sexes (Sharman 2009) although women reduce more their Systolic Blood Pressure values.

As far as race is concerned, we can establish that blood pressure decreased in Afroamerican men and black adult women although the training proved to be more effective (regarding systolic values) for Asian and Pacific Island patients than for Caucasians (Manfredini et al., 2008).

6.3 Mechanism of Action

How physical activity positively affects blood pressure is not known. The mechanisms by which aerobic physical exercise benefits people who suffer from high blood pressure are related to multiple factors including a reduction in adrenaline and noradrenalin secretion at rest and during sub-maximum effort, a release of endorphin which is produced during physical exercise and which induces a state of metal relaxation and physical well being which in turn may attenuate or eliminate the stressing factors which raise blood pressure (Chintanadilok & Lowenthal, 2002).

During physical exercise there is also a decrease in insulin secretion which causes a reduction in tubular reabsorption of sodium and a subsequent fall in blood pressure. It is worth mentioning that weight loss due to exercise also reduces blood pressure (GAFS, 2006) although the most important factors to be taken into account are mainly related to the sympathetic nervous system and the improvement of the endothelial function (Manfredini et al., 2008).

Sympathetic nervous system: Physical training improves blood pressure reaction to stress and induces modifications in the cardiovascular system. After a training session a period of hypotension follows which is associated to a lesser peripheral resistance of the blood vessels. Said resistance decreases due to the reduction in sympathetic activity which is subsequent to the physical effort, being more noticeable in patients with essential hypertension (O'Sullivan & Bell, 2000). This lower blood pressure may be maintained in time if training becomes a regular practice.

Endothelial Function: Several studies have shown that endothelial dysfunction is typical of hypertension. The endothelium lining of the blood vessels keeps a normal vascular tone, increasing blood fluidity and regulating vessel growth. Exercise produces a higher shear stress (increased blood flow in the vessel wall) and stimulates the production of nitric oxide by the endothelium (Zanesco & Antunes, 2007) Nitric oxide plays an important role in the regulation of vascular tone favoring vessel dilatation.

6.4 Physical Exercise Prescription in Hypertension

There are variations between the recommendations of different authors, although as Hagberg et al. (2000) indicates, the results show that moderate to low intensity endurance training is as efficacious as higher intensity activity. This is an important aspect to point out regarding public health, since low to moderate aerobic exercise programs are easier to perform by hypertension patients.

Intensity	Volume	Frecuency	Observationes
40-60% MHR	30-60 minutes	3-5 days/week	Possible side effects of hypertension medication (if taken) must be taken into account.

Intensity: As we already mentioned, low intensity effort has beneficial effects on blood pressure, and that is the reason why most recommendations are oriented towards low intensity. Manfredini et al. (2008) states in his work that the exercise intensity recommended by authors was 50% VO2 max, since it was obtained the same or even better results than with high intensity training. According to Wallance (2003), a training session at 50% VO2 max for 45 minutes produced better results than the same training session at 70% VO2max. In addition to this, the American College of Sport Medicine (Blaster & Blaster-Brooks, 2005) recommends aerobic exercise at intensity between 50-65% VO2 max.

Volume: There is not much consistency as far as this parameter is concerned. The general recommendation ranges from 30' to 60' of aerobic exercise. Evidence exists that an activity carried out for only 20' obtained a reduction in blood pressure. Although the relation between exercise duration and blood pressure reduction is not conclusive it can be suggested that longer duration exercise may be more effective than shorter duration exercise (Wallance, 2003). It is also important to note that interval exercising (4 10-minute fast pace walking sessions) was as effective as 40' in a continuous way (Manfredini et al. 2008). ACSM recommends starting by short duration sessions during the first (3-4) training weeks in order to achieve proper body conditioning. In a later stage time will be extended according to every person's adaptation to exercise.

Frequency: The minimum frequency for a sedentary person to be able to obtain an reduction in blood pressure is 3 days (Wallance, 2003) or approximately 60-90 minutes a week. Most authors recommend a frequency between 3-5 days a week. Higher frequencies do not decrease blood pressure significantly. We should also take into that if the patient wants to lose weight, we should increase frequency in order to optimize weight loss work.

7. Diabetes Mellitus

7.1 Disease Characteristics

There are 23.6 million people in the United States, or 8% of the population, who suffer from diabetes. The total prevalence of diabetes increased 13.5% from 2005-2007. Only 24% of diabetes is undiagnosed, down from 30% in 2005 and from 50% ten years ago. (ADA, 2009).

This illness was already known by the ancient Greek doctors who called it "diabetes" because this word in Greek means "to go through" and refers to the fast passage of water through the patient's body to be excreted as urine very shortly after it has been consumed. Almost 1,500 years after being defined the disease was named "diabetes mellitus" because "mellitus" in Greek means "honey" and describes the "sugary" tendency of diabetic urine. It was not until 1921 that insulin was discovered, a hormone obtained from animal pancreatic tissue which was directly injected into the patient's body until synthetic human insulin became available, being the common treatment nowadays. (Thibodeau & Patton, 2000).

The main feature of diabetes mellitus is lack of insulin which has negative consequences on the metabolism of carbohydrates, fats and proteins (Guyton & Hall, 2001).

This problems with insulin (either the lack or the resistance to it) make it impossible for the diabetic people's cells (except brain cells) to absorb glucose and to use it efficiently as fuel, creating a rise in blood glucose level (hyperglycemia) which is one of the most important symptoms of this illness. Glucose is filtered, as a general rule, from the blood by the renal tubes, however, when blood glucose level increases, renal tubes are unable to absorb more glucose and as a result, the exceeding amount ends up in the urine (glycosuria). The body needs more water in order to be able to handle this larger volume of sugar and therefore urine production is more abundant (polyuria). Water loss through urination generates body dehydration which becomes worse when the high blood glucose levels increase the osmotic concentration of the blood and take water from the cells. Feeling excessively and progressively thirsty (polydipsia) and drinking large amounts of liquid are also some of the main symptoms of this disease. In addition to this, diabetic patients are intensely and continuously hungry due to the inability of the cells to absorb the necessary glucose to burn as a source of energy (Thibodeau & Patton, 2000).

On the other hand, the metabolic change that involves using fats and proteins as a source of energy causes fatigue and weight loss. The metabolism of fats in diabetes increases the release of ketoacids (ketonic bodies) into the plasma. The increase in organic acid decreases blood pH inducing diabetic ketoacidosis. This can provoke a diabetic coma or even death in a very short period of time if the patient is not treated immediately with large doses of insulin. Extreme acidosis only happens in very serious cases of diabetes which are not controlled.

Another consequence of fat metabolism is that it causes higher lipid levels in the blood (hyperlipidemia) and higher cardiovascular disease risk.

There are two kinds of diabetes: Diabetes Mellitus Type 1 and Diabetes Mellitus Type 2

Diabetes Mellitus Type 1 (DM1): It is also called insulin-dependent diabetes because the patients need to inject insulin into their body in order to be able to control blood glucose levels. This kind represents 10% of the total number of diabetic people. It is also known as young diabetes as it is found in people under 30 years of age. Being diagnosed as having this illness has an influence on functional changes, sexual and psychological maturity, physical development and social adaptation (Sideraviciute et al, 2006).

This kind of diabetes is characterized by a total lack of insulin which cannot be produced by the body due to the auto-immune destruction of.-cells in the Langerhans islets (located in the pancreas) which are the ones responsible for the insulin secretion.

The best treatment for DM1 is based on three fundamental principles: insulin therapy, diet and exercise. Patients must learn to control and estimate the amount of carbohydrates that they consume in order to be able to regulate blood glucose level by adjusting their insulin doses (De Angelis et al, 2006).

Diabetes Mellitus Type 2 (DM2): Also called non insulin-dependent diabetes mellitus is the most frequent form of the disease, representing 90% of the total cases. In general, it starts gradually at 40 and often during the 50-60 decade, being known as middle-age diabetes. In susceptible people who are overweight incidence increases with age. In this kind of diabetes.-cells still produce insulin but it is insufficient to meet the patient's needs. Besides, the loss of insulin receptors in the cellular surface membrane reduces the efficiency of glucose absorption, which is known as resistance to insulin.

Non insulin-dependent patients do not need hormone injections to control the disease. In these cases, hyperglycemia usually responds positively to changes in lifestyle, but if this is not enough to reduce glucose blood levels in DM2, oral hypoglycemic drugs can be prescribed in order to stimulate .-cells activity to produce more insulin by improving the effectiveness of insulin receptors in the cell.

Genes and ethnic background are fundamental in DM2. Family history is a key factor in overweight and sedentary people. American natives have increased risk to suffer from DM2 and Hispanic and Afro-American have more chances than Caucasians to develop this kind of diabetes.

DM2 symptoms are more subtle and less noticeable than those of DM1. The American Diabetes Association (ADA) estimates that over 7 million Americans have diabetes without knowing it. This represents a risk because if hyperglycemia is not controlled it can cause numerous problems in many areas of the body. Reduced blood flow due to the accumulation of fat materials in the blood vessels (atherosclerosis) is one of the most serious complications.

The disease causes diverse problems such as heart attack, stroke and poor blood circulation in the limbs which produces a tingling sensation and numbness in the feet and in grave cases, gangrene. Retinal alterations (diabetic retinopathy) can cause blindness to some patients who have been fighting against the illness for decades. Renal disease is also a frequent diabetic complication. Almost all authors agree that a scrupulous control of blood glucose levels is the most important step that diabetics can take in order to minimize long term complications caused by the illness (Thibodeau & Patton 2000).

In both types of diabetes, diet and exercise play an important role since patients should lose weight in order to be able to reverse insulin resistance (Guyton & Hall, 2001).

7.2 Aerobic Exercise and Diabetes

DM1 incidence is lower than that of DM2 ant it is normally diagnosed in the first stages of life, which means that the patient must get used to living with the insulin treatment and with the daily control of the illness symptoms for life. Due to these complications, it is important to develop and apply strategies which allow DM1 patients to participate safely and comfortably in regular physical activities. All sports both performed with a recreational or competitive purpose are suitable for these people as long as blood glucose level is controlled (De Angelis, 2006).

Diabetes mellitus type 1:

When dealing with the problem of how much exercise should be encouraged in diabetic patients it is important to take into account the characteristics that this activity must have in order to prevent hyperglycemia, since a correct blood glucose level control enables the reduction of the disease complications and the patient's health improvement.

Aerobic exercise and resistance training have been studied and compared in order to establish which activity offers the best results to this kind of population. After 12 weeks of training both groups showed an improvement in the reduction of NPH insulin dose and a slight increase in cardio-respiratory resistance, although only the aerobic exercise group showed a decrease in the waist-hip ratio and waist circumference. There were no positive results for lipid profile of fasting food sugar either before or after the exercise program. The effect of aerobic exercise on lipid profile is a controversial matter because the results of different studies show disparate data. This fact could be related to the short duration of the training programs carried out in these studies or maybe the effect of exercise on lipid profile is only noticeable in people who have a previously altered profile before the exercise and not in those whose profile is normal. (Ramalho et al., 2008).

Most studies which have assessed the effect of physical exercise on DM1 control are based on aerobic exercise, and the results have been disparate, since metabolic control improvements have been obtained only in some cases (Kavookjian et al. 2007; Ramalho et al. 2006). 11 DM1 patients showed beneficial effects in glycated hemoglobin after a 12-week training period of aerobic exercise and resistance training. Similar results were obtained in another study of DM1 teenagers after 12 weeks of vigorous games and recreational activities. However, not every study obtained the same beneficial results despite the fact that the number of training weeks was the same in all of them (Ramalho et al. 2006).

It has been argued that one of the possible reasons for the lack of improvement in glycated hemoglobin is the fact that these studies have been carried out in a very short period of time and that it may be necessary to perform a regular exercise program with a longer span duration (a year) in order to be able to observe different results. (Ramalho et al., 2006). Another possibility is that although insulin needs decrease with physical exercise glicemic control does not improve because patients consume more carbohydrates in order to prevent exercise-associated hypoglycemia (Kavookjian et al. 2007).

Several authors (Sideraviciute et al., 2006; Komatsu et al., 2005) have reported a higher BMI value for DM1 teenagers compared to healthy adolescents. Fat mass percentage is also higher in DM1 patients although after 14 weeks of swimming training this percentage was reduced significantly (Sideraviciute et al., 2006). After the exercise program participants experienced an improvement in their aerobic capacity, which is normally lower than that of healthy people (Sideraviciute et al., 2006; Komatsu et al., 2005). This is an important fact to take into account when prescribing exercise to these populations.

Diabetes mellitus type 2

DM2 patients benefit from aerobic activity because insulin sensitivity improvement and blood glucose control produce positive changes in body composition. Despite these benefits and the encouragement of aerobic exercise by doctors, less than 30% of diabetics, which is less than the general population, participate in aerobic activities, thus not reaching the recommended minimum. This inactivity is related to the difficulties that diabetic patients have in sport practice due to being overweight and suffering from foot ailments (Plotnikoff, et al. 2008).

Kavookjian et al. (2007) in their review of numerous studies on interventions on diabetic people found that exercise could reduce Hb A1c levels in such a way that it should also reduce the risks of the illness complications. High intensity exercise obtained better results in the reduction of these levels. Cardiovascular risk is also reduced through the effect that exercise has on blood pressure, body mass index and lipid profile. They pointed out that those programs which combine resistance training and aerobic exercise can also reduce abdominal and visceral fat and obesity. This combination has shown to improve significantly insulin sensitivity when compared with aerobic exercise alone. They also emphasize the fact that the interventions on DM2 populations lasted for short periods of time, therefore, it would be necessary to carry out longer interventions in order to observe the obtained results and the practice adherence.

7.3 Mechanism of Action

In DM1 patients physical exercise along with blood glucose control reduce the thickness of the basal membrane of the muscle capillary, the record of arterial pulse volume, and increase lean body mass and effort capacity.

One of the main benefits of physical exercise is the improvement of glucose tolerance due to the increase in insulin sensitivity. When insulin receptors affinity is increased a lower amount of insulin is needed to maintain correct blood glucose levels. This higher sensitivity enables glucose to enter the muscle cells efficiently, improving glucose homeostasis and reducing medication requirements. Insulin sensitivity seems to be related to capillary growth in the muscles after repetitive exercise, which provokes muscle hypertrophy and higher glucose metabolism. These adaptations result in lower needs of basal and posprandial insulin in DM patients. In young DM1 patients a reduction in insulin requirements was observed, in some cases up to 9%, which meant obvious social benefits for them due to their participation in sports.

Diabetic people who are physically fit have also a high insulin sensitivity which can be acute (as a result of faster muscular glucose replacement) or chronic (it indicates an increase in the total amount of metabolically active muscle) and which enables glucose to enter the cells more efficiently during exercise. It is important to note that the increase in sensitivity provided by exercise (acute effect) starts to decrease after 1 or 2 inactive days and it is lost a few days later.

Regular physical activity provokes beneficial physiological changes in DM2 patients including lower resting and Sub-Max heart rate, higher expulsion volume and cardiac consumption, improved oxygen extraction and lower blood pressure both at rest and during effort. In addition to this, abdominal fat is reduced, weight is better controlled and obesity is less likely to appear.

Another benefit is lower cardiovascular risk. The increase in aerobic capacity in DM2 patients is related to a less atherogenic lipid profile. Most studies, although not all of them, have found that after physical training DM2 patients show desirable changes in triglyceride levels, total cholesterol levels and HDL cholesterol/total cholesterol ratio. Regular physical activity also reduces blood pressure in people who suffer from DM2. The high level of insulin produces hypertrophy of the tunica media of the blood vessel's wall's muscle layer. This hypertrophy produces chronic hypertension. Exercise can reduce blood pressure by lowering insulin levels and reversing the wall's hypertrophy (GAFS, 2006).

Endothelial dysfunction is related to arteriosclerosis (Kavookjian et al., 2007), since it plays an important role in keeping the blood's fluidity, vascular tone and permeability. Endothelial dysfunction has been reported in both DM1 and DM2, where blood glucose level is associated to higher oxidative stress. Increased blood flow through the muscles during exercise provokes a higher stress on vascular walls, which results in higher nitric acid release and subsequent vascular dilatation.

Lastly, it is important to point out that psychological benefits such as stress reduction can result in better blood glucose level control, since stress can be a negative factor in this respect, which in turn improves the patient's quality of life.

7.4. Physical Exercise Prescription in Diabetes

Diabetes mellitus type 1

People with this type of diabetes must be very careful with their blood glucose control in order to avoid hyperglycemia induced by a wrong adjustment between insulin dose and physical exercise.

Rabasa-Lhoret, et al. (2001), show that habitual use of insulin prior to exercise (at any intensity) is associated to a higher risk of suffering a hyperglycemia episode. They propose:

- A 50% reduction of ultra-fast prepandrial insulin dose for 60-minute-long aerobic exercise performed at 25% of VO2max.
- A 50-75% reduction for 30 to 60 minutes long exercises performed at 50% of VO2max.
- A 75% for 40-minute long exercises at 75% of VO2max.

During long duration and low intensity exercise it is recommended to consume carbohydrates (10-15g every 30 minutes) during or after the sport practice in order to prevent hypoglycemia if there has not been a reduction in the insulin dose.

According to the American College of Sport Medicine recommendations, the ideal aerobic program for DM1 is as follows:

Duration: 40 minutes

Intensity: 40-85% VO2mác or 60-90% MHR (the first weeks intensity will be 60-70% and it will increase progressively depending on the patient's adaptation to exercise)

Frecuency: 3-5 times per week.

Diabetes Mellitus Type 2

The American Collage of Sport Medicine endorses exercise as a treatment method for people with type 2 diabetes and currently recommends expending a minimum cumulative total of 1000 kcal/week of energy from aerobic activities. The American Diabetes Association has similar recommendations for at least 150 min per week of moderate intensity aerobic physical activity and/or 90 min per week of vigorous aerobic exercise. However, it is necessary to improve the strategies, looking for the most effective methods to increase adherence ratio. (Gordon et al. 2009).

According to Sigal et al. (2004) recommendations, DM2 patients should stick to this aerobic training depending on the target they want to achieve.

To improve glycemic control and reduce risk of cardiovascular disease:

- Duration: 150 min/week or, 90 min/week
- Intensity: moderate aerobic exercise 40-60% Vo2max -50-70%MHR or vigorous aerobic exercise >60% Vo2max- >70% del MHR, respectively.

- Frequency: 3 days a week at least, trying not to spend more than two consecutive days without exercising.

To reduce risk of cardiovascular disease;

- Duration: 4 hours/week
- Intensity: vigorous aerobic (>60% Vo2max- >70% del MHR) combined with resistance exercise

For long-term maintenance of major weight loss:

- Duration: 7h/week.
- Intensity: moderate or vigorous aerobic physical activity.

8. Cardiovascular Disease

8.1 Disease Characteristics

Cardiovascular diseases (CVD) are those which affect the heart and blood vessels. They can be classified into various groups:

- Coronary heart disease: Diseases which affect the blood vessels which irrigate the cardiac muscle (myocardium).
- Cerebrovascular disease: Diseases which affect the blood vessels which irrigate the brain.
- Peripheral arteriopathies: Diseases which affect the blood vessels which irrigate higher and lower limbs.
- Rheumatic cardiopathy: Injuries of the myocardium and cardiac valves due to rheumatic fever, an illness caused by streptoccocus bacteria.
- Congenital cardiopathies: Marlformations or physical anomalies of the heart present from birth.
- Deep Vein Thrombosis (DVT) and Pulmonary Embolism (PE): Blood clots in the veins of the legs (thrombuses) which may become dislodged from their site of formation (embolus) and travel to the arterial blood supply of the lungs (embolism).

The American Heart Association points out that enormous progress has currently been made in the fight against cardiovascular diseases since, during the 1990's, they were the first cause of mortality in the United States. Nowadays,about 71 million American adults suffer from one or more different cardiovascular diseases. Every year in the United States cardiovascular diseases are top on the list of the gravest health problems in the country, Coronary Heart Disease being the first cause of death among them.

The cost of cardiovascular diseases and stroke in the United States in 2009 is estimated to be $475.3 billion, according to the American Heart Association and the National Heart, Lung, and Blood Institute (NHLBI). This figure includes both direct and indirect costs. Direct costs include the cost of physicians and other professionals, hospital and nursing home services, the cost of medications, home health care and other medical durables. Indirect costs include lost productivity that results from illness and death. This is only the economic cost. The true cost in human terms of suffering and lost lives is incalculable.

However, we must point out that, in spite of these data, scientific studies show that almost all cardiovascular disease patients or people susceptible to suffer from these illnesses can use aerobic exercise as an invaluable tool to recover health (Hoekstra et al. 2008), especially if they also follow an adequate diet and give up smoking.

8.2 Aerobic Exercise and Cardiovascular Disease

Lack of exercise and sedentary life are risk factors which accentuate the possibility of developing cardiovascular diseases. Aerobic activity during free time or at work is associated to a reduction of 30% in the frequency and mortality of cardiovascular diseases.This involves an inversely proportional relationship: the more aerobic physical activity, the less incidence of cardiovascular episodes. It is important to note that aerobic exercise is beneficial for both sexes and all age groups, as long as it is regularly practiced regardless of the age at which the patient starts exercising. This indicates that it is never too late to obtain its benefits.

Olson, et al., (2006) carried out a piece of research with the aim to examine the effects of 1 year of resistance training (RT) on vascular structure and function in overweight but otherwise healthy eumenorrheic women. They included 30 student women (15 control, 15 RT) overweight (BMI > 25 kg x m(-2)) aged 24-44 yr, who were studied before and after a 1-yr RT intervention. Vascular structure and function were assessed via noninvasive ultrasound imaging of the carotid and brachial arteries, respectively. Body composition, blood pressure, fasting blood lipids and glucose were also measured. The results showed that the RT group experienced a significant mean improvement in one-repetition maximum bench press following 1 yr of RT ($P < 0.05$). There was also a significant increase in lean body mass in the RT group compared to the control group ($P = 0.04$). There were no training-associated changes in blood pressure, fasting blood lipids, glucose, or insulin levels. Although there was no change in carotid artery intimamedia thickness, peak flow-mediated dilation significantly improved in the RT group ($P < 0.05$). The principal significant finding in this study was the initial demonstration that RT alone can improve brachial artery endothelial function in overweight eumenorrheic women, and therefore resistance training reduces the possiblity of suffering from cardiovascular disease.

Murphy et al., (2006) examined the effects of 45 minutes self-paced walking, 2 d. wk(-1) on aerobic fitness, blood pressure (BP), body composition, lipids and C-Reactive Protein (CRP) in previously sedentary civil servants. Age sample group consisted of 37 subjects (24 women) aged 41.5 +/- 9.3 years who were randomly assigned to either two 45-minute walks per week group (walking group) or no training group (control group). Aerobic fitness, body composition, blood pressure (BP), CRP and lipoprotein variables were measured at baseline and following 8 weeks. Step counts were measured at baseline and during weeks 4 and 8 of the intervention. Compared to the control group, the walking group showed a significant reduction in systolic BP and maintained body fat levels ($P < 0.05$). There were no changes in other risk factors. Subjects took significantly more steps on the days when prescribed walking was performed (9303 +/- 2665) compared to rest days (5803 +/- 2749; $P < 0.001$). These findings suggest that walking twice per week for 45 minutes at approximately 62% HRmax, improves activity levels, reduces systolic BP and prevents an increase in body fat in previously sedentary adults. This walking prescription, however, failed to induce significant improvements in other markers of cardiovascular disease risk following eight weeks of training.

Harrell et al. (1998), developed a piece of research whose aim was to determine the immediate effects of two types of elementary school-based interventions on children with multiple cardiovascular disease (CVD) risk factors. Four hundred and twenty-two children aged 9 +/- 0.8 years with at least two risk factors at baseline: low aerobic power and either high serum cholesterol or obesity. Both 8-week interventions consisted of a knowledge and attitude program and an adaptation of physical education. The classroom-based intervention was given by regular teachers to all children in the 3rd and 4th grades. The risk-based intervention was given in small groups only to children with identified risk factors. Children in the control group received usual teaching and physical education. The primary outcome measure was cholesterol; additional measures were blood pressure, body mass index, body fat, eating and activity habits, and health knowledge. RESULTS: Both interventions produced large reductions in cholesterol (-10.1 mg/dL and -11.7 mg/dL) compared with a small drop (-2.3 mg/dL) in the controls. There was a trend for systolic blood pressure to increase less in both intervention groups than in the controls. Both intervention groups had a small reduction in body fat and higher health knowledge than the control group. Both brief interventions can improve the CVD risk profile of children with multiple risk factors. The classroom-based approach was easier to implement and used fewer resources. This population approach should be considered as one means of early primary prevention of CVD.

As we have been able to see in the conclusions of the previously exposed works , aerobic exercise provokes an improvement in cardiovascular disease risk factors, thus a training program especially designed taking into account the needs and limitations of the patient allows the heart to adapt itself to variable situations, performing an adequate contraction at rest and an agile response during exercise.

8.3 Mechanism of Action

Taking into account the aforementioned facts, we can conclude that regular aerobic exercise is beneficial mainly for two reasons. First, it is a fundamental pillar in the modification of cardiovascular disease risk factors (it reduces blood pressure, improves peripheral circulation and so on) and secondly, it plays an important role in the prevention and treatment of functional capacity decline, because it improves articulatory movement range and muscular strength ,especially in lower limbs, increases elasticity and tone and reduces muscular fatigue caused by insufficient postural hygiene in daily life activities. All these factors contribute to a significant improvement in people's quality of life. However, we must never forget that, although physical exercise is beneficial for cardiovascular diseases, patients must seek professional advice before taking up any kind of activity. Experts will plan and prescribe aerobic exercise and will design the guidelines for its proper performance according to the patient's physical fitness.

8.4 Physical Exercise Prescription in Cardiovascular Disease

It is a fact that those people who do aerobic exercise regularly develop a cardiac training effect, better recovery and basal heart rate which is able to respond with agility during exercise in order to increase heart performance. This is called heart-beneficial exercise because if it is combined with a serious limitation of risk factors such as smoking and excessive calorie intake, it will reduce blood pressure and cardiovascular risk profile, which enables the patient to achieve cardiovascular health. A minimum of 30 minutes of aerobic exercise 3-4 days per week is enough to keep a good physical condition. An ideal aerobic exercise program should include 5-10 minutes of warming-up, performing soft movements in order to increase heart rate. The patient should then perform gradually about 20 minutes of aerobic activity (such as aerobic gymnastics, treadmill jogging, walking, swimming) in order to reach training heart rate. Training heart rate indicates exercise intensity. At the beginning of a training program, it is advisable to stick to the lower limit of the training zone (50% of maximum HR, 40% VO2 max). If exercise is practiced regularly intensity can be raised close to the higher limit of the training zone (75% of maximum HR; 60% VO2 max) (Pescatello, 2004). Training HR must never be reached at the beginning of the training session because the muscles and the circulatory system must get ready slowly. The session should be finished with a 5-10 minute cooling down period in order to reduce HR and avoid muscle contraction.

9. Asthma

9.1 Basic Aspects of the Illness

Asthma is a chronic lung disease characterized by bronchial hyperresponsiveness, that is, an excessive constriction of the bronchial tree which causes airflow obstruction. This illness is caused, in general, by one or more factors such as exposure to a cold, humid or allergenic environment, exercise and effort in hyperreactive patients, or emotional stress. Asthma is not a new pathology. The process as a symptom is already reported in the Ebers scroll (3500 BC) and Hippocrates was the first to use the expression “panting for air” to describe these respiratory alterations.Maimonides is acknowledged as the first author to write a monography on the process of asthma. Our modern concept of asthma makes it difficult to imagine how scholars in the ancient past regarded the illness.It was not until the 17th and 18th century that asthma started to be differentiated from other respiratory diseases when doctors like

Thomas Willis and Sir John Floyer (1649-1734) in ther work “A Treatise of the Asthma” (1698) treated the disease in a way which was different from other processes but similar for all those patients who were suffering it. Asthma is a very frequent disease. Ten per cent of children and teenagers have asthma, being more frequent in boys than in girls, although this trend is reversed in adulthood when it is more frequent in women. The cause for this tendency change is still not known but some experts suggest a possible lung immaturity in boys compared to girls during the first stages of life.

Asthma has been increasing in prevalence since 1980 (Mannino et al 1998). During the1991–2001 period, the problem of asthma was the focus of programs and reports from governmental agencies (e.g., the National Heart Lung and Blood Institute’s National Asthma

Education and Prevention Program [NAEPP] (*NIH, 1993*) and the U.S. Department of Health and Human Services' Action Against Asthma report (*US-DHHS, 2001*) and nongovernmental commissions (e.g., the Pew Environmental Health Commission's Attack Asthma report (*PEHC, 2001*). A common feature of these reports and programs is a call for improved asthma surveillance. Asthma is a key component of the Healthy People 2010 objectives (*US-DHHS, 2000*).Costs generated by asthma in the United States were 6.2 billion dollars in 1990 and 12.7 billion dollars in 1998. According to estimations based on this last period, asthma costs for 2010 will exceed 20 billion dollars.

9.2 Aerobic Exercise and Asthma

Two out of three people who suffer from asthma feel unfit to perform aerobic exercise or to participate in recreational or physical activities, especially when they realise that exercise itself may provoke an asthma attack. Therefore, any kind of physical exercise performed by asthmatic patients must be adequately prescribed in order to avoid an asthma episode. However, and in spite of these possible negative consequences for the patient, aerobic exercise facilitates breathing by strengthening the respiratory muscles and improves the patient's health, therefore doctors recommend exercise to asthmatic people as long as some basic guidelines are taken into account.

Different researchers have supported the idea that aerobic exercise has a beneficial effect on the asthmatic patients' health and on their quality of life. Fanelli et al., (2007) carried out a piece of research whose aim was to check if aerobic training was effective in improving cardiopulmonary fitness in asthmatic children. However, the actual impact of physical training on clinical indicators of disease control remains controversial. The sample group consisted of thirty-eight children with moderate to severe persistent asthma who were randomly assigned to control (N=17) and training (N=21) groups. The results showed that physical training was associated with significant improvements in physiological variables at peak and submaximal exercise ($P<0.05$); in contrast, no significant changes were found in controls. Severity of exercise-induced bronchoconstriction (EIB) and postexercise breathlessness were significantly lessened in trained patients; improvement in fitness and EIB, however, were not linearly related ($P>0.05$). Consequently, we can conclude that supervised exercise training might be associated with beneficial effects on disease control and quality of life in asthmatic children. These data suggest an adjunct role of physical conditioning on clinical management of patients with more advanced disease.

Another similar piece of research was carried out by Basaran et al (2006), who assessed the effects of regular submaximal exercise on quality of life, exercise capacity and pulmonary function in asthmatic children. They included in their study sixty-two children with mild-moderate asthma (mean age 10.4 (SD 2.1) years) who were randomly allocated into exercise and control groups. The exercise group underwent a moderately intensive basketball training program for 8 weeks. A home respiratory exercise program was advised to both groups. Pediatric Asthma Quality of Life Questionnaire (PAQLQ) was used for the evaluation of activity limitation, symptoms and emotional functions. Although PAQLQ scores improved in both groups, the improvement in the exercise group was significantly higher. The exercise group performed better in the PWC 170 and 6-minute walk tests, whereas no improvement was detected in the control group at the end of the trial. Medication scores improved in both groups, but symptom scores improved only in the exercise group. No significant changes were detected in pulmonary function in either group, except for peak expiratory flow values in the exercise group. Therefore, we can claim that eight weeks of regular submaximal exercise have beneficial effects on quality of life and exercise capacity in children with asthma. Submaximal basketball training is an effective alternative exercise program for asthmatic children.

Recent reports indicate that aerobic exercise improves the overall physical fitness and health of asthmatic patients. The specific exercise-induced improvements in the pathology of asthma and the mechanisms by which these improvements occur, however, are ill-defined; thus, the therapeutic potential of exercise in the treatment of asthma remains unappreciated. Using an OVA-driven mouse model, Pastva, et al. (2004) examined the role of aerobic exercise in modulating inflammatory responses associated with atopic asthma. Data demonstrate that moderate intensity aerobic exercise training decreased leukocyte infiltration, cytokine production, adhesion molecule expression, and structural remodeling within the lungs of OVA-sensitized mice ($n = 6\text{-}10$; $p < 0.05$). Because the transcription factor NF-kappaB regulates the expression of a variety of genes that encode inflammatory mediators, we monitored changes in NF-kappaB activation in the lungs of exercised/sensitized mice. Results show that exercise decreased NF-kappaB nuclear translocation and IkappaBalpha phosphorylation, indicating that exercise decreased NF-kappaB activation in the lungs of sensitized mice ($n = 6$). Taken together, these results suggest that aerobic exercise attenuates airway inflammation in a mouse model of atopic asthma via modulation of NF-kappaB activation. Potential exists, therefore, for the amelioration of asthma-associated chronic airway inflammation through the use of aerobic exercise training as a non-drug therapeutic modality.

9.3 Mechanism of Action

Regular aerobic physical activity of adequate intensity and duration involving large muscle groups has been proved to have a number of potential beneficial effects on general health, including improvement in aerobic capacity, body composition, flexibility, muscular strength, and psychosocial measures. This improvement might be particularly true for patients who suffer from chronic diseases such as bronchial asthma. In people with asthma, physical training can improve cardiopulmonary fitness without changing lung function. This appeared to be a normal training effect and not due to an improvement in resting lung function. It is not known whether improved fitness is translated into improved quality of life. It is comforting to note that physical training does not have an adverse effect on lung function and wheeze in patients with asthma (Ram et al., 2005). Therefore, there is no reason why patients with asthma should not be able to participate in regular physical activities. When training asthmatic subjects, it would be appropriate to give them guidance about the prevention and treatment of exercise-induced asthma.

9.4 Physical Exercise Prescription in Asthma

Apart from an adequate control of asthma through medication, asthmatic patients must take into account some basic recommendations when doing exercise which include an adequate warming-up ad cooling down period in order to prevent and reduce the frequency of exercise-induced asthmatic crisis. The kind of exercise performed by the patient plays an important role to determine the degree of exercise-induced asthma. Outdoors running is the form of exercise which provokes the most exercise-induced asthma whereas indoors swimming provokes the least due to the fact that the air is hot and humid in the swimming pool and prevents cold and dryness in the airways. Another factor to take into account is the duration of physical exercise because continuous, intense and prolongued exercise causes more induced asthma than short-duration repetitive exercise. Intensity must also be taken into account because the higher the intensity of the aerobic exercise (80%-90% of maximum HR) the more likely the induced asthma will appear (Anderson, 1988). Breathing through the mouth instead of breathing slowly through the nose, not using any kind of mask when exercising in cold weather and not checking the place where exercise is going to be performed in order to eliminate irritating or allergenic substances can also bring about induced asthma. Having in mind these recommendations, an adequate selection of sport activities could help to prevent induced asthma. Swimming, wrestling, sprint racing and team sports such as football and baseball could be well tolerated (Rosimini, 2003).

Other activities which are associated to high incidence of induced asthma are particularly winter sports (except slalom ski) and those which involve long races (for example cross-country races and basketball). However,it is possible for the patients to participate in these activities by using bronchodilatators for prophylaxis.

10. Chronic Obstructive Pulmonary Disease (COPD)

10.1 Disease Characteristics

The chronic obstructive pulmonary disease (COPD) is a group of diseases of the lungs in which the airways become narrowed (A reduction in forced expiratory volume during the first second and of the relationship expiratory volume/ forced vital capacity (GOLD, 2007; Peces-Barba G, 2008)). This leads to a limitation of the flow of air to and from the lungs causing shortness of breath. In contrast to asthma, the limitation of airflow is poorly reversible and usually gets progressively worse over time. COPD is caused by noxious particles or gases, most commonly from smoking, which trigger an abnormal inflammatory response in the lung. The inflammatory response in the larger airways is known as chronic bronchitis. In the alveoli, the inflammatory response causes destruction of the tissues of the lung, a process known as emphysema. The natural course of COPD is characterized by occasional sudden worsenings of symptoms called acute exacerbations, most of which are caused by infections or air pollution.

Chronic Bronchitis (Llor et al. 2006). It is is defined clinically as a persistent cough that produces sputum (phlegm) and mucus, for at least three months in two consecutive years, as long as cough is not produced by other causes such as cystic fibrosis, bronchiecstasis, higher airways obstruction or obliterans bronchiolitis.

Enphysema (Honig, 1998) It is defined in pathological terms as the permanent widening of distal air cavities of the terminal bronchioli with alveolar wall destruction and no manifest fibrosis. Those cases of chronic asthma with irreversible airflow obstruction deserve especial consideration because their characteristics make it difficult to use differential diagnose with COPD.

Historical data report COPD since the 16th century. Hippocrates did not use this term to diagnose patients who presented cough with phlegm, dyspnea and wheezing, but he employed "asthma" for all those conditions in which the patient showed shortness of air.

In those times, the term enphysema (from the Greek word "emphysao" which means "blowing inside") started to be used to refer to the presence of air inside the tissues. In the 17th century and based on studies on autopsies, the entities that we currently describe as COPD became known. However, the term "bronchitis" was used by medical literature until the end of the18th century. In 1958 a differentiated definition of chronic bronchitis, pulmonar enphysema and COPD was established (García, 2006).

The World Health Organization has foreseen that this illness will become the fifth cause of morbidity in 2020 (it is currently the 12th) and the third cause of mortality(it is currently the 4th).World prevalence of COPD ranges from 5-10%; percentage which has considerably increased due to smoking, population ageing and greater incidence observed in women. It is estimated that around 16 million people will suffer from it in the United States and it will become the fourth cause of death between 65 and 84 years of age. The economic impact of the disease is high, approximately 30 billion dollars in the United States (20 billion for direct costs and 10 billion for indirect costs) (Akazawa et al., 2008).

Aerobic exercise presents itself as one of the treatments proposed by international experts to fight Chronic Obstructive Pulmonary Disease (COPD). Physical exercise provokes an improvement in effort tolerance and in the general health state of the patient. It has been observed that some COPD patients suffer from anxiety, depression and social isolation as a consequence of the physical limitation that the typical airflow obstruction which is characteristic of this illness involves. Exercising offers the patient an opportunity to return to social life. (Clark et al, 1996; Normandin et al, 2002).

10.2 Aerobic Exercise and Chronic Obstructive Pulmonary Disease

Skeletal muscle dysfunction is one of the most serious extrapulmonary manifestations of chronic obstructive pulmonary disease (COPD). This dysfunction limits exercise tolerance and is associated with complaints of fatigue and dyspnea even after minimal exertion (ATSERSS, 1999). Deconditioning is almost certainly a contributing factor, given that patients with COPD have symptom-limited exercise tolerance, which compromises their cardiac fitness and further limits their exercise tolerance, leading to exacerbation of their symptoms after exertion.

The efficacy of aerobic programs in COPD patients has been well established. Endurance training of the lower extremities, resulting in greater exercise tolerance, is an important component of these programs (Celli & Macnee, 2004).

Borjen et al., (2009) carried out a study whos aim was to investigate whether individual leg cycling could produce higher whole body peak oxygen uptake (VO(2peak)) than two legs cycling during aerobic high intensity interval training in chronic obstructive pulmonary disease (COPD) patients. Nineteen patients trained in 24 supervised cycling sessions either by one leg training (OLT) (n = 12) or by two legs training (TLT) (n = 7) at 4 x 4 min intervals at 85-95% of peak heart rate. Whole body VO(2peak) and peak work rate increased significantly by 12 and 23% in the OLT, and by 6 and 12% in the TLT from pre- to post-training, respectively, and were significantly greater in the OLT than the TLT ($P < 0.05$). The present study demonstrates that one leg aerobic high intensity interval cycling is superior to two legs in increasing whole body VO(2peak), indicating a muscle rather than a cardiovascular limitation to VO(2peak) in these COPD patients.

Nakamura et al (2008) evaluated whether strength or recreational activities are a useful addition to aerobic training in patients with chronic obstructive pulmonary disease (COPD). Thirty-three patients with moderate to severe COPD were randomly assigned to 12 weeks of aerobic combined with strength training (AERO+ST) or combined with recreational activities (AERO+RA). The AERO regime consisted of three weekly 20-min walking exercise sessions; the ST regime included three series of 10 repetitions of four exercises; and the RA regime consisted of training using exercise balls to perform smoothly for instrumental activity of daily living. Baseline and after-training measurements of peripheral muscular strength and endurance, cardio respiratory fitness, and 6-min walking distance were obtained, whereas quality of life was assessed with the Short Form 36 questionnaire. Change in grip strength showed a significant difference between the AERO+ST group (8.3+/-6.7%) and the control group (-1.3+/-10.5%), and AERO+RA group (-4.7+/-5.6%) ($P<0.05$). A significant increase was found in percentage change in peak (.)V(O2) between the AERO+ST group (5.1+/-11.8%) and the control group (-9.2+/-8.6%) ($P<0.05$). In the health-related quality of life scores, there was a significant difference in mean percentage change in physical functioning between the AERO+ST group (7.9+/-24.4%) and the control group (-14.8+/-19.1%) ($P<0.05$). A significant difference was found in mean percentage change in social functioning between the AERO+RA group (9.4+/-20.0%) and the control group (-14.9+/-23.2%) ($P<0.05$). A significant difference in mean percentage change in mental health was also found between the AERO+RA group (12.2+/-12.4%) and the control group (-5.0+/-7.8%) ($P<0.05$). It is preferable to introduce various forms of exercise than to use different muscles involving the whole body, such as recreational activities, as they are an appropriate approach to stimulating physical activity and to improving functional fitness gradually while improving health-related quality of life, though it is necessary to practice exercises for maintenance and improvement in patients with COPD.

Arnardóttir et al., (2006) compared the effects on exercise capacity and health-related quality of life (HRQoL) of two exercise programmes; one programme including endurance training and one including only resistance training and callisthenics. A second purpose was to find out whether the severity of chronic obstructive pulmonary disease (COPD) affected the training response and whether the interventions had a long-term effect. Sixty-three patients were stratified according to severity of COPD and randomised to two training groups. Group A had a mixed programme including endurance training. Group B had resistance training and callisthenics. All trained twice weekly for 8 weeks. A symptom-limited ergometer test, 12-min walking test, dynamic spirometry, blood gas analysis at rest and HRQoL were measured before and after the training period. Follow-up tests were conducted at 6 and 12 months after training. Forty-two patients fulfilled the trial. In group A (n=20) peak exercise capacity increased by 7W ($P<0.001$) and 12-min walking distance (12MWD) by 50 m ($P<0.01$), whereas group B (n=22) did not change in any of these variables. HRQoL did not change significantly in either group. Training response was similar in patients with moderate and severe disease. One year post-training 12MWD had returned to pre-training level in group A, and below pre-training level in group B ($P<0.05$). The conclusion was that exercise capacity in patients with severe and moderate COPD improved by intensive endurance training, two sessions a week for 8 weeks. The improvement was however small and HRQoL did not improve. Severity of illness did not affect response to training. The results indicated that the effects of a short endurance training intervention slowed down decline in baseline functional exercise capacity for 1 year.

These studies corroborate that regular physical exercise such as walking or cycling is effectively associated with a decrease in pulmonary function deterioration and with an improvement in the patient's health.

10.3 Mechanism of Action

The shortness of breath experienced by COPD patients at rest and/or during activities of daily living can lead to an increasingly sedentary lifestyle, a progressive deterioration in functional capacity, and possible isolation at home. With progressive inactivity, cardiovascular function and skeletal muscle mass decline. The deterioration in aerobic fitness and strength creates a vicious cycle that leads to greater breathlessness with exertion, muscular fatigue, eventual loss of functional independence and depression. A major goal of aerobic exercise programs is, therefore, to reverse the physical disability resulting from inactivity. Aerobic Exercise, at almost any level, improves the oxygen utilization, work capacity, and state of mind of COPD patients. Low-impact activities place minimum stress on joints and are easier to perform than high-intensity activities.

Many physiological and psychological benefits have been reported in COPD patients after participation in prescribed exercise involving upper and lower body aerobic and resistance training.

Major benefits include increased physical capacity, decreased anxiety about breathlessness, greater independence in daily activities, reduced fatigue and improved quality of life. These positive outcomes occur even through impaired lung function continues to persist after exercise training. Regular exercise thus enables COPD patients to do more recreational and vocational activities despite their lung disease. Importantly, the gain in fitness and confidence with exercise reverses the spiral of deconditioning associated with COPD. One reason of the decreased exercise anxiety is that patients become desensitized to the shortness of breath that they live with on a daily basis. Furthermore, researchers have shown that COPD patients who exercise may also show better performance on tests of verbal fluency (Emery et al., 1998)., suggesting that regular exercise increases blood flow to the brain to enhance cognitive function.

10.4 Physical Exercise Prescription in COPD

Exercise guidelines for COPD patients include 30-minute sessions 3-4 times a week for a period of 6-8 weeks (Cooper, 2001) for the patient to be able to notice an improvement, althought the patient's perception of his improvement will be conditioned by his disease status. However, other studies show an improvement in the patient from the fourth week on (Cochrane, 2002). As far as intensity is concerned, there is no unanimity among researchers. Casaburi et al. (1997) and Ries et al (1995) showed that patients trained at a higher intensity presented better physiological responses such as lactate decrease, minute ventilation, HR and VO2, but they required a closer supervision and stimulus. By contrast, other researchers obtained better responses to low to moderate intensity training in COPD patients.

According to the British Thoracic Society stamdards (BTS, 2001), in order to obtain the desired results an aerobic program must last at least for 4 to 12 weeks, 2-5 times a week, in 20-30 minute sessions and at an intensity of 60% of VO2 max. The plan must be progressively adjusted in duration and intensity, taking into account the fact that the higher intensity, the more lasting the effects. According to GOLD (2003) the optimal duration of an exercise program has not been established in randomized and controlled clinical studies, so this depends on available resources; however, they suggest a duration varying from 4 to 10 weeks, with longer lasting effects in those patients who participate in longer training programs.

11. Multiple Sclerosis

11.1 Disease Characteristics

Multiple Sclerosis (MS) is an inflammatory disease of the central nervous system (CNS) which was discovered by Dr. Charcot in 1868. There are about 300,000 patients suffering from Multiple Sclerosis in North America today. The peak onset is between 20 and 30 years of age . Almost 70% of patients manifest symptoms between ages 21 and 40. This disease rarely occurs prior to 10 or after 60 years of age. Multiple Sclerosis affects young and genetically predisposed people who have been exposed during their childhood to one or more adverse environmental conditions, probably viruses. It causes a dysfunction in the immune system, which develops a self-damaging action, mainly directed against the white substance. A series of plaque-shaped scars appear in different zones on the CNS and hence the disease's name, Multiple Sclerosis (multiple scars) or plaque sclerosis (Cambier, 2003). The typical symptoms of the illness are varied, but the commonest are visual disorder, fatigue, balance and coordination problems and muscular weakness among others. Due to this variability, the criteria for its diagnosis include complex neurological tests, such as evoked potential, magnetic resonance and analysis of the cephalorachidian fluid. Multiple Sclerosis can present itself in outbreaks or progressively, provoking a degenerative disability to those who suffer from it, and in some cases even death. There is no completely effective treatment against it, although some drugs like "Interferón" have demonstrated some efficacy in slowing down the advance of the illness. Although for many years MS patients were advised to avoid exercise, nowadays physical activity is regarded as a useful tool that should be part of every neurological rehabilitation program.

11.2 Aerobic Exercise and Multiple Sclerosis

For years, the relationship between MS and physical exercise was considered very harmful. Neurologists thought that MS patients should direct their energies to the performance of everyday activities, and keep away from physical exercise, since the rising in body temperature produced by it could exacerbate the signs of the illness. Besides, it was also taken into account the fact that other typical illness symptoms were likely to appear, such as Lhermitte's (an electric discharge which runs along the spine), or to become acute, such as fatigue.

According to the bibliography on the matter (Ayán, 2007), it was not before the 1970's when a former American Olympic champion, Jimmie Heuga was diagnosed with MS. Far from following the medical advice, this elite sportsman kept on training and exercising as much as his illness allowed him to do it, thus altering the scientific community's traditional point of view on the issue, and founding a centre in Colorado, The Jimmie Heuga Center, to offer an opportunity to those people willing to get involved in scientific research aimed at determining the role of exercise in SM patients.

In the early 1980's research on the effects of aerobic exercise on MS began to shape up, and it was based on aquatic activities, because floating enables the performance of movements and water temperature decreases the risk of temperature regulation problems. However, the most important reason to advise exercising in water is the recreational possibilities that this element offers. When a person suffers from MS, fatigue and muscular weakness prevent him or her to perform physical and recreational activities, thus missing the satisfaction of enjoying exercises and games in the company of friends and relatives. These inconveniences increase the time that the individuals spend stuck at home and therefore, their mood gets worse, and they end up with depression, which in turn makes the patients to isolate themselves even more. Nevertheless, given that an MS patient can move through water, and their muscular weakness is a less important handicap in water than on land, swimming pools and aquatic parks are ideal places for them not only to exercise, but also to be able to participate and enjoy recreational activities in the company of their loved ones, thus fighting off the negative psychological effects previously mentioned.

One of the first pieces of research which aimed at examining fitness improvement in MS patients after the performance of aquatic exercises was carried out by Gehslen et al. (1984), who recruited ten physically autonomous patients to participate in an aquatic training program which lasted for ten weeks, with the objective of studying the changes in their muscular resistance and strength. The training sessions were based on the performance of basic gymnastic exercises combined with several swimming styles, in three one-hour sessions per week. Intensity was established around 60%-75% of the maximum heart rate and water temperature oscillated between 25ºC and 27ºC. At the end of the program, it was observed, through dynamometric tests, an increase in muscular strength in all of the patients, along with a reduction in fatigue, which reinforced the hypothesis of the potential benefits of aquatic exercise. In another similar study (Sutherland et al, 2001) 22 patients were recruited, 11 of whom received aerobic training in a swimming pool three times a week for a period of ten weeks. When comparing their health state with that of the other individuals through several questionnaires, the researchers found that those patients who had participated in the training sessions not only presented less fatigue and a greater feeling of good health, but also confessed to have improved their sexual and social lives.

As far as the effectiveness of aerobic exercise outside the water is concerned, Olgiati et al., (1986), recruited 11 MS patients and submitted them to a rehabilitation program which lasted for four weeks and which consisted of light aerobic exercises. By the end of the program, the individuals proved to be able to walk faster and to cover longer distances before fatigue appeared when comparing them to a control group. These results suggest a possible cardiorespiratory improvement provoked by exercise, and they constitute an important antecedent for later research. Aerobic training became a very common tool in this kind of research. However, it could not be applied to everyone, due to the inability to walk that many MS patients present. Thus, new adapted cyclo-ergometers were created, designed to exercise upper and lower limbs, such as those used by Gappmaier et al.,(1994), who designed an aerobic program to determine the effects of 15 weeks of training, structured in 3-4 40-minute sessions a week. MS patients pedalled at an intensity around 60% of their VO2 max. After finishing the intervention, their aerobic capacity improved up to 21% and their epidermis thickness decreased down to 15%.

Similar research showed that this kind of patients can benefit from aerobic training regardless of their physical disability, and that its effects do not only affect them at a conditional level. In fact, the most recent scientific works point out that short aerobic training programs (lasting for less than 3 months) can help to improve MS patients' quality of life (Motl, 2008) and even reduce their level of fatigue (Newman, 2007). For these reasons, aerobic exercise should be included in the neurorehabilitation process of the illness.

11.3 Mechanism of Action

Aerobic exercise can be beneficial for MS patients for several reasons. First, this kind of patients experience fatigue and muscular weakness and tend to adopt a sedentary behaviour which aggravates their problems even more. When they participate in a training program, they abandon their sedentary routine and break that vicious circle, improving their well-being. Besides, the conditional improvements allow them to cope more efficiently with everyday routines and duties, reduce their level of fatigue and make them feel better. All these effects bring about a physical, psychological and social improvement that provokes an increase in the patient's quality of life.

Because of this, it has been stated that the effect of aerobic exercise training on the quality of life in MS is comparable in magnitude to the positive effects of disease modifying medications on the rate of exacerbations in MS and chronic exercise on mental health outcomes of cognitive function and feelings of energy and fatigue.

11.4 Physical Exercise Prescription in MS

In order to plan and carry out an exercise program for MS patients it must be taken into account that fatigue and increased body temperature will be the major limiting factors. After a thorough neurological examination to find out the individual's level of disability, the training program will be customized for the patient, paying attention to possible specific problems in coordination, ataxia, spasticity and motivation of every patient. The following table proposes an example of exercise prescription:

Example of protocol for aerobic walking-based training.

AGE	DISABILITY LEVEL	EXERCISE	CHARGE
20-35	Mild and sensory.	Running	15-20 min. 120 beats/min
20-45	Respects lower limb	Walking-running	1-5 min. walk / 5-10 min. run
------	Affects lower limb	Mild walk	60 min. Individual rest

Protocol for the performance of aerobic exercise in exercise bycicle

INTENSITY	VOLUME	FREQUENCY
50-60% de max. HR	20 min.	4 days/week
60-75% de max. HR	30 min.	3 days/week

12. Crohn's Disease

12.1 Basic Aspects of the Illness

Crohn's disease is defined as a chronic, relapsing inflammatory disorder of the alimentary canal which may involve anywhere from the mouth to the anus. Although it was first described by Giovanni Battista in the 18th century and by the Polish surgeon Dr. Lesniowski in the 20th century, it was named after the American gastroenterologist Bernard Crohn, who described fourteen cases in 1932 and gave the illness a new clinical identity (Blumberg, 2008).

Crohn's disease affects approximately 380,000 to 480,000 people in the United States. Although it may occur at any age, the incidence is bimodal with a peak in the third decade of life and a smaller peak in the fifth decade. The etiology of Crohn's disease is unknown, but suggested possibilities include genetic, environmental, immunologic, and infectious causes. An imbalance in local mucosal production of pro-inflammatory cytokines over anti-inflammatory cytokines is theorized to cause the well-demarcated, discontinuous, transmural, ulcerative lesions characteristic of the disease (Knutson, 2003). The diagnosis of Crohn's disease is based on a combination of exams: endoscopy, X-rays and histologic blood and tissue tests. The illness alternates flare-ups with states of remission and its most frequent symptoms are diarrhoeal bowel movements, abdominal pain and fever, among others. The current pharmacologic treatment can achieve the illness' remission in the long term, although acute cases are treated with steroids and surgery. Some lifestyle modifications such as changing some dietary habits and taking up some kind of activity have been suggested as factors which could induce an improvement in the patients' quality of life. Therefore, physical exercise may play an important role in this respect.

12.2 Aerobic Exercise and Crohn Disease

Although different epidemiological investigations have found and inverse relationship between CD development and occupational and recreational physical activity (Sonenberg, 1990), very few clinical relevant studies have evaluated the effects of an aerobic exercise intervention in patients experiencing CD. In this regard, Loudon et al. (1999) evaluated the effects of a 12-week mild walking program in 16 CD patients with inactive or mildly active disease. Once the intervention ended, physical health, general well-being, quality of life and perceived stress improved in some patients without disease exacerbation. Although the study presented some methodological flaws that can limit its findings, such as lack of a control group and small sample size (only 12 patients finished the program), a 6-month post study intervention showed that 50% of the completers were continuing to exercise between two and six days per week, suggesting that CD patients obtain some benefit from exercising. Separately, D'Inca et al. (1999), evaluated the effect of one-hour's exercise at a maximum of 60% oxygen in six males with ileal Crohn's disease in remission. Although a biochemical analysis showed that the patients at rest had primed neutrophils with increased activation after exercise, the proposed physical training did not elicit subjective symptoms or changes in intestinal permeability and lipoperoxidation. Since without symptom correlation, the clinical impact of this activation is hard to asses, this study shows that short-term exercise appeared to be well tolerated by CD patients in remission.

Finally, Ng et al. (2007) built on the preliminary work done by Loudon et al by including a control group and proposing and independent walking program. In this study patients were instructed to walk 30 for minutes at a low intensity, three times per week during three months. All of the sixteen subjects included in the exercise group completed the program, without suffering any disease exacerbation. Once the intervention finished, the obtained data showed that a low-intensity exercise program was enough to elicit improvements in quality of life and to decrease Crohn's disease-related symptoms.

In the light all of this, it seems intuitively appealing to promote participation in regular exercise in the management of CD.

12.3 Mechanism of Action

The aerobic training works by breaking a vicious cycle. Fatigue and low energy feeling together with muscle weakness limit the patient's physical functioning. The training aims to improve fitness, thereby reducing fatigue. Besides aerobic activities can enhance muscle performance, thereby enabling the patient to better manage daily life. In addition, it is likely that the patient benefits psychologically from experiencing these fitness improvements. However, it is important to note that Crohn's disease involves an immune system dysfunction. Research has implicated the proinflammatory cytokines interleukin-6 (IL-6) and tumour necrosis factor-alpha (TNF-α) in the intestinal inflammation inherent to CD (Lee et al. 2005). Although physical activity appears to reduce these inflammation markers, the results of several studies involving cycling, running, swimming and resistance exercises are controversial and no clear pattern emerges from them, so in this regard, more research is needed.

In spite of all this, physical exercise has been regarded as a useful tool when treating some of the symptoms that are strongly related to CD, such as pain, fatigue, bone mineral loss, sleep disturbances, bone mineral density, body composition and even intestitnal problems. It may be that physical exercise could improve quality of life in this kind of patients by means of attenuating some or all of this symptoms.

12.4 Physical Exercise Prescription in CD

When considering including physical activity in CD treatment, physicians need to know the different types of recommendable exercises that exist, as well as the determining aspects of duration, intensity, frequency and progression involved in them, in order to be able to prescribe them safely to CD patients. Some basic guidelines for carrying out aerobic exercise interventions with people suffering from CD can be found in the findings of the reviewed clinical studies.

According to several physical exercise interventions carried out with people suffering from different inflammatory pathologies, walking appears to be a safe, practical and easy-to-do form or aerobic exercise. Because of that, and giving its effects on the QoL of CD patients, walking is the main type of aerobic activity that should be recommended. Regarding the level of effort, it has been found that aerobic activity performed at an intensity between 40% and 60% of maximal oxygen consumption does not affect intestinal impermeability. Simultaneously, it has been shown that CD patients can walk and average distance of 3.5 kilometres without experiencing symptoms' exacerbation. Giving all that, physicians can prescribe 20 to 30 minutes of low intensity walking at 60% of individual's maximal heart rate, three days per week to start with. Once the patients get used to this exercise prescription, they should be encouraged to perform the same schedule during most days of the week. However, aerobic activity must be stopped whenever the patient feels that fatigue or CD related symptoms show some sign of exacerbation. Moreover, if CD patients cannot follow the exercise regime proposed, they should walk continuously at their own pace during bouts of 4 or 5 minutes, in order to obtain a minimum of 20 minutes of activity per day.

Finally, it must be noted that currently there is not available information regarding the effects of different types of aerobic exercise on CD patients such as cycling, swimming or weight-bearing walking. In this regard, further research is needed before any advice can be given.

References

Ablin, J., Neumann, L. B. & Buskila, D. (2008) Pathogenesis of fibromyalgia – a review. *Joint Bone Spine*, *75*, 273-279.

Aceves-Avila, F. J., Medina, F. & Fraga, A. (2001). The antiquity of rheumatoid arthritis: a reappraisal. *J Rheumatol.*, *28(4)*, 691-693.

Agre, J. C., Pierce, L. E., Raab, D. M., McAdams, M. & Smith, E. L. (1988). Light resistente and stretching exercise in elderly women: effect upon strenth. *Arch Phys Med Rehabil*, 273-276.

Ahlborg, H. G., Johnell, O., Turner, C. H., et al. (2003). Bone loss and bone size after menopause. *N Engl J Med.*, *349*, 327–34.

Akazawa, M., Halpern, R., Riedel, A. A., et al. (2008). Economic burden prior to COPD diagnosis: a matched case-control study in the United States. *Respir Med.*, *102*(12), 1744-52.

Alastair, J. J. Wood. (1998). Treatment of postmenopausal osteoporosis. *NEJM.*, *338*,736-746.

American College of Sports Medicine. (1990). The recommended quantity and quality of exercise for developing and maintaining cardiorespiratory and muscular fitness in healthy adults. *Med Sci Sports Exerc.*, *22*, 265-74.

American College of Sports Medicine. (1999). *Manual ACSM para la valoración y prescripción del ejercicio.* Barcelona: Paidotribo.

American Diabetes Association, www.diabetes.org. [Accesed march 10th 2009].

American Thoracic Society-European Respiratory Society Statement. (1999). Skeletal muscle dysfunction in chronic obstructive pulmonary disease. *Am J Respir Crit Care Med.*, *159*, 1s-28s.

Anderson, S. D. (1998). Exercise-induced asthma. En: E., Middleton, C., Reed, E., Ellis, N. F., Adkinson, J. W., Yunginger, (eds). *Allergy: Principles and practice.* (3rd. Edition). St. Louis: CV Mosby C°.

Andreoli, A., Monteleone, M., van Loan, M., et al. (2001). Effects of different sports on bone density and muscle mass in highly trained athletes. *Med Sci Sports Exerc.*, *33*, 507-11.

Arnardóttir, R. H., Sörensen, S., Ringqvist, I. & Larsson, K. (2006). Two different training programmes for patients with COPD: a randomised study with 1-year follow-up. *Respir Med.*, *100*(1), 130-9.

Arnett, F. C., Edworthy, S. M., Bloch, D. A., et al. (1988) The American Rheumatism Association 1987 revised criteria for the classification of rheumatoid arthritis. *Arthritis Rheum.*, *31*,315-24.

Assis, M. R. Silva, L.E., Alves, A.M., Pessanha, A.P., Valim, V., Feldman, D., et al. (2006). A randomized controlled trial of deep water running: clinical effectiveness of aquatic exercise to treat fibromyalgia. *Arthritis & Rheumatism.*, *55*, 57-65.

Ayán, C. (2007). *Esclerosis Múltiple y Ejercicio Físico.* Sevilla: Wanceulen.

Ayán, C. & Martín, V. (2007). Systemic lupus erythematosus and exercise. *Lupus.*, *16*, 5-9.

Bacon, S. L., Sherwood, A., Hinderliter, A., et al. (2004). Effects of exercise, diet and weight loss on high blood pressure. *Sports Med, 34 (5)*, 307-316.

Bailey, D. A., McKay, H. A., Mirwald, R. L., Crocker, P. R., et al. (1999). A six-year longitudinal study of the relationship of physical activity to bone mineral accrual in growing children: the university of Saskatchewan bone mineral accrual study. *J Bone Miner Res.*, *14*, 1672-9.

Barbado, C. (2001). *Revisión bibliográfica sobre osteoporosis y actividad física.* www.sectorfitness.com.

Basaran, S., Guler-Uysal, F., Ergen, N., et al. (2006). Effects of physical exercise on quality of life, exercise capacity and pulmonary function in children with asthma. *J Rehabil Med.*, *38*(2),130-5.

Baster, T. & Baster-Brooks, C. (2005). Exercise and hypertension. *Australian Family Physician.*, *34* (6), 419-424.

Bellver, M. & Pujol, P. (1997).*Osteoporosis y Ejercicio Físico.* CAR, Sant Cugat del Vallés en Temas actuales en Actividad Física y Salud. Menarini. Barcelona.

Birge, S. L., Daisky, G. (1989). The role of exercise in preventing osteoporosis. *Public Health Rep.*,*104*, 54-58.

Bjørgen, S., Hoff, J., Husby, V. S., et al. (2009). Aerobic high intensity one and two legs interval cycling in chronic obstructive pulmonary disease: the sum of the parts is greater than the whole. *Eur J Appl Physiol*, Apr 1.

Blumberg, R. S. (2008). Crohn disease. *Journal of American Medical Association., 300*,439-440.

British Thoracic Society Standards of Care Subcommittee on Pulmonary Rehabilitation. (2001). BTS Statement: Pulmonary Rehabilitation. *Thorax., 56*, 827-834.

Busch, A. J., Barber, K. A., Overend, T. J., Peloso, P. M. & Schachter, C. L. (2007). Exercise for treating fibromyalgia syndrome. *Cochrane Databases Systemic Review., 4*, CD003786

Cambier, J., Masson, M. & Dehen, H. (2003). *Esclerosis en Placas.*Barcelona: Masso.

Cancela, J. M. & Ayán, C. (2007). Effects of High-Intensity Combined Training on Women over 65. *Gerontology., 53*, 340-346.

Carvalho, M., Sato, E., Tebexreni, A., Heidecher, R. T., Schenkman, S. & Neto, T. L. (2005). Effects of supervised cardiovascular training programme on exercise tolerance, aerobic capacity and quality of life in patients with systemic lupus erythematosus. *Arthritis & Rheumatism., 53*, 838-844.

Casaburi, R., Porszasz, J., Burns, M. R., et al. (1997). Physiologic benefits of exercise training in rehabilitation of patients with chronic obstructive pulmonary disease. *Am J Respir Crit Care Med., 155*, 1541-51.

Celli, B. R. & MacNee, W. (2004). Standards for the diagnosis and treatment of patients with COPD: a summary of the ATS/ERS position paper. *Eur Respir J., 23*, 932-946.

Centers for Disease Control and Prevention (CDC).(1994). Arthritis prevalence and activity limitation: United States, 1990. *MMWR Morb Mortal Wkly Rep., 43*, 433-8.

Chintanadilok, J. & Lowenthal, D. T. (2002). Exercise in treating hypertension (tailoring therapies for active patients). *Phys Sportsmed., 30*, 11-23.

Church, T. S., Earnest, C. P., Skinner, J. S. et al. (2007). Effects of differente doses of physical activity on cardiorespiratory fitness among sedentary, overweight or obese postmenopausal women with elevated blood pressure: a randomized controlled trial. *JAMA., 297*(19), 2081-2091.

Clark, C. J., Cochrane, L. & Mackay, E. (1996). Low intensity peripheral muscle conditioning improves exercise tolerance and breathlessness in COPD. *Eur Respir J., 9*, 2590-2596.

Clarke-Jenssen, A., Fredriksen, P., Lilleby, L. & Menghsoel, A. (2005). Effects of supervised aerobic exercise in patients with systemic lupus erythematosus: a pilot study. *Arhtritis& Rheumatism., 53*, 308-312.

Compston, E. (1992). HRT and osteoporosis. *British Medical Bulletin., 48*, 309-344.

Cooper, C., Campion, G. & Melton, L. J. (1992). 3rd Hip fractures in the elderly: a world-wide projection. *Osteoporos Int., 2*, 285-9.

Cooper, C. B. (2001). Exercise in chronic pulmonary disease: aerobic exercise prescription. *Med Sci Sports Exerc., 33*(7) Suppl, 671-79

Courteix, D., et al. (1998). Effects of Physical Training on Bone Mineral Density in Prepuberal Girls: A Comparative Study Between Impact-Loading and Non-Impact-Loading Sports. *Osteoporosis International., 8*(2), 152-158.

Cranney, A., Papaioannou, A., Zytaruk, N., et al. (2006). Clinical Guidelines Committee of Osteoporosis Canada. Parathyroid hormone for the treatment of osteoporosis: a systematic review. *CMAJ., 175*(1) ,52-9.

D'Inca, R., Varnier, M., Mestriner, C., Martines, D., D'Odorico, A. & Sturniolo, G. (1999). Effects of moderate exercise on Crohn's disease patients in remission. *Italian Journal of Gastroenterology Hepatology., 31*, 205-210.

De Angelis, K., da Pureza, L. J. F., Rodrigues, B., et al. (2006). Efeitos Fisiológicos do Treinamento Físico em Pacientes Portadores de Diabetes Tipo 1. *Arq Bras Endocrinol Metab.*, *50* (6), 1005-1013.

Del Rio, L. & Roig, D. (2001). Actividad Física y Calidad Ósea. *Archivos de Medicina del Deporte .,18(*83), 211-21.

Duppe, H., Gardsell, P., Johnell, O., et al. (1997). Bone mineral density, muscle strength and physical activity. A population-based study of 332 subjects aged 15-42 years. *Acta Orthop Scand.*, *68*, 97-103.

Ekdahl, C. & Broman, G. (1992). Muscle strength, endurance, and aerobic capacity in rheumatoid arthritis: a comparative study with healthy subjects. *Ann Rheum Dis.*, *51*, 35-40.

Emery, C. F., Schein, R. L., Hauck, E. R. & MacIntyre, N. R. (1998) Psychological and cognitive outcomes of a randomized trial of exercise among patients with chronic obstructive pulmonary disease. *Health Psychol.*, *17*(3), 232-40.

Fanelli, A., Cabral, A. L., Neder, J. A., et al. (2007).Exercise training on disease control and quality of life in asthmatic children. *Med Sci Sports Exerc.*, *39*(9), 1474-80.

Fenster, C. P., Weinsier, R. L., Darley-Usmar, V. M. et al. (2002). Obesity, Aerobic exercise and vascular disease: the role of oxidant stress. *Obesity Research.*, *10*(9), 964-968.

Finckh, A., Iversen, M. & Liang, M. H. (2003) The exercise prescription in rheumatoid arthritis: primum non nocere. *Arthritis Rheum.*, *48*, 2393-5.

Gappmaier, E., Spencer, M., White, A., et al. (1994). Fifteen weeks of aerobic training improves multiple sclerosis patients' fitness. *Medicine and Science in Sport and Exercise.*, *26*, 432-441.

García, M. A. (2006). Setenta y un años de historia de la EPOC en el Instituto Nacional de Enfermedades Respiratorias Ismael Cosío Villegas (1935-2006). *Rev Inst Nal Enf Resp Mex.*, *19*(4), 316-20.

Gaudin, P., Leguen-Guegan, S., Allenet, B., et al. (2008) Is dynamic exercise beneficial in patients with rheumatoid arthritis? *Joint Bone Spine.*, *75*, 11-17.

Ghelsen , G., Grisby, S. & Winant, D. (1984). Effects of an aquatic fitness program on the muscular strength and endurance of patients with multiple sclerosis. *Physical Therapy.*, *64*, 635-657.

Global Initiative for Chronic Obstructive Lung Disease (GOLD). (2007). Global strategy for the diagnosis, management, and prevention of chronic obstructive pulmonary disease. Bethesda (MD): Global Initiative for Chronic Obstructive Lung Disease, World Health Organization, National Heart, Lung and Blood Institute.

Global Initiative for Obstructive Lung Disease (GOLD). www.goldcopd.com, (Citado 18 Marzo de 2003).

Goran, M. I., Reynolds, K. D. & Lindquist, C. H. (1999). Role of physical activity in the prevention of obesity in children. *International Journal of Obesity.*, *23*, S18±S33.

Gordon, B. A., Benson, A. C., Bird, S. R. et al. (2009). Resistance training improves metabolic health in type 2 diabetes: a systematic review. *Diabetes Research and clinical practice.*, *83*, 157-175.

Grupo de trabajo de Actividad Física y Salud (GAFS). (2006). *Prescripción de ejercicio en el tratamiento de enfermedades crónicas.* Barcelona: Semfyc.

Guyton, A. C. & Hall, J. E. (2001). *Tratado de fisiología médica.* Madrid: McGraw Hill/ Interamericana.

Hagberg, J. M.; Park, J. J. & Brown, M. D. (2000). The role of exercise training in the treatment of hypertension. *Sports Med 30*(3), 193-206.

Halbert, J. A., Silagy, C. A., Finucane, P. et al. (1997). The effectiveness of exercise training in lowering blood pressure: a meta-analysis of randomised controlled trials of 4 weeks or longer. *J Hum Hypertens.*, *11*, 641-649.

Harkcom, T. M., Lampman, R. M., Banwell, B. F. & Castor, C. W. (1985). Therapeutic value of graded aerobic exercise training in rheumatoid arthritis. *Arthritis Rheum.*, *28*,32-9.

Harrell, J. S., Gansky, S. A., McMurray, et al. (1998). School-based interventions improve heart health in children with multiple cardiovascular disease risk factors. *Pediatrics.*,*102*, 371-80.

Harris, E. D. Jr., Budd, R. C., Genovese, M. C., et al. eds. (2005) *Kelley's Textbook of Rheumatology.* (7th ed). Philadelphia: Saunders Elsevier.

Harris, M. I., Flegal, K. M., Cowie, C. C., et al. (1998).Prevalence of diabetes, impaired fasting glucose, and impaired glucose tolerance in US adults: the Third National Health and Nutrition Examination Survey, 1988-1994. *Diabetes Care.*,*21*,518-524.

Henderson, N. K., White, C. P. & Eisman, J. A. (1998). The Roles of Exercise and Fall Risk Reduction in the Prevention of Osteoporosis. *Endocrinal Metab Clin North Am.*, *27*, 369-87.

Honda, A., Umemura, Y. & Nagasawa, S. (2001). Effect of high-impact and low-repetition training on bones in ovariectomized rats. *J Bone Miner Re.*,*16*, 1688-93.

Honig, E. G. & Ingram, R. H. Jr. (1998). Chronic bronchitis, emphysema, and airways obstruction. En: Isselbacher Kl, Braunwald E, Wilson SD, et al, editors. *Harrison's principles of internal medicine.* (14th ed, pp. 1451-9). New York: McGraw-Hill.

Hui, S. L., Slemenda, C. W. & Johnston, C. C. (1990). The contribution of bone loss to postmenopausal osteoporosis. *Osteoporos Int.*, *1*, 30-4.

Impallomeni, M., Santodirocco, A. (2003). Osteoporosis en el anciano. *Revista Española de Geriatría y Gerontología.*, *38*(1), 54-59.

Irwin, M. L., Yasui, Y., Ulrico, C. M. et al. Effect of exercise on total and intra-abdominal body fat in postmenopausal women. A randomized controlled trial. *JAMA.*, *289*, 323-330.

Jakicic, J. M. & Otto, A. D. (2005). Physical activity considerations for the treatment and prevention of obesity. *Am J Clin Nutr.*, *82*, 226S-229S.

Jakicic, J. M., Marcus, B. H., Gallagher, K. I. et al. (2003). Effect of exercise duration and Intensity on weight loss in overweight, sedentary women: a randomized trial. *JAMA.*, *290*(19), 1323-1330.

Karlsson, M. K., Nordqvist, A. & Karlsson, C. (2008). Physical activity increases bone mass during growth. *Food Nutr Res.*, *52,* 10.

Katz, R. S., Wolfe, F. & Michaud, K. (2006). Fibromyalgia diagnosis: a comparison of clinical, survey, and American College of Rheumatology criteria. *Arthritis & Rheumatism.*, *54*, 169-176.

Kavookjian, J., Elswick, B. M. & Whetsel, T. (2007). Interventions for being active among individuals with diabetes: a systematic review of the literature. *The Diabetes Educator.*, *33*, 962-988.

Kelley, G. A., Kelley, K. S. & Tran, Z. V. (2005). Aerobic exercise, lipids and lipoproteins in iverweight and obese adults: a meta-nalysis of randomized controlled trials. *Int J Obes (Lond) 29* (8), 881-893.

Komatsu, W. R., Gabbay, M. A. L., Castro, M. L., et al. (2005). Aerobic exercise capacity in normal adolescents and those with type 1 diabetes mellitus. *Pediatric Diabetes.*, *6*, 145-149.

Krall, E. A., Garcia, R. I. & Dawson-Hughes, B. (1996). Increased risk of tooth loss is related to bone loss at the whole body, hip, and spine. *Calcif Tissue Int.*, *59*, 433-437.

Landre Beauvais, A. J. (2001). The first description of rheumatoid arthritis. Unabridged text of the doctoral dissertation presented in 1800. *Joint Bone Spine.*, *68*(2), 130-143.

Lee, N., Radford-Smith, G. & Taaffe, D. (2005). Bone loss in Crohn's disease: exercise as a potential countermeasure. *Inflammatory Bowel Disease.*, *11*, 1108-1118.

Lewis, R. D. & Modlesky, C. M. (1998). Nutrition, Physical Activity and Bone Health in Women. *Int J Sport Nutr.*, *8*, 250-84.

Lindroth, Y., Strombeck, B., Brosner, M., Gullberg, B. & Wollheim, F. (1994). Learned helplesnes and to impairment, paint, anxiety on depresion, in rheumatoid arthritis. *Scandinavian Journal Rheumatology .*, *23*, 299-304.

Llor, C., Naberan, K., Cots, J. M., et al. (2006). Estudio EFEMAP. Risk factors for increased cost of exacerbations of chronic bronchitis and chronic obstructive pulmonary disease. *Arch Bronconeumol.*, *42*(4), 175-82.

Loudon, C., Coroll, V., Butcher, J., Pawsthorne, P. & Berstein, C. (1999). The effects of physical exercise on patients with Crohn's disease. *American Journal of Gastroenterology.*, 697-703.

Mallavarapu, R. & Grimsley, E. W. (2007). The history of lupus erythematosus. *Southern Medical Journal.*, *100*, 896-896.

Manfredini, F., Malagoni, A. M., Mandini, S. et al. (2008), Sport Therapy for Hypertension: why, how and how much?. *Angiology*. Doi: 10.1177/0003319708316012.

Mannerkorpi, K. (2005). Exercise in fibromyalgia. *Current Opinion in Rheumathology.*, *17*, 190-194.

Mannino, D. M., Homa, D. M., Pertowski, C. A., et al. (1998). Surveillance for asthma—United States, 1960-1995. In: CDC Surveillance Summaries, *MMWR.*, *47*(SS-1), 1-28.

Matsumoto, T. y cols. (1997). Bone Density and Bone Metabolic Markers in Active Collegiate Athletes: Findings in Long-Distance Runners, Judoists and Swimmers. *Int J Sport Med.*, *18*(6), 408-12.

Minor, M. (1996). Arthritis and exercise: 'the times they are a-changin'. *Arthritis Care Res.*, *9*, 79-81.

Minor, M. A., Hewett, J. E., Webel, R. R., et al. (1989). Efficacy of physical conditioning exercise in patients with rheumatoid arthritis and osteoarthritis. *Arthritis Rheum.*, *32*, 1396-1405.

Motl, R. W. & Gosney, J. L. (2008). Effect of exercise training on quality of life in multiple sclerosis: a meta-analysis. *Multiple Sclerosis.*, *14*, 129-35.

Murphy, M. H., Murtagh, E. M., Boreham, C. A., Hare, L. G., Nevill, A. M. (2006), The effect of a worksite based walking programme on cardiovascular risk in previously sedentary civil servants. *BMC Public Health.*, *22*.

Nakamura, Y., Tanaka, K., Shigematsu, R., et al. (2008). Effects of aerobic training and recreational activities in patients with chronic obstructive pulmonary disease. *Int J Rehabil Res.*, *31*(4),275-83.

National Institutes of Health, National Asthma Education Program. (1993). *Expert panel report 2: guidelines for the diagnosis and management of asthma*. Bethesda, MD:

National Institutes of Health, National Heart, Lung, and Blood Institute, 1-153. Available at www.nhlbi.nih.gov/guidelines/asthma/asthgdln.htm. Accessed November 19, 2001.

Newman, M. A., Dawes, H., van den Berg, M., et al. (2007). Can aerobic treadmill training reduce the effort of walking and fatigue in people with multiple sclerosis: a pilot study. *Multiple Sclerosis.*, *13*, 113-9.

Ng, V., Millard, W., Lebrun, C. & Howard, J. (2007). Low-intensity exercise improves quality of life in patients with Crohn's disease. *Clinical Journal of Sport Medicine.*, *17*, 384-388.

Nordin, B. E. (2009). The definition and diagnosis of osteoporosis. *Salud Publica Mex.,51* Suppl 1,S132-3.

Normandin, E. A., McCusker, C., Connors, M., et al. (2002). An evaluation of two approaches to exercise conditioning in pulmonary rehabilitation. *Chest.*, *121*, 1085-1091.

O' Sullivan, S. E. & Bell, C. (2000). The effects of exercise and training on human cardiovascular reflex control. *Journal of the Autonomic Nervous System.*, *81*, 16-24.

Olgiati, R. & Di Prampero P. (1986). Effects of physical exercise on adaptation to energy expenditure in multiple sclerosis. *Schweiz Med Wochenser.*, *116*, 374-377

Olson, T. P., Dengel, D. R., Leon, A. S. & Schmitz, K. H. (2006). Moderate resistance training and vascular health in overweight women. *Med Sci Sports Exerc.*, *38*(9), 1558-64.

Pastva, A., Estell, K., Schoeb, T. R., et al. (2004).Aerobic exercise attenuates airway inflammatory responses in a mouse model of atopic asthma. *J Immunol 2004, 172*(7),4520-6.

Peces-Barba, G., Barberà, J. A., Agustí, A., et al. (2008). Diagnosis and management of chronic obstructive pulmonary disease: joint guidelines of the Spanish Society of Pulmonology and Thoracic Surgery (SEPAR) and the Latin American Thoracic Society (ALAT). *Arch Bronconeumol.*, *44*(5),271-81.

Pescatello, L. S., Franklin, B. A., Fagard, R., et al. (2004) American College of Sports Medicine. American College of Sports Medicine position stand. Exercise and hypertension. *Med Sci Sports Exerc.*, *36*(3), 533-53.

Plotnikoff, R. C., Courneya, K. S., Trinh, L., et al. (2008). Aerobic physical actvity and resistance training: an application of the theory of planned behaviour among adults with type 2 diabetes in a random, nationale sample of Canadians. *International Journal of Behavioral Nutrition and Physical Activity.*, *5*.

Pool, A. J., Axford, J. S. (2001). The effects of exercise on the hormonal and immune systems in rheumatoid arthritis. *Rheumatology.*, *40*, 610-614.

Prince, R. L., Smith, M., Dick, I. M., et al. (1991). Prevention of postmenopausal osteoporosis. A comparative study of exercise, calcium supplementation and hormone-replacement therapy. *N Engl J Med.*, *325*, 1.189-1.195.

Rabasa-Lhoret, R., Bourque, J., Ducros, F., et al. (2001). Guidelines for premeal insuline dose reduction for post-prandial exercise of differents intensities and durations in type 1 diabetic subjects treated intensively with a basalbolus insulin regimen (ultralente-lispro). *Diabetes Care.*, *24*, 625-630.

Ram, F. S., Robinson, S. M., Black, P. N., Picot, J. (2005). Physical training for asthma. *Cochrane Database Syst Rev.*, *9*(4),CD00111.

Ramalho, A. C. & Soares, S. (2008). The role of exercise in the treatment of type 1 diabetes. *Arq Bras Endocrinol Metabol.*, *52*(2), 260-267.

Ramalho, A. C., de Lourdes Lima, M., Nunes, F., et al. (2006) The effect of resistance versus aerobic training on metabolic control in patients with type-1 diabetes mellitus. *Diabetes Res Clin Pract., 72*(3),271-6.

Ries, A. L., Kaplan, R. M. & Limberg, T. M. (1995). Effects of pulmonary rehabilitation on physiologic and psychosocial outcomes in patients with chronic obstructive pulmonary disease. *Ann Intern Med., 122*, 823-32.

Robinson, R., Krzywicki, T., Almond, L., et al. (1998). Effect o a low impact exercise program on bone mineral density in CD: a randomized controlled trial. *Gastroenterology., 115*, 36-41.

Robling, A. G., Hinant, F. M., Burr, D. B., et al. (2002). Shorter, more frequent mechanical loading sessions enhance bone mass. *Med Sci Sports Exerc., 34*, 196-202.

Rosimini, C. (2003). Benefits of swim training for children and adolescents with asthma. *J Am Acad Nurse Pract., 15*(6), 247-52.

Santora, A. C. (1987). Role of nutrition and exercise in osteoporosis. *Am J Med., 13*,73-79.

Schachter, C. L., Busch, A. J., Peloso, P. M. & Sheppard, M. S. (2003). Effects of short versus long bouts of aerobic exercise in sedentary women with fibromyalgia: a randomized controlled trial. *Physical Therapy., 83*, 340-358

Sharman, J. E., Stowasser, M. (2009) Australian association for exercise ans sports science position statement on exercise and hypertension. *J sci Med Sport.* Doi:10.1016/j.jsams. 2008. 10.009.

Short, C. L. (1974). The antiquity of rheumatoid arthritis. *Arthritis Rheum., 17*(3), 193-205.

Sideravičiūtė, S., Gailiūnienė, A., Visagurskienė, K., et al. (2006). The effect off log-term swimming program on body composition, aerobic capacity and blood lipids in 14-19 year aged healthy girls and girls with type 1 diabetes mellitus. *Medicina (Kaunas)., 42*(8), 661-666.

Sigal, R. J., Kenny, G. P., Wasserman, D. H. et al. (2004). Physical activity/exercise and type 2 diabetes. *Diabetes Care., 27*(10), 2518-2539.

Smolen, J. S., Aletaha, D., Koeller, M., et al. (2007). New therapies for treatment of rheumatoid arthritis. *Lancet., 370*(9602), 1861-74.

Soneneberg, A. (1990). Occupational distribution of inflammatory bowel disease among German employees. *Gut., 31*, 1037-1040.

Stenstrom, C. H., Minor, M. A. (2003) Evidence for the benefit of aerobic and strengthening exercise in rheumatoid arthritis. *Arthritis Care Res., 49*, 428-34.

Sueiro, F., Estévez, I., Ayán, C., Cancela, J. & Martín, V. (2008). Potential benefits of non-pharmacological therapies in fibromyalgia. *The Open Rheumatology Journal., 2*, 1-6.

Sutherland, G. & Andersen, M. (2001). Exercise and multiple sclerosis: physiological, psychological and quality of life issues. *Journal of Sports Medical Physical Fitness., 41*, 421-423

Tench, C., McCarthy, J., McCurdle, I., White, P. & D'Cruz D.(2003). Fatigue in systemic lupus erythematosus: a randomized controlled trial of exercise. *Rheumatology (Oxford)., 42*, 1050-1054.

The Cochrane Database of Systematic Reviews. Pulmonary Rehabilitation for COPD. Chrocane Library, The Cochrane collaboration. Vol(issue3) 2002.

The Pew Environmental Health Commission. (2001). *Attack asthma: why America needs a public health defense system to battle environmental threats*. Baltimore, MD: John

Hopkins School of Public Health, Pew Environmental Health Commission. Available at http://pewenvirohealth.jhsph.edu/html/home/home.html. Accessed November 19, 2001.

Thibodeau, G. A. & Patton K. T. (2000). *Anatomia y Fisiología*. Madrid: Harcourt.

Thompson, W. G., Cook, D. A., Clark, M. M. et al. (2007). Treatment of Obesity. *Mayo Clinic Proc.*, *82* (1), 93-102.

US Department of Health and Human Services. (2000). Action against asthma: a strategic plan for the Department of Health and Human Services. Rockville, MD: US Department of Health and Human Services, Office of the Assistant Secretary for Planning and Evaluation, 2000. Available at http://aspe.hhs.gov/sp/asthma. Accessed November 19, 2001.

US Department of Health and Human Services. (2000). Respiratory diseases [Goal 24]. In: Healthy people 2010 (conference ed., vol II). Washington, DC: US Department of Health and Human Services, *24*,1-27.

Valencia, M., Alonso, B., Alvarez, M. J., Barrientos, M. J., Ayán, C. & Martín, V. (2009). Effects of 2 physiotherapy programs on pain perception, muscular flexibility, and illness impact in women with fibromyalgia: a pilot study. *Journal of Manipulative and Physiological Therapeutics.*, *32*, 84-92.

Van den Ende, C. H., Vliet Vlieland, T. P., Munneke, M., et al. (1998). Dynamic exercise therapy in rheumatoid arthritis: a systematic review. *Br J Rheumatol.*, *37*(6), 677-87.

Van der Laan, L. & Goris, R. J. (1997). Sudeck's syndrome. Was Sudeck right?. *Unfallchirurg.*, *100*(2), 90-9.

Wallance, J. P. (2003). Exercise in hypertension: a clinical review. *Sports Med.*, *33* (8), 585-598.

Ward, M. J. (2004). Prevalence of physician-diagnosed systemic lupus erythematosus in the United States: results from the third national health and nutrition examination survey. *Womens Health (Larchmt).*, *13*, 712-718

Westby, M. D., Wade, J. P., Rangno, K. K., et al. (2000) A randomized controlled trial to evaluate the effectiveness of an exercise program in women with rheumatoid arthritis taking low dose prednisone. *J Rheumatol.*, *27*(7), 1674-80.

Westerterp, K.R. & Goram, M.I. (1997). Relationship between physical activity related energy expenditure and body composition: a gender difference. *Int J Clin Obes.*, *21*, 184-188.

Whalen, R.T., Carter, D.R., Steele, C.R. (1988). Influence of physical activity on the regulation of bone density. *J Biomech*, *21*, 825-37.

Woo, R. & Pi Sunyer, F.X. (1982). Effect of exercise on spontaneous calories intake in obesity. *Am J Clin Nutr.*, *36*, 470-477.

Xhardez, Y. (1995). *Vademécum de Kinesioterapia y de Reeducación Funcional*. Barcelona: El Ateneo.

Zanesco, A. & Antunes, E. (2007). Effects of exercise training on the cardiovascular system: pharmacological approaches. *Pharmacology & Therapeutics.*, *114*, 307-317.

In: Encyclopedia of Sports and Athletics
Editors: Jack L. Murray and Emily O. Watson

ISBN: 978-1-61209-959-0

Chapter II

The Anti-Inflammatory Effects of Exercise

***Pedro Tauler*[1] *and Antoni Aguiló*[2]**

[1]Departament de Biologia Fonamental i Ciències de la Salut. Universitat de les Illes Balears. E-07122 Palma de Mallorca. Spain.

[2]Departament d'Infermeria i Fisioteràpia. Universitat de les Illes Balears. E-07122 Palma de Mallorca, Spain

Abstract

Public health physical activity recommendations state that moderate-intensity aerobic physical activity for a minimum of 30 min on at least five days each week confers substantial protection against chronic diseases such as cardiovascular disease, atherosclerosis, type 2 diabetes, insulin resistance, colon cancer and breast cancer. The mechanisms responsible for the protective effects of exercise are not completely clear. Nowadays it is well-known that these diseases are associated with chronic low-grade systemic inflammation. Thus, it has been suggested that the modification of the levels of the inflammation markers may have therapeutic potential.

In general, the plasma cytokines found following acute bouts of exercise suggest that exercise induces a strong anti-inflammatory effect. This finding may provide, in part, a mechanism as to why physical exercise either reduces the susceptibility to, or improves the symptoms of diseases associated with low-grade inflammation. In fact, muscle contraction induced factors with anti-inflammatory actions, which are released to the circulation during exercise, may be involved in mediating the health beneficial effects of exercise and play important roles in the protection against these diseases associated with low-grade inflammation. Furthermore, cross-sectional studies demonstrate an association between physical inactivity and low-grade systemic inflammation in healthy subjects, in elderly people, as well as in patients with intermittent claudication. However, it is not clear how chronic moderate exercise could perform its anti-inflammatory effects. It has been hypothesized that the long-term healthy effect of exercise may to some extend be ascribed to the anti-inflammatory response elicited by acute bouts of moderate exercise. In addition, it has been suggested that following acute exercise, there is a transient increase in circulating levels of anti-inflammatory factors, whereas chronic exercise reduces basal levels of pro-inflammatory cytokines. Recent studies have suggested that continuous an additional subtle changes resulting in reductions in fat and body mass or in improved lipid and glycemic profiles could induce the anti-inflammatory effect of regular moderate-intensity exercise.

The aim of this review is to examine the anti-inflammatory effects of aerobic exercise and to discuss to what extend the exercise induced anti-inflammatory response may play a therapeutic role in chronic diseases associated with low-grade inflammation.

Introduction

Public health physical activity recommendations state that moderate-intensity aerobic physical activity for a minimum of 30 min on at least five days each week confers substantial protection against chronic diseases such as cardiovascular disease, type 2 diabetes and others [1, 2]. Regular physical activity was, independently of body mass index (BMI), associated with lower risk of both cardiovascular mortality and cancer mortality [3].

On the other hand, physical inactivity has been recently suggested to be a disease in itself and proposed to be the most important behavioral cause of insulin resistance [4]. In fact, physical inactivity accelerates the development of major chronic disease, with studies showing a particularly marked and consistent effect on cardiovascular disease [5]. Several studies have demonstrated a BMI–independent association between low fitness level and all-cause mortality [6-11], as well as between a low level of self-reported physical activity and premature mortality [12-20]. Moreover, physical inactivity has been identified as a stronger predictor of these chronic diseases than risk factors such as hypertension, hyperlipidemia, diabetes, and obesity for all-cause mortality [6]. It should be highlighted that chronic diseases are the largest cause of death in the world, led by cardiovascular disease followed by cancer, chronic lung diseases, and diabetes mellitus [21]. Regular exercise offers protection against all-cause mortality, primarily protection against atherosclerosis, type 2 diabetes, colon cancer, and breast cancer [21]. In fact, there is clinical general evidence for a beneficial effect of continuous moderate physical activity in patients with chronic diseases. The evidence for prescribing exercise in patients with chronic diseases was reviewed in an excellent work [22]. Randomized intervention studies have shown that physical training is effective in the treatment of patients with, among others, ischemic heart disease, insulin resistance, type 2 diabetes, dyslipemias, chronic obstructive pulmonary disease (COPD), cancer [22] and heart failure [23, 24].

Over the past decade, there has been an increasing focus on the role of inflammation in the pathogenesis of atherosclerosis [25]. Furthermore, inflammation has been suggested to be a key factor in insulin resistance [26]. In this sense, the term low grade chronic inflammation, which is characterised by increased systemic levels of some cytokines and C-reactive protein (CRP) [27], has been introduced to describe the inflammatory picture found in several chronic diseases. Some reports investigating various markers of inflammation have confirmed an association between low-grade systemic inflammation on one hand and atherosclerosis and type 2 diabetes on the other [28]. Recent findings demonstrate that physical activity induces an increase in the systemic levels of a number of cytokines with anti-inflammatory properties [29] and skeletal muscle has recently been identified as an endocrine organ, which produces and releases cytokines [29-32].

Given that chronic low-grade systemic inflammation may be involved in several chronic diseases and given the finding that physical exercise induces an increase in levels of some cytokines with anti-inflammatory properties, we discuss whether physical activity exerts anti-inflammatory effects and, as a consequence, could protect against chronic diseases associated with low-grade systemic inflammation.

Components of the Inflammatory Response

The local response to infections or tissue injury involves the production of cytokines that are released at the site of inflammation [29]. Cytokines are small polypeptides, which were originally discovered to have immuno-regulatory roles [33, 34]. Some of these cytokines facilitate an influx of lymphocytes, neutrophils, monocytes, and other cells to the site of inflammation [29]. The local inflammatory response is accompanied by a systemic response known as the acute-phase response. This response includes the production of several acute phase proteins, such as C reactive protein (CRP), produced by the liver, and can be mimicked by the injection of the cytokines tumour necrosis factor α (TNF-α), interleukin (IL)-1β, and IL-6 into laboratory animals or humans [33-35]. The initial cytokines in the cytokine cascade are, in order of appearance, TNF-α, IL-1β, IL-6, IL-1 receptor antagonist (IL-1ra), and soluble TNF-α receptors (sTNF-R). IL-1ra inhibits IL-1 signal transduction and sTNF-R represents the naturally occurring inhibitor of TNF-α [33-35]. In response to an acute infection or trauma, the cytokines and cytokine inhibitors may increase several folds and decrease when the infection or trauma is healed [29]. Some of the cytokines involved in the inflammatory response are clearly pro-inflammatory (e.g. IL-1, TNF-α) but others are mainly anti-inflammatory (e.g. IL-10, IL-1ra). Whereas IL-10 influences multiple cytokines inhibiting their production [36-38], the biological role of IL-1ra is to inhibit signalling transduction through the IL-1 receptor complex [39]. In fact, both pro- and anti-inflammatory cytokines play an essential role after tissue injury or infection. For example, it has been recently suggested that during skeletal muscle regeneration an inflammatory stage followed by an anti-inflammatory one are essential in order to complete tissue regeneration [40]. Whereas the inflammatory environment stage is characterized by removing necrotic tissue, during the anti-inflammatory one the myogenic differentiation and muscle repair is produced [40].

The particularities of each cytokine will not be discussed in this chapter. However, it could be interesting to highlight several aspects regarding cytokine production and roles. As in has been indicated above, there is an interesting, but also complex, relation between immune system and cytokines. For example, it has been indicated that T lymphocytes can be classified as type 1 or type 2 cells, depending on which cytokines they predominantly produce [41]. Type 1 T lymphocytes produce mainly TNF-α, and their actions activate macrophages and induce killer mechanisms, including T-cytotoxic cells, thus driving the immune system toward cell-mediated immune responses, which primarily provide protection against intracellular pathogens such as viruses. Type 2 lymphocytes mainly synthesize IL-4, IL-5, IL-10 and IL-13, which are necessary for promotion of humoral immunity, IgE-mediated allergic reactions, and activation of potentially tissue-damaging eosinophils. IL-4 and IL-13 primarily drive B-cell differentiation to antibody production, while IL-5 stimulates and primes eosinophils. Together with IL-4, IL-10 (which is also produced by monocytes and B cells) can inhibit type 1 T-cell cytokine production.

However, most of the recent research has been focused on IL-6 and its production by muscle. Skeletal muscle, the largest organ in the human body, has recently been identified as an endocrine organ which produces and releases cytokines [29-32]. In fact, during physical exercise IL-6 is predominantly produced within the working skeletal muscles [42-44]. Muscle contraction is supposed to activate this production and release of cytokines, which could influence metabolism and modify cytokine production in tissue and organs as well as in immune cells. IL-6 is induced in skeletal muscle via a Ca^{2+} dependent pathway [45] and acts through AMP-activated kinase [46-48]. Due to its complex role in both metabolism and inflammation, IL-6 has been proposed as the key factor during exercise [32].

As it is indicated above, the production of cytokines is influenced, among other factors, by myokine release. Furthermore, once released transiently into the blood stream, myokines mediate some of the systemic and beneficial effects of exercise in non-muscle tissue, e.g. modulation of hepatic glucose production through IL-6. Thus, the transient fluctuations of myokines following physical activity, that will be discussed later, might contribute to the beneficial effects of exercise on organs other than muscle in a hormone-like fashion, whereas chronic elevation of many of these same molecules is almost certainly pro-inflammatory and detrimental. It has been suggested that because systemic markers of inflammation are elevated in several chronic diseases, modifying their levels through exercise may have therapeutic potential [49].

Evidences for Inflammation in Chronic Diseases: Low-Grade Systemic Inflammation

Inflammation has been considered as the natural host response to an acute infectious episode, whereas chronic inflammation has been considered a sign of chronic infection. It has now become clear that low-grade chronic inflammation is a key player in the pathogenesis of most chronic diseases [50]. In this sense, the concept of low-grade chronic inflammation has been introduced and it is now widely used [29]. Low-grade chronic inflammation is characterized by increased systemic levels of some cytokines and, specially, C-reactive protein (CRP) [27]. Chronic low-grade systemic inflammation has been introduced as a term for conditions in which a two to three-fold increase in the systemic concentrations of TNF-α, IL-1, IL-6, IL-1ra, sTNF-R, and CRP is reflected [29]. In this sense, chronically elevated levels of systemic IL-6, IL-8, IL-10, IL-1 or TNF-α have been linked to the development of many diseases associated with inflammation including cancer, COPD, rheumatoid arthritis and other age-associated diseases such as sarcopenia [51-57]. In addition, chronic elevation of IL-6 and TNF-α results in skeletal muscle atrophy and inhibition of muscle regeneration, respectively [58, 59]. Furthermore, chronically elevated serum IL-6 levels have a predictive value for obesity and type 2 diabetes [60]. Plasma IL-6, TNF-α and CRP have emerged as strong independent risk factors for cardiovascular diseases development [61].

As it has been suggested above, recent findings indicate that many chronic diseases have been found to be associated with this sterile, persistent, low-grade systemic inflammation. For example, the development of insulin resistance [26, 62] and type 2 diabetes is closely correlated with immune cell infiltration and inflammation in white adipose tissue [51]. In cardiovascular diseases, activated immune cells and inflammation play a major role, particularly in the aetiology of atherosclerosis [25, 49, 52, 63]. Furthermore, COPD is characterised by chronic inflammation, with high levels of TNF-α both in blood [55] and in the muscle [57]. Several reports investigating various markers of inflammation have confirmed an association between low-grade systemic inflammation, on one hand, and atherosclerosis and type 2 diabetes, on the other [28]. Inflammation has been also observed in rheumatoid arthritis, characterised by permanent high levels of circulating TNF-α levels [56]. Increasing evidence suggests that TNF-α plays a direct role in the metabolic syndrome [64], pointing to an effect of TNF-α on insulin signalling. TNF-α impairs insulin-stimulated rates of glucose storage in cultured human muscle cells and impairs insulin-mediated glucose uptake in rats. TNF-α protein is elevated locally and systemically in diabetes model animals [65]. Furthermore, neutralization of TNF-α in obese rats caused a significant increase in the peripheral uptake of glucose in response to insulin [65]. These results point to a role for TNF-α in the insulin resistance and diabetes that often accompany obesity. After adjustment for multiple confounders, including IL-6, high plasma TNF-α concentrations have been associated with insulin resistance [66] and evidence for a direct role of TNF-α in insulin resistance in humans in vivo has been obtained [64]. It was demonstrated that TNF-α infusion in healthy humans induces insulin resistance in skeletal muscle without an effect on endogenous glucose production. TNF-α directly impaired glucose uptake and metabolism by altering insulin signal transduction. These data provide a possible molecular link between low-grade systemic inflammation and insulin resistance [64]. Patients with diabetes showed high mRNA and protein expression of TNF-α in skeletal muscle and increased TNF-α levels in plasma, and it is likely that adipose tissue, which produces TNF-α, is the main source of the circulating TNF-α in chronic inflammation [65]. Because TNF-α mainly works locally, TNF-α transcription may not always be reflected in enhanced systemic levels of TNF-α [67]. In this sense, it has been suggested that chronically elevated levels of IL-6, IL-1ra, and CRP are likely to reflect local ongoing TNF-α production [68].

When IL-6 findings are analysed, results showed in the bibliography are, at least, controversial. Several studies suggest a link between IL-6 and insulin resistance. However, the evaluation of the metabolic effects of physiological concentrations of IL-6 in humans demonstrates that IL-6 enhances glucose uptake and induces fat oxidation. It has been suggested that IL-6 promotes insulin resistance due to the observation that plasma IL-6 is often elevated in patients with metabolic disease [50]. At resting conditions, acute IL-6 administration at physiological concentrations did not impair whole-body glucose disposal, net leg-glucose uptake, or increased endogenous glucose production in resting healthy young humans [69-71]. In patients with type 2 diabetes, plasma-insulin decreased in response to IL-6 infusion, suggesting an insulin-sensitizing effect of IL-6 [71]. Carey *et al.* demonstrated that IL-6 increased the glucose infusion rate and glucose oxidation without affecting the suppression of endogenous glucose production during a hyperinsulinemic euglycemic clamp in healthy humans [47]. Infusion of recombinant human IL-6 into healthy humans to obtain physiological concentrations of IL-6 increased lipolysis in the absence of high triacylglyceride levels or changes in catecholamines, glucagon, insulin, or any adverse effects in healthy individuals [70-72] and in patients with type 2 diabetes [71]. These findings, as well as others demonstrating that IL-6 alone markedly increases both lipolysis and fat oxidation in cell cultures, suggest that IL-6 could be considered as a novel lipolytic factor. Blocking IL-6 in clinical trials with patients with rheumatoid arthritis leads to enhanced cholesterol and plasma glucose levels, indicating that functional lack of IL-6 may lead to insulin resistance and an atherogenic lipid profile rather than the opposite [73, 74]. Thus, more studies are necessary in order to clarify the relationship between high permanent IL-6 plasma levels and the incidence or development of chronic diseases.

Interestingly, tumour initiation, promotion, and progression are stimulated by systemic elevation of pro-inflammatory cytokines [53]. In addition, evidence exists to suggest that inflammation accelerates cancer cell growth [75]. The association between inflammation and cancer has been clearly illustrated by epidemiologic and clinical studies [75-77]. For instance, the risk of colorectal cancer was 10-fold greater when linked with inflammatory bowel disease, such as ulcerative colitis and Crohn's disease [78, 79]. Moreover, the control of colitis by a number of anti-inflammatory agents reduced colon cancer incidence [80, 81], and people who have taken non steroidal anti-inflammatory drugs are at reduced risk of colon cancer [82, 83]. Direct evidence for the involvement of TNF-α in malignancy comes from the observation that mice lacking the gene for TNF-α are resistant to skin carcinogenesis [84]. TNF-α activates nuclear factor KB (NF-KB) and more recently, it has become clear that NF-KB signalling also has a critical role in cancer development and progression. NF-KB could suppose the link between inflammation and cancer and is a major factor controlling the ability of both pre-neoplastic and malignant cells to resist apoptosis based tumour surveillance mechanisms [85].

Acute Effects of Exercise on Immune Function

Physical activity, inflammation and immunity are tightly linked in an interesting and complex way [86]. Regular, moderate exercise reduces systemic inflammation [41]. The mediators of this beneficial effect of exercise are unclear; however, several candidate mechanisms have been identified. First, exercise increases the release of epinephrine, cortisol, growth hormone and other factors that have immuno-modulatory effects [87]. Furthermore, exercise results in decreased expression of Toll-like receptor on monocytes suggested being involved in mediating whole body inflammation [88]. In contrast to the reduction of chronic inflammation by regular, moderate exercise, prolonged, high intensity training results in increased systemic inflammation and elevated risk of infection [41]. In fact, subsequent to this type of exercise, athletes exhibit a transient exercise-induced immuno-depression [89]. The anti-inflammatory effects of exercise will be discussed later in this chapter.

It is well recognized that intense exercise causes perturbations to the immune system. Long-duration or damaging exercise initiates reactions that resemble the acute-phase response to infection [41, 90]. It has been suggested that this immune response is necessary for muscular regeneration and adaptation to physical exercise [91, 92]. Although results regarding effects of exercise on immune cells functionality are controversial, the effects of exercise on the circulating number of these immunocompetent cells during the acute phase response have been well described. An increase in neurophil number (neutrophilia) is well documented after an acute bout of exercise [41, 93-96]. However, lymphocyte concentration increases during exercise but falls below basal values after intense or long duration exercises

[41, 87, 93-95, 97]. Furthermore, exercise induces redistribution in lymphocyte populations [90]. The magnitude of these changes is basically related to both the intensity and duration of exercise [93].

Although moderate exercise stimulates the immune system, strenuous exercise induces a temporary immune depression in the recovery period and may explain the increased risk of infection in athletes [98]. In a few studies involving strenuous (marathons) or very extreme exercise (such as ultra-marathons), this immune depression has been associated with an increased incidence of infection in the weeks following the event [99-102]. The mechanisms underlying exercise-associated immune changes are multi-factorial and include neuroendocrinological factors such as adrenaline, noradrenaline, epinephrine, growth hormone, and cortisol [41, 98, 103]. In fact, the response to exercise includes hormonal changes which could influence immune function [41, 93]. These hormonal changes include increases in the plasma concentration of adrenaline, cortisol and growth hormone, which are known to have immuno-modulatory effects [93].

Exercise also induces increases in the plasma concentrations of various non-hormonal substances that are known to influence leukocyte functions, including inflammatory cytokines, such as macrophage inflammatory protein-1, and IL-1β; anti-inflammatory cytokines IL-6, IL-10, and IL-1ra; and acute phase proteins, including CRP [41]. As it will be discussed later, the large increase in plasma IL-6 concentration observed during exercise can be entirely attributed to the release of this cytokine from exercising muscle [42-44]. This IL-6 release could play an essential role as the key factor in the anti-inflammatory effects of exercise.

Though an acute bout of physical activity is accompanied by responses that in many aspects are similar to those induced by infection and sepsis, there are some important differences in the cytokine response to exercise from that induced by severe infection [41, 98, 104, 105]. These differences could be essential in order to understand the possible anti-inflammatory effects of exercise. As it has been indicated previously, the initial cytokines as they appear in the circulation in relation to an acute infection consist of (named in order): TNF-α, IL-1β, IL-6, IL-1ra, sTNF-R and IL-10. The most important, and essential, difference between exercise and sepsis with regard to cytokine responses is that the pro-inflammatory cytokines, TNF-α and IL-1β, in general do not increase with exercise.

Acute Exercise and Circulating Cytokine Levels

The fact that the pro-inflammatory cytokines, TNF-α and IL-1β, in general do not increase with exercise, suggests that, as it has been indicated before, the cytokine cascade induced by exercise markedly differs from the cytokine cascade induced by infections. IL-6 is the first cytokine present in the circulation during exercise, and the appearance of IL-6 in the circulation is, by far, the most marked and its appearance precedes that of the other cytokines [104]. The level of circulating IL-6 increases in an exponential way (up to 100 fold) in response to exercise, and declines in the post-exercise period [98, 104]. The magnitude by which plasma IL-6 increases is related to exercise duration, intensity, endurance capacity and muscle mass involved in the mechanical work [32, 98, 104, 106]. However, it is not related to muscle damage because a marked increase in circulating levels of IL-6 after exercise without muscle damage has been a remarkably consistent finding [32, 98, 104, 106]. Another finding in relation to exercise is increased circulating levels of well-known anti-inflammatory cytokines, cytokine inhibitors such as IL-1ra and sTNF-R [105, 107]. Thus, it has been shown that, in general, exercise provokes an increase primarily in IL-6, followed by an increase mainly in sTNF-R, IL-1ra and IL-10 [32, 49, 104, 108, 109]. A small increase of CRP levels is seen the day after exhaustive exercises [98].

Regarding the response of other cytokines to exercise, changes observed are not as consistent as the ones indicated above. Plasma concentration of IL-8 increases in response to exhaustive exercise such as running, which involves eccentric muscle contractions [110, 111]. However, concentric exercise, such as bicycle ergometry [112] or rowing [113] of moderate intensity, does not increase plasma IL-8 concentration. In a study by Nieman *et al.*, an increase in IL-8 mRNA was found in skeletal muscle biopsies from subjects having completed a three-hour treadmill run concomitant with increased plasma levels of IL-8 [111]. Similarly, IL-8 mRNA increased in response to 1 hour of exercise in a cycle-ergometer, but with no change in the plasma concentration of IL-8 [112]. Akerstom *et al.* found that IL-8 protein was clearly expressed in human skeletal muscle in response to concentric exercise [114]. The finding of a marked increase of IL-8 mRNA in muscle biopsies during and following exercise and IL-8 protein expression within skeletal muscle fibers in the recovery from exercise indicates that exercise stimulates muscle cells to produce IL-8, which, in addition, exerts its effects locally [114]. These results are in accordance with the finding that muscle cells in vitro have the capacity to express IL-8, both at the mRNA and protein levels [115]. In fact, it has been proposed that IL-8 should be classified as a myokine [114].

The physiological function of IL-8 within the muscle is still unknown. It is well know that IL-8 attracts primarily neutrophils and, in addition, IL-8 acts as an angiogenic factor [116]. The main part of the systemic increase in IL-8 as seen during exercise with an eccentric component is most likely because of an inflammatory response. In fact, not all the studies found increases in plasma IL-8 concentration during or after concentric exercise [111-114]. However, when the arterio-venous concentration difference across a concentrically exercising limb was measured, a small and transient net release of IL-8, which does not result in an increase in the systemic IL-8 plasma concentration has been detected [114]. The high local IL-8 expression taking place in working muscle with only a small and transient release could indicate that muscle-derived IL-8 acts locally and exerts its effect in an endocrine or paracrine fashion. Taking into account these results, it has been suggested that a plausible function of the muscle-derived IL-8 would be chemo attraction of neutrophils and macrophages when, in fact, in concentric exercise there is little or no accumulation of neutrophils or macrophages in skeletal muscle.

Levels of IL-15 mRNA were found to be higher in human skeletal muscles dominated by type-2 muscle fibres than in muscles dominated by type-1 muscle fibres, and that IL-15 mRNA content increased 24 hours following a bout of resistance exercise [117]. The increase in IL-15 mRNA levels was not accompanied by an increase in muscular IL-15 protein expression, neither was plasma IL-15 protein increased after a bout of resistance exercise. This was in contrast to Riechman *et al.* [118] who demonstrated a small, but significant increase in plasma IL-15 protein following resistance exercise. They found an increase in plasma IL-15 immediately after the end of a resistance exercise bout. A third study in humans did not find any change in IL-15 mRNA level in muscle biopsies obtained immediately after exercise. However, the strength training in this study influenced vastus lateralis to only a minor degree [119], possibly explaining the discrepancy. IL-15 has anabolic effects on muscle cell culture and decreases the muscle degradation rate in a cachexia model, suggesting that IL-15 might be of importance in muscle growth [120]. Furthermore, IL-15 has been suggested to play a role in muscle-adipose tissue interaction [121]. Thus, it is not known if IL-15 is an essential component in exercise-induced immuno-regulation. However, the findings that IL-15 is constitutively expressed by skeletal muscle and regulated by strength training, together with the finding that IL-15 has anabolic effects and seems to play a role in reducing adipose tissue mass, could indicate that IL-15 may play a role in muscle-fat cross talk [117], possibly reducing inflammation by means of a decrease in circulating lipids.

Several studies have examined the effects of both acute and chronic exercise on serum CRP levels. Regarding changes induced by an acute bout of exercise, studies in marathon runners have found that strenuous acute exercise produces large transient increases in CRP [122]. CRP highest levels are usually found 24 hours after exercise. The finding of increased circulating CRP levels after exercise is consistent across most studies and is probably due to the exercise-induced release of IL-6 and other pro-inflammatory cytokines from skeletal muscle that regulate CRP production in the liver [29].

Anti-inflammatory Response Induced by Acute Exercise: Role of IL-6

Extensive research has shown that during and immediately after exercise, there is a significant increase in plasma IL-6, which, in the hours following exercise, is accompanied by an increase in the anti-inflammatory cytokines IL-10 [105, 123] and IL-1ra [32, 49, 104, 108, 109]. Furthermore, acute prolonged exercise has been shown to increase the expression of the oxidant-responsive anti-inflammatory gene HO-1 in lymphocytes [124, 125]. During acute exercise, working muscles release a number of cytokines into the circulation, including IL-6 that may modulate systemic low-level inflammation [107]. The exercise-induced increase in IL-6 stimulates the appearance of other anti-inflammatory cytokines, including IL-1ra, sTNF-R and IL-10, whereas circulating levels of pro-inflammatory cytokines, such as TNF-α and IL-1, are generally not increased by acute exercise [29].

As it has been indicated, the increase of IL-6 is independent on concomitant muscle damage and the magnitude by which plasma IL-6 increases is related to exercise duration, intensity, the muscle mass involved in the mechanical work, and the endurance capacity. Even moderate exercise has major effects on muscle-derived IL-6 [126, 127]. The IL-6 mRNA is up-regulated in contracting skeletal muscle [42, 111, 128-132] and the transcriptional rate of the IL-6 gene is markedly enhanced by exercise, especially when muscle glycogen levels are low [133]. It has also been demonstrated that the IL-6 protein is expressed after exercise in muscle fibers [134], and that IL-6 is released from skeletal muscle during exercise [44]. Exercise was also found to increase IL-6 receptor production in human skeletal muscle, suggesting a possible post-exercise sensitizing mechanism to IL-6 [48]. It has been suggested that IL-6 acts as an autocrine factor up-regulating its mRNA levels, thereby supporting its function as an exercise activated factor in skeletal muscle cells [45]. Unlike IL-6 signalling in macrophages, intramuscular IL-6 expression is regulated by a network of signalling events that among other pathways are likely to involve the production of nitric oxide (NO) [135] and Ca^{2+} [136] following muscle contraction and p38 MAPK pathways regarding reduction of the glycogen content [137].

In spite of IL-6 was classified as a pro-inflammatory cytokine, recent data suggest that IL-6 and IL-6-regulated acute phase proteins are anti-inflammatory and immuno-suppressive, and may negatively regulate the acute phase response [138]. It has been shown that the exercise induced increase in plasma IL-6 is followed by increased circulating levels of well-known anti-inflammatory cytokines such as IL-1ra and IL-10 [107]. The cytokine response to exercise has been replicated by using an infusion of IL-6 to healthy donors, increasing also the systemic levels of cortisol [139].

Some studies have found results pointing to inhibitory effects of IL-6 on TNF-α and IL-1β production. It has been shown that IL-6 inhibits lipopolysaccharide (LPS)-induced TNF-α production both in cultured human monocytes and in the human monocytic line U937 [140], indicating that circulating IL-6 is involved in the regulation of TNF-α levels. Furthermore, Starkie *et al.* showed that IL-6 stimulates the release of soluble TNF-α receptors, but not IL-1β and TNF-α [141]. They also suggested that IL-6 was the primary inducer of the hepatocyte-derived acute-phase proteins, many of which have anti-inflammatory properties. Interestingly, both exercise and IL-6 infusion suppress TNF-α production in humans [141]. Both, in vitro [142] and animal [143, 144] studies have also suggested the role of IL-6 inhibiting TNF-α production.

The appearance of IL-10 and IL-1ra in the circulation after exercise contributes to the anti-inflammatory effects of exercise [29]. The anti-inflammatory properties of IL-10 derived from the ability to inhibit the production of the pro-inflammatory cytokines IL-1α, IL-1β and TNF-α, as well as the production of several pro-inflammatory chemokynes, especially in monocytes and neutrophils [36, 37, 145]. Interestingly, it has been shown that while IL-10 inhibits cytokine synthesis in mononuclear cells acting mainly at the level of cytokine gene transcription [37], the IL-8 production is prevented by affecting both gene transcription and mRNA stability [36]. All these compounds are essential in the activation of most of the immune cells and their recruitment to the sites of inflammation. Then, it can be suggested that the exercise induced increase in IL-10 limits the inflammatory response by preventing the appearance of several pro-inflammatory cytokines and chemokynes. The IL-1ra appearance in circulation after exercise could contribute to the anti-inflammatory effects of exercise because, as it has been indicated previously, the role of IL1-ra is to inhibit signalling transduction through the IL-1 receptor complex, preventing the production of the pro-inflammatory cytokines IL-1α, IL-1β [39]. CRP has been also described as an anti-inflammatory compound because of its role in both the induction of anti-inflammatory cytokines and in the suppression of the synthesis of pro-inflammatory cytokines [146]. As well as IL-10 and IL-1ra, CRP has been suggested to increase after exercise, at least in part, due to IL-6 induction [29].

Taking into account these results, we can conclude that exercise induces, via IL-6, an anti-inflammatory environment by inducing the production of IL-1ra and IL-10, and the inhibition of the TNF-α production. However, exercise is likely to suppress TNF-α also via IL-6-independent pathways, as demonstrated by the finding of a modest decrease of TNF-α following exercise in IL-6 KO mice [147]. As it has been indicated previously (Chapter 5), exercise induces high levels of epinephrine, and epinephrine infusion has been shown to prevent the appearance of TNF-α in response to endotoxin in vivo [148]. As epinephrine infusion induces only a small increase in IL-6 [149], the mechanism whereby epinephrine inhibits TNF-α production is not clear. However, authors of these works suggested that epinephrine and IL-6 inhibit the endotoxin-induced appearance of TNF-α via independent mechanisms. Interestingly, it has recently been demonstrated that epinephrine infusion also increased IL-10 release [148], indicating a possible contribution of epinephrine to the anti-inflammatory environment after exercise.

In a very interesting and innovative study, the existence of a true anti-inflammatory response to exercise, as well as the role of IL-6, was analysed in a model of "low-grade inflammation" based on the administration of a low dose of Escherichia coli endotoxin to healthy volunteers [141]. To test the hypotheses that IL-6 as well as physical exercise inhibits TNF-α production, eight healthy males participated in three experiments where they rested or performed bicycling for three hours or were infused with recombinant IL-6 (rhIL-6) for three hours while they rested. After 2.5 hours, the volunteers received a bolus of E. Coli lipopolysaccharide endotoxin intravenously to induce low grade inflammation. In the control study, plasma TNF-α increased significantly in response to endotoxin. In contrast, in subjects with high levels of IL-6, induced by the exercise or by the rhIL-6 infusion, the endotoxin-induced increase in TNF-α was completely abolished. Thus, this study demonstrated that physical exercise inhibits the production of TNF-α elicited by low-grade endotoxemia in humans and suggested that exercise-induced IL-6 production may contribute to mediate the effect of exercise on endotoxin-induced TNF-α production. Finally, authors of the study suggested that IL-6 plays an essential role mediating the anti-inflammatory effects of exercise [141].

Influence of Exercise Intensity and Duration

Some studies utilizing moderate-intensity exercise have shown that exercise elicits changes in certain inflammatory markers, and others have found no effect [150-152]. Nieman *et al.* [150] demonstrated a modest increase in total leukocyte count and plasma IL-6 concentration one hour following a 30-min treadmill walk at 60-65% VO_2max in young women who were accustomed to regular walking. It is not clear whether differences in subject characteristics (sex, age, or fitness) or exercise intensity (50% vs. 60-65% VO_2max) explain this apparent discrepancy. Only a few studies have investigated the effect of moderate-intensity exercise on plasma concentrations of the anti-inflammatory cytokine IL-10. As an example, the systemic concentration of IL-10 in young well-trained male runners did not change following one hour of running at 60% VO_2max [153]. However, and it has been indicated before, even moderate exercise induces increases in plasma IL-6 [126, 127].

No effect on the expression of the anti-inflammatory protein HO-1 in lymphocytes or in lymphocyte adhesion to cultured endothelial cells was found after a protocol of moderate exercise [154]. Lymphocyte HO-1 expression is up-regulated in response to prolonged demanding exercise [124, 125], but eccentric contractions and a short exhaustive run have been shown to have no effect on HO-1 protein expression in leukocytes [1]. In vitro adhesion assays have been used to demonstrate a reduction in lymphocyte adhesion to human umbilical venous endothelial cells in middle-age healthy individuals following a short cycle ergometer exercise at 75% VO_2max, which was accompanied by a significant increase in serum IL-6 concentrations immediately after finishing exercise [152]. It seems that exercise intensity and duration are both important in determining the inflammatory response to exercise, with intensity being particularly important. Markovitch *et al.* did not observe an inflammatory response following a 30-min walking protocol at 50% VO_2max [154]. Other studies show that exercise of a shorter or similar duration can elicit an inflammatory response, but only if the intensity is higher [155, 156]. Similarly, low-intensity protocols that are very prolonged in duration (1-legged dynamic knee extensor exercise for five hours at 40% VO_2max) also induce an inflammatory response [44]. In their work, Markovitch *et al.* pointed that studies using more intense exercise protocols tend to use younger and fitter individuals, and this means that not only is there a difference in terms of relative work rate (e.g., 50% VO_2max vs. 60% VO_2max), but there will be an even more pronounced difference in absolute work rate because of an age-related decline in capacity (e.g., in absolute running speeds or METs). The conclusion of this interesting work is that a single bout of moderate-intensity exercise of a duration that would meet public health recommendations in middle-aged men was insufficient to induce a pro- or anti-inflammatory response [154]. Taking into account their and other results revised, they suggested that some kind of intensity or duration threshold must be achieved to elicit an acute change in measures such as IL-6 and IL-10 [154].

Anti-Inflammatory Effects of Chronic Moderate Exercise

As it has been indicated previously, there is clinical general evidence for a beneficial effect of continuous moderate physical activity in patients with chronic diseases or metabolic disorders [22]. However, it would be interesting to clarify to what extend the benefits of regular moderate exercise in patients with chronic diseases are due to the anti-inflammatory exercise effects. Studies examining the effects of chronic exercise on cytokine production and circulating cytokine levels present contradictory results [49] and, in general, do not clarify the possible mechanisms involved.

Several chronic diseases and metabolism related disorders involve high TNF-α levels. TNF-α reduces muscle strength by affecting myocite differentiation and inducing cachexia [157]. Both COPD and rheumatoid arthritis are characterized by high circulating TNF-α levels and muscle strength lost [56, 57]. It has been suggested that exercise training could prevent muscle strength lost in these patients because of the exercise induced release of IL-6 [22]. Furthermore, the IL-6 inhibition of TNF-α production and, in general, the IL-6 induced anti-inflammatory environment [106] could be the responsible for the positive effects of exercise in patients with chronic diseases characterized by high levels of inflammatory cytokines. In fact, cross-sectional studies show that increasing levels of physical activity and/or fitness are generally associated with modest decreases in circulating levels of CRP, TNF-α and IL-6, and increased levels of IL-10 [158, 159]. In agreement with these results, Smith *et al.* [160] observed a significant reduction in the production of the pro-inflammatory cytokines IFN-γ, TNF-α and IL-1β, and a significant increase in the production of the anti-inflammatory cytokines TGF-β (transforming growth factor-β), IL-4 and IL-10, by cultured mononuclear cells from persons at risk of developing ischemic heart disease after six months of programmed physical activity when compared with production before exercise. Subjects in this study followed an individualized, supervised exercise program, with a mean of 2.5 hours of exercise per week. Smith *et al.* also observed a possible dose-response relationship between some of the changes observed and the time subjects spent performing some types of exercise [160]. However, in order to discuss this last result, it should be noted that only 43 subjects completed the study. Recently, Sanders *et al.* evaluated the associations between physical activity and inflammatory markers (CRP and IL-1β) in patients with periodontitis as well as in healthy subjects [161]. They found that increased physical activity was associated with lower levels of CRP in subjects with periodontitis; however, they indicated that this association was not apparent in healthy subjects [161]. Some more studies demonstrate reduced circulating levels of TNF-α, IL-6, IFN-γ and other markers of systemic inflammation after exercise training programs, but others did not find any effect [159]. It has been suggested that these discrepancies may be due to a number of factors, including differences in subject characteristics, the type and intensity of the exercise intervention, the timing of the blood samples taken and inherent variability in the assays used to measure many of these cytokines [49]. However, it has been also indicated that the preponderance of evidence suggests that both acute and chronic exercise is associated with modest improvements in markers of systemic low-grade inflammation [49]. In this sense, chronic exercise has been hypothesized to reduce circulating levels of CRP and other inflammatory markers. In fact, most of the studies focused on the effects of continuous moderate exercise on inflammation have used plasma CRP as inflammatory marker. A decrease in plasma CRP levels is considered an indicator of decreased systemic inflammation. Cross-sectional studies demonstrate an association between physical inactivity and low-grade systemic inflammation in healthy subjects [160, 162-168], in elderly people [169], and in patients with intermittent claudication [170]. These correlational data do not, however, provide any information with regard to a possible causal relationship. However, the finding in longitudinal studies that regular training induces a reduction in CRP level suggests that physical activity may suppress systemic low grade inflammation [162, 163, 171, 172].

Data from prospective studies examining the effect of exercise training on CRP levels have been inconclusive. Smith *et al.* found a 35% decrease in serum levels of CRP after a 6-month exercise program [160]. Authors suggested that the decrease observed was as a result of changes in blood mononuclear cells function observed after the six month of exercise (as it has been commented previously) [160]. In a meta-analysis of randomized controlled clinical trials published in 2006, Kelley *et al.* concluded that aerobic exercise training does not reduce basal CRP levels [173]. This meta-analysis included data from 323 male and female subjects in five independent trials in which subjects were randomized to either a control group or an aerobic exercise intervention (171 exercise and 152 control) lasting at least 4 weeks. Results showed a non-significant reduction of about 3% in CRP levels in the exercise groups after exercise training. Kohut *et al.* [174] randomly assigned adults (64 years old) to either an aerobic exercise program or a flexibility/strength exercise treatment for 10 months. They found that the aerobic exercise program significantly reduced serum CRP by 10-15% [174]. Furthermore, the aerobic program resulted in significant reductions when compared with the decrease observed after the flexibility/strength exercise. Both, IL-6 and IL-18 in this study followed the same pattern of change as CRP. After reviewing data from several longitudinal studies, Plaisance and Grandjean [158] suggested that long-term exercise training significantly reduces plasma CRP levels. They suggested that this positive effect could be independent of baseline CRP levels, body composition and weight loss [158], which could be some of the confounding factors in these studies regarding the mechanisms for the positive effects of exercise. It has been suggested that the clinical significance of these improvements is uncertain because they may not reflect changes occurring at the tissue level. But, on the other hand, it has been also suggested that a change in the tissue concentration of certain chemokynes, which work at local level, could not be reflected in the circulating levels but could produce either positive or negative effects [68].

In addition to the previous ones, several studies have demonstrated, also, interesting and healthy relations between different programs of regular physical activity or training programs and inflammatory markers (CRP and others). In this sense both epidemiological and clinical data evidenced positive effects of physical activity [165, 167, 175-177]. In a cohort of 5,888 men and women over 65 years of age, higher levels of self-reported physical activity were associated with lower serum concentrations of several markers of inflammation, including CRP and fibrinogen, as well as lower white blood cell counts, after adjusting for age, sex, race, presence of cardiovascular disease, smoking, BMI, diabetes, and hypertension [165]. These data suggest that increased exercise is associated with reduced inflammation [165]. Cross-sectional studies consistently demonstrate an inverse relationship between plasma CRP and both physical activity level and cardio-respiratory fitness [178]. These associations remain after controlling for potential confounders in some studies [175], although others suggest they may be influenced by factors, such as gender, body composition and the type of physical activity among others.

As it has been suggested earlier, no relationship between physical activity levels and CRP is found in some studies after adjusting for BMI (body mass index) and other risk factors [181, 182]. In this sense, Arsenault *et al.* [183] recently showed that after adjusting for visceral adipose tissue, fitness was not associated with variation in inflammatory markers. Authors of this study suggested that the previously reported association between poor fitness and low-grade inflammation may be largely attributable to increased visceral adipose tissue accumulation and its associated state of insulin resistance, conditions frequently observed in subjects with poor cardiorespiratory fitness [183]. As it has been highlighted previously, weight loss could be an important confounding factor in these studies. In fact, it has been consistently reported that weight loss induces a decrease in CRP levels [184]. Most exercise training interventions have shown modest or no effects on CRP after statistically correcting for weight loss, but few studies have assessed the effect of exercise on CRP in the absence of weight loss [184]. In the same way, Hammet *et al.* [188] studied the effects of exercise training on five inflammatory markers associated with cardiovascular risk (including fibrinogen and CRP) in 152 healthy female smokers. The exercise group took part in three 45-minute supervised exercise sessions per week using different ergometers (cycle, treadmill and rowing). They found that the exercise training improved cardio-respiratory fitness but had no consistent effect on inflammatory marker levels. Because they found that baseline associations between physical fitness and inflammatory markers were largely explained by differences in body fat, they suggested that associations between greater physical fitness and lower inflammatory markers may be explained by long-term regular exercise reducing body and visceral fat [188], which is the main reason some authors have suggested for decreased inflammation after an exercise training program.

Several studies have shown a significant inverse relationship between physical fitness and plasma IL-6 [185], whereas plasma IL-10, an anti-inflammatory cytokine, is positively related to fitness [186]. As in CRP, and in spite of IL-6 has been recognised as an anti-inflammatory cytokine, continuous increased IL-6 levels are considered as a marker of low-grade systemic inflammation. Thus, a decrease in basal IL-6 circulating levels would be a healthy achievement. In an analysis of 880 participants aged between 70 and 79 years, Taaffe *et al.* showed found that both serum IL-6 and CRP concentrations were inversely associated with the hours per year undertaking moderate and strenuous physical activity and, also, with aerobic fitness as measured by the distance covered in six minutes of fast walking [167]. Survival seven years later was associated with lower baseline IL-6 concentrations and also greater baseline six-minute walking distances [167]. The effects of physical activity on inflammatory cytokine activity persist even when obesity is considered. It is well known that obesity is associated with increased production of pro-inflammatory cytokines [65, 67]. Hotamisligil *et al.* [65] showed first in animal models that TNF-α protein was elevated locally and systemically in obese animal models, indicating a role for TNF-α in obesity. In an analysis of 27,158 apparently healthy adult women (mean age 54.7 years) from the Women's Health Study, which found significant associations between BMI and several inflammatory and lipid markers, including serum concentrations of CRP, fibrinogen, soluble intracellular adhesion molecule-1 (sICAM-1), total cholesterol, and low-density lipoprotein [177]. As expected, high density lipoprotein cholesterol (HDL-C) concentrations decreased with increasing BMI [177]. However, physical activity was associated with small but significant reductions in the serum concentrations of these biomarkers compared with inactive individuals, (except HDL-C, which increased slightly), independent of BMI [177]. This beneficial effect was strongest on inflammatory markers, such as CRP and fibrinogen, as compared to lipid biomarkers [177]. In a study involving high-intensity training, Mattusch *et al.* examined the effects of a nine-month increased training program in preparation for a marathon [163]. CRP was reduced about 31% in highly trained runners after the nine months of increased training but did not change significantly in non-training control subjects. Although the reduction in CRP in the training group in this study was statistically significant, authors indicated that the physiological relevance of such a small absolute change in CRP levels is unknown [163]. Furthermore, it was suggested that because the subjects in the 'training' group were already highly fit runners, the significance of these findings to the general population is also uncertain [49]. In a cohort of 3,075 elderly men and women (aged 70-79) from the Health, Aging and Body Composition Study, higher levels of exercise were associated with lower concentrations of CRP, IL-6, and TNF-α in subjects not taking antioxidant supplements [187]. However, in one of the longest randomized controlled trial Rauramaa *et al.* did not find any significant effect of low to moderate intensity training on plasma CRP levels [180]. After six years of exercise training they found a non-significant decrease in plasma CRP levels in the exercise group in spite of the increase observed in the ventilatory aerobic threshold [180].

As indicated previously, the type of physical activity could be one of the confounding factors when results of these studies are analysed. Some studies have examined and compared the relationship between different types of exercise and CRP levels. King *et al.* (in the Third National Health and Nutrition Examination Survey) [166], found that different aerobic exercises (e.g. jogging, swimming, cycling, aerobic dancing) were associated with lower CRP levels. However, after controlling for possible confounding factors such as age, race, sex and BMI, only regular participants in jogging and aerobic dancing showed still significant lower CRP levels [166]. Dufaux *et al.* [179] concluded that exercise training induces a decrease in CRP circulating levels in both male and female swimmers when compared to controls. However, they find non-significant lower levels in rowers, cyclists and football players [179]. Kohut *et al.* [174] found that both, an aerobic and a flexibility/strength exercise program induced significant decreases in TNF-α plasma levels after ten months of exercise training. Sloan *et al.* [189] examined the anti-inflammatory effects of exercise by measuring monocyte TNF-α production after a 12-week aerobic training program. Blood was taken before and after a moderate or high intensity training schedule and, then, it was stimulated ex vivo by addition of lipopolysaccharide. The authors found that exercise training induced a decrease in TNF-α production only in the high intensity training group. However, authors of the study did not measure any other inflammatory or anti-inflammatory marker or possible mediators in the mechanism involved.

Finally, it is also possible that gender influences effects of exercise on inflammatory markers. Several studies have found differences between the effects of training on CRP levels in males and females [179, 190, 191]. Some of these observational studies indicate that chronic physical activity reduces CRP levels more in males than females [179, 190, 191]. However, Arsenault *et al.* [183] reported that fitness did not correlate with any of the individual inflammatory markers in men, whereas it was negatively associated with CRP and IL-6 in women. They indicate that more studies are necessary to explain the basis of gender differences.

Mechanisms Involved in the Anti-Inflammatory Effect of Moderate Exercise

It has been suggested that regular physical activity is anti-inflammatory partly because of the changes induced by each individual bout of exercise [29, 138]. In this sense, with regular exercise, the anti-inflammatory effects of an acute bout of exercise will protect against chronic systemic low-grade inflammation, but such a link between the acute effects of exercise and the long-term benefits has not yet been proven. Vigorous exercise elevates serum IL-6 concentration, which may be anti-inflammatory through the increased production of IL-1ra and IL-10 [29]. Furthermore, vigorous exercise increases the lymphocyte expression of the anti-inflammatory enzyme HO-1 [124, 125]. However, several studies did not find any anti-inflammatory response after an acute bout of moderate-intensity exercise protocols. For example, Markovitch *et al.* did not find any change in CRP, IL-6, IL-10, lymphocyte HO-1, or lymphocyte adhesion levels over a 7-day period in response to a single bout of moderate-intensity exercise [154].

The authors of this last study [154] indicated that, as it had been suggested previously, it was possible that some of the benefits derived from such activity are largely related to acute changes induced by the last bout of activity. For example, the regular up-regulation of anti-inflammatory molecules such as HO-1 may contribute to an overall down-regulation of pro-atherogenic inflammatory pathways in the same way that acute regular changes in lipid metabolism may play a role in the long-term benefits of regular exercise [192]. This hypothesis seems to be adequate when demanding exercise is performed because, as it has discussed previously in this chapter, an anti-inflammatory environment is generated after an acute bout of demanding exercise. However, there is less evidence that this is relevant to moderate-intensity physical activity as described in most physical activity recommendations. Taking into account their results, Markovitch *et al.* concluded that even though regular moderate-intensity exercise appears to be associated with reduced markers of inflammation in cross-sectional comparisons [185, 193, 194], this does not appear to be explained by acute inflammatory changes induced by each exercise bout because they did not find any change after an acute bout of moderate exercise. Authors of this study suggested that other mechanisms inducing the anti-inflammatory effect of long-term, moderate-intensity exercise should be considered and examined in future studies. They also suggested that it seems that other changes associated with regular moderate-intensity exercise ultimately explain the anti-inflammatory effect. For example, a reduction in body mass following a controlled physical activity program [195] or fat mass through dietary intervention [196] can be anti-inflammatory and reduce chronic inflammation. Furthermore, positive changes in lipid and glycemic profiles could also explain the anti-inflammatory effect of regular moderate-intensity exercise [197]. In fact, there is considerable evidence that independently of weight loss, physical activity has beneficial effects on patients with dyslipidemia, improving the blood lipid profile [22]. In training studies, an increase in high-density lipoprotein (HDL) and a decrease in low-density lipoprotein (LDL) are consistent findings [22]. The decrease in LDL could be an essential event in the anti-inflammatory effects of exercise in the prevention of atherosclerosis. High LDL levels are an important cardiovascular risk factor which can initiate the development of atherosclerosis even in the absence of other risk factors [49]. When circulating levels are elevated, LDL can accumulate in the sub-endothelial space, where it becomes oxidized [49]. The oxidative modification of LDL (ox-LDL) promotes an inflammatory response, recruitment of macrophages and the development of atherosclerotic lesions. The inflammation initiated by ox-LDL is mediated by the local production of pro-inflammatory cytokines in the artery wall [49]. Thus, if exercise reduces LDL circulating levels, it also could reduce LDL oxidation, ox-LDL induced inflammatory response and, as a consequence, atherosclerosis development.

Conclusion

There is important evidence regarding the positive effects of regular exercise in patients with chronic diseases but also in the prevention of the diseases. Low grade systemic inflammation has been found to be involved in several chronic diseases which suppose the largest cause of death in the world. Recent findings have demonstrated that an acute bout of physical activity induces an anti-inflammatory response, with the muscle playing an essential role in this response via IL-6 production. Furthermore, there is increasing evidence regarding the anti-inflammatory effects of continuous moderate-intensity physical activity. However, the mechanisms underlying these positive effects remain unclear.

References

[1] Fehrenbach, E; Niess, AM; Passek, F; Sorichter, S; Schwirtz, A; Berg, A; Dickhuth, HH; Northoff, H. Influence of different types of exercise on the expression of haem oxygenase-1 in leukocytes. J Sports Sci, 2003, 21, 383-9.

[2] Department of Health and Human Services, CfDCaP, National Center for Chronic Disease Prevention and Health Promotion. Physical Activity and Health: A Report of the Surgeon General. Atlanta: GA: DHHS, 1996.

[3] Hu, G; Tuomilehto, J; Silventoinen, K; Barengo, NC; Peltonen, M; Jousilahti, P. The effects of physical activity and body mass index on cardiovascular, cancer and all-cause mortality among 47 212 middle-aged Finnish men and women. Int J Obes (Lond), 2005, 29, 894-902.

[4] Lees, SJ; Booth, FW. Physical inactivity is a disease. World Rev Nutr Diet, 2005, 95, 73-9.

[5] Thompson, PD; Buchner, D; Pina, IL; Balady, GJ; Williams, MA; Marcus, BH; Berra, K; Blair, SN; Costa, F; Franklin, B; Fletcher, GF; Gordon, NF; Pate, RR; Rodriguez, BL; Yancey, AK; Wenger, NK. Exercise and physical activity in the prevention and treatment of atherosclerotic cardiovascular disease: a statement from the Council on Clinical Cardiology (Subcommittee on Exercise, Rehabilitation, and Prevention) and the Council on Nutrition, Physical Activity, and Metabolism (Subcommittee on Physical Activity). Circulation, 2003, 107, 3109-16.

[6] Myers, J; Kaykha, A; George, S; Abella, J; Zaheer, N; Lear, S; Yamazaki, T; Froelicher, V. Fitness versus physical activity patterns in predicting mortality in men. Am J Med, 2004, 117, 912-8.

[7] Church, TS; Cheng, YJ; Earnest, CP; Barlow, CE; Gibbons, LW; Priest, EL; Blair, SN. Exercise capacity and body composition as predictors of mortality among men with diabetes. Diabetes Care, 2004, 27, 83-8.

[8] Farrell, SW; Braun, L; Barlow, CE; Cheng, YJ; Blair, SN. The relation of body mass index, cardiorespiratory fitness, and all-cause mortality in women. Obes Res, 2002, 10, 417-23.

[9] Sandvik, L; Erikssen, J; Thaulow, E; Erikssen, G; Mundal, R; Rodahl, K. Physical fitness as a predictor of mortality among healthy, middle-aged Norwegian men. N Engl J Med, 1993, 328, 533-7.

[10] Stevens, J; Cai, J; Evenson, KR; Thomas, R. Fitness and fatness as predictors of mortality from all causes and from cardiovascular disease in men and women in the lipid research clinics study. Am J Epidemiol, 2002, 156, 832-41.

[11] Stevens, J; Evenson, KR; Thomas, O; Cai, J; Thomas, R. Associations of fitness and fatness with mortality in Russian and American men in the lipids research clinics study. Int J Obes Relat Metab Disord, 2004, 28, 1463-70.

[12] Crespo, CJ; Palmieri, MR; Perdomo, RP; McGee, DL; Smit, E; Sempos, CT; Lee, IM; Sorlie, PD. The relationship of physical activity and body weight with all-cause mortality: results from the Puerto Rico Heart Health Program. Ann Epidemiol, 2002, 12, 543-52.

[13] Andersen, LB; Schnohr, P; Schroll, M; Hein, HO. All-cause mortality associated with physical activity during leisure time, work, sports, and cycling to work. Arch Intern Med, 2000, 160, 1621-8.
[14] Batty, GD; Shipley, MJ; Marmot, M; Smith, GD. Physical activity and cause-specific mortality in men: further evidence from the Whitehall study. Eur J Epidemiol, 2001, 17, 863-9.
[15] Batty, GD; Shipley, MJ; Marmot, M; Smith, GD. Physical activity and cause-specific mortality in men with Type 2 diabetes/impaired glucose tolerance: evidence from the Whitehall study. Diabet Med, 2002, 19, 580-8.
[16] Hu, FB; Willett, WC; Li, T; Stampfer, MJ; Colditz, GA; Manson, JE. Adiposity as compared with physical activity in predicting mortality among women. N Engl J Med, 2004, 351, 2694-703.
[17] Arraiz, GA; Wigle, DT; Mao, Y. Risk assessment of physical activity and physical fitness in the Canada Health Survey mortality follow-up study. J Clin Epidemiol, 1992, 45, 419-28.
[18] Gregg, EW; Cauley, JA; Stone, K; Thompson, TJ; Bauer, DC; Cummings, SR; Ensrud, KE. Relationship of changes in physical activity and mortality among older women. Jama, 2003, 289, 2379-86.
[19] Sundquist, K; Qvist, J; Sundquist, J; Johansson, SE. Frequent and occasional physical activity in the elderly: a 12-year follow-up study of mortality. Am J Prev Med, 2004, 27, 22-7.
[20] Haapanen-Niemi, N; Miilunpalo, S; Pasanen, M; Vuori, I; Oja, P; Malmberg, J. Body mass index, physical inactivity and low level of physical fitness as determinants of all-cause and cardiovascular disease mortality--16 y follow-up of middle-aged and elderly men and women. Int J Obes Relat Metab Disord, 2000, 24, 1465-74.
[21] Murray, CJ; Lopez, AD. Global mortality, disability, and the contribution of risk factors: Global Burden of Disease Study. Lancet, 1997, 349, 1436-42.
[22] Pedersen, BK; Saltin, B. Evidence for prescribing exercise as therapy in chronic disease. Scand J Med Sci Sports, 2006, 16 Suppl 1, 3-63.
[23] Flynn, KE; Pina, IL; Whellan, DJ; Lin, L; Blumenthal, JA; Ellis, SJ; Fine, LJ; Howlett, JG; Keteyian, SJ; Kitzman, DW; Kraus, WE; Miller, NH; Schulman, KA; Spertus, JA; O'Connor, CM; Weinfurt, KP. Effects of exercise training on health status in patients with chronic heart failure: HF-ACTION randomized controlled trial. Jama, 2009, 301, 1451-9.
[24] O'Connor, CM; Whellan, DJ; Lee, KL; Keteyian, SJ; Cooper, LS; Ellis, SJ; Leifer, ES; Kraus, WE; Kitzman, DW; Blumenthal, JA; Rendall, DS; Miller, NH; Fleg, JL; Schulman, KA; McKelvie, RS; Zannad, F; Pina, IL. Efficacy and safety of exercise training in patients with chronic heart failure: HF-ACTION randomized controlled trial. Jama, 2009, 301, 1439-50.
[25] Libby, P. Inflammation in atherosclerosis. Nature, 2002, 420, 868-74.
[26] Dandona, P; Aljada, A; Bandyopadhyay, A. Inflammation: the link between insulin resistance, obesity and diabetes. Trends Immunol, 2004, 25, 4-7.
[27] Ross, R. Atherosclerosis--an inflammatory disease. N Engl J Med, 1999, 340, 115-26.
[28] Festa, A; D'Agostino, R, Jr.; Tracy, RP; Haffner, SM. Elevated levels of acute-phase proteins and plasminogen activator inhibitor-1 predict the development of type 2 diabetes: the insulin resistance atherosclerosis study. Diabetes, 2002, 51, 1131-7.

[29] Petersen, AM; Pedersen, BK. The anti-inflammatory effect of exercise. J Appl Physiol, 2005, 98, 1154-62.
[30] Pedersen, BK; Febbraio, M. Muscle-derived interleukin-6--a possible link between skeletal muscle, adipose tissue, liver, and brain. Brain Behav Immun, 2005, 19, 371-6.
[31] Pedersen, BK; Steensberg, A; Fischer, C; Keller, C; Keller, P; Plomgaard, P; Wolsk-Petersen, E; Febbraio, M. The metabolic role of IL-6 produced during exercise: is IL-6 an exercise factor? Proc Nutr Soc, 2004, 63, 263-7.
[32] Pedersen, BK; Steensberg, A; Fischer, C; Keller, C; Keller, P; Plomgaard, P; Febbraio, M; Saltin, B. Searching for the exercise factor: is IL-6 a candidate? J Muscle Res Cell Motil, 2003, 24, 113-9.
[33] Akira, S; Kishimoto, T. IL-6 and NF-IL6 in acute-phase response and viral infection. Immunol Rev, 1992, 127, 25-50.
[34] Akira, S; Taga, T; Kishimoto, T. Interleukin-6 in biology and medicine. Adv Immunol, 1993, 54, 1-78.
[35] Dinarello, CA. Interleukin-1 and interleukin-1 antagonism. Blood, 1991, 77, 1627-52.
[36] Wang, P; Wu, P; Anthes, JC; Siegel, MI; Egan, RW; Billah, MM. Interleukin-10 inhibits interleukin-8 production in human neutrophils. Blood, 1994, 83, 2678-83.
[37] Wang, P; Wu, P; Siegel, MI; Egan, RW; Billah, MM. IL-10 inhibits transcription of cytokine genes in human peripheral blood mononuclear cells. J Immunol, 1994, 153, 811-6.
[38] Bogdan, C; Paik, J; Vodovotz, Y; Nathan, C. Contrasting mechanisms for suppression of macrophage cytokine release by transforming growth factor-beta and interleukin-10. J Biol Chem, 1992, 267, 23301-8.
[39] Dinarello, CA. The role of the interleukin-1-receptor antagonist in blocking inflammation mediated by interleukin-1. N Engl J Med, 2000, 343, 732-4.
[40] Chazaud, B; Brigitte, M; Yacoub-Youssef, H; Arnold, L; Gherardi, R; Sonnet, C; Lafuste, P; Chretien, F. Dual and beneficial roles of macrophages during skeletal muscle regeneration. Exerc Sport Sci Rev, 2009, 37, 18-22.
[41] Gleeson, M. Immune function in sport and exercise. J Appl Physiol, 2007, 103, 693-9.
[42] Jonsdottir, IH; Schjerling, P; Ostrowski, K; Asp, S; Richter, EA; Pedersen, BK. Muscle contractions induce interleukin-6 mRNA production in rat skeletal muscles. J Physiol, 2000, 528 Pt 1, 157-63.
[43] Starkie, RL; Arkinstall, MJ; Koukoulas, I; Hawley, JA; Febbraio, MA. Carbohydrate ingestion attenuates the increase in plasma interleukin-6, but not skeletal muscle interleukin-6 mRNA, during exercise in humans. J Physiol, 2001, 533, 585-91.
[44] Steensberg, A; van Hall, G; Osada, T; Sacchetti, M; Saltin, B; Klarlund Pedersen, B. Production of interleukin-6 in contracting human skeletal muscles can account for the exercise-induced increase in plasma interleukin-6. J Physiol, 2000, 529 Pt 1, 237-42.
[45] Weigert, C; Dufer, M; Simon, P; Debre, E; Runge, H; Brodbeck, K; Haring, HU; Schleicher, ED. Upregulation of IL-6 mRNA by IL-6 in skeletal muscle cells: role of IL-6 mRNA stabilization and Ca^{2+}-dependent mechanisms. Am J Physiol Cell Physiol, 2007, 293, C1139-47.
[46] Glund, S; Deshmukh, A; Long, YC; Moller, T; Koistinen, HA; Caidahl, K; Zierath, JR; Krook, A. Interleukin-6 directly increases glucose metabolism in resting human skeletal muscle. Diabetes, 2007, 56, 1630-7.

[47] Carey, AL; Steinberg, GR; Macaulay, SL; Thomas, WG; Holmes, AG; Ramm, G; Prelovsek, O; Hohnen-Behrens, C; Watt, MJ; James, DE; Kemp, BE; Pedersen, BK; Febbraio, MA. Interleukin-6 increases insulin-stimulated glucose disposal in humans and glucose uptake and fatty acid oxidation in vitro via AMP-activated protein kinase. Diabetes, 2006, 55, 2688-97.
[48] Keller, P; Penkowa, M; Keller, C; Steensberg, A; Fischer, CP; Giralt, M; Hidalgo, J; Pedersen, BK. Interleukin-6 receptor expression in contracting human skeletal muscle: regulating role of IL-6. Faseb J, 2005, 19, 1181-3.
[49] Wilund, KR. Is the anti-inflammatory effect of regular exercise responsible for reduced cardiovascular disease? Clin Sci (Lond), 2007, 112, 543-55.
[50] Mathur, N; Pedersen, BK. Exercise as a mean to control low-grade systemic inflammation. Mediators Inflamm, 2008, 2008, Article identification 109502.
[51] Hotamisligil, GS. Inflammation and metabolic disorders. Nature, 2006, 444, 860-7.
[52] Haffner, SM. The metabolic syndrome: inflammation, diabetes mellitus, and cardiovascular disease. Am J Cardiol, 2006, 97, 3A-11A.
[53] Lin, WW; Karin, M. A cytokine-mediated link between innate immunity, inflammation, and cancer. J Clin Invest, 2007, 117, 1175-83.
[54] Roubenoff, R. Physical activity, inflammation, and muscle loss. Nutr Rev, 2007, 65, S208-12.
[55] Eid, AA; Ionescu, AA; Nixon, LS; Lewis-Jenkins, V; Matthews, SB; Griffiths, TL; Shale, DJ. Inflammatory response and body composition in chronic obstructive pulmonary disease. Am J Respir Crit Care Med, 2001, 164, 1414-8.
[56] Brennan, FM; Maini, RN; Feldmann, M. TNF alpha--a pivotal role in rheumatoid arthritis? Br J Rheumatol, 1992, 31, 293-8.
[57] Palacio, J; Galdiz, JB; Bech, JJ; Marinan, M; Casadevall, C; Martinez, P; Gea, J. Interleukin 10 and tumor necrosis factor alpha gene expression in respiratory and peripheral muscles. Relation to sarcolemmal damage. Arch Bronconeumol, 2002, 38, 311-6.
[58] Haddad, F; Zaldivar, F; Cooper, DM; Adams, GR. IL-6-induced skeletal muscle atrophy. J Appl Physiol, 2005, 98, 911-7.
[59] Coletti, D; Moresi, V; Adamo, S; Molinaro, M; Sassoon, D. Tumor necrosis factor-alpha gene transfer induces cachexia and inhibits muscle regeneration. Genesis, 2005, 43, 120-8.
[60] Handschin, C; Spiegelman, B. The role of exercise and PGC1α in inflammation and chronic disease. Nature, 2008, 454, 463-469.
[61] Cesari, M; Penninx, BW; Newman, AB; Kritchevsky, SB; Nicklas, BJ; Sutton-Tyrrell, K; Rubin, SM; Ding, J; Simonsick, EM; Harris, TB; Pahor, M. Inflammatory markers and onset of cardiovascular events: results from the Health ABC study. Circulation, 2003, 108, 2317-22.
[62] Meyerhardt, JA; Heseltine, D; Niedzwiecki, D; Hollis, D; Saltz, LB; Mayer, RJ; Thomas, J; Nelson, H; Whittom, R; Hantel, A; Schilsky, RL; Fuchs, CS. Impact of physical activity on cancer recurrence and survival in patients with stage III colon cancer: findings from CALGB 89803. J Clin Oncol, 2006, 24, 3535-41.
[63] Packard, RR; Libby, P. Inflammation in atherosclerosis: from vascular biology to biomarker discovery and risk prediction. Clin Chem, 2008, 54, 24-38.

[64] Plomgaard, P; Bouzakri, K; Krogh-Madsen, R; Mittendorfer, B; Zierath, JR; Pedersen, BK. Tumor necrosis factor-alpha induces skeletal muscle insulin resistance in healthy human subjects via inhibition of Akt substrate 160 phosphorylation. Diabetes, 2005, 54, 2939-45.
[65] Hotamisligil, GS; Shargill, NS; Spiegelman, BM. Adipose expression of tumor necrosis factor-alpha: direct role in obesity-linked insulin resistance. Science, 1993, 259, 87-91.
[66] Plomgaard, P; Nielsen, AR; Fischer, CP; Mortensen, OH; Broholm, C; Penkowa, M; Krogh-Madsen, R; Erikstrup, C; Lindegaard, B; Petersen, AM; Taudorf, S; Pedersen, BK. Associations between insulin resistance and TNF-alpha in plasma, skeletal muscle and adipose tissue in humans with and without type 2 diabetes. Diabetologia, 2007, 50, 2562-71.
[67] Hotamisligil, GS; Arner, P; Caro, JF; Atkinson, RL; Spiegelman, BM. Increased adipose tissue expression of tumor necrosis factor-alpha in human obesity and insulin resistance. J Clin Invest, 1995, 95, 2409-15.
[68] Pedersen, BK; Febbraio, MA. Point: Interleukin-6 does have a beneficial role in insulin sensitivity and glucose homeostasis. J Appl Physiol, 2007, 102, 814-6.
[69] Steensberg, A; Fischer, CP; Sacchetti, M; Keller, C; Osada, T; Schjerling, P; van Hall, G; Febbraio, MA; Pedersen, BK. Acute interleukin-6 administration does not impair muscle glucose uptake or whole-body glucose disposal in healthy humans. J Physiol, 2003, 548, 631-8.
[70] Lyngso, D; Simonsen, L; Bulow, J. Interleukin-6 production in human subcutaneous abdominal adipose tissue: the effect of exercise. J Physiol, 2002, 543, 373-8.
[71] Petersen, EW; Carey, AL; Sacchetti, M; Steinberg, GR; Macaulay, SL; Febbraio, MA; Pedersen, BK. Acute IL-6 treatment increases fatty acid turnover in elderly humans in vivo and in tissue culture in vitro. Am J Physiol Endocrinol Metab, 2005, 288, E155-62.
[72] van Hall, G; Steensberg, A; Sacchetti, M; Fischer, C; Keller, C; Schjerling, P; Hiscock, N; Moller, K; Saltin, B; Febbraio, MA; Pedersen, BK. Interleukin-6 stimulates lipolysis and fat oxidation in humans. J Clin Endocrinol Metab, 2003, 88, 3005-10.
[73] Nishimoto, N; Yoshizaki, K; Miyasaka, N; Yamamoto, K; Kawai, S; Takeuchi, T; Hashimoto, J; Azuma, J; Kishimoto, T. Treatment of rheumatoid arthritis with humanized anti-interleukin-6 receptor antibody: a multicenter, double-blind, placebo-controlled trial. Arthritis Rheum, 2004, 50, 1761-9.
[74] Choy, EH; Isenberg, DA; Garrood, T; Farrow, S; Ioannou, Y; Bird, H; Cheung, N; Williams, B; Hazleman, B; Price, R; Yoshizaki, K; Nishimoto, N; Kishimoto, T; Panayi, GS. Therapeutic benefit of blocking interleukin-6 activity with an anti-interleukin-6 receptor monoclonal antibody in rheumatoid arthritis: a randomized, double-blind, placebo-controlled, dose-escalation trial. Arthritis Rheum, 2002, 46, 3143-50.
[75] Coussens, LM; Werb, Z. Inflammation and cancer. Nature, 2002, 420, 860-7.
[76] Balkwill, F; Mantovani, A. Inflammation and cancer: back to Virchow? Lancet, 2001, 357, 539-45.
[77] Lu, H; Ouyang, W; Huang, C. Inflammation, a key event in cancer development. Mol Cancer Res, 2006, 4, 221-33.
[78] Itzkowitz, SH; Yio, X. Inflammation and cancer IV. Colorectal cancer in inflammatory bowel disease: the role of inflammation. Am J Physiol Gastrointest Liver Physiol, 2004, 287, G7-17.

[79] Seril, DN; Liao, J; Yang, GY; Yang, CS. Oxidative stress and ulcerative colitis-associated carcinogenesis: studies in humans and animal models. Carcinogenesis, 2003, 24, 353-62.
[80] Moody, GA; Jayanthi, V; Probert, CS; Mac Kay, H; Mayberry, JF. Long-term therapy with sulphasalazine protects against colorectal cancer in ulcerative colitis: a retrospective study of colorectal cancer risk and compliance with treatment in Leicestershire. Eur J Gastroenterol Hepatol, 1996, 8, 1179-83.
[81] Eaden, J; Abrams, K; Ekbom, A; Jackson, E; Mayberry, J. Colorectal cancer prevention in ulcerative colitis: a case-control study. Aliment Pharmacol Ther, 2000, 14, 145-53.
[82] Thun, MJ; Namboodiri, MM; Calle, EE; Flanders, WD; Heath, CW, Jr. Aspirin use and risk of fatal cancer. Cancer Res, 1993, 53, 1322-7.
[83] Langman, MJ; Cheng, KK; Gilman, EA; Lancashire, RJ. Effect of anti-inflammatory drugs on overall risk of common cancer: case-control study in general practice research database. Bmj, 2000, 320, 1642-6.
[84] Moore, RJ; Owens, DM; Stamp, G; Arnott, C; Burke, F; East, N; Holdsworth, H; Turner, L; Rollins, B; Pasparakis, M; Kollias, G; Balkwill, F. Mice deficient in tumor necrosis factor-alpha are resistant to skin carcinogenesis. Nat Med, 1999, 5, 828-31.
[85] Karin, M. Nuclear factor-kappaB in cancer development and progression. Nature, 2006, 441, 431-6.
[86] Febbraio, MA. Exercise and inflammation. J Appl Physiol, 2007, 103, 376-7.
[87] Nieman, DC. Current perspective on exercise immunology. Curr Sports Med Rep, 2003, 2, 239-42.
[88] Gleeson, M; McFarlin, B; Flynn, M. Exercise and Toll-like receptors. Exerc Immunol Rev, 2006, 12, 34-53.
[89] Gleeson, M; Nieman, DC; Pedersen, BK. Exercise, nutrition and immune function. J Sports Sci, 2004, 22, 115-25.
[90] Cannon, J; Blumberg, JB. Acute phase immune response in exercise. In: Sen CK, Packer L, Hänninen O, eds. Handbook of Oxidants and Antioxidants in Exercise. Amsterdam: Elsevier Science B.V., 2000:177-194.
[91] Pizza, FX; Davis, BH; Henrickson, SD; Mitchell, JB; Pace, JF; Bigelow, N; DiLauro, P; Naglieri, T. Adaptation to eccentric exercise: effect on CD64 and CD11b/CD18 expression. J Appl Physiol, 1996, 80, 47-55.
[92] Tidball, JG. Inflammatory cell response to acute muscle injury. Med Sci Sports Exerc, 1995, 27, 1022-32.
[93] Nieman, DC. Exercise immunology: integration and regulation. Int J Sports Med, 1998, 19 Suppl 3, S171.
[94] Tauler, P; Aguilo, A; Gimeno, I; Noguera, A; Agusti, A; Tur, JA; Pons, A. Differential response of lymphocytes and neutrophils to high intensity physical activity and to vitamin C diet supplementation. Free Radic Res, 2003, 37, 931-8.
[95] Tauler, P; Aguilo, A; Gimeno, I; Guix, P; Tur, JA; Pons, A. Different effects of exercise tests on the antioxidant enzyme activities in lymphocytes and neutrophils. J Nutr Biochem, 2004, 15, 479-84.
[96] Hessel, E; Haberland, A; Muller, M; Lerche, D; Schimke, I. Oxygen radical generation of neutrophils: a reason for oxidative stress during marathon running? Clin Chim Acta, 2000, 298, 145-56.

[97] McCarthy, DA; Dale, MM. The leucocytosis of exercise. A review and model. Sports Med, 1988, 6, 333-63.

[98] Pedersen, BK; Hoffman-Goetz, L. Exercise and the immune system: regulation, integration, and adaptation. Physiol Rev, 2000, 80, 1055-81.

[99] Nieman, DC; Johanssen, LM; Lee, JW; Arabatzis, K. Infectious episodes in runners before and after the Los Angeles Marathon. J Sports Med Phys Fitness, 1990, 30, 316-28.

[100] Peters, EM; Bateman, ED. Ultramarathon running and upper respiratory tract infections. An epidemiological survey. S Afr Med J, 1983, 64, 582-4.

[101] Peters, EM; Goetzsche, JM; Grobbelaar, B; Noakes, TD. Vitamin C supplementation reduces the incidence of postrace symptoms of upper-respiratory-tract infection in ultramarathon runners. Am J Clin Nutr, 1993, 57, 170-4.

[102] Nieman, DC. Exercise, upper respiratory tract infection, and the immune system. Med Sci Sports Exerc, 1994, 26, 128-39.

[103] Pedersen, BK; Nieman, DC. Exercise immunology: integration and regulation. Immunol Today, 1998, 19, 204-6.

[104] Febbraio, MA; Pedersen, BK. Muscle-derived interleukin-6: mechanisms for activation and possible biological roles. Faseb J, 2002, 16, 1335-47.

[105] Ostrowski, K; Rohde, T; Asp, S; Schjerling, P; Pedersen, BK. Pro- and anti-inflammatory cytokine balance in strenuous exercise in humans. J Physiol, 1999, 515 (Pt 1), 287-91.

[106] Pedersen, BK; Steensberg, A; Schjerling, P. Muscle-derived interleukin-6: possible biological effects. J Physiol, 2001, 536, 329-37.

[107] Ostrowski, K; Schjerling, P; Pedersen, BK. Physical activity and plasma interleukin-6 in humans--effect of intensity of exercise. Eur J Appl Physiol, 2000, 83, 512-5.

[108] Pedersen, BK; Steensberg, A; Schjerling, P. Exercise and interleukin-6. Curr Opin Hematol, 2001, 8, 137-41.

[109] Pedersen, BK. IL-6 signalling in exercise and disease. Biochem Soc Trans, 2007, 35, 1295-7.

[110] Ostrowski, K; Rohde, T; Asp, S; Schjerling, P; Pedersen, BK. Chemokines are elevated in plasma after strenuous exercise in humans. Eur J Appl Physiol, 2001, 84, 244-5.

[111] Nieman, DC; Davis, JM; Henson, DA; Walberg-Rankin, J; Shute, M; Dumke, CL; Utter, AC; Vinci, DM; Carson, JA; Brown, A; Lee, WJ; McAnulty, SR; McAnulty, LS. Carbohydrate ingestion influences skeletal muscle cytokine mRNA and plasma cytokine levels after a 3-h run. J Appl Physiol, 2003, 94, 1917-25.

[112] Chan, MH; Carey, AL; Watt, MJ; Febbraio, MA. Cytokine gene expression in human skeletal muscle during concentric contraction: evidence that IL-8, like IL-6, is influenced by glycogen availability. Am J Physiol Regul Integr Comp Physiol, 2004, 287, R322-7.

[113] Henson, DA; Nieman, DC; Nehlsen-Cannarella, SL; Fagoaga, OR; Shannon, M; Bolton, MR; Davis, JM; Gaffney, CT; Kelln, WJ; Austin, MD; Hjertman, JM; Schilling, BK. Influence of carbohydrate on cytokine and phagocytic responses to 2 h of rowing. Med Sci Sports Exerc, 2000, 32, 1384-9.

[114] Akerstrom, T; Steensberg, A; Keller, P; Keller, C; Penkowa, M; Pedersen, BK. Exercise induces interleukin-8 expression in human skeletal muscle. J Physiol, 2005, 563, 507-16.

[115] De Rossi, M; Bernasconi, P; Baggi, F; de Waal Malefyt, R; Mantegazza, R. Cytokines and chemokines are both expressed by human myoblasts: possible relevance for the immune pathogenesis of muscle inflammation. Int Immunol, 2000, 12, 1329-35.
[116] Baggiolini, M. Chemokines in pathology and medicine. J Intern Med, 2001, 250, 91-104.
[117] Nielsen, AR; Mounier, R; Plomgaard, P; Mortensen, OH; Penkowa, M; Speerschneider, T; Pilegaard, H; Pedersen, BK. Expression of interleukin-15 in human skeletal muscle effect of exercise and muscle fibre type composition. J Physiol, 2007, 584, 305-12.
[118] Riechman, SE; Balasekaran, G; Roth, SM; Ferrell, RE. Association of interleukin-15 protein and interleukin-15 receptor genetic variation with resistance exercise training responses. J Appl Physiol, 2004, 97, 2214-9.
[119] Nieman, DC; Davis, JM; Brown, VA; Henson, DA; Dumke, CL; Utter, AC; Vinci, DM; Downs, MF; Smith, JC; Carson, J; Brown, A; McAnulty, SR; McAnulty, LS. Influence of carbohydrate ingestion on immune changes after 2 h of intensive resistance training. J Appl Physiol, 2004, 96, 1292-8.
[120] Grabstein, KH; Eisenman, J; Shanebeck, K; Rauch, C; Srinivasan, S; Fung, V; Beers, C; Richardson, J; Schoenborn, MA; Ahdieh, M; et al. Cloning of a T cell growth factor that interacts with the beta chain of the interleukin-2 receptor. Science, 1994, 264, 965-8.
[121] Argiles, JM; Lopez-Soriano, J; Almendro, V; Busquets, S; Lopez-Soriano, FJ. Cross-talk between skeletal muscle and adipose tissue: a link with obesity? Med Res Rev, 2005, 25, 49-65.
[122] Weight, LM; Alexander, D; Jacobs, P. Strenuous exercise: analogous to the acute-phase response? Clin Sci (Lond), 1991, 81, 677-83.
[123] Das, UN. Anti-inflammatory nature of exercise. Nutrition, 2004, 20, 323-6.
[124] Niess, AM; Passek, F; Lorenz, I; Schneider, EM; Dickhuth, HH; Northoff, H; Fehrenbach, E. Expression of the antioxidant stress protein heme oxygenase-1 (HO-1) in human leukocytes. Free Radic Biol Med, 1999, 26, 184-92.
[125] Thompson, D; Basu-Modak, S; Gordon, M; Poore, S; Markovitch, D; Tyrrell, RM. Exercise-induced expression of heme oxygenase-1 in human lymphocytes. Free Radic Res, 2005, 39, 63-9.
[126] Pedersen, M; Steensberg, A; Keller, C; Osada, T; Zacho, M; Saltin, B; Febbraio, MA; Pedersen, BK. Does the aging skeletal muscle maintain its endocrine function? Exerc Immunol Rev, 2004, 10, 42-55.
[127] Fischer, CP; Hiscock, NJ; Penkowa, M; Basu, S; Vessby, B; Kallner, A; Sjoberg, LB; Pedersen, BK. Supplementation with vitamins C and E inhibits the release of interleukin-6 from contracting human skeletal muscle. J Physiol, 2004, 558, 633-45.
[128] Ostrowski, K; Rohde, T; Zacho, M; Asp, S; Pedersen, BK. Evidence that interleukin-6 is produced in human skeletal muscle during prolonged running. J Physiol, 1998, 508 (Pt 3), 949-53.
[129] Steensberg, A; Febbraio, MA; Osada, T; Schjerling, P; van Hall, G; Saltin, B; Pedersen, BK. Interleukin-6 production in contracting human skeletal muscle is influenced by pre-exercise muscle glycogen content. J Physiol, 2001, 537, 633-9.
[130] Steensberg, A; Keller, C; Starkie, RL; Osada, T; Febbraio, MA; Pedersen, BK. IL-6 and TNF-alpha expression in, and release from, contracting human skeletal muscle. Am J Physiol Endocrinol Metab, 2002, 283, E1272-8.

[131] Febbraio, MA; Steensberg, A; Keller, C; Starkie, RL; Nielsen, HB; Krustrup, P; Ott, P; Secher, NH; Pedersen, BK. Glucose ingestion attenuates interleukin-6 release from contracting skeletal muscle in humans. J Physiol, 2003, 549, 607-12.

[132] Pedersen, BK; Akerstrom, TC; Nielsen, AR; Fischer, CP. Role of myokines in exercise and metabolism. J Appl Physiol, 2007, 103, 1093-8.

[133] Keller, C; Steensberg, A; Pilegaard, H; Osada, T; Saltin, B; Pedersen, BK; Neufer, PD. Transcriptional activation of the IL-6 gene in human contracting skeletal muscle: influence of muscle glycogen content. Faseb J, 2001, 15, 2748-50.

[134] Hiscock, N; Chan, MH; Bisucci, T; Darby, IA; Febbraio, MA. Skeletal myocytes are a source of interleukin-6 mRNA expression and protein release during contraction: evidence of fiber type specificity. Faseb J, 2004, 18, 992-4.

[135] Steensberg, A; Keller, C; Hillig, T; Frosig, C; Wojtaszewski, JF; Pedersen, BK; Pilegaard, H; Sander, M. Nitric oxide production is a proximal signaling event controlling exercise-induced mRNA expression in human skeletal muscle. Faseb J, 2007, 21, 2683-94.

[136] Keller, C; Hellsten, Y; Steensberg, A; Pedersen, BK. Differential regulation of IL-6 and TNF-alpha via calcineurin in human skeletal muscle cells. Cytokine, 2006, 36, 141-7.

[137] Chan, MH; McGee, SL; Watt, MJ; Hargreaves, M; Febbraio, MA. Altering dietary nutrient intake that reduces glycogen content leads to phosphorylation of nuclear p38 MAP kinase in human skeletal muscle: association with IL-6 gene transcription during contraction. Faseb J, 2004, 18, 1785-7.

[138] Pedersen, BK. The anti-inflammatory effect of exercise: its role in diabetes and cardiovascular disease control. Essays Biochem, 2006, 42, 105-17.

[139] Steensberg, A; Fischer, CP; Keller, C; Moller, K; Pedersen, BK. IL-6 enhances plasma IL-1ra, IL-10, and cortisol in humans. Am J Physiol Endocrinol Metab, 2003, 285, E433-7.

[140] Schindler, R; Mancilla, J; Endres, S; Ghorbani, R; Clark, SC; Dinarello, CA. Correlations and interactions in the production of interleukin-6 (IL-6), IL-1, and tumor necrosis factor (TNF) in human blood mononuclear cells: IL-6 suppresses IL-1 and TNF. Blood, 1990, 75, 40-7.

[141] Starkie, R; Ostrowski, SR; Jauffred, S; Febbraio, M; Pedersen, BK. Exercise and IL-6 infusion inhibit endotoxin-induced TNF-alpha production in humans. Faseb J, 2003, 17, 884-6.

[142] Fiers, W. Tumor necrosis factor. Characterization at the molecular, cellular and in vivo level. FEBS Lett, 1991, 285, 199-212.

[143] Matthys, P; Mitera, T; Heremans, H; Van Damme, J; Billiau, A. Anti-gamma interferon and anti-interleukin-6 antibodies affect staphylococcal enterotoxin B-induced weight loss, hypoglycemia, and cytokine release in D-galactosamine-sensitized and unsensitized mice. Infect Immun, 1995, 63, 1158-64.

[144] Mizuhara, H; O'Neill, E; Seki, N; Ogawa, T; Kusunoki, C; Otsuka, K; Satoh, S; Niwa, M; Senoh, H; Fujiwara, H. T cell activation-associated hepatic injury: mediation by tumor necrosis factors and protection by interleukin 6. J Exp Med, 1994, 179, 1529-37.

[145] Pretolani, M. Interleukin-10: an anti-inflammatory cytokine with therapeutic potential. Clin Exp Allergy, 1999, 29, 1164–1171.

[146] Pue, C; Mortensen, R; Marsh, C; Pope, H; Wewers, M. Acute phase levels of C-reactive protein enhance IL-1 beta and IL-1ra production by human blood monocytes

but inhibit IL-1 beta and IL-1ra production by alveolar macrophages. J Immunol, 1996, 156, 1594–1600.
[147] Keller, C; Keller, P; Giralt, M; Hidalgo, J; Pedersen, BK. Exercise normalises overexpression of TNF-alpha in knockout mice. Biochem Biophys Res Commun, 2004, 321, 179-82.
[148] van der Poll, T; Coyle, SM; Barbosa, K; Braxton, CC; Lowry, SF. Epinephrine inhibits tumor necrosis factor-alpha and potentiates interleukin 10 production during human endotoxemia. J Clin Invest, 1996, 97, 713-9.
[149] Steensberg, A; Toft, AD; Schjerling, P; Halkjaer-Kristensen, J; Pedersen, BK. Plasma interleukin-6 during strenuous exercise: role of epinephrine. Am J Physiol Cell Physiol, 2001, 281, C1001-4.
[150] Nieman, DC; Henson, DA; Austin, MD; Brown, VA. Immune response to a 30-minute walk. Med Sci Sports Exerc, 2005, 37, 57-62.
[151] Plaisance, EP; Taylor, JK; Alhassan, S; Abebe, A; Mestek, ML; Grandjean, PW. Cardiovascular fitness and vascular inflammatory markers after acute aerobic exercise. Int J Sport Nutr Exerc Metab, 2007, 17, 152-62.
[152] Mills, PJ; Maisel, AS; Ziegler, MG; Dimsdale, JE; Carter, S; Kennedy, B; Woods, VL, Jr. Peripheral blood mononuclear cell-endothelial adhesion in human hypertension following exercise. J Hypertens, 2000, 18, 1801-6.
[153] Peake, JM; Suzuki, K; Hordern, M; Wilson, G; Nosaka, K; Coombes, JS. Plasma cytokine changes in relation to exercise intensity and muscle damage. Eur J Appl Physiol, 2005, 95, 514-21.
[154] Markovitch, D; Tyrrell, RM; Thompson, D. Acute moderate-intensity exercise in middle-aged men has neither an anti- nor proinflammatory effect. J Appl Physiol, 2008, 105, 260-5.
[155] Steinberg, JG; Ba, A; Bregeon, F; Delliaux, S; Jammes, Y. Cytokine and oxidative responses to maximal cycling exercise in sedentary subjects. Med Sci Sports Exerc, 2007, 39, 964-8.
[156] Zaldivar, F; Wang-Rodriguez, J; Nemet, D; Schwindt, C; Galassetti, P; Mills, PJ; Wilson, LD; Cooper, DM. Constitutive pro- and anti-inflammatory cytokine and growth factor response to exercise in leukocytes. J Appl Physiol, 2006, 100, 1124-33.
[157] Li, YP; Reid, MB. Effect of tumor necrosis factor-alpha on skeletal muscle metabolism. Curr Opin Rheumatol, 2001, 13, 483-7.
[158] Plaisance, EP; Grandjean, PW. Physical activity and high-sensitivity C-reactive protein. Sports Med, 2006, 36, 443-58.
[159] Bruunsgaard, H. Physical activity and modulation of systemic low-level inflammation. J Leukoc Biol, 2005, 78, 819-35.
[160] Smith, JK; Dykes, R; Douglas, JE; Krishnaswamy, G; Berk, S. Long-term exercise and atherogenic activity of blood mononuclear cells in persons at risk of developing ischemic heart disease. Jama, 1999, 281, 1722-7.
[161] Sanders, AE; Slade, GD; Fitzsimmons, TR; Bartold, PM. Physical activity, inflammatory biomarkers in gingival crevicular fluid and periodontitis. J Clin Periodontol, 2009, 36, 388-95.
[162] Fallon, KE; Fallon, SK; Boston, T. The acute phase response and exercise: court and field sports. Br J Sports Med, 2001, 35, 170-3.

[163] Mattusch, F; Dufaux, B; Heine, O; Mertens, I; Rost, R. Reduction of the plasma concentration of C-reactive protein following nine months of endurance training. Int J Sports Med, 2000, 21, 21-4.
[164] Abramson, JL; Vaccarino, V. Relationship between physical activity and inflammation among apparently healthy middle-aged and older US adults. Arch Intern Med, 2002, 162, 1286-92.
[165] Geffken, DF; Cushman, M; Burke, GL; Polak, JF; Sakkinen, PA; Tracy, RP. Association between physical activity and markers of inflammation in a healthy elderly population. Am J Epidemiol, 2001, 153, 242-50.
[166] King, DE; Carek, P; Mainous, AG, 3rd; Pearson, WS. Inflammatory markers and exercise: differences related to exercise type. Med Sci Sports Exerc, 2003, 35, 575-81.
[167] Taaffe, DR; Harris, TB; Ferrucci, L; Rowe, J; Seeman, TE. Cross-sectional and prospective relationships of interleukin-6 and C-reactive protein with physical performance in elderly persons: MacArthur studies of successful aging. J Gerontol A Biol Sci Med Sci, 2000, 55, M709-15.
[168] Wannamethee, SG; Lowe, GD; Whincup, PH; Rumley, A; Walker, M; Lennon, L. Physical activity and hemostatic and inflammatory variables in elderly men. Circulation, 2002, 105, 1785-90.
[169] Bruunsgaard, H; Ladelund, S; Pedersen, AN; Schroll, M; Jorgensen, T; Pedersen, BK. Predicting death from tumour necrosis factor-alpha and interleukin-6 in 80-year-old people. Clin Exp Immunol, 2003, 132, 24-31.
[170] Tisi, PV; Hulse, M; Chulakadabba, A; Gosling, P; Shearman, CP. Exercise training for intermittent claudication: does it adversely affect biochemical markers of the exercise-induced inflammatory response? Eur J Vasc Endovasc Surg, 1997, 14, 344-50.
[171] Stewart, LK; Flynn, MG; Campbell, WW; Craig, BA; Robinson, JP; Timmerman, KL; McFarlin, BK; Coen, PM; Talbert, E. The influence of exercise training on inflammatory cytokines and C-reactive protein. Med Sci Sports Exerc, 2007, 39, 1714-9.
[172] Goldhammer, E; Tanchilevitch, A; Maor, I; Beniamini, Y; Rosenschein, U; Sagiv, M. Exercise training modulates cytokines activity in coronary heart disease patients. Int J Cardiol, 2005, 100, 93-9.
[173] Kelley, GA; Kelley, KS. Effects of aerobic exercise on C-reactive protein, body composition, and maximum oxygen consumption in adults: a meta-analysis of randomized controlled trials. Metabolism, 2006, 55, 1500-7.
[174] Kohut, ML; McCann, DA; Russell, DW; Konopka, DN; Cunnick, JE; Franke, WD; Castillo, MC; Reighard, AE; Vanderah, E. Aerobic exercise, but not flexibility/resistance exercise, reduces serum IL-18, CRP, and IL-6 independent of beta-blockers, BMI, and psychosocial factors in older adults. Brain Behav Immun, 2006, 20, 201-9.
[175] Ford, ES. Does exercise reduce inflammation? Physical activity and C-reactive protein among U.S. adults. Epidemiology, 2002, 13, 561-8.
[176] Fischer, CP; Berntsen, A; Perstrup, LB; Eskildsen, P; Pedersen, BK. Plasma levels of interleukin-6 and C-reactive protein are associated with physical inactivity independent of obesity. Scand J Med Sci Sports, 2007, 17, 580-7.

[177] Mora, S; Lee, IM; Buring, JE; Ridker, PM. Association of physical activity and body mass index with novel and traditional cardiovascular biomarkers in women. Jama, 2006, 295, 1412-9.

[178] Kasapis, C; Thompson, PD. The effects of physical activity on serum C-reactive protein and inflammatory markers: a systematic review. J Am Coll Cardiol, 2005, 45, 1563-9.

[179] Verdaet, D; Dendale, P; De Bacquer, D; Delanghe, J; Block, P; De Backer, G. Association between leisure time physical activity and markers of chronic inflammation related to coronary heart disease. Atherosclerosis, 2004, 176, 303-10.

[180] Rawson, ES; Freedson, PS; Osganian, SK; Matthews, CE; Reed, G; Ockene, IS. Body mass index, but not physical activity, is associated with C-reactive protein. Med Sci Sports Exerc, 2003, 35, 1160-6.

[181] Arsenault, BJ; Cartier, A; Cote, M; Lemieux, I; Tremblay, A; Bouchard, C; Perusse, L; Despres, JP. Body composition, cardiorespiratory fitness, and low-grade inflammation in middle-aged men and women. Am J Cardiol, 2009, 104, 240-6.

[182] Selvin, E; Paynter, NP; Erlinger, TP. The effect of weight loss on C-reactive protein: a systematic review. Arch Intern Med, 2007, 167, 31-9.

[183] Hammett, CJ; Prapavessis, H; Baldi, JC; Varo, N; Schoenbeck, U; Ameratunga, R; French, JK; White, HD; Stewart, RA. Effects of exercise training on 5 inflammatory markers associated with cardiovascular risk. Am Heart J, 2006, 151, 367 e7-367 e16.

[184] Kondo, N; Nomura, M; Nakaya, Y; Ito, S; Ohguro, T. Association of inflammatory marker and highly sensitive C-reactive protein with aerobic exercise capacity, maximum oxygen uptake and insulin resistance in healthy middle-aged volunteers. Circ J, 2005, 69, 452-7.

[185] Jankord, R; Jemiolo, B. Influence of physical activity on serum IL-6 and IL-10 levels in healthy older men. Med Sci Sports Exerc, 2004, 36, 960-4.

[186] Colbert, LH; Visser, M; Simonsick, EM; Tracy, RP; Newman, AB; Kritchevsky, SB; Pahor, M; Taaffe, DR; Brach, J; Rubin, S; Harris, TB. Physical activity, exercise, and inflammatory markers in older adults: findings from the Health, Aging and Body Composition Study. J Am Geriatr Soc, 2004, 52, 1098-104.

[187] Rauramaa, R; Halonen, P; Vaisanen, SB; Lakka, TA; Schmidt-Trucksass, A; Berg, A; Penttila, IM; Rankinen, T; Bouchard, C. Effects of aerobic physical exercise on inflammation and atherosclerosis in men: the DNASCO Study: a six-year randomized, controlled trial. Ann Intern Med, 2004, 140, 1007-14.

[188] Dufaux, B; Order, U; Geyer, H; Hollmann, W. C-reactive protein serum concentrations in well-trained athletes. Int J Sports Med, 1984, 5, 102-6.

[189] Sloan, RP; Shapiro, PA; Demeersman, RE; McKinley, PS; Tracey, KJ; Slavov, I; Fang, Y; Flood, PD. Aerobic exercise attenuates inducible TNF production in humans. J Appl Physiol, 2007, 103, 1007-11.

[190] Albert, MA; Glynn, RJ; Ridker, PM. Effect of physical activity on serum C-reactive protein. Am J Cardiol, 2004, 93, 221-5.

[191] Isasi, CR; Deckelbaum, RJ; Tracy, RP; Starc, TJ; Berglund, L; Shea, S. Physical fitness and C-reactive protein level in children and young adults: the Columbia University BioMarkers Study. Pediatrics, 2003, 111, 332-8.

[192] Hardman, AE. The influence of exercise on postprandial triacylglycerol metabolism. Atherosclerosis, 1998, 141 Suppl 1, S93-100.

[193] LaMonte, MJ; Durstine, JL; Yanowitz, FG; Lim, T; DuBose, KD; Davis, P; Ainsworth, BE. Cardiorespiratory fitness and C-reactive protein among a tri-ethnic sample of women. Circulation, 2002, 106, 403-6.
[194] Pitsavos, C; Panagiotakos, DB; Chrysohoou, C; Kavouras, S; Stefanadis, C. The associations between physical activity, inflammation, and coagulation markers, in people with metabolic syndrome: the ATTICA study. Eur J Cardiovasc Prev Rehabil, 2005, 12, 151-8.
[195] Okita, K; Nishijima, H; Murakami, T; Nagai, T; Morita, N; Yonezawa, K; Iizuka, K; Kawaguchi, H; Kitabatake, A. Can exercise training with weight loss lower serum C-reactive protein levels? Arterioscler Thromb Vasc Biol, 2004, 24, 1868-73.
[196] Nicklas, BJ; Ambrosius, W; Messier, SP; Miller, GD; Penninx, BW; Loeser, RF; Palla, S; Bleecker, E; Pahor, M. Diet-induced weight loss, exercise, and chronic inflammation in older, obese adults: a randomized controlled clinical trial. Am J Clin Nutr, 2004, 79, 544-51.
[197] Shojaee-Moradie, F; Baynes, KC; Pentecost, C; Bell, JD; Thomas, EL; Jackson, NC; Stolinski, M; Whyte, M; Lovell, D; Bowes, SB; Gibney, J; Jones, RH; Umpleby, AM. Exercise training reduces fatty acid availability and improves the insulin sensitivity of glucose metabolism. Diabetologia, 2007, 50, 404-13.

In: Encyclopedia of Sports and Athletics
Editors: Jack L. Murray and Emily O. Watson

ISBN: 978-1-61209-959-0

Chapter III

Brain in Movement: The Role of Physical Exercise in Parkinson's Disease

Aderbal S. Aguiar Jr. [*] ***and Rui D. S. Prediger***
Laboratório Experimental de Doenças Neurodegenerativas, Departamento de Farmacologia, Universidade Federal de Santa Catarina (UFSC), Florianópolis-SC, Brazil

Abstract

Parkinson's disease is the second most common neurodegenerative disorder, following Alzheimer's disease, affecting approximately 1% of the population older than 50 years. Since the incidence of the disease increases with age (the most important risk factor), it is likely that the number of people suffering from Parkinson's disease will rise as improved health care lengthens the average life span. Classically, Parkinson's disease is considered to be a motor system disease and its diagnosis is based on the presence of a set of cardinal motor signs (e.g. rigidity, bradykinesia, rest tremor and postural reflex disturbance). These symptoms of Parkinson's disease mainly result from the progressive degeneration of dopamine neurons of the *substantia nigra pars compacta* (SNpc) that project predominantly to the striatum. Nowadays there is considerable evidence showing that deficits in olfactory and cognitive functions precede the classical motor symptoms seen in Parkinson's disease. The beneficial effects of the drugs currently available for the treatment of Parkinson's disease (such as levodopa) on improving the cognitive function affected in this disease is controversial. Thus, the management of non-motor symptoms of Parkinson's disease remains a challenge. Over the last decade, regular physical exercise has been implicated to an increased plasticity in the adult brain (such as increase in neurogenesis and cognitive processes and neurotrophic factors production). Research is now emerging on a possible influence of physical exercise in the neurodegenerative process associated to Parkinson's disease. The present chapter attempts to review results reported in different clinical studies and animal models to provide a comprehensive

[*] Corresponding autor: Laboratório Experimental de Doenças Neurodegenerativas, Departamento de Farmacologia, Universidade Federal de Santa Catarina, Campus Trindade, 88049-900, Florianópolis, SC, Brazil., Phone (55) 48 3721 9491 – Fax (55) 48 3337 5479., E-mail address: aderbalaguiar@gmail.com

picture of the role of physical exercise in Parkinson's disease. Although many of the training programs investigated were accompanied by some degree of oxidative stress, which should be taken into account in physical training programs for this population, it is important to emphasize that this response did not promote any negative impact on the rehabilitation aspects of Parkinson's disease patients. Taken together, the current literature suggests that regular physical exercise can present beneficial effects in Parkinson's disease patients evaluated through different tests. It might also afford protection against dopaminergic neurons death and motor dysfunction elicited in experimental models. Finally, this chapter shows recent findings from our laboratory indicating that moderate physical exercise plays an important role into improvement cognitive deficits in an experimental model of Parkinson's disease, reinforcing the potential of physical exercise in the management of non-motor symptoms of Parkinson's disease.

Introduction

At the beginning of the nineteenth century, when James Parkinson published the book entitled "Essay on the Shaking Palsy", life expectation was no longer than 45 years old. The "shaking palsy", later named Parkinson's disease by Charcot, affects mainly aged people. Nowadays, 0.3 % of the whole population and 1% of the population over 60 years old have Parkinson's disease. This percentage increases with age. Besides, now in the beginning of the XXI century, life expectancy is near 80 years old. Therefore, there are much more parkinsonian patients nowadays than two centuries ago and with the increasing age of the general population, the prevalence of Parkinson's disease will rise steadily in the future.

At least, a century ago one could say that the Parkinson's disease caused only motor disabilities such as bradykinesia/hypokinesia, muscular rigidity and resting tremor, but preserved sensorial and cognitive functions. Unfortunately, more recent studies have shown that is not the truth, since olfactory dysfunction and cognitive impairments are often present during the earlier stages of Parkinson's disease even before the development of its classical symptoms. The non-motor symptoms that include memory deficits can be more important than the motor deficits to determine the patients' quality of life and represent an important factor to determine the need for nursing home care. The beneficial effects of the drugs currently available for the treatment of Parkinson's disease (such as levodopa, L-DOPA) on improving the olfactory and cognitive function affected in Parkinson's disease is controversial. Thus, the management of non-motor symptoms of Parkinson's disease remains a challenge.

Over the last decade, several lines of evidence have suggested that preventive strategies such as a physically active lifestyle may help to delay the onset of cognitive decline and reduce the risk for age-related neurological diseases. Regular exercise attenuated the age-associated decline in memory and reduced the accumulation of proteins affected by oxidative damage in the brain. Moreover, regular physical exercise has been implicated to an increased number of new neurons, brain plasticity and the production of neurotrophic factors. Of high importance, physical exercise has been identified with one therapeutic alternative to minimize motor and non-motor symptoms of Parkinson's disease and it might also afford protection against dopaminergic neurons death and motor dysfunction elicited in rodent models of Parkinson's disease. The present chapter attempts to review results reported in different clinical studies and animal models to provide a comprehensive picture of the role of physical exercise in Parkinson's disease.

Parkinson's Disease – New Insights for an old Disease

More than 180 years ago, James Parkinson first described the disorder that bears his name, in "An Essay on the Shaking Palsy"(1) and 30 years ago L-DOPA, still the most effective therapy in the management of Parkinson's disease symptoms, was introduced. Parkinson's disease is a neurodegenerative disorder of unknown cause that affects over 1 million people in North America. The prevalence of Parkinson's disease in industrialized countries is generally estimated at 0.3% of the entire population and about 1% in people over 60 years of age (2), and with the increasing age of the general population, the prevalence of Parkinson's disease will rise steadily in the future (2-4). Annual disease incidence ranges from 110 to 330 per 100,000 individuals over age 50 and it incidence increases with increasing age throughout the life span (4, 5). After age 80 years, the incidence rate increases to 400 to 500 individuals per 100,000 annually (4).

The primary, idiopathic or sporadic is the most common variant of Parkinson's disease (86%), followed by drug-induced parkinsonism (7%) (6). Parkinson's disease is characterized clinically by bradykinesia, rest tremor, muscle rigidity, and postural reflex impairment (7, 8), as well as a host of other motor and non-motor signs (9-11). Increasing age is the only unequivocal risk factor for Parkinson's disease (5) and the average age-at-onset of motor symptoms is 60 years, with a slowly progressive course.

A minimum criterion for the diagnosis generally requires identification of some combination of the cardinal motor signs of bradykinesia, rigidity, tremor, and postural instability (4, 12-14). Probable Parkinson's disease has been defined as the presence of at least two of the key signs, at least one of which must be either resting tremor or bradykinesia: resting tremor, cogwheel rigidity, bradykinesia, postural reflex impairment (14, 15). No other cause of parkinsonism should be present, and other signs such as dementia or autonomic dysfunction should be absent. A history of a beneficial response to L-DOPA also increases the assurance of the diagnosis (14, 15). Possible Parkinson's disease is reserved for persons who meet many of the same criteria described above but in the absence of either bradykinesia or resting tremor. The response to L-DOPA may also be unknown and other clinical symptoms or signs may be present. A reliable and easily applicable diagnostic test or marker for Parkinson's disease is not yet available. Thus, the diagnosis is clinical. Currently, only about 75% of clinical diagnoses of Parkinson's disease are confirmed at autopsy (12, 14, 16), largely because the cardinal signs can also occur in conditions other than Parkinson's disease; they are then termed "extrapyramidal signs," "parkinsonian features" or "parkinsonism".

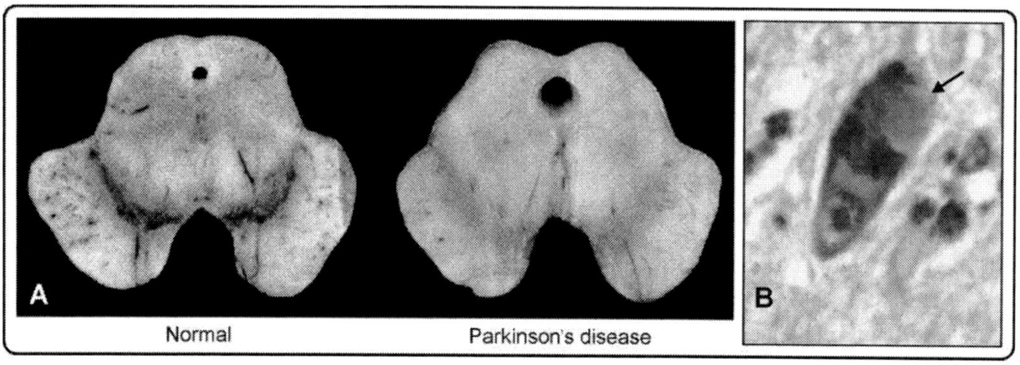

Figure 1. The loss of the neuromelanin-pigmented neurons of the SNpc in the midbrain (A), and the occurrence of intracellular proteinaceous inclusions known as Lewy bodies, revealed here by a hematoxinin-eosin staining (B), are the main hallmarks of Parkinson's disease.

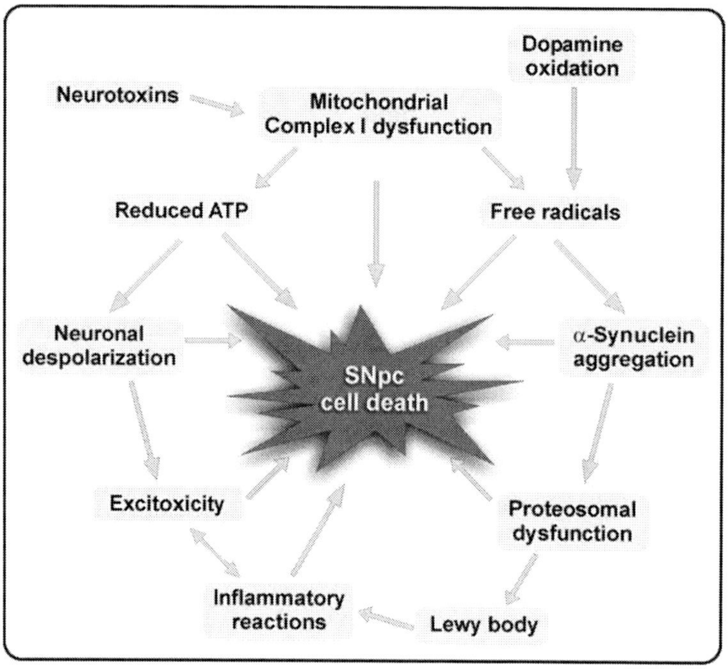

Figure 2. Multifactorial causes for *substantia nigra pars compacta* (SNpc) neurodegeneration in Parkinson's disease.

The pathological hallmarks of Parkinson's disease are the neurodegeneration of specific subnuclei of the *substantia nigra pars compacta* (SNpc), with severe obliteration of their neuromelanin-laden projection neurons – frequently is considered to be the most important hallmark of Parkinson's disease – and the presence specific α-synuclein-immunoreactive inclusion bodies, which develop as spindle- or thread-like Lewy neurites in cellular processes, and in the form of globular Lewy bodies in neuronal perikarya (17-19) (see Figure 1). A major component Lewy neurites and Lewy bodies is an aggregated form of the normally presynaptic protein α-synuclein (17-19).

However, it is important to emphasize that the neurodegenerative processes that lead to sporadic Parkinson's disease begin many years before the appearance of the characteristic motor symptoms. It seems that the pathological process start with the formation of Lewy bodies and Lewy neurites in the anterior olfactory structures as well as in regions of the medulla oblongata and pontine tegmentum, including the noradrenergic neurons of the *locus coeruleus* and the serotonergic neurons of the caudal raphe nuclei (stages 1-2). Later, the cholinergic nucleus basalis of Meynert also becomes affected (stage 3). By the time somatomotor disabilities are evident (stage 4 and beyond), there is considerable loss of dopaminergic neurons in the SNpc. Cortical Lewy bodies and Lewy neurites occur initially in the temporal mesocortex (stage 4) and, thereafter, in the neocortex (stages 5-6) (18).

Although dopaminergic neuron loss is characteristic for Parkinson's disease, the neurodegeneration extends well beyond dopaminergic neurons. Neurodegeneration and Lewy bodies formation are found in noradrenergic (locus coeruleus), serotonergic (raphe nuclei), and cholinergic (nucleus basalis of Meynert, dorsal motor nucleus of vagus) systems, and in the cerebral cortex (especially the cingulate and entorhinal cortices), olfactory bulb, and autonomic nervous system (17-19). The degeneration of hippocampal structures and cholinergic cortical inputs most likely explains the high rate of dementia that accompanies Parkinson's disease, particularly in older patients (17-19). However, the lesions in cholinergic, serotonergic, and noradrenergic pathways are not as clearly characterized as those in the dopaminergic systems (17-19). Whereas involvement of these neurochemical systems is generally thought to occur in more severe or late-stage disease, the temporal relationship of damage to specific neurochemical systems is not well established (17-19).

In addition to the characteristic motor symptoms, Parkinson's disease can also cause a host of other motor and non-motor signs, such as early olfactory dysfunction, depression, personality changes, dementia, sleep disturbance, speech impairment, and sexual dysfunction. Within a few years after the onset of disease, all of these manifestations may be present. Subtle cognitive impairments are often present even during the earlier phases of Parkinson's disease. Such impairments include a dysexecutive syndrome that involves attentional and working memory deficits accompanied by secondary deficits in the internal representation of visuospatial stimuli (9, 20). Skill and habit learning is also impaired in these patients (21). In about 20-40% of patients, these problems may eventually proceed to dementia, which constitutes an important risk factor for caregiver distress, decreased quality of life, and nursing home placement (22). Although there are reports of declarative (or episodic) memory impairments in Parkinson's disease, they are less severe in comparison to other neurodegenerative disorders such as Alzheimer's disease (23). In humans, the beneficial effects of the drugs currently available for the treatment of Parkinson's disease (such as L-DOPA) on improving the cognitive function affected in Parkinson's disease is controversial. While some studies indicate an improvement of cognitive functions in PD patients treated with Parkinson's disease (24, 25), others have shown that this treatment may cause no or only mild improvement (26-28), or may even aggravate Parkinson's disease cognitive impairments (29, 30).

Moreover, approximately 90% of Parkinson's disease patients at early-stage exhibit olfactory dysfunction unrelated to the use of medications (e.g., L-DOPA, DA agonists, anticholinergic compounds) (31, 32) and the olfactory bulb is among the first brain structures to exhibit Parkinson's disease-related pathology (18). Although olfactory disturbances, i.e., odor detection, discrimination and identification, are not specific for Parkinson's disease and sense of smell can be affected by different disorders or habits, such as rhinitis, smoking or toxic agents, it has been shown that olfactory testing may discriminate Parkinson's disease patients from healthy controls with a sensitivity of 88% and a specificity of 83% (33). Consequently, olfactory dysfunction might be an early indicator of Parkinson's disease and the development of specific olfactory testing may represent an important tool in the clinical diagnosis of early stages of this disease (18, 32, 34).

Etiopathogenesis of Parkinson's Disease

As stated in the previous section, Lewy bodies are intracitoplasmatic incrustations composed mainly by the proteins α-synuclein and ubiquitin. Many studies suggest that the death of dopamine cells in Parkinson's disease is linked to protein aggregation and dysfunction of the ubiquitin proteasome pathway. An altered form of the α-synuclein gene has been found in a case of family inherited Parkinson's disease with early onset. However, this abnormal gene was not found in most cases of the so called idiopathic Parkinson's disease that affects aged people. In these cases, no apparent genetic pattern of inheritance was found. Since the polymerization of this protein, as well as many neurotoxins that cause parkinsonism, produce free radical species, they are often pointed as the trigger of the neurodegenerative process that leads to the disease. The inhibition of the mitochondrial complex I, oxidative stress, and inflammation have also been pointed as important steps leading to neurodegeneration in Parkinson's disease (see Figure 2). Indeed, the midbrain dopamine cells are among the most vulnerable cells to degenerative processes in the brain. However, the primary event that starts the neurodegeneration cascade and how to stop the disease progression are not precisely known.

A genetic hypothesis for Parkinson's disease

At least 10 distinct loci are responsible for rare Mendelian forms of Parkinson's disease: PARK1 to PARK10, including Parkinson's disease-associated genes to synapse (35) and mitochondria (36-39). As the name already implies α-synuclein (α-SYN, SNCA, PARK1) was initially identified as a synaptic and nuclear protein (40). Despite intensive studies the exact role of α-synuclein at the synapse remains elusive. There is evidence that the protein plays a role in maintenance of synaptic vesicle pools (41) and activity-dependent dopamine release (42). A role for α-synuclein in Parkinson's disease was fueled by the discovery of missense mutations in the α-synuclein gene as a cause of autosomal dominantly inherited Parkinson's disease (35). An Ala53→Thr (A53T) mutation resulting from a G to A transition at position 209 was identified in large Italian-American Greek kindred, and an Ala30→Pro (A30P) mutation resulting from a G to C transition at position 88 was identified in small German kindred (35, 43). A genomic triplication of wild-type α-synuclein leading to over expression of wild-type α-synuclein is the disease-causing mutation in familial Parkinson's disease in the Iowan kindred and the PARK4 locus (35, 44). Genetic variability in the α-synuclein gene is also a risk factor for the development of Parkinson's disease (45-48). Even though mutations in α-synuclein are a very rare cause of hereditary Parkinson's disease, its apparent role as the major structural feature of the LB has placed α-synuclein at center stage in the pathophysiology of Parkinson's disease (49-53). The mutated α-synuclein is rare, but it is thought to be prone to fibrillogenesis and aggregation, which, in turn, may cause neuronal injury and synaptic loss and is a major characteristic of the disease (49-53). Alternatively, mutated α-synuclein may disrupt vesicular dopamine storage leading to its accumulation in the cytoplasm, which could promote oxidative stress as it undergoes metabolism in the nigral neurons (54, 55).

The Parkin gene mutation was first identified in a Japanese family with autosomal recessive, levodopa-responsive disease characterized by degeneration in the SNpc and the absence of Lewy bodies (56-58). A number of families from diverse backgrounds have been observed with Parkin mutations (59, 60). Over 20 different mutations have been identified, and these mutations are now considered to be the most common cause of familial Parkinson's disease (46-50). The average age-at-onset of symptoms is between 35 and 40 years but has ranged from 7 to 58 years (46-50). Most mutations described in Parkin have been deletions or missense mutations, but nonsense and deletions have also been observed and each affects protein degradation (61, 62). Parkin and ubiquitin carboxy-terminal hydrolase L1 (UCHL1) PD-related genes are related to the ubiquitin-proteasome system (UPS) (63). Parkin functions as an ubiquitin-protein ligase, E3, and acts along with ubiquitin-conjugating enzymes (63). Familial Parkinson's disease-associated mutations in Parkin result in loss of function through defects in E3 ligase activity, solubility, or substrate binding (63). UCH-L1 is a 230-amino acid and 26-kDa protein, a highly abundant, neuron-specific protein that belongs to a family of deubiquitinating enzymes, which are responsible for hydrolyzing polymeric ubiquitin chains to free ubiquitin monomers (63). Moreover, synphilin-1, a protein that interacts with α-synuclein, also interacts with Parkin. Mutations in one allele of Parkin have also been observed in patients with Parkinson's disease, which suggests a dominant pattern of inheritance or haploinsufficiency (61, 62, 64).

Mutations in the DJ-1 gene, located on chromosome 1p36, were recently identified in families with autosomal recessive early-onset Parkinsonism (37, 38). The normal function of DJ-1 and its role in dopamine cell degeneration is unknown, but there is evidence-linking DJ-1 to oxidative stress response and mitochondrial function (36, 39).

Environmental Neurotoxins

Although the specific etiology of Parkinson's disease remains unknown, recent epidemiological studies indicate that exposure to environmental agents, including well water, a number of industrial and agricultural chemicals, pesticides, and/or herbicides may contribute to the pathogenesis of such disorder (65-70). A number of exogenous toxins have been associated with the development of parkinsonism, including trace metals, cyanide, lacquer thinner, organic solvents, carbon monoxide, and carbon disulfide (71). However, no specific toxin has been found in the brain of Parkinson's disease patients, and in many instances the parkinsonism seen in association with toxins is not that of typical Lewy body of Parkinson's disease. The most compelling evidence for an environmental factor in Parkinson's disease relates to the toxin 1-methyl-4-phenyl-1,2,3,6-tetrahydropyridine (MPTP). In 1982, young heroin users developed a rapidly progressive parkinsonian syndrome traced to intravenous use of a street preparation of 1-methyl-4-phenyl-4-propionoxypiperidine (MPPP), an analog of the narcotic meperidine (Demerol) (72). MPTP was the responsible neurotoxic contaminant, inadvertently produced during the illicit synthesis of MPPP in a basement laboratory. In humans and monkeys, MPTP produces an irreversible and severe parkinsonian syndrome characterized by all of the features of Parkinson's disease, including tremor, rigidity, slowness movement, postural instability, and freezing (73-77). In MPTP-intoxicated humans and nonhuman primates, the beneficial response to L-DOPA and development of long-term motor complications to medical therapy are virtually identical to that seen in Parkinson's disease patients (78-81). Also similar to Parkinson's disease, the susceptibility to MPTP increases with age in both primates and rodents (82-87).

Burning Neurons

Oxidative stress is a deleterious condition that results from insufficient scavenging of reactive oxygen species (ROS), which are generated by a myriad of biochemical reactions. Normally, these species are eliminated by intracellular antioxidant systems, which might be impaired as a result of the ageing process or in disease states. Studies in human post-mortem material indicate that ROS are important in the pathogenesis of sporadic Parkinson's disease (88-90). A selective 30–40% decrease in complex I activity of the mitochondrial respiratory chain has been found in the SNpc of Parkinson's disease patients (91-93). The cause of the decreased complex I activity in Parkinson's disease remains a mystery. No specific abnormality has been detected in the subunits of complex I or in the mitochondrial or nuclear genes that encode complex I proteins. In a recent study, a complex I defect was found in cybrids carrying mtDNA derived from Parkinson's disease platelets (94). This indicates the presence of a defect in the mitochondrial genome that can be transferred through multiple passages. Such a defect could be due to an inherited mutation or to a toxic insult, possibly secondary to oxidant stress, although disease-related mtDNA mutations have not been detected in Parkinson's disease and oxidative stress typically affects both complexes IV and I. A mitochondrial complex I defect could contribute to cell degeneration in Parkinson's disease through decreased ATP synthesis and a bioenergetic defect.

Moreover, dopamine has a great potential to yield hydrogen peroxide (H_2O_2) and other ROS (71, 82, 89, 95). Oxidant stress and consequent cell death could develop in the SNpc under circumstances in which there is (*a*) increased dopamine turnover, resulting in excess peroxide formation; (*b*) a deficiency in glutathione (GSH), thereby diminishing the brain's capacity to clear H_2O_2; or (*c*) an increase in reactive iron, which can promote hydroxyl radical ($OH^{\cdot}$) formation (71, 82, 89, 95). Indeed, postmortem studies in Parkinson's disease brains demonstrate increased iron, decreased GSH, and oxidative damage to lipids, proteins, and DNA, suggesting that the SNpc is in a state of oxidant stress (71, 82, 95).

Further evidence that oxidative stress participates in the loss of nigral neurons in Parkinson's disease comes from studies using parkinsonism-inducing toxins. The toxin 6-hydroxydopamine (6-OHDA) was introduced more than 30 years ago such as the first pharmacological tool associated with SNpc dopaminergic neuronal death (82, 96), because 6-OHDA is 22 fold more oxidant than dopamine. Although 6-OHDA-induced pathology differs from PD, it is still extensively used as a valid experimental model of Parkinson's disease. 6-OHDA-induced toxicity is relatively selective for monoaminergic neurons, resulting from preferential uptake by DA and noradrenergic transporters (82, 97, 98). Inside neurons, 6-

OHDA accumulates in the cytosol, generating ROS and inactivating biological macromolecules by generating quinones that attack nucleophilic groups (82, 99, 100). Moreover, the active metabolite of MPTP, 1-methyl-4-pyridinium (MPP^+) (101-103), was found to be a mitochondrial poison that inhibits mitochondrial respiration at complex I of the electron transport chain (102, 104). The selectivity of MPP^+ for dopaminergic neurons is due to the fact that it is an excellent substrate for the dopamine transporter, and is thereby accumulated preferentially in cells that transport dopamine. Following recognition of MPTP's toxicity and its mechanism of action, several laboratories reported a selective defect in complex I of the electron transport chain in Parkinson's disease (91-93, 105-110).

Impaired complex I activity leads to free radical stress and makes neurons vulnerable to glutamate excitotoxicity. Excitotoxicity refers to a process of neuronal death caused by excessive or prolonged activation of receptors for the excitatory amino acid neurotransmitter glutamate (111) and is an established cause of neurodegeneration that has been implicated in Parkinson's disease (112-117) based on two possible mechanisms. The first involves "strong" excitotoxicity resulting from increased glutamate formation. SNpc dopaminergic neurons are rich in glutamate receptors, receive extensive glutamate innervation from the cortex and the subthalamic nucleus (STN), and demonstrate a pattern of burst firing in response to exogenously administered glutamate (71, 118). Dopamine lesions desinhibit the STN and increase the firing rate of its excitatory output neurons (119, 120). It can be postulated that as STN fibers project to the SNpc, dopamine lesions promote further excitotoxic damage (71, 121, 122). Indeed, STN lesions protect nigral neurons from 6-OHDA toxicity. A second hypothesis involves the "weak" excitotoxic mechanism (71, 112). This theory suggests that a reduction in energy metabolism due to a defect in mitochondrial function results in a loss of the ATP-dependent Mg-blockade of N-methyl-D-aspartate (NMDA) receptors and allows physiological concentrations of glutamate to mediate a calcium influx into the cell (71). In support of a role of excitotoxicity in Parkinson's disease are reports that NMDA antagonists protect against dopamine cell loss resulting from MPP^+ infusion into the SNpc of rats (123, 124) and MPTP treatment in primates (71, 125-127).

Treatment of Parkinson's Disease

The treatment of Parkinson's disease is very complex due to the progressive nature of the disease and the array of motor and non-motor features combined with early and late side effects associated with therapeutic interventions. While no treatments have yet been shown conclusively to slow the progression of the disease, a growing number of symptomatic pharmacologic therapies are available, as well as several forms of surgery and numerous non-pharmacological approaches.

Among dopaminergic drugs, L-DOPA standard and controlled release formulations are marketed as fixed associations with a dopa-decarboxylase inhibitor carbidopa or benzeraside. There are several dopamine agonists, with different receptor binding, pharmacokinetic profiles, and routes of administration, and two types of indirect dopamine transmission enhancers, monoamine oxidase B (MAO-B) and catechol-O-methyltransferase (COMT) inhibitors. Among non-dopaminergic medications there are several anticholinergics, although amantadine is the only drug widely available for anti-glutamatergic effects. Functional neurosurgery for Parkinson's disease attempts to restore functional balance in basal ganglia relays. There are currently three targets: the ventral intermediate nucleus of the thalamus, the internal segment of the Globus Pallidus, and the subthalamic nucleus. Either CNS lesions (thalamotomy, pallidotomy, or subthalamic nucleus lesions) or implants of chronic stimulating electrodes at these sites (deep brain stimulation) can be used. Reconstructive surgery involves the implantation of human fetal mesencephalic cells (fetal transplant) or other dopamine producing cells into the striatum. Rehabilitation for Parkinson's disease (speech, occupational, and physical therapies) has been applied empirically based on its accepted use in other chronic disorders.

Pharmacological Treatment

It is important to consider that while drug treatment available for Parkinson's disease increased in the last 30 years, the first dopaminergic drug L-DOPA remains the more effective. Actually, the more recent drugs refined the treatment but they do not altered the clinical aspect and the evolution of the disease, and everyone can only temporary control and ameliorate the motor symptoms. The increasing evidences that cognitive dysfunctions, depression, constipation, pain and nocturnal incapacity can play important role in the quality of life of patients and the benefits of any new treatment should be evaluated in their impact in the well-bearing, mental health and others deficiencies of the patients. A summarized review of the pharmacological approaches currently available for Parkinson's disease is illustrated in the Figure 3.

L-dopa

Since dopamine does not cross the blood-brain barrier, it is replaced by giving its precursor L-DOPA, which does (128-131) (Figure 1). L-DOPA was introduced in the Parkinson's disease therapy in the 1960s, and remains the most effective therapy for motor symptoms. It alleviates all the cardinal motor symptoms of Parkinson's disease, including bradykinesia, which is generally the most disabling motor feature of the disease (129-131). Carbidopa (in the United States) or benserazide (not available in the United States) are included in the standard oral formulation to inhibit conversion of L-DOPA to dopamine outside of the brain (in the periphery) because these drugs do not cross the blood-brain-barrier (129-131) (Figure 3).

L-DOPA is a large neutral amino acid, which is absorbed in the gut and transported across the blood-brain barrier by the large neutral amino acid transporter (129-131). Thus, it competes with dietary amino acids for transport, and patients with advanced Parkinson's disease may need to schedule the administration of their doses far from meal times, or reduce the protein content of their meals (129-131).

As well as occasional early nausea or vomiting, to which tolerance usually develops rapidly, the side effects of L-DOPA can include postural hypotension, aggravation of peptic ulcers, sweating attacks, and dark discoloration of urine and sweat (132, 133). The most problematic adverse effects are the motor fluctuations and dyskinesia that constitute the long-term L-DOPA syndrome (see later) (132, 134-136) and neuropsychiatric symptoms (133, 137-139). Finally, although concerns have been voiced about the theoretical possibility that

L-DOPA could accelerate the disease process, there is no conclusive evidence to support this view (140-147).

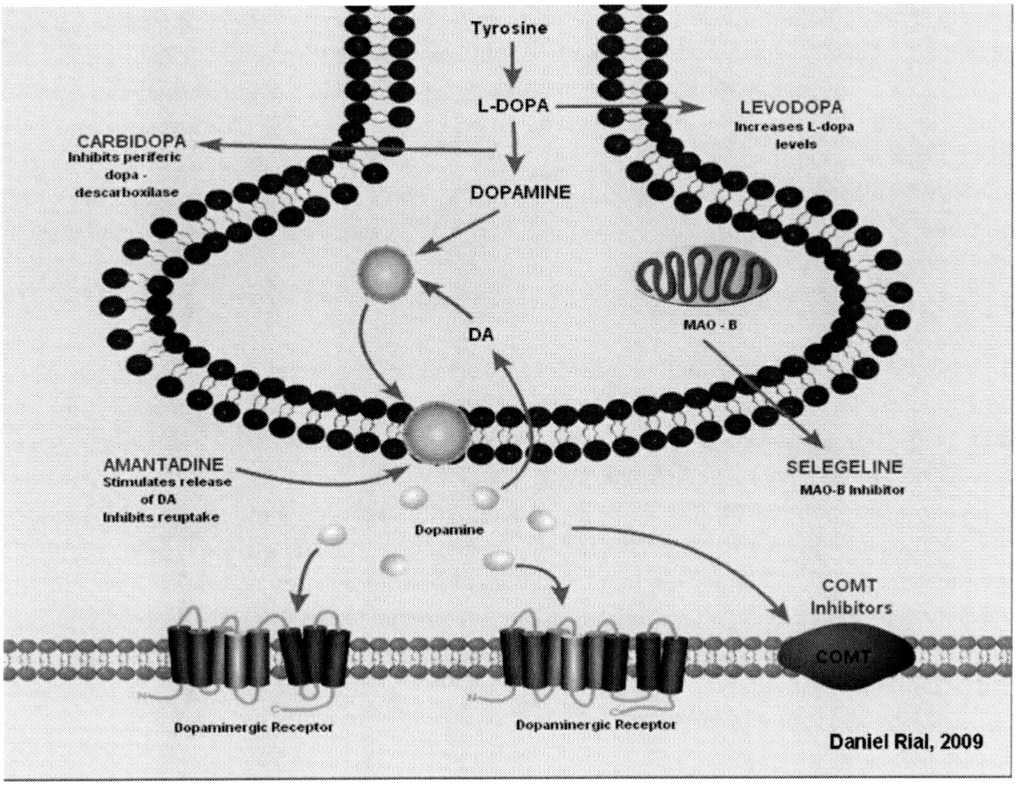

Figure 3. The pharmacological approaches currently available for Parkinson's disease: L-DOPA, Carbidopa, Amantadine and COMT and MAO-B inhibitors. Generally, these drugs reverts temporarily the dopamine dysfunction caused by dopaminergic neurodegeneration in the basal ganglia of Parkinson's disease patients.

Dopamine agonists

Dopamine agonists directly stimulate dopamine receptors, and do not require metabolic conversion within the degenerating cells of the substantia nigra. The use of dopamine agonists as add-on to L-DOPA in patients with fluctuating Parkinson's disease is nowadays a well accepted therapeutic approach (148-150). In the most recent literature, however, the choice of dopamine agonist for initial dopaminomimetic treatment of Parkinson's disease has become controversial (151). There are evidences that monotherapy with dopamine agonists in early Parkinson's disease is a newer strategy developed to prevent the motor fluctuations and dyskinesias which occur within a few years following the start of L-DOPA treatment (150, 152, 153). A large evidence-based review of the use of dopamine agonists in early Parkinson's disease endorses the fact that this strategy has long-term benefits. Bromocriptine, cabergoline, pergolide, pramipexole, and ropinirole were all shown to be superior to levodopa in delaying motor fluctuations and dyskinesias, at the expense of smaller motor benefit (150, 152, 153). The use of dopamine agonists has been thought to be neuroprotective, measured by imaged striatal dopaminergic function. This point is also open to discussion since these results could be a pharmacological effect of proteins that interact with imaging ligands and not a true reflection of striatal neuroprotection.

Since dopamine agonist act in the periphery as well as centrally, they often cause initial sickness by stimulating dopamine receptors in the vomiting centre in the medulla, which is functionally outside the blood-brain barrier. Unlike other anti-emetics, which all worsen parkinsonism, the peripherally acting dopamine receptor blocker domperidone can prevent, reduce, or abolish sickness without blocking striatal receptors (154). All agonists can cause postural hypotension, and all cause psychiatric side effects (155, 156) more commonly than L-DOPA. Unlike L-DOPA, dopamine agonists sometimes cause vasospasm (157), erythromelalgia (128, 158), ankle swelling (128, 159), and (rarely) pleuropulmonary or retroperitoneal fibrosis (160).

Comt inhibitors

Inhibition of catechol O-methyltransferase (COMT) prevents conversion of L-DOPA to 3 O-methyldopa in the periphery, thus increasing the L-DOPA available for transport into the brain (161-163) (Figure 3). Two COMT inhibitors are approved in the United States, entacapone and tolcapone. Neither has significant activity in the CNS. Both have been shown to decrease the duration of "off" time in patients with significant off time (163). Frequent liver function monitoring is required for patients commencing therapy (161). This requires a blood test every 2-4 weeks for the first 6 months; to be sure that certain critical liver function values are not rising. After that, blood tests are recommended at intervals deemed clinically relevant. Treatment should be discontinued if the ALT/AST levels rise above twice the upper limit of normal.

Mao-b inhibitors

Monoamine oxidase B (MAO-B) acts in the brain to degrade dopamine (164) (Figure 3). Thus, inhibiting MAO-B is a therapeutic strategy for treatment of Parkinson's disease (165). Two selective MAO-B inhibitors are available in the United States and elsewhere: selegiline and rasagiline. Both are irreversible inhibitors of the enzyme and they are approved for the treatment of signs and symptoms of Parkinson's disease as initial monotherapy and as adjunct therapy to L-DOPA (166, 167). As monotherapy, it may reduce parkinsonian disability. As adjunctive therapy, it may reduce off time and increase dyskinesia-free on time (166, 167). Rasagiline side effects include insomnia, hallucinations, and orthostatic hypotension. Selegiline, as adjunctive therapy, it may reduce off time and increase dyskinesia-free on time.

Anticholinergics

Anticholinergics have a limited role in the treatment of Parkinson's disease (168). They are primarily effective against tremor and rigidity, and their side effects may be especially significant in elderly patients (168). Doses should begin low and increase slowly. Common side effects are memory loss, dry mouth, urinary retention, constipation, sedation, delirium, and hallucinations (168-170).

Amantadine

Amantadine (Figure 3) has a mild symptomatic effect on the motor symptoms of PD, but a more significant effect on the reduction of dyskinesias (171, 172). It is believed to act through blockade of N-methyl-D-aspartate (NMDA) receptors (173, 174). Side effects include hallucinations, insomnia, agitation, and difficulty concentrating, as well as ankle edema, dry mouth and mottled skin.

Surgery

Brain surgery is an option for advanced Parkinson's disease patients whose symptoms can no longer be adequately managed pharmacologically (175, 176). The best surgical candidate is someone who responds well to dopaminergic therapy but has motor complications (off periods and dyskinesias and with increasing equilibrium and speech dysfunction) that are limiting factors to patients, and who is otherwise healthy and a good surgical risk (177). Advanced age is not necessarily a barrier to surgery; however, impaired cognition and brain atrophy increase surgical risk and decrease the likelihood of an optimal outcome. Depending on the patient, procedure, and skill of the operating team, cognition may be mildly impaired or largely unaffected. The most commonly reported adverse neuropsychiatric effects are reduced executive function (178-180) and language impairments (181, 182).

There are two surgical procedures—lesioning and deep brain stimulation—and three target locations in Parkinson's disease surgery: thalamus, globus pallidum internus (GPi), and subthalamic nucleus (STN) (175, 176). Deep brain stimulation (DBS) uses implanted electrodes to create a functional and "reversible" thalamotomy, pallidotomy or subthalamotomy (183-185). Lesion procedures— thalamotomy (176, 184, 186), pallidotomy (176, 187-189)—deliver radio-frequency energy to heat and ablate a pea-sized region within the target.

Stem cell transplants (190, 191), gene therapy (192), neurotrophic factor delivery (193, 194), and mitochondrial medicine (195) remain experimental procedures for the treatment of Parkinson's disease.

Rehabilitation

A wide variety of health professionals - physical therapists, occupational therapists, speech-language pathologists, gerontologists, neurologists, psychologists, and others - may be involved in the rehabilitation of Parkinson's disease patients. Often physical therapy focuses on the impairments (e.g., neurological symptoms), functional limitations (e.g., walking, stair climbing, reaching, grasping), and disabilities (e.g., hobbies, sport, social activities) and is comprised of mobility exercises, gait training (with and without the application of external cues), training of daily activities, relaxation therapy, and breathing exercises (196). Another goal is to educate the individual (as well as partner and family) about the disease process and the benefits of exercise therapy (196). Goals of occupational therapy include maximizing fine motor coordination, especially of the upper extremities, reducing energy expenditure, increasing safety and independence, and improving quality of life and efficiency of activities of daily living (197). Moreover, it has been suggested that physical therapy is an important adjunct to the anti-parkinsonian medication (196).

Physical Exercise and Brain Health

In 1890, William James first recognized that one of the most important features of human behavior is the ability to carry out meaningful change (198). He broadly defined this under the rubric of 'behavioral plasticity'. Since then, this concept of plasticity has been further developed to include structural change in the brain at the cellular, molecular, and system levels, with the convergence of these mechanisms ultimately supporting behavioral plasticity. Maintaining brain health and plasticity throughout life is an important public health goal, and it is increasingly clear that behavioral stimulation and exercise can help us to achieve it. Such intervention is particularly crucial from middle age onwards, when the brain faces a series of challenges that can include the pathogenesis of neurodegenerative diseases like Alzheimer's disease (198). Over the past decade, a number of studies on humans have shown the benefits of exercise on brain health and function, particularly in aging populations. Several molecular systems could potentially participate in the benefits of exercise on the brain. Neurotrophic factors (such as the brain-derived neurotrophic factor – BDND) have most of the properties that could underlie such beneficial effects because they support the survival and growth of many neuronal subtypes, including glutamatergic neurons (198-200).

Physical Exercise and Parkinson's Disease

Clinical Findings of the Role of Physical Exercise in Parkinson's Disease

There are numerous studies evaluating the effects of physical exercise on patients with Parkinson's disease that are summarized on Table 1. Despite some inconsistencies in the literature (that can be largely attributed to methodological issues), the preponderant results would suggest that physical exercise is beneficial for PD patients. The exercise protocols include range of motion (ROM) and flexibility exercises, gait and equilibrium training, and exercises of mobility and coordination (201). These studies reported positive results for the groups that received the intervention, such as improvement in gait (202, 203), increased spinal flexibility (204), better functional reach (205, 206), improved axial mobility (204, 205), improved motor ability (205), increased muscle strength, and reduction in number of falls (207). These improvements are important for daily activities such as turning over, moving in bed, standing from a sitting position, reaching forward while sitting or standing, turning while standing, and walking. Interesting, the body weight supported treadmill training (BWSTT) was found to be superior to regular physiotherapy, especially as far as short step gait is concerned (201, 203).

In terms of aerobic capacity, maximal oxygen uptake (VO_2max) achieved by subjects with Parkinson's disease was not significantly different from normal rest values, so that evidences of decreased latency to achieve exercise-induced fatigue (208, 209), increased heart rat response (210) and decrease maximal ventilatory levels during the exercise (211). However, all of these variables were modified by physical training in Parkinson's disease patients (210-213).

Moreover, it was hypothesized that physical therapy is an important adjunct to pharmacologic treatment in patients with Parkinson's disease, with regard to neurologic symptoms (e.g., tremor, bradykinesia, rigidity), walking ability, ADLs (activities of daily living), and QOL (196). The literature support the hypothesis that patients with Parkinson's disease benefit from physical therapy in terms of ADLs and walking ability (walking speed, stride length), but not in terms of neurologic signs (196). However, the mobility can be more easily influenced by physical therapy than by neurologic symptoms. It should be noticed, however, that physical therapy is mainly focused on mobility rather than neurologic symptoms, such as rigidity and tremor (196).

In addition, there are some evidences about the effect of a physical therapy group treatment program (196). Gauthier et al. (1987) (212) and Palmer et al. (1986) (213) reported improvement of psychological well-being. Gauthier et al. (1987) (212) also reported facilitation of several positive behavioral changes as additional effects of group treatment.

Effects of Physical Exercise in Animal Models of Parkinson's Disease

Several studies have demonstrated the positive effects of physical exercise in animal models of Parkinson's disease (214-216). Tillerson et al. (2003) (214) reported behavioral improvement after treadmill exercise in two rodent models of basal ganglia injury (the 6-OHDA rat and MPTP-lesioned mouse), which was associated with attenuation of dopamine loss. These investigators concluded that exercise might work largely through neuroprotective mechanisms because exercise was started within 12 hours of lesioning, and MPTP and 6-OHDA may take several days to complete cell death (113, 217). Exercise resulted also in decreased dopamine transporter (DAT) compared to non-exercised groups in mice exposed to MPTP (218). In the basal ganglia, the biosynthesis of dopamine is dependent on the enzyme tyrosine hydroxylase (TH) and the primary mechanism of clearance of dopamine from the extracellular space is through the DAT (219, 220). Several mechanisms have been shown to regulate DAT activity including: (1) gene and protein expression of transporter number; (2) phosphorylation activated through glutamate receptors such as the mGluR5 metabotropic receptor; and (3) internalization within endosomes mediated by dopamine (221). Alterations in DAT activity can influence the synaptic occupancy of dopamine. An intervention (such as exercise) that downregulates DAT expression may therefore lead to behavioral improvement by increasing synaptic occupancy of dopamine. The down regulation of DAT in exercised animals could also account for the superior running capabilities of both the MPTP and control groups compared to the non-exercised groups (218). Moreover, there are evidences of exercise-induced decreased activity of TH in the MPTP mice model of Parkinson's disease (222). The expression of DAT and TH proteins, as well as the level of striatal dopamine, is closely linked. For example, DAT knockout mice have been shown to express reduced striatal TH protein (223). Although the precise link between DAT and TH is still unclear, it is speculated that the increased synaptic bioavailability of dopamine, through the down regulation of DAT, may lead to increased activation of the dopamine autoreceptor, leading to the down regulation of TH (224). A similar down regulation of DAT with activity can be induced in young mice exposed to environmental enrichment and this can in fact prove neuroprotective against MPTP toxicity (225).

Table 1. Overview of clinical outcomes in patients with Parkinson's disease submitted to physical exercise

Reference	Disease stage (H&Y)	Intervention	Significative outcomes
Kamsma et al. 1995	2-4	Training program involving sitting, stand-ing and gait activities in relation to bed	↑ turning in bed, ↑ rising from a chair, ↓ falling.
Schenkman et al. 1998	2-3	Exercise to improve axial rotation, functional reach, time supine and stand, 360° turn, 6-min walking distance and 10-min walking time	↑ functional axial rotation, ↑ functional reach, ↓ time to complete 360° return
Marchese et al. 2000	1.5-3	Physical therapy	↑ UPDRS after follow-up
Comella et al. 1993	2-3	Exercises to improve ROM, endurance, balance, gait and fine motor dexterity	↑ UPDRS
Miyai et al. 2002	2.5-3	BWSTT	↑ gait
Protas et al. 2005	2-3	Gait and step training	↑ gait speed, cadence and step test
Toole et al. 2000	1-3	Lower body resistance training and balance training	↑ equilibrium composite score
Bergen et al. 2002	2	Cycling and treadmill	↑ VO_2max, ↑ movement initiation
Hass et al. 2007	1-3	Muscle strengthening	↑ 1RM, ↑ fat-free mass
Kuroda et al. 1992	3 or higher	Exercise	↓ mortality

Abbreviations: ↑: increase; ↓: decrease; BWSTT: Body Weight-Supported Treadmill Training; H&Y: Hoehn and Yahr; ROM: Range of Motion; UPDRS: Unified Parkinson's Disease Rating Scale; 1RM: maximal muscle contraction.

Table 2. Overview of basic outcomes in experimental models of Parkinson's disease associating physical exercise

Study	Animal model	Intervention	Outcomes
Tillerson et al. 2003	intra-striatal 6-OHDA in Fisher rats and i.p. MPTP in C57BL/6 mice	Treadmill	↑ striatal DA, DOPAC and HVA; ↑ TH in the SNpc; ↑ gait
Fisher et al. 2004	i.p. MPTP in C57BL/6 mice	Treadmill	↓ striatal DAT ↑ striatal DA D_2 receptors
Petzinger et al. 2007	i.p. MPTP in C57BL/6 mice	Treadmill	↑ coordination ↑ striatal DA ↓ striatal TH and DAT
Poulton and Muir 2005	i.c.v. 6-OHDA in Long Evan rats	Treadmill	↑ striatal DA No motor improvement
Mabandla et al. 2003	Intra-medial forebrain bundle 6-OHDA in Long Evan rats	Running wheel	↓ rotations following apomorphine challenge

Abbreviations: ↑: increase; ↓: decrease; 6-OHDA: 6-hydroxydopamine; MPTP: 1-methyl-4-phenyl-1,2,3,6-tetrahydropyridine; i.p.: intraperitoneal; i.c.v.: intracerebroventricular; DA: dopamine; DOPAC: 3,4-dihydroxyphenylacetic acid; HVA: homovallinic acid; SNpc: substantia nigra pars compacta; TH: tyrosine hydroxylase.

This chapter provides additional evidences that moderate physical exercise plays an important role into improvement of motor and cognitive deficits verified in an experimental model of PD. Four consecutive weeks in running wheel or treadmill attenuated the motor disruption induced by 5 mg/kg subcutaneous injection of reserpine in rats (see Figure 4), corroborating previous observations that physical exercise ameliorates motor performance in neurointoxicants rodent models of PD, such as 6-OHDA (214, 218) and MPTP (214, 217, 218, 222) (see Table 2). Moreover, our findings demonstrate that physical exercise improve selectively social recognition memory deficits induced by 1 mg/kg subcutaneous injection of reserpine in rats, reinforcing the potential of physical exercise in the management of non-motor symptoms of Parkinson's disease.

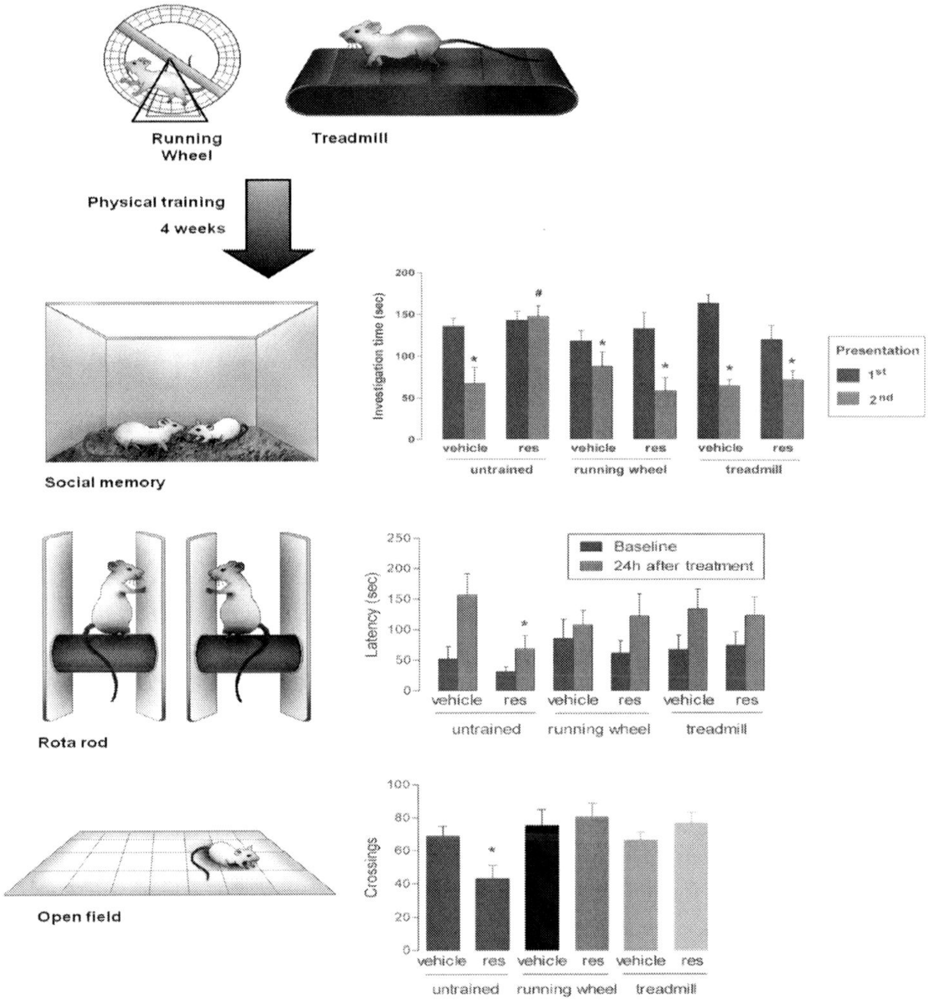

Figure 4. Four weeks of moderate physical training running wheel or treadmill reversed the cognitive (social memory test) and motor (open field and rota rod test) impairments induced by reserpine in rats. In the social memory test, sedentary reserpinized rats did not recognize the pup during the second exposition. In the rota rod and open field tests, reserpine administration induced, respectively, coordination and locomotion deficits in sedentary rats. In all tests, the running wheel and treadmill training reversed the impairments induced by reserpine. Figure 1.

Normally, when rodents are placed in a novel environment, they initially display a high level of exploratory activity, of which locomotion is an important, although not an exclusive component (226). This class of spatial exploration is a complex cognitive process, modulated by the state of arousal, sensory processing, and a vast array of motivational factors (e.g. hunger, fear, curiosity, etc.) (226). The systemic administration of reserpine to rodents is frequently used as a model of the motor disturbance of PD (227-229), and several clinically used anti-parkinsonian drugs (e.g., dopamine receptor agonists, L-DOPA plus benzerazide, amantadine and trihexyphenidyl) have been shown to improve this motor impairment (230). In accordance with these previous studies, we observed that the locomotion and exploratory activity were highly reduced in reserpine-treated (5 mg/kg) rats (Figure 4), probably due to the depletion of dopamine (and other monoamines) in the basal ganglia nuclei (227, 231). Of high interest, both types (running wheel and treadmill) of moderate exercise induced a full recovery of the locomotor performance of reserpinized animals in the open field and rota-rod tests (Figure 4).

Based on the extensive literature reporting the benefits that physical exercise can produce in motor function of rodents submitted to animal models of PD such as 6-OHDA and MPTP (214, 218, 222, 232) (see Table 2), a speculative hypothesis can be given. The positive effects of exercise on motor function seem to be mediated, at least in part, by adaptive changes of dopaminergic system in basal ganglia and motor circuitry. For instance, Petzinger et al. (2007) (222) have recently published a highlight study demonstrating a pronounced dopamine release in dorsolateral striatum of MPTP-treated mice submitted to treadmill for 28 days. In this same study, the authors reported that exercise leads to the downregulation of both DAT and TH. A possible explanation for these regional specific effects may be because of use-dependent forms of synaptic plasticity. The high degree of engagement required from the dorsolateral striatum for forelimb and hind limb movement during treadmill exercise is supported by studies demonstrating a selective increase in blood flow and metabolic activity within the dorsolateral striatum during treadmill exercise (233-236).

To date, the majority of studies performed with animal models of Parkinson's disease have focused upon their ability to induce nigrostriatal dopaminergic pathway damage and motor alterations associated with advanced phases of Parkinson's disease. Since Parkinson's disease is accompanied by alterations in a variety of functions including memory deficits (9, 20) and olfactory dysfunction (31, 237, 238), it seems important to evaluate whether the proposed animal models alter any of these functions. We therefore investigated the occurrence of cognitive alterations in rats after a single administration of a low dose of reserpine (1 mg/kg).

The data presented in Figure 4 demonstrates that the acute treatment with reserpine (1 mg/kg) induced pronounced deficits in the social recognition memory in rats. The social recognition memory is a particular model of olfactory memory mediated by olfactory cues (239) and may involve a non-procedural form of a short-term working memory based upon the olfactory discriminative ability of rats. The persistence with which an adult rat investigates a juvenile can be enhanced or decreased in a predictive manner by using inhibition and facilitation procedures (240). It can be facilitated by memory-enhancing drugs and disrupted by pharmacological and pathophysiological models known to impair memory in rodents (241-243). We found that rats treated with reserpine spent as much time investigating the familiar juvenile rat during the second presentation as they did on the first encounter, suggesting impairment in their ability to recognize the juvenile after a short period of time (30 min). Of high interest, the moderate physical training induced a full reversion of the short-term social memory deficits induced by reserpine in rats (Figure 2). Classically, exercise is knowledge to improve learning and memory in both humans and rodents (198, 244, 245). However, the mechanisms are not yet completely understood. In line with this, regular physical exercise has been related to an increase in the number of new hippocampal cells (246, 247), an increase in brain plasticity (198), an increase in the production of neurotrophic factors (248-250), and an increase in learning and memory (218, 247, 250-252).

Conclusion

The findings reviewed in this chapter suggest that physical exercise significantly improve the motor impairments of Parkinson's disease patients. Data obtained in basic research has indicated the potential neuroprotective of physical exercise in neurointoxicant models of Parkinson's disease. In particular, our new findings indicate that moderate physical exercise might afford protection against memory dysfunction elicited in reserpinized rats, reinforcing it cognitive enhancing properties that may be of interest in the management of cognitive declines associated to Parkinson's disease. Finally, a better evaluation of the potential of combining physical exercise and the current drugs available in Parkinson's disease therapy is also indicated.

References

[1] Parkinson, J. An essay on the shaking palsy. 1817. *J Neuropsychiatry Clin Neurosci.*, 2002, (14), 223-36; discussion 2.

[2] Nussbaum, RL; Ellis, CE. Alzheimer's disease and Parkinson's disease. *N Engl J Med.*, 2003, (348), 1356-64.

[3] MacDonald, BK; Cockerell, OC; Sander, JW; Shorvon, SD. The incidence and lifetime prevalence of neurological disorders in a prospective community-based study in the UK. *Brain.*, 2000, (123 (Pt 4)), 665-76.

[4] Mayeux, R. Epidemiology of neurodegeneration. *Annu Rev Neurosci.*, 2003, (26), 81-104.

[5] Tanner, CM; Goldman, SM. Epidemiology of Parkinson's disease. *Neurol Clin.*, 1996, (14), 317-35.

[6] Rajput, AH; Offord, KP; Beard, CM; Kurland, LT. Epidemiology of parkinsonism: incidence, classification, and mortality. *Ann Neurol.*, 1984 (16), 278-82.

[7] Lang, AE; Lozano, AM. Parkinson's disease. First of two parts. *N Engl J Med.*, 1998, (339), 1044-53.

[8] Lang, AE; Lozano, AM. Parkinson's disease. Second of two parts. *N Engl J Med.*, 1998, (339), 1130-43.

[9] Dubois, B; Pillon, B. Cognitive deficits in Parkinson's disease. *J Neurol.*, 1997, (244), 2-8.

[10] Gunal, DI; Nurichalichi, K; Tuncer, N; Bekiroglu, N; Aktan, S. The clinical profile of nonmotor fluctuations in Parkinson's disease patients. *Can J Neurol Sci*, 2002, (29), 61-4.

[11] Weintraub, D; Moberg, PJ; Duda, JE; Katz, IR; Stern, MB. Effect of psychiatric and other nonmotor symptoms on disability in Parkinson's disease. *J Am Geriatr Soc*, 2004, (52), 784-8.

[12] Gibb, WR. Accuracy in the clinical diagnosis of parkinsonian syndromes. *Postgrad Med J*, 1988, (64), 345-51.

[13] Gelb, DJ; Oliver, E; Gilman, S. Diagnostic criteria for Parkinson disease. *Arch Neurol*, 1999, (56), 33-9.

[14] Hughes, AJ; Daniel, SE; Kilford, L; Lees, AJ. Accuracy of clinical diagnosis of idiopathic Parkinson's disease: a clinico-pathological study of 100 cases. *J Neurol Neurosurg Psychiatry*, 1992, (55), 181-4.

[15] Louis, ED; Klatka, LA; Liu, Y; Fahn, S. Comparison of extrapyramidal features in 31 pathologically confirmed cases of diffuse Lewy body disease and 34 pathologically confirmed cases of Parkinson's disease. *Neurology*, 1997 (48), 376-80.

[16] Jellinger, KA. The neuropathologic diagnosis of secondary parkinsonian syndromes. *Adv Neurol*, 1996, (69), 293-303.

[17] Braak, H; Del Tredici, K; Rub, U; de Vos, RA; Jansen Steur, EN; Braak, E. Staging of brain pathology related to sporadic Parkinson's disease. *Neurobiol Aging*, 2003, (24), 197-211.

[18] Braak, H; Ghebremedhin, E; Rub, U; Bratzke, H; Del Tredici, K. Stages in the development of Parkinson's disease-related pathology. *Cell Tissue Res*, 2004, (318), 121-34.

[19] Schulz, JB. Neuronal pathology in Parkinson's disease. *Cell Tissue Res*, 2005, (320), 211.

[20] Bosboom, JL; Stoffers, D; Wolters, E. Cognitive dysfunction and dementia in Parkinson's disease. *J Neural Transm*, 2004, (111), 1303-15.

[21] Knowlton, BJ; Mangels, JA; Squire, LR. A neostriatal habit learning system in humans. *Science*, 1996, (273), 1399-402.

[22] Aarsland, D; Tandberg, E; Larsen, JP; Cummings, JL. Frequency of dementia in Parkinson disease. *Arch Neurol*, 1996, (53), 538-42.

[23] Bondi, MW; Kaszniak, AW. Implicit and explicit memory in Alzheimer's disease and Parkinson's disease. *J Clin Exp Neuropsychol*, 1991, (13), 339-58.

[24] Cooper, JA; Sagar, HJ; Doherty, SM; Jordan, N; Tidswell, P; Sullivan, EV. Different effects of dopaminergic and anticholinergic therapies on cognitive and motor function in Parkinson's disease. A follow-up study of untreated patients. *Brain*, 1992, (115, (Pt 6)), 1701-25.

[25] Loranger, AW; Goodell, H; Lee, JE; McDowell, F. Levodopa treatment of Parkinson's syndrome. Improved intellectual functioning. *Arch Gen Psychiatry*, 1972, (26), 163-8.

[26] Growdon, JH; Kieburtz, K; McDermott, MP; Panisset, M; Friedman, JH. Levodopa improves motor function without impairing cognition in mild non-demented Parkinson's disease patients. Parkinson Study Group. *Neurology*, 1998, (50), 1327-31.

[27] Pillon, B; Dubois, B; Bonnet, AM; Esteguy, M; Guimaraes, J; Vigouret, JM; Lhermitte, F; Agid, Y. Cognitive slowing in Parkinson's disease fails to respond to levodopa treatment: the 15-objects test. *Neurology*, 1989, (39), 762-8.

[28] Rektorova, I; Rektor, I; Bares, M; Dostal, V; Ehler, E; Fanfrdlova, Z; Fiedler, J; Klajblova, H; Kulist'ak, P; Ressner, P; Svatova, J; Urbanek, K; Veliskova, J. Cognitive performance in people with Parkinson's disease and mild or moderate depression: effects of dopamine agonists in an add-on to L-dopa therapy. *Eur J Neurol*, 2005, (12), 9-15.

[29] Huber, SJ; Shulman, HG; Paulson, GW; Shuttleworth, EC. Dose-dependent memory impairment in Parkinson's disease. *Neurology*, 1989, (39), 438-40.

[30] Poewe, W; Berger, W; Benke, T; Schelosky, L. High-speed memory scanning in Parkinson's disease: adverse effects of levodopa. *Ann Neurol*, 1991, (29), 670-3.

[31] Doty, RL. The olfactory vector hypothesis of neurodegenerative disease: is it viable? *Ann Neurol*, 2008, (63), 7-15.

[32] Doty, RL; Bromley, SM; Stern, MB. Olfactory testing as an aid in the diagnosis of Parkinson's disease: development of optimal discrimination criteria. *Neurodegeneration*, 1995, (4), 93-7.

[33] Tissingh, G; Berendse, HW; Bergmans, P; DeWaard, R; Drukarch, B; Stoof, JC; Wolters, EC. Loss of olfaction in de novo and treated Parkinson's disease: possible implications for early diagnosis. *Mov Disord*, 2001, (16), 41-6.

[34] Becker, G; Muller, A; Braune, S; Buttner, T; Benecke, R; Greulich, W; Klein, W; Mark, G; Rieke, J; Thumler, R. Early diagnosis of Parkinson's disease. *J Neurol*, 2002, (249 Suppl 3), III/40-8.

[35] Polymeropoulos, MH; Lavedan, C; Leroy, E; Ide, SE; Dehejia, A; Dutra, A; Pike, B; Root, H; Rubenstein, J; Boyer, R; Stenroos, ES; Chandrasekharappa, S; Athanassiadou, A; Papapetropoulos, T; Johnson, WG; Lazzarini, AM; Duvoisin, RC; Di Iorio, G; Golbe, LI; Nussbaum, RL. Mutation in the alpha-synuclein gene identified in families with Parkinson's disease. *Science*, 1997, (276), 2045-7.

[36] Biskup, S; Gerlach, M; Kupsch, A; Reichmann, H; Riederer, P; Vieregge, P; Wullner, U; Gasser, T. Genes associated with Parkinson syndrome. *J Neurol*, 2008, (255 Suppl 5), 8-17.

[37] Bonifati, V; Rizzu, P; Squitieri, F; Krieger, E; Vanacore, N; van Swieten, JC; Brice, A; van Duijn, CM; Oostra, B; Meco, G; Heutink, P. DJ-1(PARK7), a novel gene for autosomal recessive, early onset parkinsonism. *Neurol Sci*, 2003, (24), 159-60.

[38] Bonifati, V; Rizzu, P; van Baren, MJ; Schaap, O; Breedveld, GJ; Krieger, E; Dekker, MC; Squitieri, F; Ibanez, P; Joosse, M; van Dongen, JW; Vanacore, N; van Swieten, JC; Brice, A; Meco, G; van Duijn, CM; Oostra, BA; Heutink, P. Mutations in the DJ-1 gene associated with autosomal recessive early-onset parkinsonism. *Science*, 2003, (299), 256-9.

[39] Dawson, TM; Dawson, VL. Molecular pathways of neurodegeneration in Parkinson's disease. *Science*, 2003, (302), 819-22.

[40] Maroteaux, L; Campanelli, JT; Scheller, RH. Synuclein: a neuron-specific protein localized to the nucleus and presynaptic nerve terminal. *J Neurosci*, 1988, (8), 2804-15.

[41] Murphy, DD; Rueter, SM; Trojanowski, JQ; Lee, VM. Synucleins are developmentally expressed, and alpha-synuclein regulates the size of the presynaptic vesicular pool in primary hippocampal neurons. *J Neurosci*, 2000, (20), 3214-20.

[42] Abeliovich, A; Schmitz, Y; Farinas, I; Choi-Lundberg, D; Ho, WH; Castillo, PE; Shinsky, N; Verdugo, JM; Armanini, M; Ryan, A; Hynes, M; Phillips, H; Sulzer, D;

Rosenthal, A. Mice lacking alpha-synuclein display functional deficits in the nigrostriatal dopamine system. *Neuron*, 2000, (25), 239-52.

[43] Kruger, R; Kuhn, W; Muller, T; Woitalla, D; Graeber, M; Kosel, S; Przuntek, H; Epplen, JT; Schols, L; Riess, O. Ala30Pro mutation in the gene encoding alpha-synuclein in Parkinson's disease. *Nat Genet*, 1998, (18), 106-8.

[44] Singleton, AB; Farrer, M; Johnson, J; Singleton, A; Hague, S; Kachergus, J; Hulihan, M; Peuralinna, T; Dutra, A; Nussbaum, R; Lincoln, S; Crawley, A; Hanson, M; Maraganore, D; Adler, C; Cookson, MR; Muenter, M; Baptista, M; Miller, D; Blancato, J; Hardy, J; Gwinn-Hardy, K. alpha-Synuclein locus triplication causes Parkinson's disease. *Science*, 2003, (302), 841.

[45] Farrer, M; Maraganore, DM; Lockhart, P; Singleton, A; Lesnick, TG; de Andrade, M; West, A; de Silva, R; Hardy, J; Hernandez, D. alpha-Synuclein gene haplotypes are associated with Parkinson's disease. *Hum Mol Genet*, 2001, (10), 1847-51.

[46] Maraganore, DM; de Andrade, M; Elbaz, A; Farrer, MJ; Ioannidis, JP; Kruger, R; Rocca, WA; Schneider, NK; Lesnick, TG; Lincoln, SJ; Hulihan, MM; Aasly, JO; Ashizawa, T; Chartier-Harlin, MC; Checkoway, H; Ferrarese, C; Hadjigeorgiou, G; Hattori, N; Kawakami, H; Lambert, JC; Lynch, T; Mellick, GD; Papapetropoulos, S; Parsian, A; Quattrone, A; Riess, O; Tan, EK; Van Broeckhoven, C. Collaborative analysis of alpha-synuclein gene promoter variability and Parkinson disease. *JAMA*, 2006, (296), 661-70.

[47] Myhre, R; Toft, M; Kachergus, J; Hulihan, MM; Aasly, JO; Klungland, H; Farrer, MJ. Multiple alpha-synuclein gene polymorphisms are associated with Parkinson's disease in a Norwegian population. *Acta Neurol Scand*, 2008, (118), 320-7.

[48] Winkler, S; Hagenah, J; Lincoln, S; Heckman, M; Haugarvoll, K; Lohmann-Hedrich, K; Kostic, V; Farrer, M; Klein, C. alpha-Synuclein and Parkinson disease susceptibility. *Neurology*, 2007, (69), 1745-50.

[49] Goedert, M; Spillantini, MG. Lewy body diseases and multiple system atrophy as alpha-synucleinopathies. *Mol Psychiatry*, 1998, (3), 462-5.

[50] Spillantini, MG; Schmidt, ML; Lee, VM; Trojanowski, JQ; Jakes, R; Goedert, M. Alpha-synuclein in Lewy bodies. *Nature*, 1997, (388), 839-40.

[51] Tofaris, GK; Layfield, R; Spillantini, MG. alpha-synuclein metabolism and aggregation is linked to ubiquitin-independent degradation by the proteasome. *FEBS Lett*, 2001, (509), 22-6.

[52] Tofaris, GK; Spillantini, MG. Alpha-synuclein dysfunction in Lewy body diseases. *Mov Disord*, 2005, (20 Suppl 12), S37-44.

[53] Tofaris, GK; Spillantini, MG. Physiological and pathological properties of alpha-synuclein. *Cell Mol Life Sci*, 2007, (64), 2194-201.

[54] Yu, S; Ueda, K; Chan, P. Alpha-synuclein and dopamine metabolism. *Mol Neurobiol*, 2005, (31), 243-54.

[55] Lee, FJ; Liu, F. Genetic factors involved in the pathogenesis of Parkinson's disease. *Brain Res Rev*, 2008, (58), 354-64.

[56] Kitada, T; Asakawa, S; Matsumine, H; Hattori, N; Shimura, H; Minoshima, S; Shimizu, N; Mizuno, Y. Progress in the clinical and molecular genetics of familial parkinsonism. *Neurogenetics*, 2000, (2), 207-18.

[57] Hattori, N; Kitada, T; Matsumine, H; Asakawa, S; Yamamura, Y; Yoshino, H; Kobayashi, T; Yokochi, M; Wang, M; Yoritaka, A; Kondo, T; Kuzuhara, S; Nakamura,

S; Shimizu, N; Mizuno, Y. Molecular genetic analysis of a novel Parkin gene in Japanese families with autosomal recessive juvenile parkinsonism: evidence for variable homozygous deletions in the Parkin gene in affected individuals. *Ann Neurol*, 1998, (44), 935-41.

[58] Kitada, T; Asakawa, S; Hattori, N; Matsumine, H; Yamamura, Y; Minoshima, S; Yokochi, M; Mizuno, Y; Shimizu, N. Mutations in the parkin gene cause autosomal recessive juvenile parkinsonism. *Nature*, 1998, (392), 605-8.

[59] Mizuno, Y; Hattori, N; Kitada, T; Matsumine, H; Mori, H; Shimura, H; Kubo, S; Kobayashi, H; Asakawa, S; Minoshima, S; Shimizu, N. Familial Parkinson's disease. Alpha-synuclein and parkin. *Adv Neurol*, 2001, (86), 13-21.

[60] Shimura, H; Hattori, N; Kubo, S; Mizuno, Y; Asakawa, S; Minoshima, S; Shimizu, N; Iwai, K; Chiba, T; Tanaka, K; Suzuki, T. Familial Parkinson disease gene product, parkin, is a ubiquitin-protein ligase. *Nat Genet*, 2000, (25), 302-5.

[61] Abbas, N; Lucking, CB; Ricard, S; Durr, A; Bonifati, V; De Michele, G; Bouley, S; Vaughan, JR; Gasser, T; Marconi, R; Broussolle, E; Brefel-Courbon, C; Harhangi, BS; Oostra, BA; Fabrizio, E; Bohme, GA; Pradier, L; Wood, NW; Filla, A; Meco, G; Denefle, P; Agid, Y; Brice, A. A wide variety of mutations in the parkin gene are responsible for autosomal recessive parkinsonism in Europe. French Parkinson's Disease Genetics Study Group and the European Consortium on Genetic Susceptibility in Parkinson's Disease. *Hum Mol Genet*, 1999, (8), 567-74.

[62] Chung, KK; Zhang, Y; Lim, KL; Tanaka, Y; Huang, H; Gao, J; Ross, CA; Dawson, VL; Dawson, TM. Parkin ubiquitinates the alpha-synuclein-interacting protein, synphilin-1: implications for Lewy-body formation in Parkinson disease. *Nat Med*, 2001, (7), 1144-50.

[63] Domingues, AF; Arduino, DM; Esteves, AR; Swerdlow, RH; Oliveira, CR; Cardoso, SM. Mitochondria and ubiquitin-proteasomal system interplay: relevance to Parkinson's disease. *Free Radic Biol Med*, 2008, (45), 820-5.

[64] Ciechanover, A; Brundin, P. The ubiquitin proteasome system in neurodegenerative diseases: sometimes the chicken, sometimes the egg. *Neuron*, 2003, (40), 427-46.

[65] Gorell, JM; Johnson, CC; Rybicki, BA; Peterson, EL; Richardson, RJ. The risk of Parkinson's disease with exposure to pesticides, farming, well water, and rural living. *Neurology*, 1998, (50), 1346-50.

[66] Koller, W; Vetere-Overfield, B; Gray, C; Alexander, C; Chin, T; Dolezal, J; Hassanein, R; Tanner, C. Environmental risk factors in Parkinson's disease. *Neurology*, 1990, (40), 1218-21.

[67] Liou, HH; Tsai, MC; Chen, CJ; Jeng, JS; Chang, YC; Chen, SY; Chen, RC. Environmental risk factors and Parkinson's disease: a case-control study in Taiwan. *Neurology*, 1997, (48), 1583-8.

[68] Marder, K; Logroscino, G; Alfaro, B; Mejia, H; Halim, A; Louis, E; Cote, L; Mayeux, R. Environmental risk factors for Parkinson's disease in an urban multiethnic community. *Neurology*, 1998, (50), 279-81.

[69] Priyadarshi, A; Khuder, SA; Schaub, EA; Priyadarshi, SS. Environmental risk factors and Parkinson's disease: a metaanalysis. *Environ Res*, 2001, (86), 122-7.

[70] Wong, GF; Gray, CS; Hassanein, RS; Koller, WC. Environmental risk factors in siblings with Parkinson's disease. *Arch Neurol*, 1991, (48), 287-9.

[71] Olanow, CW; Tatton, WG. Etiology and pathogenesis of Parkinson's disease. *Annu Rev Neurosci*, 1999, (22), 123-44.

[72] Langston, JW; Ballard, P; Tetrud, JW; Irwin, I. Chronic Parkinsonism in humans due to a product of meperidine-analog synthesis. *Science*, 1983, (219), 979-80.

[73] Kolata, G. Monkey model of Parkinson's disease. *Science*, 1983, (220), 705.

[74] Chiueh, CC; Markey, SP; Burns, RS; Johannessen, JN; Jacobowitz, DM; Kopin, IJ. Neurochemical and behavioral effects of 1-methyl-4-phenyl-1,2,3,6- tetrahydropyridine (MPTP) in rat, guinea pig, and monkey. *Psychopharmacol Bull*, 1984, (20), 548-53.

[75] Jacobowitz, DM; Burns, RS; Chiueh, CC; Kopin, IJ. N-methyl-4-phenyl-1,2,3,6-tetrahydropyridine (MPTP) causes destruction of the nigrostriatal but not the mesolimbic dopamine system in the monkey. *Psychopharmacol Bull*, 1984, (20), 416-22.

[76] Langston, JW; Langston, EB; Irwin, I. MPTP-induced parkinsonism in human and non-human primates--clinical and experimental aspects. *Acta Neurol Scand Suppl*, 1984, (100), 49-54.

[77] Lyden, A; Bondesson, U; Larsson, BS; Lindquist, NG. Melanin affinity of 1-methyl-4-phenyl-1,2,5,6-tetrahydropyridine, an inducer of chronic parkinsonism in humans. *Acta Pharmacol Toxicol, (Copenh)*, 1983, (53), 429-32.

[78] Crossman, AR; Peggs, D; Boyce, S; Luquin, MR; Sambrook, MA. Effect of the NMDA antagonist MK-801 on MPTP-induced parkinsonism in the monkey. *Neuropharmacology*, 1989, (28), 1271-3.

[79] Lang, AE; Blair, RD. Parkinson's disease in 1984: an update. *Can Med Assoc J*, 1984, (131), 1031-7.

[80] Jenner, P; Rupniak, NM; Rose, S; Kelly, E; Kilpatrick, G; Lees, A; Marsden, CD. 1-Methyl-4-phenyl-1,2,3,6-tetrahydropyridine-induced parkinsonism in the common marmoset. *Neurosci Lett*, 1984, (50), 85-90.

[81] Langston, JW; Ballard, P. Parkinsonism induced by 1-methyl-4-phenyl-1,2,3,6-tetrahydropyridine (MPTP): implications for treatment and the pathogenesis of Parkinson's disease. *Can J Neurol Sci*, 1984, (11), 160-5.

[82] Dauer, W; Przedborski, S. Parkinson's disease: mechanisms and models. *Neuron*, 2003, (39), 889-909.

[83] Prediger, RD; Fernandes, MS; Rial, D; Wopereis, S; Pereira, VS; Bosse, TS; Da Silva, CB; Carradore, RS; Machado, MS; Cechinel-Filho, V; Costa-Campos, L. Effects of acute administration of the hydroalcoholic extract of mate tea leaves (Ilex paraguariensis) in animal models of learning and memory. *J Ethnopharmacol*, 2008, (120), 465-73.

[84] Franco, J; Prediger, RD; Pandolfo, P; Takahashi, RN; Farina, M; Dafre, AL. Antioxidant responses and lipid peroxidation following intranasal 1-methyl-4-phenyl-1,2,3,6-tetrahydropyridine (MPTP) administration in rats: increased susceptibility of olfactory bulb. *Life Sci*, 2007, (80), 1906-14.

[85] Prediger, RD; Batista, LC; Medeiros, R; Pandolfo, P; Florio, JC; Takahashi, RN. The risk is in the air: Intranasal administration of MPTP to rats reproducing clinical features of Parkinson's disease. *Exp Neurol*, 2006, (202), 391-403.

[86] Aziz, TZ; Peggs, D; Agarwal, E; Sambrook, MA; Crossman, AR. Subthalamic nucleotomy alleviates parkinsonism in the 1-methyl-4-phenyl-1,2,3,6-tetrahydropyridine (MPTP)-exposed primate. *Br J Neurosurg*, 1992, (6), 575-82.

[87] Bergman, H; Wichmann, T; DeLong, MR. Reversal of experimental parkinsonism by lesions of the subthalamic nucleus. *Science*, 1990, (249), 1436-8.

[88] Jenner, P; Olanow, CW. Understanding cell death in Parkinson's disease. *Ann Neurol*, 1998, (44), S72-84.

[89] Jenner, P; Olanow, CW. Oxidative stress and the pathogenesis of Parkinson's disease. *Neurology*, 1996, (47), S161-70.

[90] Hunot, S; Brugg, B; Ricard, D; Michel, PP; Muriel, MP; Ruberg, M; Faucheux, BA; Agid, Y; Hirsch, EC. Nuclear translocation of NF-kappaB is increased in dopaminergic neurons of patients with parkinson disease. *Proc Natl Acad Sci U S A*, 1997, (94), 7531-6.

[91] Schapira, AH. Mitochondrial complex I deficiency in Parkinson's disease. *Adv Neurol*, 1993, (60), 288-91.

[92] Cooper, JM; Mann, VM; Krige, D; Schapira, AH. Human mitochondrial complex I dysfunction. *Biochim Biophys Acta*, 1992, (1101), 198-203.

[93] Parker, WD, Jr.; Boyson, SJ; Parks, JK. Abnormalities of the electron transport chain in idiopathic Parkinson's disease. *Ann Neurol*, 1989, (26), 719-23.

[94] Swerdlow, RH; Parks, JK; Miller, SW; Tuttle, JB; Trimmer, PA; Sheehan, JP; Bennett, JP, Jr.; Davis, RE; Parker, WD, Jr. Origin and functional consequences of the complex I defect in Parkinson's disease. *Ann Neurol*, 1996, (40), 663-71.

[95] Halliwell, B. Oxidants and the central nervous system: some fundamental questions. Is oxidant damage relevant to Parkinson's disease, Alzheimer's disease, traumatic injury or stroke? *Acta Neurol Scand Suppl*, 1989, (126), 23-33.

[96] Hokfelt, T; Ungerstedt, U. Specificity of 6-hydroxydopamine induced degeneration of central monoamine neurones: an electron and fluorescence microscopic study with special reference to intracerebral injection on the nigro-striatal dopamine system. *Brain Res*, 1973, (60), 269-97.

[97] Luthman, J; Fredriksson, A; Sundstrom, E; Jonsson, G; Archer, T. Selective lesion of central dopamine or noradrenaline neuron systems in the neonatal rat: motor behavior and monoamine alterations at adult stage. *Behav Brain Res*, 1989, (33), 267-77.

[98] Archer, T; Danysz, W; Fredriksson, A; Jonsson, G; Luthman, J; Sundstrom, E; Teiling, A. Neonatal 6-hydroxydopamine-induced dopamine depletions: motor activity and performance in maze learning. *Pharmacol Biochem Behav*, 1988, (31), 357-64.

[99] Stack, EC; Ferro, JL; Kim, J; Del Signore, SJ; Goodrich, S; Matson, S; Hunt, BB; Cormier, K; Smith, K; Matson, WR; Ryu, H; Ferrante, RJ. Therapeutic attenuation of mitochondrial dysfunction and oxidative stress in neurotoxin models of Parkinson's disease. *Biochim Biophys Acta*, 2008, (1782), 151-62.

[100] Glinka, Y; Gassen, M; Youdim, MB. Mechanism of 6-hydroxydopamine neurotoxicity. *J Neural Transm Suppl*, 1997, (50), 55-66.

[101] Javitch, JA; D'Amato, RJ; Strittmatter, SM; Snyder, SH. Parkinsonism-inducing neurotoxin, N-methyl-4-phenyl-1,2,3,6 -tetrahydropyridine: uptake of the metabolite N-methyl-4-phenylpyridine by dopamine neurons explains selective toxicity. *Proc Natl Acad Sci U S A*, 1985, (82), 2173-7.

[102] Nicklas, WJ; Vyas, I; Heikkila, RE. Inhibition of NADH-linked oxidation in brain mitochondria by 1-methyl-4-phenyl-pyridine, a metabolite of the neurotoxin, 1-methyl-4-phenyl-1,2,5,6-tetrahydropyridine. *Life Sci*, 1985, (36), 2503-8.

[103] Przedborski, S; Jackson-Lewis, V; Yokoyama, R; Shibata, T; Dawson, VL; Dawson, TM. Role of neuronal nitric oxide in 1-methyl-4-phenyl-1,2,3,6-tetrahydropyridine (MPTP)-induced dopaminergic neurotoxicity. *Proc Natl Acad Sci U S A*, 1996, (93), 4565-71.

[104] Tipton, KF; Singer, TP. Advances in our understanding of the mechanisms of the neurotoxicity of MPTP and related compounds. *J Neurochem*, 1993, (61), 1191-206.

[105] Schapira, AH. Evidence for mitochondrial dysfunction in Parkinson's disease--a critical appraisal. *Mov Disord*, 1994, (9), 125-38.

[106] Cooper, JM; Schapira, AH. Mitochondrial dysfunction in neurodegeneration. *J Bioenerg Biomembr*, 1997, (29), 175-83.

[107] Jenner, P; Schapira, AH; Marsden, CD. New insights into the cause of Parkinson's disease. *Neurology*, 1992, (42), 2241-50.

[108] Schapira, AH. Oxidative stress in Parkinson's disease. *Neuropathol Appl Neurobiol*, 1995, (21), 3-9.

[109] Schapira, AH; Cooper, JM; Dexter, D; Clark, JB; Jenner, P; Marsden, CD. Mitochondrial complex I deficiency in Parkinson's disease. *J Neurochem*, 1990, (54), 823-7.

[110] Seaton, TA; Cooper, JM; Schapira, AH. Free radical scavengers protect dopaminergic cell lines from apoptosis induced by complex I inhibitors. *Brain Res*, 1997, (777), 110-8.

[111] Doble, A. The role of excitotoxicity in neurodegenerative disease: implications for therapy. *Pharmacol Ther*, 1999, (81), 163-221.

[112] Beal, MF. Excitotoxicity and nitric oxide in Parkinson's disease pathogenesis. *Ann Neurol*, 1998, (44), S110-4.

[113] Jackson-Lewis, V; Smeyne, RJ. MPTP and SNpc DA neuronal vulnerability: role of dopamine, superoxide and nitric oxide in neurotoxicity. Minireview. *Neurotox Res*, 2005, (7), 193-202.

[114] Koutsilieri, E; Riederer, P. Excitotoxicity and new antiglutamatergic strategies in Parkinson's disease and Alzheimer's disease. *Parkinsonism Relat Disord*, 2007, (13 Suppl 3), S329-31.

[115] Luquin, MR; Saldise, L; Guillen, J; Belzunegui, S; San Sebastian, W; Izal, A; Garrido, P; Vazquez, M. Does increased excitatory drive from the subthalamic nucleus contribute to dopaminergic neuronal death in Parkinson's disease? *Exp Neurol*, 2006, (201), 407-15.

[116] Olney, JW; Zorumski, CF; Stewart, GR; Price, MT; Wang, GJ; Labruyere, J. Excitotoxicity of L-dopa and 6-OH-dopa: implications for Parkinson's and Huntington's diseases. *Exp Neurol*, 1990, (108), 269-72.

[117] Shaw, PJ. Excitatory amino acid neurotransmission, excitotoxicity and excitotoxins. *Curr Opin Neurol Neurosurg*, 1992, (5), 383-90.

[118] Rothstein, JD; Bristol, LA; Hosler, B; Brown, RH, Jr.; Kuncl, RW. Chronic inhibition of superoxide dismutase produces apoptotic death of spinal neurons. *Proc Natl Acad Sci U S A*, 1994, (91), 4155-9.

[119] Bergman, H; Deuschl, G. Pathophysiology of Parkinson's disease: from clinical neurology to basic neuroscience and back. *Mov Disord*, 2002, (17 Suppl 3), S28-40.

[120] DeLong, MR. Primate models of movement disorders of basal ganglia origin. *Trends Neurosci*, 1990, (13), 281-5.

[121] Rodriguez, MC; Obeso, JA; Olanow, CW. Subthalamic nucleus-mediated excitotoxicity in Parkinson's disease: a target for neuroprotection. *Ann Neurol*, 1998, (44), S175-88.
[122] Obeso, JA; Rodriguez-Oroz, MC; Rodriguez, M; Lanciego, JL; Artieda, J; Gonzalo, N; Olanow, CW. Pathophysiology of the basal ganglia in Parkinson's disease. *Trends Neurosci*, 2000, (23), S8-19.
[123] Mazzio, E; Huber, J; Darling, S; Harris, N; Soliman, KF. Effect of antioxidants on L-glutamate and N-methyl-4-phenylpyridinium ion induced-neurotoxicity in PC12 cells. *Neurotoxicology*, 2001, (22), 283-8.
[124] Turski, L; Bressler, K; Rettig, KJ; Loschmann, PA; Wachtel, H. Protection of substantia nigra from MPP+ neurotoxicity by N-methyl-D-aspartate antagonists. *Nature*, 1991, (349), 414-8.
[125] Morissette, M; Dridi, M; Calon, F; Hadj Tahar, A; Meltzer, LT; Bedard, PJ; Di Paolo, T. Prevention of dyskinesia by an NMDA receptor antagonist in MPTP monkeys: effect on adenosine A2A receptors. *Synapse*, 2006, (60), 239-50.
[126] Loschmann, PA; De Groote, C; Smith, L; Wullner, U; Fischer, G; Kemp, JA; Jenner, P; Klockgether, T. Antiparkinsonian activity of Ro 25-6981, a NR2B subunit specific NMDA receptor antagonist, in animal models of Parkinson's disease. *Exp Neurol*, 2004, (187), 86-93.
[127] Przuntek, H. Non-dopaminergic therapy in Parkinson's disease. *J Neurol*, 2000, (247 Suppl 2), II19-24.
[128] Calne, DB. Treatment of Parkinson's disease. *N Engl J Med*, 1993, (329), 1021-7.
[129] Horstink, M; Tolosa, E; Bonuccelli, U; Deuschl, G; Friedman, A; Kanovsky, P; Larsen, JP; Lees, A; Oertel, W; Poewe, W; Rascol, O; Sampaio, C. Review of the therapeutic management of Parkinson's disease. Report of a joint task force of the European Federation of Neurological Societies and the Movement Disorder Society-European Section. Part I: early (uncomplicated) Parkinson's disease. *Eur J Neurol*, 2006, (13), 1170-85.
[130] Kieburtz, K. Issues in neuroprotection clinical trials in Parkinson's disease. *Neurology*, 2006, (66), S50-7.
[131] Rascol, O; Goetz, C; Koller, W; Poewe, W; Sampaio, C. Treatment interventions for Parkinson's disease: an evidence based assessment. *Lancet*, 2002, (359), 1589-98.
[132] Fahn, S; Oakes, D; Shoulson, I; Kieburtz, K; Rudolph, A; Lang, A; Olanow, CW; Tanner, C; Marek, K. Levodopa and the progression of Parkinson's disease. *N Engl J Med*, 2004, (351), 2498-508.
[133] Nausieda, PA; Weiner, WJ; Kaplan, LR; Weber, S; Klawans, HL. Sleep disruption in the course of chronic levodopa therapy: an early feature of the levodopa psychosis. *Clin Neuropharmacol*, 1982, (5), 183-94.
[134] Ahlskog, JE; Muenter, MD. Frequency of levodopa-related dyskinesias and motor fluctuations as estimated from the cumulative literature. *Mov Disord*, 2001, (16), 448-58.
[135] Bhidayasiri, R; Truong, DD. Motor complications in Parkinson disease: clinical manifestations and management. *J Neurol Sci*, 2008, (266), 204-15.
[136] Jankovic, J. Motor fluctuations and dyskinesias in Parkinson's disease: clinical manifestations. *Mov Disord*, 2005, (20 Suppl 11), S11-6.
[137] Factor, SA; Molho, ES; Podskalny, GD; Brown, D. Parkinson's disease: drug-induced psychiatric states. *Adv Neurol*, 1995, (65), 115-38.

[138] Friedman, JH; Factor, SA. Atypical antipsychotics in the treatment of drug-induced psychosis in Parkinson's disease. *Mov Disord*, 2000, (15), 201-11.
[139] Moskovitz, C; Moses, H, 3rd; Klawans, HL. Levodopa-induced psychosis: a kindling phenomenon. *Am J Psychiatry*, 1978, (135), 669-75.
[140] Murer, MG; Dziewczapolski, G; Menalled, LB; Garcia, MC; Agid, Y; Gershanik, O; Raisman-Vozari, R. Chronic levodopa is not toxic for remaining dopamine neurons, but instead promotes their recovery, in rats with moderate nigrostriatal lesions. *Ann Neurol*, 1998, (43), 561-75.
[141] Agid, Y. Levodopa: is toxicity a myth? *Neurology*, 1998, (50), 858-63.
[142] Agid, Y; Chase, T; Marsden, D. Adverse reactions to levodopa: drug toxicity or progression of disease? *Lancet*, 1998, (351), 851-2.
[143] Mytilineou, C; Walker, RH; JnoBaptiste, R; Olanow, CW. Levodopa is toxic to dopamine neurons in an in vitro but not an in vivo model of oxidative stress. *J Pharmacol Exp Ther*, 2003, (304), 792-800.
[144] Ogawa, N. Levodopa and dopamine agonists in the treatment of Parkinson's disease: advantages and disadvantages. *Eur Neurol*, 1994, (34 Suppl 3), 20-8.
[145] Kostrzewa, RM; Kostrzewa, JP; Brus, R. Neuroprotective and neurotoxic roles of levodopa (L-DOPA) in neurodegenerative disorders relating to Parkinson's disease. *Amino Acids*, 2002, (23), 57-63.
[146] Murer, MG; Raisman-Vozari, R; Gershanik, O. Levodopa in Parkinson's disease: neurotoxicity issue laid to rest? *Drug Saf*, 1999, (21), 339-52.
[147] Simuni, T; Stern, MB. Does levodopa accelerate Parkinson's disease? *Drugs Aging*, 1999, (14), 399-408.
[148] Rascol, O; Brooks, DJ; Korczyn, AD; De Deyn, PP; Clarke, CE; Lang, AE. A five-year study of the incidence of dyskinesia in patients with early Parkinson's disease who were treated with ropinirole or levodopa. 056 Study Group. *N Engl J Med*, 2000, (342), 1484-91.
[149] Holloway, RG; Shoulson, I; Fahn, S; Kieburtz, K; Lang, A; Marek, K; McDermott, M; Seibyl, J; Weiner, W; Musch, B; Kamp, C; Welsh, M; Shinaman, A; Pahwa, R; Barclay, L; Hubble, J; LeWitt, P; Miyasaki, J; Suchowersky, O; Stacy, M; Russell, DS; Ford, B; Hammerstad, J; Riley, D; Standaert, D; Wooten, F; Factor, S; Jankovic, J; Atassi, F; Kurlan, R; Panisset, M; Rajput, A; Rodnitzky, R; Shults, C; Petsinger, G; Waters, C; Pfeiffer, R; Biglan, K; Borchert, L; Montgomery, A; Sutherland, L; Weeks, C; DeAngelis, M; Sime, E; Wood, S; Pantella, C; Harrigan, M; Fussell, B; Dillon, S; Alexander-Brown, B; Rainey, P; Tennis, M; Rost-Ruffner, E; Brown, D; Evans, S; Berry, D; Hall, J; Shirley, T; Dobson, J; Fontaine, D; Pfeiffer, B; Brocht, A; Bennett, S; Daigneault, S; Hodgeman, K; O'Connell, C; Ross, T; Richard, K; Watts, A. Pramipexole vs levodopa as initial treatment for Parkinson disease: a 4-year randomized controlled trial. *Arch Neurol*, 2004, (61), 1044-53.
[150] Rinne, UK; Bracco, F; Chouza, C; Dupont, E; Gershanik, O; Marti Masso, JF; Montastruc, JL; Marsden, CD. Early treatment of Parkinson's disease with cabergoline delays the onset of motor complications. Results of a double-blind levodopa controlled trial. The PKDS009 Study Group. *Drugs*, 1998, (55 Suppl 1), 23-30.
[151] Schade, R; Andersohn, F; Suissa, S; Haverkamp, W; Garbe, E. Dopamine agonists and the risk of cardiac-valve regurgitation. *N Engl J Med*, 2007, (356), 29-38.

[152] Shannon, KM; Bennett, JP, Jr.; Friedman, JH. Efficacy of pramipexole, a novel dopamine agonist, as monotherapy in mild to moderate Parkinson's disease. The Pramipexole Study Group. *Neurology*, 1997, (49), 724-8.
[153] A controlled trial of rotigotine monotherapy in early Parkinson's disease. *Arch Neurol*, 2003, (60), 1721-8.
[154] Quinn, N; Illas, A; Lhermitte, F; Agid, Y. Bromocriptine and domperidone in the treatment of Parkinson disease. *Neurology*, 1981, (31), 662-7.
[155] Friedman, JH; Fernandez, HH. Atypical antipsychotics in Parkinson-sensitive populations. *J Geriatr Psychiatry Neurol*, 2002, (15), 156-70.
[156] Nirenberg, MJ; Waters, C. Compulsive eating and weight gain related to dopamine agonist use. *Mov Disord*, 2006, (21), 524-9.
[157] Korczyn, AD; Nussbaum, M. Emerging therapies in the pharmacological treatment of Parkinson's disease. *Drugs*, 2002, (62), 775-86.
[158] Pinter, MM; Pogarell, O; Oertel, WH. Efficacy, safety, and tolerance of the non-ergoline dopamine agonist pramipexole in the treatment of advanced Parkinson's disease: a double blind, placebo controlled, randomised, multicentre study. *J Neurol Neurosurg Psychiatry*, 1999, (66), 436-41.
[159] Quinn, N. Drug treatment of Parkinson's disease. *BMJ*, 1995, (310), 575-9.
[160] Gerlach, M; Double, K; Reichmann, H; Riederer, P. Arguments for the use of dopamine receptor agonists in clinical and preclinical Parkinson's disease. *J Neural Transm Suppl*, 2003 167-83.
[161] Mannisto, PT; Kaakkola, S. Catechol-O-methyltransferase (COMT): biochemistry, molecular biology, pharmacology, and clinical efficacy of the new selective COMT inhibitors. *Pharmacol Rev*, 1999, (51), 593-628.
[162] Guldberg, HC; Marsden, CA. Catechol-O-methyl transferase: pharmacological aspects and physiological role. *Pharmacol Rev*, 1975, (27), 135-206.
[163] Rinne, UK; Larsen, JP; Siden, A; Worm-Petersen, J. Entacapone enhances the response to levodopa in parkinsonian patients with motor fluctuations. Nomecomt Study Group. *Neurology*, 1998, (51), 1309-14.
[164] Fowler, JS; Volkow, ND; Wang, GJ; Pappas, N; Logan, J; MacGregor, R; Alexoff, D; Shea, C; Schlyer, D; Wolf, AP; Warner, D; Zezulkova, I; Cilento, R. Inhibition of monoamine oxidase B in the brains of smokers. *Nature*, 1996, (379), 733-6.
[165] Talati, R; Reinhart, K; Baker, W; White, CM; Coleman, CI. Pharmacologic treatment of advanced Parkinson's disease: A meta-analysis of COMT inhibitors and MAO-B inhibitors. *Parkinsonism Relat Disord*, 2009.
[166] Ravina, BM; Fagan, SC; Hart, RG; Hovinga, CA; Murphy, DD; Dawson, TM; Marler, JR. Neuroprotective agents for clinical trials in Parkinson's disease: a systematic assessment. *Neurology*, 2003, (60), 1234-40.
[167] Pahwa, R; Factor, SA; Lyons, KE; Ondo, WG; Gronseth, G; Bronte-Stewart, H; Hallett, M; Miyasaki, J; Stevens, J; Weiner, WJ. Practice Parameter: treatment of Parkinson disease with motor fluctuations and dyskinesia (an evidence-based review): report of the Quality Standards Subcommittee of the American Academy of Neurology. *Neurology*, 2006, (66), 983-95.
[168] Goetz, CG; Poewe, W; Rascol, O; Sampaio, C. Evidence-based medical review update: pharmacological and surgical treatments of Parkinson's disease: 2001 to 2004. *Mov Disord*, 2005, (20), 523-39.

[169] de Smet, Y; Ruberg, M; Serdaru, M; Dubois, B; Lhermitte, F; Agid, Y. Confusion, dementia and anticholinergics in Parkinson's disease. *J Neurol Neurosurg Psychiatry*, 1982, (45), 1161-4.

[170] Van Spaendonck, KP; Berger, HJ; Horstink, MW; Buytenhuijs, EL; Cools, AR. Impaired cognitive shifting in parkinsonian patients on anticholinergic therapy. *Neuropsychologia*, 1993, (31), 407-11.

[171] Crosby, N; Deane, KH; Clarke, CE. Amantadine in Parkinson's disease. *Cochrane Database Syst Rev*, 2003 CD003468.

[172] Crosby, NJ; Deane, KH; Clarke, CE. Amantadine for dyskinesia in Parkinson's disease. *Cochrane Database Syst Rev*, 2003, CD003467.

[173] Dingledine, R; Borges, K; Bowie, D; Traynelis, SF. The glutamate receptor ion channels. *Pharmacol Rev*, 1999, (51), 7-61.

[174] Kornhuber, J; Weller, M; Schoppmeyer, K; Riederer, P. Amantadine and memantine are NMDA receptor antagonists with neuroprotective properties. *J Neural Transm Suppl*, 1994, (43), 91-104.

[175] Limousin, P; Krack, P; Pollak, P; Benazzouz, A; Ardouin, C; Hoffmann, D; Benabid, AL. Electrical stimulation of the subthalamic nucleus in advanced Parkinson's disease. *N Engl J Med*, 1998, (339), 1105-11.

[176] Laitinen, LV; Bergenheim, AT; Hariz, MI. Leksell's posteroventral pallidotomy in the treatment of Parkinson's disease. *J Neurosurg*, 1992, (76), 53-61.

[177] Forno, LS. Neuropathology of Parkinson's disease. *J Neuropathol Exp Neurol*, 1996, (55), 259-72.

[178] Pillon, B; Ardouin, C; Damier, P; Krack, P; Houeto, JL; Klinger, H; Bonnet, AM; Pollak, P; Benabid, AL; Agid, Y. Neuropsychological changes between "off" and "on" STN or GPi stimulation in Parkinson's disease. *Neurology*, 2000, (55), 411-8.

[179] Funkiewiez, A; Ardouin, C; Caputo, E; Krack, P; Fraix, V; Klinger, H; Chabardes, S; Foote, K; Benabid, AL; Pollak, P. Long term effects of bilateral subthalamic nucleus stimulation on cognitive function, mood, and behaviour in Parkinson's disease. *J Neurol Neurosurg Psychiatry*, 2004, (75), 834-9.

[180] Trepanier, LL; Saint-Cyr, JA; Lozano, AM; Lang, AE. Neuropsychological consequences of posteroventral pallidotomy for the treatment of Parkinson's disease. *Neurology*, 1998, (51), 207-15.

[181] Rettig, GM; York, MK; Lai, EC; Jankovic, J; Krauss, JK; Grossman, RG; Levin, HS. Neuropsychological outcome after unilateral pallidotomy for the treatment of Parkinson's disease. *J Neurol Neurosurg Psychiatry*, 2000, (69), 326-36.

[182] Obwegeser, AA; Uitti, RJ; Lucas, JA; Witte, RJ; Turk, MF; Wharen, RE, Jr. Predictors of neuropsychological outcome in patients following microelectrode-guided pallidotomy for Parkinson's disease. *J Neurosurg*, 2000, (93), 410-20.

[183] Deep-brain stimulation of the subthalamic nucleus or the pars interna of the globus pallidus in Parkinson's disease. *N Engl J Med*, 2001, (345), 956-63.

[184] Benabid, AL; Pollak, P; Gao, D; Hoffmann, D; Limousin, P; Gay, E; Payen, I; Benazzouz, A. Chronic electrical stimulation of the ventralis intermedius nucleus of the thalamus as a treatment of movement disorders. *J Neurosurg*, 1996, (84), 203-14.

[185] Schuurman, PR; Bosch, DA; Bossuyt, PM; Bonsel, GJ; van Someren, EJ; de Bie, RM; Merkus, MP; Speelman, JD. A comparison of continuous thalamic stimulation and thalamotomy for suppression of severe tremor. *N Engl J Med*, 2000, (342), 461-8.

[186] Benabid, AL; Pollak, P; Gervason, C; Hoffmann, D; Gao, DM; Hommel, M; Perret, JE; de Rougemont, J. Long-term suppression of tremor by chronic stimulation of the ventral intermediate thalamic nucleus. *Lancet*, 1991, (337), 403-6.
[187] Lozano, AM; Lang, AE; Galvez-Jimenez, N; Miyasaki, J; Duff, J; Hutchinson, WD; Dostrovsky, JO. Effect of GPi pallidotomy on motor function in Parkinson's disease. *Lancet*, 1995, (346), 1383-7.
[188] Baron, MS; Vitek, JL; Bakay, RA; Green, J; Kaneoke, Y; Hashimoto, T; Turner, RS; Woodard, JL; Cole, SA; McDonald, WM; DeLong, MR. Treatment of advanced Parkinson's disease by posterior GPi pallidotomy: 1-year results of a pilot study. *Ann Neurol*, 1996, (40), 355-66.
[189] Baron, MS; Vitek, JL; Bakay, RA; Green, J; McDonald, WM; Cole, SA; DeLong, MR. Treatment of advanced Parkinson's disease by unilateral posterior GPi pallidotomy: 4-year results of a pilot study. *Mov Disord*, 2000, (15), 230-7.
[190] Lindvall, O; Bjorklund, A. Cell therapy in Parkinson's disease. *NeuroRx*, 2004, (1), 382-93.
[191] McLaren, FH; Svendsen, CN; Van der Meide, P; Joly, E. Analysis of neural stem cells by flow cytometry: cellular differentiation modifies patterns of MHC expression. *J Neuroimmunol*, 2001, (112), 35-46.
[192] Dunnett, SB; Bjorklund, A. Prospects for new restorative and neuroprotective treatments in Parkinson's disease. *Nature*, 1999, (399), A32-9.
[193] Kordower, JH; Emborg, ME; Bloch, J; Ma, SY; Chu, Y; Leventhal, L; McBride, J; Chen, EY; Palfi, S; Roitberg, BZ; Brown, WD; Holden, JE; Pyzalski, R; Taylor, MD; Carvey, P; Ling, Z; Trono, D; Hantraye, P; Deglon, N; Aebischer, P. Neurodegeneration prevented by lentiviral vector delivery of GDNF in primate models of Parkinson's disease. *Science*, 2000, (290), 767-73.
[194] Gill, SS; Patel, NK; Hotton, GR; O'Sullivan, K; McCarter, R; Bunnage, M; Brooks, DJ; Svendsen, CN; Heywood, P. Direct brain infusion of glial cell line-derived neurotrophic factor in Parkinson disease. *Nat Med*, 2003, (9), 589-95.
[195] Lin, MT; Beal, MF. Mitochondrial dysfunction and oxidative stress in neurodegenerative diseases. *Nature*, 2006, (443), 787-95.
[196] de Goede, CJ; Keus, SH; Kwakkel, G; Wagenaar, RC. The effects of physical therapy in Parkinson's disease: a research synthesis. *Arch Phys Med Rehabil*, 2001, (82), 509-15.
[197] Mutch, WJ; Strudwick, A; Roy, SK; Downie, AW. Parkinson's disease: disability, review, and management. *Br Med J (Clin Res Ed)*, 1986, (293), 675-7.
[198] Cotman, CW; Berchtold, NC. Exercise: a behavioral intervention to enhance brain health and plasticity. *Trends Neurosci*, 2002, (25), 295-301.
[199] Barde, YA. Neurotrophins: a family of proteins supporting the survival of neurons. *Prog Clin Biol Res*, 1994, (390), 45-56.
[200] Lindvall, O; Kokaia, Z; Bengzon, J; Elmer, E; Kokaia, M. Neurotrophins and brain insults. *Trends Neurosci*, 1994, (17), 490-6.
[201] Crizzle, AM; Newhouse, IJ. Is physical exercise beneficial for persons with Parkinson's disease? *Clin J Sport Med*, 2006, (16), 422-5.
[202] Miyai, I; Fujimoto, Y; Ueda, Y; Yamamoto, H; Nozaki, S; Saito, T; Kang, J. Treadmill training with body weight support: its effect on Parkinson's disease. *Arch Phys Med Rehabil*, 2000, (81), 849-52.

[203] Miyai, I; Fujimoto, Y; Yamamoto, H; Ueda, Y; Saito, T; Nozaki, S; Kang, J. Long-term effect of body weight-supported treadmill training in Parkinson's disease: a randomized controlled trial. *Arch Phys Med Rehabil*, 2002, (83), 1370-3.
[204] Schenkman, M; Cutson, TM; Kuchibhatla, M; Chandler, J; Pieper, CF; Ray, L; Laub, KC. Exercise to improve spinal flexibility and function for people with Parkinson's disease: a randomized, controlled trial. *J Am Geriatr Soc*, 1998, (46), 1207-16.
[205] Baatile, J; Langbein, WE; Weaver, F; Maloney, C; Jost, MB. Effect of exercise on perceived quality of life of individuals with Parkinson's disease. *J Rehabil Res Dev*, 2000, (37), 529-34.
[206] Kuroda, K; Tatara, K; Takatorige, T; Shinsho, F. Effect of physical exercise on mortality in patients with Parkinson's disease. *Acta Neurol Scand*, 1992, (86), 55-9.
[207] Hirsch, MA; Toole, T; Maitland, CG; Rider, RA. The effects of balance training and high-intensity resistance training on persons with idiopathic Parkinson's disease. *Arch Phys Med Rehabil*, 2003, (84), 1109-17.
[208] Canning, CG; Alison, JA; Allen, NE; Groeller, H. Parkinson's disease: an investigation of exercise capacity, respiratory function, and gait. *Arch Phys Med Rehabil*, 1997, (78), 199-207.
[209] Stanley, RK; Protas, EJ; Jankovic, J. Exercise performance in those having Parkinson's disease and healthy normals. *Med Sci Sports Exerc*, 1999, (31), 761-6.
[210] Reuter, I; Engelhardt, M; Stecker, K; Baas, H. Therapeutic value of exercise training in Parkinson's disease. *Med Sci Sports Exerc*, 1999, (31), 1544-9.
[211] Koseoglu, F; Inan, L; Ozel, S; Deviren, SD; Karabiyikoglu, G; Yorgancioglu, R; Atasoy, T; Ozturk, A. The effects of a pulmonary rehabilitation program on pulmonary function tests and exercise tolerance in patients with Parkinson's disease. *Funct Neurol*, 1997, (12), 319-25.
[212] Gauthier, L; Dalziel, S; Gauthier, S. The benefits of group occupational therapy for patients with Parkinson's disease. *Am J Occup Ther*, 1987, (41), 360-5.
[213] Palmer, SS; Mortimer, JA; Webster, DD; Bistevins, R; Dickinson, GL. Exercise therapy for Parkinson's disease. *Arch Phys Med Rehabil*, 1986, (67), 741-5.
[214] Tillerson, JL; Caudle, WM; Reveron, ME; Miller, GW. Exercise induces behavioral recovery and attenuates neurochemical deficits in rodent models of Parkinson's disease. *Neuroscience*, 2003, (119), 899-911.
[215] Jones, TA; Schallert, T. Use-dependent growth of pyramidal neurons after neocortical damage. *J Neurosci*, 1994, (14), 2140-52.
[216] Stroemer, RP; Kent, TA; Hulsebosch, CE. Neocortical neural sprouting, synaptogenesis, and behavioral recovery after neocortical infarction in rats. *Stroke*, 1995, (26), 2135-44.
[217] Jackson-Lewis, V; Jakowec, M; Burke, RE; Przedborski, S. Time course and morphology of dopaminergic neuronal death caused by the neurotoxin 1-methyl-4-phenyl-1,2,3,6-tetrahydropyridine. *Neurodegeneration*, 1995, (4), 257-69.
[218] Fisher, BE; Petzinger, GM; Nixon, K; Hogg, E; Bremmer, S; Meshul, CK; Jakowec, MW. Exercise-induced behavioral recovery and neuroplasticity in the 1-methyl-4-phenyl-1,2,3,6-tetrahydropyridine-lesioned mouse basal ganglia. *J Neurosci Res*, 2004, (77), 378-90.
[219] Gainetdinov, RR; Sotnikova, TD; Caron, MG. Monoamine transporter pharmacology and mutant mice. *Trends Pharmacol Sci*, 2002, (23), 367-73.

[220] Mortensen, OV; Amara, SG. Dynamic regulation of the dopamine transporter. *Eur J Pharmacol*, 2003, (479), 159-70.
[221] Page, G; Peeters, M; Najimi, M; Maloteaux, JM; Hermans, E. Modulation of the neuronal dopamine transporter activity by the metabotropic glutamate receptor mGluR5 in rat striatal synaptosomes through phosphorylation mediated processes. *J Neurochem*, 2001, (76), 1282-90.
[222] Petzinger, GM; Walsh, JP; Akopian, G; Hogg, E; Abernathy, A; Arevalo, P; Turnquist, P; Vuckovic, M; Fisher, BE; Togasaki, DM; Jakowec, MW. Effects of treadmill exercise on dopaminergic transmission in the 1-methyl-4-phenyl-1,2,3,6-tetrahydropyridine-lesioned mouse model of basal ganglia injury. *J Neurosci*, 2007, (27), 5291-300.
[223] Jaber, M; Dumartin, B; Sagne, C; Haycock, JW; Roubert, C; Giros, B; Bloch, B; Caron, MG. Differential regulation of tyrosine hydroxylase in the basal ganglia of mice lacking the dopamine transporter. *Eur J Neurosci*, 1999, (11), 3499-511.
[224] Fauchey, V; Jaber, M; Caron, MG; Bloch, B; Le Moine, C. Differential regulation of the dopamine D1, D2 and D3 receptor gene expression and changes in the phenotype of the striatal neurons in mice lacking the dopamine transporter. *Eur J Neurosci*, 2000, (12), 19-26.
[225] Bezard, E; Jaber, M; Gonon, F; Boireau, A; Bloch, B; Gross, CE. Adaptive changes in the nigrostriatal pathway in response to increased 1-methyl-4-phenyl-1,2,3,6-tetrahydropyridine-induced neurodegeneration in the mouse. *Eur J Neurosci*, 2000, (12), 2892-900.
[226] Kelley, AE; Cador, M; Stinus, L. Behavioral analysis of the effect of substance P injected into the ventral mesencephalon on investigatory and spontaneous motor behavior in the rat. *Psychopharmacology (Berl)*, 1985, (85), 37-46.
[227] Carlsson, A. Monoamine-depleting drugs. *Pharmacol Ther [B]*, 1975, (1), 393-400.
[228] Colpaert, FC. Pharmacological characteristics of tremor, rigidity and hypokinesia induced by reserpine in rat. *Neuropharmacology*, 1987, (26), 1431-40.
[229] Kaur, S; Starr, MS. Antiparkinsonian action of dextromethorphan in the reserpine-treated mouse. *Eur J Pharmacol*, 1995, (280), 159-66.
[230] Menzaghi, F; Whelan, KT; Risbrough, VB; Rao, TS; Lloyd, GK. Interactions between a novel cholinergic ion channel agonist, SIB-1765F and L-DOPA in the reserpine model of Parkinson's disease in rats. *J Pharmacol Exp Ther*, 1997, (280), 393-401.
[231] Elverfors, A; Nissbrandt, H. Reserpine-insensitive dopamine release in the substantia nigra? *Brain Res*, 1991, (557), 5-12.
[232] Zhang, WQ; Tilson, HA; Nanry, KP; Hudson, PM; Hong, JS; Stachowiak, MK. Increased dopamine release from striata of rats after unilateral nigrostriatal bundle damage. *Brain Res*, 1988, (461), 335-42.
[233] Brown, LL; Sharp, FR. Metabolic mapping of rat striatum: somatotopic organization of sensorimotor activity. *Brain Res*, 1995, (686), 207-22.
[234] Cospito, JA; Kultas-Ilinsky, K. Synaptic organization of motor corticostriatal projections in the rat. *Exp Neurol*, 1981, (72), 257-66.
[235] Ebrahimi, A; Pochet, R; Roger, M. Topographical organization of the projections from physiologically identified areas of the motor cortex to the striatum in the rat. *Neurosci Res*, 1992, (14), 39-60.

[236] Holschneider, DP; Maarek, JM; Yang, J; Harimoto, J; Scremin, OU. Functional brain mapping in freely moving rats during treadmill walking. *J Cereb Blood Flow Metab*, 2003, (23), 925-32.
[237] Hawkes, CH; Shephard, BC; Daniel, SE. Olfactory dysfunction in Parkinson's disease. *J Neurol Neurosurg Psychiatry*, 1997, (62), 436-46.
[238] Hawkes, CH; Shephard, BC; Daniel, SE. Is Parkinson's disease a primary olfactory disorder? *QJM*, 1999, (92), 473-80.
[239] Sawyer, TF; Hengehold, AK; Perez, WA. Chemosensory and hormonal mediation of social memory in male rats. *Behav Neurosci*, 1984, (98), 908-13.
[240] Dantzer, R; Bluthe, RM; Koob, GF; Le Moal, M. Modulation of social memory in male rats by neurohypophyseal peptides. *Psychopharmacology (Berl)*, 1987, (91), 363-8.
[241] Perio, A; Terranova, JP; Worms, P; Bluthe, RM; Dantzer, R; Biziere, K. Specific modulation of social memory in rats by cholinomimetic and nootropic drugs, by benzodiazepine inverse agonists, but not by psychostimulants. *Psychopharmacology (Berl)*, 1989, (97), 262-8.
[242] Prediger, RD; Takahashi, RN. Ethanol improves short-term social memory in rats. Involvement of opioid and muscarinic receptors. *Eur J Pharmacol*, 2003, (462), 115-23.
[243] Terranova, JP; Perio, A; Worms, P; Le Fur, G; Soubrie, P. Social olfactory recognition in rodents: deterioration with age, cerebral ischaemia and septal lesion. *Behav Pharmacol*, 1994, (5), 90-8.
[244] Cotman, CW; Berchtold, NC; Christie, LA. Exercise builds brain health: key roles of growth factor cascades and inflammation. *Trends Neurosci*, 2007, (30), 464-72.
[245] Cotman, CW; Engesser-Cesar, C. Exercise enhances and protects brain function. *Exerc Sport Sci Rev*, 2002, (30), 75-9.
[246] van Praag, H; Christie, BR; Sejnowski, TJ; Gage, FH. Running enhances neurogenesis, learning, and long-term potentiation in mice. *Proc Natl Acad Sci U S A*, 1999, (96), 13427-31.
[247] van Praag, H; Kempermann, G; Gage, FH. Running increases cell proliferation and neurogenesis in the adult mouse dentate gyrus. *Nat Neurosci*, 1999, (2), 266-70.
[248] Aguiar, AS, Jr.; Speck, AE; Prediger, RD; Kapczinski, F; Pinho, RA. Downhill training upregulates mice hippocampal and striatal brain-derived neurotrophic factor levels. *J Neural Transm*, 2008, (115), 1251-5.
[249] Neeper, SA; Gomez-Pinilla, F; Choi, J; Cotman, CW. Physical activity increases mRNA for brain-derived neurotrophic factor and nerve growth factor in rat brain. *Brain Res*, 1996, (726), 49-56.
[250] Ogonovszky, H; Berkes, I; Kumagai, S; Kaneko, T; Tahara, S; Goto, S; Radak, Z. The effects of moderate-, strenuous- and over-training on oxidative stress markers, DNA repair, and memory, in rat brain. *Neurochem Int*, 2005, (46), 635-40.
[251] Radak, Z; Kaneko, T; Tahara, S; Nakamoto, H; Pucsok, J; Sasvari, M; Nyakas, C; Goto, S. Regular exercise improves cognitive function and decreases oxidative damage in rat brain. *Neurochem Int*, 2001, (38), 17-23.
[252] Radak, Z; Toldy, A; Szabo, Z; Siamilis, S; Nyakas, C; Silye, G; Jakus, J; Goto, S. The effects of training and detraining on memory, neurotrophins and oxidative stress markers in rat brain. *Neurochem Int*, 2006, (49), 387-92.

In: Encyclopedia of Sports and Athletics
Editors: Jack L. Murray and Emily O. Watson

ISBN: 978-1-61209-959-0

Chapter IV

Nutrition Strategy during an Eight–Day Mountainbike Stage Race – A Case Study

Katharina C. Wirnitzer*
Department of Sport Science, University of Innsbruck, Innsbruck, Austria

Abstract

Introduction

The Transalp Challenge (TAC) is one of the most difficult mountainbike (MTB) stage races in the world. Professional and amateur cyclists are required to cope with an altitude difference of 22500 m and a distance of 662 km within eight successive stages. Therefore, the purpose of this study was to determine the nutrient intake during the TAC.

Method

The subject was a female vegan MTBer (age: 30 years, height: 1.61 m, body mass: 49 ± 1 kg) finishing the TAC 2004 (41 hours 59 minutes 45 seconds, final ranking of 16th place). The athlete has been successfully following a vegan lifestyle for five years. Dietary intake was completely recorded over the full period of competition. Fluid intake (FI) and energy intake (EI) were calculated and subdivided into macronutrients carbohydrate (CHO), protein and fat.

Results

The exercise intensity of 88 ± 2 % of HR_{MAX} determined in the field was maintained over eight days. EI was found to be 24.61 MJ/day. Total calories contribute to 83.3 %

* Corresponding author: Berchat 302/2, A – 6135 Stans, Phone: +43 (650) 590 17 94, E–mail: katharina@wirnitzer.at

from CHO, 7.5 % from protein and 9.2 % from fat. The female ingested 17.4 % pre–race, 35.2 % while racing and 47.4 % post–race.

Discussion

This was the first study showing a well planned vegan diet to adequately meet the nutritional demands of severe MTB stage racing. The dietary requirements of a TAC are challenging for several reasons. Opportunities and time available for FI and EI are restricted by a great diversity of terrains and traits (difficult nature of course profile) simultaneously with aggressive riding tactics. After many years of research, mainly focused on health aspects, the effects of a plant–based diet on athletic performance are still unclear. However, any athlete, regardless of whether omnivore or vegan, should plan his/her diet carefully to avoid the risk of nutritional deficiencies and adverse effects on performance. It is broadly accepted that athletes involved in heavy endurance exercise should ingest a higher amount of energy from CHO to maximize muscle glycogen synthesis. The main advantages of vegetarian diets are the higher amount of CHO, lower fat and adequate protein. Especially vegans consume the majority of their energy from CHO. Therefore, endurance athletes may adopt vegetarian diets as an optimum strategy. Generally, endurance training and competition tend to reduce iron stores. However, iron deficiency occurs in 20 % of the world population, reflecting a similar incidence among vegetarians or vegans compared to omnivores.

Keywords: Mountainbiking; marathon; stage race; nutrition; female; vegan

Introduction

Protein – A Historical Review

In 1839 the Dutch chemist Gerhard Mulder discovered the nitrogen–containing chemical substance protein (Greek: proteios, “of premium importance“). Early scientists such as the German Carl Voit were staunch advocates of protein. He stated that “man” cannot get too much protein. Voit was the mentor of several nutritional scientists in the early 1900s, such as W. O. Atwater (organizer and director of the first nutrition laboratory at the United States Department of Agriculture/USA). The British physician Major McCay was stationed in the colony of India (1912). By identifying good fighting men in the Indian tribes, he commented that people who consumed less protein were found to be of worse physique (Campbell and Campbell 2006).

To date, protein is still the most misunderstood and misinterpreted of all nutrients. In the nineteenth century protein was synonymous with animal protein. Protein was, and today still is, equated with meat. The vital force was suggested to be exclusively inserted into meat. Therefore, the people were encouraged to eat as much meat as possible. The belief in this connection is still held by many people. Most people immediately think of meat, when they consider protein. That is why vegetarians and vegans still have to face the question of how they will obtain their protein requirements, because plant based protein is even thought to be execrable (Campbell and Campbell 2006).

Following the accumulated scientific knowledge of former times, someone ate plenty of protein (meat), if he/she was civilized and rich. When a person was poor and belonged to the lower social classes, they ate plant based foods such as potatoes and bread. They were considered to be indolent and less capable, as a result of not eating sufficient amounts of animal protein. As a consequence, this leaded to a fundamental cultural bias that had become firmly entrenched (Campbell and Campbell 2006).

Scientific Studies Considering Plant Based Nutrition Connected to Sports

The relationship between nutrition and exercise has been a major area of scientific interest for over 150 years (Febbraio 2002).

In the late 1800s the London Vegetarian Society formed an athletic and cycling club to compete against their meat eating counterparts which outperformed them in most cases during athletic competition (Niemann 1988). In 1893 such a cycling race was conducted from Berlin to Vienna (599 km) in which the first two finishers were vegetarian (Whorton 1982).

At the beginning of the 20th century, Russell H. Chittenden, a well established scientist in the field of nutrition at the Yale University Medical School, studied whether the consumption of plant based diets influences physical capacities. The physical performance of the male subjects (students, fellow faculty members, himself) was measured during laboratory testing. He found that ingesting a plant based diet enables the subject to exercise more, with less fatigue, compared with a diet based on animal protein (Chittenden 1904/1907). Simultaneously and also at Yale, Irving Fisher (having a wide range of interests including diet and nutrition) designed a series of tests to compare the stamina and strength of meat–eaters against those of vegetarians. Male subjects were selected from three groups: meat–eating athletes, vegetarian athletes and vegetarian sedentary subjects. The results have shown that vegetarians have twice the stamina of meat eaters, showing the latter to have far less endurance than the vegetarians (even in sedentary subjects). He reasoned that the difference in endurance was entirely due to the difference in their diet. He provided strong evidence that a vegetarian diet raises endurance (Fisher 1907).

In 1968, a Danish team of researchers re–popularized Fishers classic Yale study. A variety of diets were tested on male subjects by using a stationary bicycle to measure their strength and endurance. First, the men were fed a mixed diet of meat and vegetables for a period of time, and then tested on the bicycle. The average time they could pedal before muscle failure was 114 minutes. Later, they were fed a diet rich in meat, milk and eggs for a similar period and were then re–tested. On the high animal protein diet, their pedalling time dropped dramatically to 57 minutes. Finally, the group was switched to a strictly vegetarian diet, composed of grains, vegetables and fruits. Following a diet lacking in animal products, they pedalled for an average of 167 minutes (Astrand 1968).

Growing Interest in Vegetarian Diets

Since the 1960s, there has been a growth in professional interest in vegetarian nutrition. As shown in Figure 1, the number of articles in the scientific literature related to vegetarism has increased (Sabate et. al. 1999). Additionally, the main focus of the articles is changing. In the late 1960s, articles primarily tended to question the nutritional adequacy of vegetarian diets. More recently, the predominant issue has been the use of vegetarian diets in the prevention and treatment of chronic disease. There is a growing appreciation of the clear benefits of plant–based diets (Campbell and Campbell 2006, ADA 2003).

In 1978, the earliest major report on five studies which measured the diets of a cohort of individuals and monitored their subsequent death was published. It compared disease mortality in pure vegetarians (vegans) with that in other vegetarians and meat–eaters. The results showed the vegans to have had the lowest rates of mortality due to heart disease. Along with other studies, this confirmed the vegetarian diets to be beneficial against heart disease (Phillips et. al. 1978).

Mountainbike Stage Racing

In July 1998, the first Transalp Challenge (TAC) was organized, based on the model of the major road cycling tours. The TAC is considered to be one of the most difficult mountainbike (MTB) races in the world. Professional and amateur cyclists are required to cross the Central Alps (Figure 2) during eight successive stages, each consisting of an ultraendurance MTB marathon (> 4 hours of exercise: Peters 2003).

To finish this MTB event, tremendous strains have to be accomplished and vast amounts of energy have to be replaced. Therefore, careful planning and monitoring of nutrient intake is required to meet the energy demands of stage racing. Although MTB stage events are still growing in popularity, to the best of author`s knowledge, no studies have yet examined dietary intake during this kind of competition. Moreover, as increasing numbers of women are participating in road cycling and MTB sports, recommendations for their dietary intake in order to improve performance have become important, in addition to information about the requirements of the vegetarian and vegan cyclist. The use of current dietary recommendations for female athletes is limited as they have been developed from male athletic populations (Gabel 2002). In general, data on female cyclists is sparse and insufficient, if available at all (Burke 2001).

Recently, Wirnitzer and Kornexl (2008) were the first to study exercise intensity during the TAC 2004. The knowledge of the exercise intensity and the nutritional requirements of cross–country marathon (XCM) races is essential to develop appropriate training interventions and adequate nutritional strategies in order to sustain the physical demands of MTB stage races.

Therefore, the purpose of this study was i) to quantify the exercise intensity of the TAC 2004 by measuring the heart rate (HR) response and ii) to determine the energy intake of a female vegan athlete during the TAC 2004.

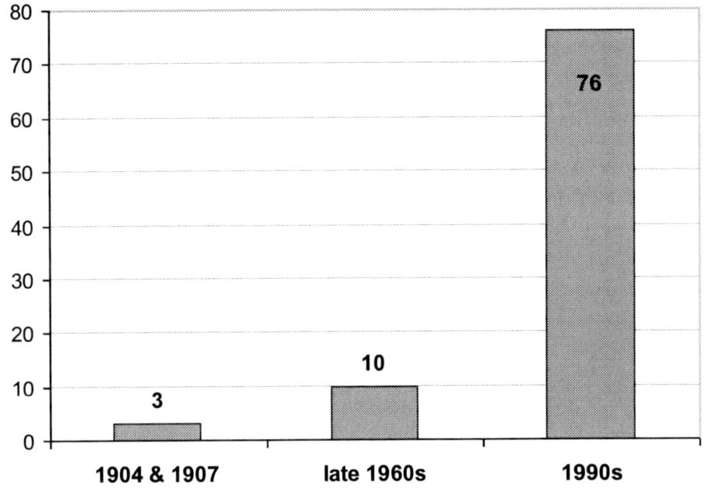

Figure 1. Development of scientific interest in vegetarian nutrition, showing the number of articles published per year, drawn from Chittenden (1904/1097), Fisher (1907) as well as Sabate et. al. (1999).

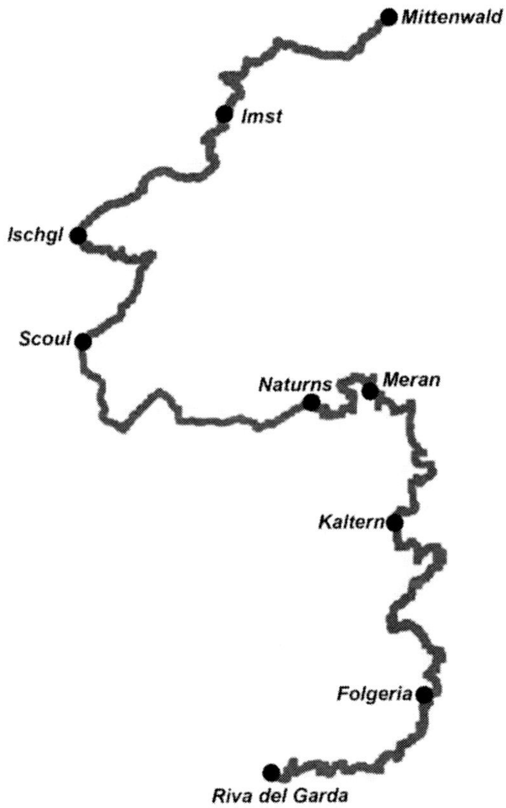

©Uli Stanciu

Figure 2. Course of Transalp Challenge 2004 (with permission of the organizer) covering an altitude difference of 22.500 m along with a distance of 662 km, starting at Mittenwald, Germany, passing the Tyrol, Austria and finishing at Riva del Garda, Italy.

Table 1. Characteristics of the female vegan mountainbiker and results of incremental laboratory test prior to the start of the Transalp Challenge 2004 (starting at 100 W, steps of 30 W every 5 min) are mean. PO = power output, PPO = peak PO, LT = fixed lactate threshold of 2 (LT2), 4 (LT4), 6 (LT6) mmol/L, HR = heart rate, bpm = beats/min

	Unit	Female Mountainbiker
Anthropological characteristics		
Age	years	30.0
Body mass	kg	47.0
Height	cm	161
Hematological characteristics		
Iron	µg/dl	105
Transferrin	mg/dl	238
Transferrin saturation	%	31
Hemoglobin	g/dl	14
Hematocrit	%	41
Vitamin B 12	pg/ml	280
Physiological Characteristics		
PPO	W	214
	W/kg	4.6
PO at LT2	W	174
	W/kg	3.5
	% max	76.1
PO at LT4	W	199
	W/kg	4.0
	% max	87.0
PO at LT6	W	213
	W/kg	4.3
	% max	93.5
Maximal HR	bpm	182
HR at LT2	bpm	154
	% max	84.6
HR at LT4	bpm	166
	% max	91.2
HR at LT6	bpm	168
	% max	92.3

Methods

Subject

One female amateur, a well experienced endurance off–road cyclist, was recruited for this case report. Table 1 shows the anthropological and physiological characteristics of the female subject. In 2004 she participated in the TAC for the second time, having previously completed the TAC in 2003. The MTB used was a front suspension bike (10.2 kg). To prepare for this eight day stage race, the subject trained for between 20 – 25 hours a week (including several ultraendurance MTB marathon races) over almost a year. The female rider had successfully followed a vegan lifestyle (a dietary pattern exclusively sourced from plant based nutrition, rejecting all products directly or indirectly sourced from or tested on animals) both as a daily lifestyle and during endurance training and competition for five years (and to date, still does in 2009). The study was approved by the Institutional Review Board and, according to the Declaration of Helsinki, was performed during the TAC 2004. Written informed consent was obtained after explanation of the procedures.

Laboratory Testing

Two weeks prior to the TAC 2004 a standardized blood test was conducted (samples drawn by a physician and analyzed at a professional diagnostics laboratory, both at the athlete`s hometown) to determine the micronutrient levels of iron, iron stores, hemoglobin, hematocrit and vitamin B 12.

Seven days before the start of the TAC 2004 the subject performed an incremental laboratory cycling test on an electromagnetically braked ergometer (Schoberer Rad Messtechnik SRM GmbH, Jülich, Germany). Exhaustive exercise had been avoided for at least 15 hours prior to the test. After 15 min of warm up with freely chosen workload and cadence, the test started at 100 W and workload was increased by 30 W every 5 min. The subject was instructed to maintain the cadence at 90 revolutions/min (rpm; range 85 – 95 rpm; Takaishi et al. 1996). The test was terminated upon voluntary exhaustion or incapacity to maintain the given cadence. When the final work load was not maintained for the full period peak power output (PPO) was calculated using the equation of Kuipers et. al. (1985): $PPO = PO_{FINAL} + (t/300s \times 30W)$, where PO_{FINAL} is the value for the last complete workload, 300 is the duration of each step in seconds, 30 W is the power output (PO) increment, and t is the time in seconds of the incomplete workload. In the last 30 s of each step, capillary blood samples (10 μL) were taken from the ear lobe and immediately analyzed (Vario Photometer, Diaglobal GmbH, Berlin, BRD). During the test, heart rate (HR) and PO were continuously recorded.

Following the first study during the TAC 2004 recently published by Wirnitzer and Kornexl (2008), the intensity zones were defined using the HR corresponding to the lactate thresholds (LTs). For the female, the HR at a fixed concentration of 2 mmol/L (LT2) and 4 mmol/L (LT4) was determined. In addition, in order to obtain an exercise intensity zone which better reflects very high–demanding efforts, the HR at 6 mmol/L (LT6) was measured. At and above this level energy supply is increasingly met by anaerobic sources (growing recruitment of type IIa fibres: Gilman 1996, Gilman and Wells 1993). HR values at LTs were identified by straight line interpolation between the two closest points. According to Wirnitzer and Kornexl (2008), four intensity zones were identified which describe the exercise intensity profile of the Transalp Challenge 2004:

1. LOW zone for intensity below the HR corresponding to LT2
2. MODERATE zone for intensity between the HR corresponding to LT2 and LT4
3. HIGH zone for intensity between the HR corresponding to LT4 and LT6
4. VERY HIGH zone for intensity above the HR corresponding to LT6

Characteristics of the Race

1074 athletes participated in the TAC 2004. The total altitude climbed was 22500 m and the total distance covered by the riders was 662 km. This resulted in a daily average altitude climbed of about 2810 m over a distance of 83 km. In terms of the total daily load, single stages were comparable to these of the mountainous Vuelta a Espana. The longest uphill climb and downhill section as one unit was 1700 m and 1400 m in altitude difference, respectively. The total distance climbed uphill was 315 km and was 275 km in downhill section. The course profile of the TAC 2004 (Stage 1 to 8) is presented in Figures 3 to 10. Peak values of temperature and relative humidity were taken from meteorological stations nearest to competitive waypoints of the TAC 2004 (ZAMG, Innsbruck, Austria). The characteristics of the TAC 2004 are presented in Table 2.

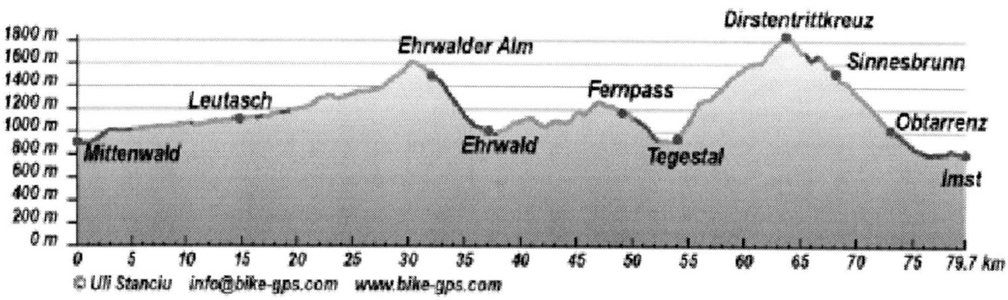

Figure 3. Stage 1 (Mittenwald, Germany to Imst, Austria).

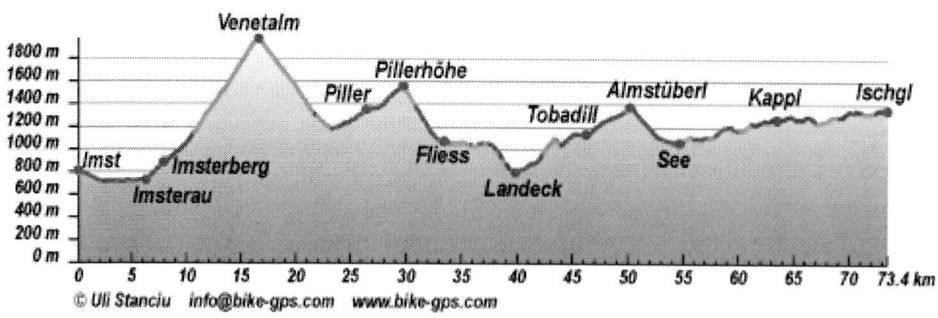

Figure 4. Stage 2 (Imst, Austria to Ischgl, Austria).

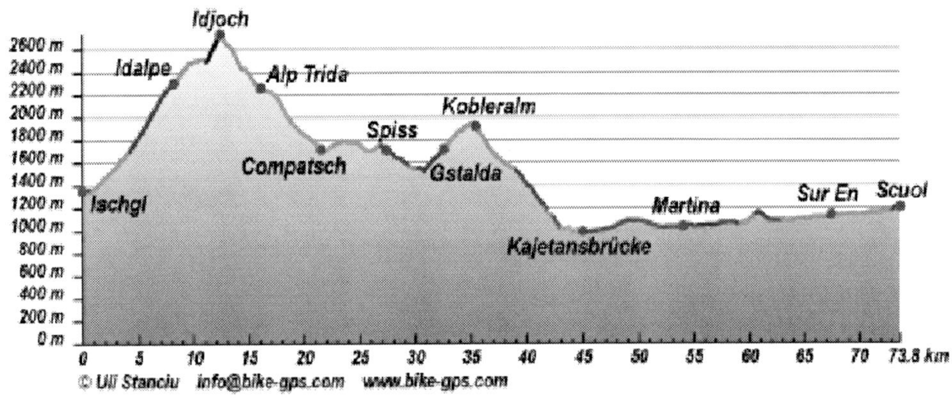

Figure 5. Stage 3 (Ischgl, Austria to Scuol, Switzerland).

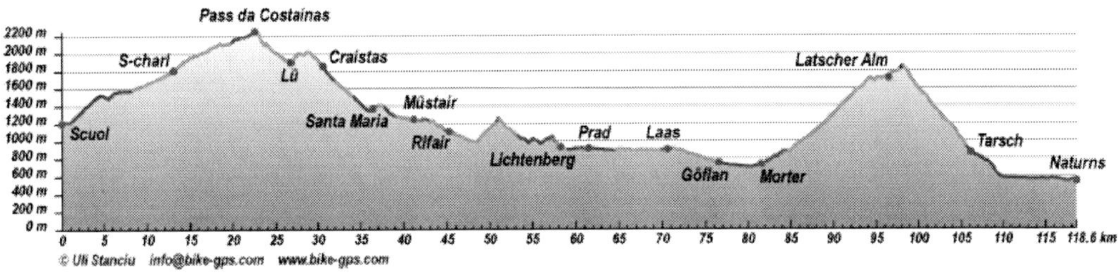

Figure 6. Stage 4 (Scuol, Switzerland to Naturns, Italy).

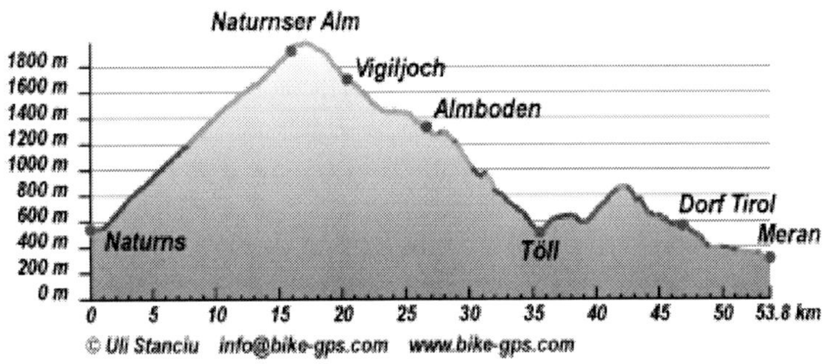

Figure 7. Stage 5 (Naturns, Italy to Meran, Italy).

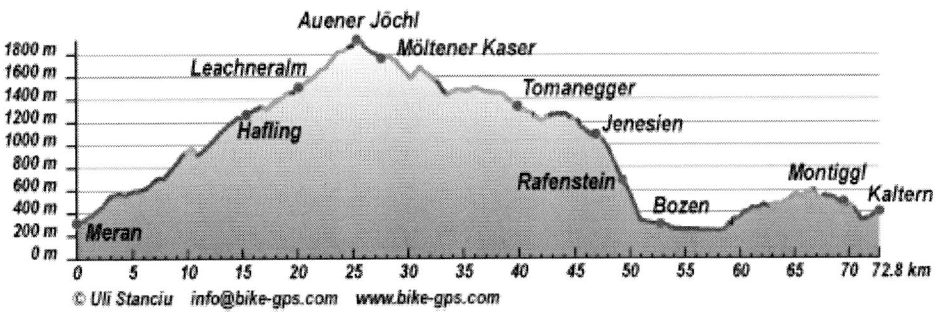

Figure 8. Stage 6 (Meran, Italy to Kaltern, Italy).

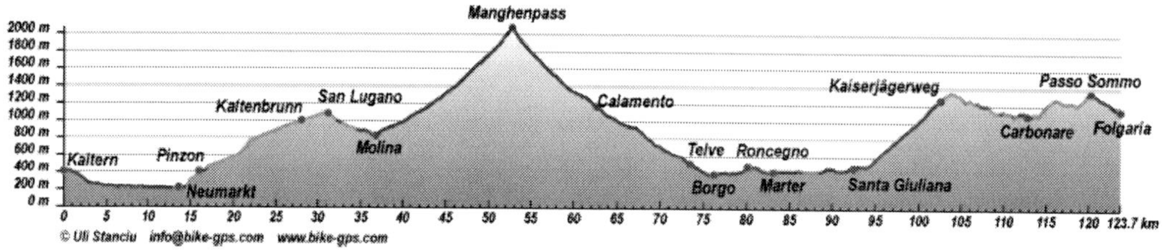

Figure 9. Stage 7 (Kaltern, Italy to Folgaria, Italy).

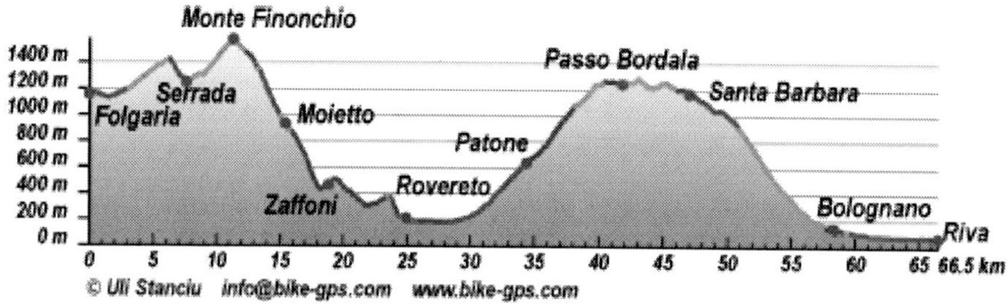

Figure 10. Final and rainy Stage 8 (Folgaria, Italy to Riva del Garda, Italy).

Collection of Field Data

During the TAC 2004, the HR response was continuously monitored using a short range HR telemetry system (S710, Polar Electro Oy, Kempele, Finland). The HR was recorded using a sample rate of 60 s in order to be able to store the HR data of the entire MTB event. At the end of this stage race the data set was analysed using a specific software (Polar Precision Performance 4 SW, Polar Electro Oy, Kempele, Finland), excluding from the analysis HR files which contained more than 5 % of sample data outside a range of 60 – 220 beats/min (bpm). The relative intensity of exercise was expressed as percentage of maximum HR reached in each stage (HR_{MAX}Field) and of laboratory determined maximum HR (HR_{MAX}Lab).

Immediately after finishing the daily stage, the cyclist rated how hard the entire stage had been overall, by reporting the rate of perceived exertion (RPE scale 6–20: Borg 1998). Furthermore, the body mass was measured including bike uniform but without MTB shoes (Medica, Soehnle, Germany).

The female was instructed to maintain adequate fluid and nutritional intake (high in carbohydrates). Recommendations for fluid intake were assumed from Maughan (2002) and Jeukendrup (2002a). Current guidelines for carbohydrate (CHO) intake were adopted (Burke 2002, Hargreaves 2002, Jentjens 2002, Jeukendrup 2002a). Using a self–reported survey, the dietary intake was continuously recorded in detail with the maximum possible accuracy for all fluid and food consumed over the full period of eight consecutive days. Fluid intake (FI) and energy intake (EI) were calculated for three occasions and subdivided into macronutrients CHO, protein and fat:

1. Pre race (breakfast)
2. Race (sports drink, solid energy bars and energy gels)
3. Post race (including snacks and dinner)

The recorded daily FI took into consideration the kind of fluid and was calculated from both the reported number and content of ingested cups, glasses and bottles of fluid and drinking bottles of sport drinks down to an accuracy of 125 ml. The energy value and contents of ingested sport drinks of prepared and packed commercial substrate was available from their food labels. Furthermore, the energy value and nutritional data of any alcohol consumed was derived from manufacturer`s declarations. Based on the personal conversations with the head waiter, the latter information was received by respectively contacting the producers.

Energy content and composition of prepared and packed commercial energy food (solid bars and gels) were taken from the manufacturer`s declaration. The energy content and detailed information for pieced and/or portioned food (such as bread, pate, fresh or dried fruit, snacks) were taken directly from food labels, where available. Otherwise, the mass of pieces and/or portions of food was weighed using kitchen scales (accuracy of 10 g: Culina Plus, Soehnle, Germany). Based on personal communication with the chef of any bed & breakfast or restaurant, the EI was then calculated from the detailed nutritional information of standardized portions (e. g. type of bread, ingredients, distribution of macronutrients). Similarly, the analysis and calculation of EI of a specific dish of combined food (such as standardized portions of pizza and pasta,) was derived from nutritional data (as described above) after personal conversation with the relevant chef. From this information, if no food label or further description of nutritional content from other sources was available (which could be totalled to a negligible magnitude), the calculation of total EI and the respective macronutrients for each piece, portion or combined dish of food was determined by using the nutritional information chart of Petter and Pohlmann (2007) as well as some standardized food composition databases available online (www.dge.de, www.naehrwerttabelle.de, www.bleibfit.at).

The translation of units was calculated according to the Systeme International d` Unites (SI: www.bipm.org, www.bipm.org/en/CGPM/db/11/12/). Following this concept, the energy of 1 kcal equates to 4.1868 kJ (http://ester). The quantity of energy ingested was calculated according to Geiss and Hamm (1992): 1 gram of CHO equates to 4.1 kcal, 1 gram of protein to 4.1 kcal and 1 gram of fat to 9.3 kcal.

Results

Given the technical, physical and mental difficulties of a Transalp Challenge, the drop out rate after eight days of competition was 18.81 % for whole bulk of TAC 2004, also including professional riders.

Performance

The subject showed a relative PPO of 4.6 W/kg during laboratory testing. The female MTBer finished the TAC 2004 in 41 hours 59 minutes 45 seconds, achieving a final ranking of 16th place (with the world elite of professional MTB marathon and cross–country (XC) athletes on occupying the higher rankings). The average daily runtime was 5 hours 15 minutes (ranging between 4 – 7 hours) with an average speed of 15.6 km/h.

The mean exercise intensity expressed as percentage of HR_{MAX} determined in the field was 88 ± 2 %. The time spent in the respective intensity zones low, moderate, high and very high – determined using the HR_{MAX}Field – was 15.1 %, 32.5 %, 41.6 % and 10.8 % of total race time, respectively. The results of exercise intensity during the eight stages are presented in Table 3.

Dietary Intake

During the TAC 2004, dietary intake reached maximum values with a FI of 4.5 L and an EI of 3116 kcal during "king size" Stage 7. In contrast, values were minimal during the cool and rainy Stage 8 (FI was 1.5 L, EI was 1409 kcal). Tables 4 – 6 depict the dietary intake during the whole period of TAC 2004.

The full period of 24 hours was accounted for by pre race period (6 – 8 a. m.), daily runtime, time for sleep (10 p. m. – 6 a. m.) and post exercise recovery period, which was found on average to be 8 hours 45 minutes.

Environmental Conditions and Fluid Intake

The athlete had to cope with high temperatures for almost two third of the whole race (28 – 33 °C) with an average temperature of 28 °C. Six of the eight stages were competed under dry conditions (44 – 50 % relative humidity). Daily FI ranged from 4.25 L to 7.75 L, reflecting a daily average of 5.48 L. Fluid ingested during breakfast, averaging of 200 ml/day (3.7 % of total FI), came exclusively from tea (English or Green) without sugar. The fluid ingested while racing came exclusively from isotonic sport drinks rich in CHO, accounting for 24 L (3 L/stage). This volume amounts to 54.7 % of the total FI ingested during the whole TAC 2004. Expressed as relative terms, the female consumed 12 ml/kg*h during racing, which is 570 ml/h runtime. The MTBer ingested 59 g of CHO/L during racing (6 % solution). The total energy consumed exclusively from sport drinks was 20.1 MJ, reflecting 30.6 % of CHO intake during daily racing. Furthermore, 12.3 % of the total CHO intake during the entire TAC 2004 came from CHO consumed with isotonic sport drinks. FI during post race period came exclusively from water (tap, table and mineral) accounting for 17.1 L. Alcoholic drinks, solely consumed after the finish of TAC 2004, accounted for 1.125 L. Together, post exercise FI derived from water and alcohol contributed 41.6 % of total FI.

Energy and Macronutrient Intake

The average EI was found to be 24.61 MJ/day. When total EI is separated by occasions, the female ingested 17.4 % during breakfast and 35.2 % during racing. The most important occasions to eat were post race, accounting for 47.4 % of total EI. The distribution of total calories was 83.3 % from CHO, 7.5 % from protein and 9.2 % from fat.

EI during daily racing was found to be 94.9 % (65.76 MJ) derived from CHO, reflecting 40.1 % of total CHO intake during the entire TAC 2004. Similarly, 44.2 % of total CHO intake was consumed during the post race period (72.6 MJ) while breakfast only accounted for a smaller amount of 15.7 % (25.8 MJ) of total CHO intake during the full period of TAC 2004.

Relative CHO intake was calculated to be 24.4 g/kg*day (100 kcal/kg*day). An average of 188 g CHO (3.8 g CHO/kg) was ingested daily during breakfast. The relative amounts of CHO ingested daily during racing were 9.8 g CHO/kg body mass and 91.2 g CHO/h runtime. Relative EI from CHO during daily racing was calculated to be 7.63 kcal/kg*h. Relative daily post race ingestion from CHO was 1.2 g/kg*h (60.4 g CHO/h).

Daily amounts consumed of fat and protein consumed totalled 58 g/day (1.2 g/kg*day) and 107 g/day (2.2 g/kg*day), respectively. With respect to the total EI during TAC 2004, fat and protein contributed 9.2 % and 7.5 %, respectively.

Food Groups

Energy exclusively from solid energy bars and gels accounted for 49.1 MJ (6.1 MJ/day). Taken together, 25 % of total EI during the whole period of TAC 2004 came from solid energy food. Energy from bread was found to have provided 26.9 % of total energy ingested (52.9 MJ), whilst combined food together accounted for 17.6 % of total EI (34.6 MJ). A total of 6.14 % (12.1 MJ) came from sweets. Calories from fruit was calculated to be 4.29 % (8.4 MJ), including 2.8 % of total EI (5.56 MJ) coming from bananas. The main source of CHO, besides energy food, was bread, pizza and pasta as well as sweets. EI from the most important food groups are shown in Table 6.

Discussion

Nutritional treatment is well known to play a major role in endurance performance, especially during competition. It is well documented that optimum performance cannot be maintained without adequate glycogen stores based on appropriate diet.

Since vegetarian and vegan nutrition strategies were introduced to high performance sports, along with women competing in the same MTB races as men, this is the first report i) showing that a well planned vegan diet can adequately meet the nutritional demands of severe MTB stage racing and ii) studying a female cyclist during one of the most difficult MTB stage races in the world, previously shown to be physiologically very demanding (Wirnitzer and Kornexl 2008).

Table 2. Characteristics of Transalp Challenge 2004. Mean value is presented ± standard deviation (SD)g22

	Unit	Stage 1	Stage 2	Stage 3	Stage 4	Stage 5	Stage 6	Stage 7	Stage 8	Mean (±SD)
Temperature	°C	28	24	24	29	32	33	28	22	28 (±4)
Humidity	%	45	45	44	50	45	60	50	94	69 (±17)
Stage distance	km	80	73	74	119	54	73	124	67	83 (±25)
Stage time	min	293	328	287	402	225	280	426	278	315 (±60)
Speed	km/h	16.4	13.4	15.5	17.8	14.4	15.6	17.5	14.5	15.6 (±1.5)
Nature of course profile										
Asphalt	%	18.3	39.8	16.8	4.4	14.3	10.8	10.8	25	17.5 (±11)
Cycle track	%	8.1	20.2	24.5	32.6	26.6	40	60	25.3	29.7 (±15)
Gravel track/trail	%	51.1	27	54.3	52.1	32	29.2	19.3	34.1	37.4 (±13)
Forest–/meadow trail	%	18.3	5	1.2	3.3	16.9	8.8	7.6	0.5	7.7 (±7)
Alpine trail	%	4.2	8	1.6	7.4	10.2	9.7	2.3	15.1	7.3 (±5)
Push and/or carry	%	0	0	1.6	0.2	0	1.5	0	0	0.4 (±1)
Uphill cycling										
Total altitude climbed	m	2398	3099	2619	3366	2103	2732	3995	2141	2807 (±650)
Distance	km	43.8	43.9	39.7	46.3	23.1	34.7	69.1	14.7	39 (±16)
Time	min	228	252	210	220	150	197	233	179	209 (±33)
Speed	km/h	11.5	10.5	11.3	12.6	9.2	10.6	17.8	4.9	11.1 (±3.6)
Downhill cycling										
Total altitude climbed	m	2512	2556	2770	4030	2333	2633	3264	3234	2917 (±560)
Distance	km	29.1	26.4	26.8	67.1	27.5	34.6	28.2	34.9	34 (±14)
Time	min	60	61	63	110	75	83	79	88	77 (±17)
Speed	km/h	29.1	26.0	25.5	36.6	22.0	25.0	21.4	23.8	26.2 (±4.9)

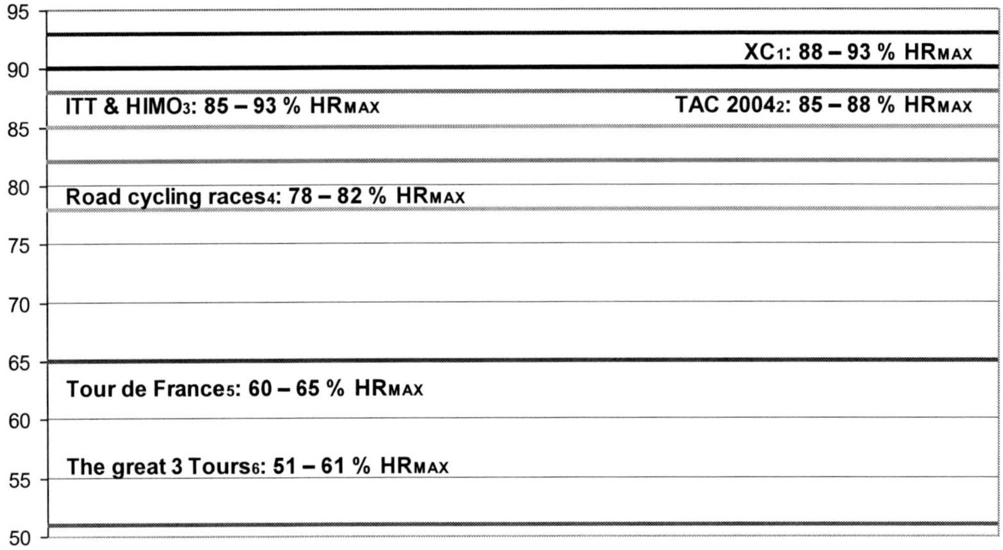

$_1$(Impellizzeri et. al. 2002/2005a+b, Stapelfeldt et. al. 2004), $_2$(Wirnitzer and Kornexl 2008), $_3$(Lucia et. al. 2003, Palmer et. al. 1994), $_4$(Palmer et. al. 1994), $_5$(Saris et. al. 1989), $_6$(Padilla et. al. 2001)

Figure 11. Exercise intensity in mountainbike sports (single performance) compared to road cycling (single performance, mass start races with bunch building, the great 3 Tours) as percentage of maximum heart rate (HR). XC = cross–country, TAC = Transalp Challenge. HR_{MAX} = maximum HR, ITT & HIMO = individual time trial & high mountain stages (road cycling races).

The main finding of this study is that a female vegan MTBer is able to maintain eight days of stage racing, with an average exercise intensity of 88 % of HR_{MAX}Field.

Performance

Stapelfeldt et. al. (2004) reported a relative PPO of 4.5 W/kg in one female elite MTBer of the German national team (age: 30 years, height: 1.70 m, body mass: 62 kg). From personal communication with coaches of national and international MTB team members also as several time winners of UCI (Union Cycliste Internationale: www.uci.ch) XCM races as well as winners and vice–winners of the overall XCM world cup, the bench mark for obtaining professional status in female MTB sports might be stated to be 4.7 W/kg. However, the subject (relative PPO: 4.6 W/kg) could be classified as a very well endurance trained non–professional MTBer.

The present exercise intensity is high compared to recent findings during TAC 2004 (85 % of HR_{MAX}Field: Wirnitzer and Kornexl 2008), but low compared to previous studies of one days XC races (90 – 91 % of maximum: Impellizzeri et. al. 2002/2005a, Stapelfeldt et. al. 2004). Furthermore, 52.4 % of total runtime (22 hours) was spent in high and very high intensity zones. The female maintained a very positive mood and each day was highly motivated to compete and perform at her maximum to reach the best possible final ranking. Therefore, sparing behaviour might (but ultimately cannot) be excluded.

The decline in HR_{MAX}Field during the TAC 2004 was recently reported by Wirnitzer and Kornexl (2008). The HR decline found in the present study might be explained by a secondary hypervolemia occurring as a consequence of acute high intensity exercise in already trained subjects (Wirnitzer and Faulhaber 2007, Richardson et. al. 1996). Another possible mechanism might be an incomplete restoration of muscle glycogen stores. Especially during stage races, when CHO intake is crucially very high and the next activity starts within the following 8 – 16 hours, glycogen levels will be suboptimal (Jentjens 2002, Jeukendrup 2002a). As a result, an incomplete restoration of glycogen stores might be excluded based on a total recovery time of 16 hours 45 minutes (post race period and time of sleep).

Generally, the exercise intensity during mass start stages of a road cycling race, characterized by bunch building and drafting, clearly is lower (Palmer et. al. 1994: 78 – 82 % HR_{MAX}) than during MTB races, in particular for the great 3 Tours (daily runtime of 4 – 7 h over 2 – 3 weeks) ranging from 51 – 65 % HR_{MAX} (Padilla et. al. 2001, Saris et. al. 1989). Mean exercise intensity during the Tour de France was shown to be 60 – 65 % HR_{MAX} (range: 40 – 80 % HR_{MAX}) in two cyclists by HR measurements (Saris et. al. 1989). Figure 11 presents an overview of the exercise intensity in MTB sports as compared to road cycling.

Racing in the Heat

When exercising in the heat as well as endogenous heat is produced, thermoregulatory mechanisms of the body are heavily stressed by heat loss. As a result fatigue prior to CHO depletion occurs. Therefore, fluid ingestion is of major importance in order to postpone a rise in body core temperature and to prevent impaired exercise performance resulting from several factors (Febbraio 2002). Any athlete who is exposed to heat may require different levels of some nutrients from those recommended by current guidelines (Knechtle et. al. 2005). It is generally accepted that exercise in the heat results in a substrate shift towards increased CHO utilization (Febbraio 2002).

FI not only attenuates the rise in body core temperature, it also reduces the likelihood of CHO depletion by reducing the muscle glycogen use during prolonged exercise (Hargreaves et. al. 1996a+b). Together, both CHO and fluid availability are vital when exposed to heat during severe exercise and result in an improved exercise performance in a hot environment (Febbraio 2002, Below et. al. 1995). Therefore, especially during racing, it is important to maintain appropriate FI and adequate energy supply to fuel muscle contraction and to prevent both hyperthermia and exercise induced dehydration.

The results for exercise induced FI, as well as the markedly high values of CHO intake during daily racing and whole TAC 2004, seem to be appropriate to sustain the high effort of this stage race, considering the hot and dry conditions faced by the subject together with the high exercise intensity.

Table 3. Heart rate (HR) and rate of perceived exertion (RPE) during the Transalp Challenge 2004. Mean value is presented ± standard deviation (SD). HRave = average HR, HR_{MAX} = maximal HR, % HR_{MAX}Field = values of HR expressed as percentage of maximal HR during race, % HR_{MAX}Lab = values of HR expressed as percentage of maximal HR during laboratory testing, bpm = beats/min

	Unit	Stage 1	Stage 2	Stage 3	Stage 4	Stage 5	Stage 6	Stage 7	Stage 8	Mean (±SD)
HRave	bpm	164	142	142	143	143	140	138	132	143 (±9)
HRave	% HR_{MAX}Field	91	87	87	88	88	86	87	86	88 (±2)
HRave	% HR_{MAX}Lab	90	78	78	79	79	77	76	73	79 (±5)
HR_{MAX}	bpm	181	164	164	162	163	162	158	154	164 (±8)
HR_{MAX}	% HR_{MAX}Lab	99	90	90	89	90	89	87	85	90 (±4)
RPE (6–20)	points	15	17	19	14	15	17	17	18	16.5 (±1.7)

Table 4. Energy intake (EI) and fluid intake (FI) for each occasion. Mean value is presented ± standard deviation (SD)

	Unit	Stage 1	Stage 2	Stage 3	Stage 4	Stage 5	Stage 6	Stage 7	Stage 8	Total	Mean (±SD)
Breakfast											
EI	kcal	1512.5	983.2	804.6	1782	737.4	782.5	491.6	1085.6	8179	1022 (±429)
FI	L	0.125	0.25	0.25	0.25	0.25	0.125	0.25	0.125	1.625	0.20 (±0.06)
Race											
EI	kcal	1929.6	2151.6	2373.6	1930	1930	1711	3116	1408.8	16550	2069 (±510)
FI	L	3	3	3	3	3	3	4.5	1.5	24	3 (±0.8)
Post Race											
EI	kcal	2594.8	2536.4	1586.8	1309	3192	2943	3844	4024.1	22300	2787 (±925)
FI	L	1.8	1.8	1.0	1.5	3.0	2.5	3.0	3.63	18.23	2.28 (±0.9)
Total TAC 2004											
EI	kcal	6036.9	5671.2	5035	5021	5859.4	5436.5	7451.6	6518.5	47030	5878 (±810)
	MJ	25.28	23.74	21.08	21.02	24.53	22.76	31.2	27.29	196.91	24.61 (±3.39)
FI	L	4.93	5.05	4.25	4.75	6.25	5.63	7.75	5.25	43.85	5.48 (±1.1)
Body mass	kg	48	50	48	49	50	50	50	50	–	49 (±1)

Off-Road Cycling

Ultraendurance cycling and stage racing poses an increased demand for energy and CHO. Meeting these demands requires careful planning and monitoring of dietary intake (Lindemann 1991).

In addition to heat exposure, the high EI found during the TAC 2004 can be explained by the characteristics of XC competitions as recently discussed (Wirnitzer and Kornexl 2008). Particularly during MTB races, FI and EI are usually limited by the practical situation. The nutritional requirements of a TAC are challenging for several reasons. Opportunities and time available for FI and EI are restricted by a great diversity of terrains and traits (difficult nature of course profile during both uphill and downhill sections) simultaneously with aggressive riding tactics (Wirnitzer and Kornexl 2008). In contrast to road cycling, downhill sections are not sections of either low intensity or recovery (Hurst and Atkins 2002/2006, Stapelfeldt et. al. 2004) and therefore dietary intake is almost impossible. Despite these factors combining to prevent the athlete from consuming more food and drinks, the nutritional requirements necessarily had to be met by appropriate dietary intake. As a consequence, a greater reliance was put on post race replenishment to provide EI, mainly through CHO as the most important fuel in ultraendurance and cycling (stage) races.

Information of dietary interventions on MTB performance is scarce. Recently, Rose and Peters (2008) studied amateur MTBers during a three days MTB race (Sani2C MTB Race, South Africa) in cool conditions (6 – 21 °C). Wingo et. al. (2004) examined the influence of pre–exercise glycerol beverage on performance and physiologic function in a one day XC MTB race in the heat. Cramp et. al. (2004) conducted a simulated MTB race in the laboratory (93 min) to study the effects of consuming different CHO treatments on metabolic effects and performance. Mastroianni et. al. (2000) studied the differences in energy expenditure between off–road cyclists and runners while voluntarily pacing. Seifert el. al. (1997) investigated the energy cost of riding a full versus front suspended MTB. In these studies all the subjects were male. Due to the wide range of purposes, conditions and design of these few studies available, the current findings are difficult to use for comparative purposes.

Major Stage Races and Ultraendurance Cycling

Several authors have described the dietary practice of athletes during major cycling tours. The few studies available report mean daily EIs of 23.3 MJ (Erp van–Baart et. al. 1989: Tour l`Avenir), 23.5 MJ (Garcia–Roves et al. 1998) and 24.7 MJ (Saris et al. 1989) for male athletes competing in the major stage races. Maximum values of EI were found of 28.2 MJ/day were found during the Vuelta a Espana (Garcia–Roves et al. 1998) and of 32.4 MJ/day during the Tour de France (Saris et al. 1989). The relative contributions of energy from CHO, protein and fat was similar during both the Tour de France (Saris et al. 1989: 62 %, 15 % and 23 %) and the Vuelta a Espana (Garcia–Roves et al. 1998: 60 %, 14.5 % and 25.5 %). Contrary to the TAC 2004, cyclists in the Tour de France consumed 49 % of their total EI during the race. Moreover, 58 % of daily CHO ingested was taken during daily stages. About 30 % of total CHO intake came from CHO rich liquids. Mean daily FI was 6.7 L with 61 % (4.1 L) of total fluid consumed during daily racing in the Tour de France (Saris et. al. 1989).

During the Race Across America (RAAM) the relative contribution of total calories consumed from CHO as the main source of energy was found to be 75.2 % (Knechtle et al. 2005) and 78 % (Lindemann 1991). Since environmental conditions were similar for the RAAM (Lindemann 1991: 21 – 35 °C) and TAC 2004, mean FI resulted in 0.72 L/h runtime and 0.57 L/h runtime, respectively.

The relative contribution of CHO to total EI in the TAC 2004 exceeds the results of the Tour de France and Vuelta a Espana, but was quite comparable to those of RAAM.

Dietary Intake during TAC 2004

In the course of the TAC 2004 the subject gradually become weary of the sweet taste of energy food and drinks ingested during the race. Therefore, spicy food and dishes were preferred, especially post race. Even though the cyclist permanently felt sated, she tried to eat constantly to provide energy replenishment and to restore muscle glycogen. Since the energy cost of cycling is an exponential function of speed (Jeukendrup 2002b) the average speed during TAC 2004 (15.6 km/h) is connected to the high EI of 24.6 MJ/day. The body mass measured after daily stages remained stable after oscillating from stages 1 to 4. This indicates that CHO replacement and hydration strategies were adequate.

Pre race. Except for Stage 1, which had a unique start time of 12 a. m., breakfast was daily taken at 6.30 a. m. due to the early start times of 8 a. m. It is suprising that only once gastrointenstinal discomfort did occur, during breakfast of Stage 7, resulting in the lowest EI. Compared to the major stage races of road cycling, where start times are fixed at around noon, the time for dietary intake prior to the race was very limited. As a consequence, pre race values for EI and FI were documented to be lower in the current study. Fluid consumed was approximately half the volume of 300 – 400 ml recommended to be consumed pre race (Jeukendrup 2002a). CHO intake during breakfast fitted well with the pre race recommendations of Burke (2002: 1 – 4 g CHO/kg) with 49 – 196 g CHO derived for the subject.

Race. The fluid ingested during the race, exclusively coming from sport drinks rich in CHO, fits well with the current recommendations for both CHO solution (Maughan 2002: 2 – 8 %) and relative FI during races lasting more than 90 min (Jeukendrup 2002a: 8 – 12 ml/kg*h), with volumes of 400 – 600 ml/h ingested for the MTBer. On the one hand, the findings for CHO intake during daily racing (479 g) exceed the recommendations of 60 – 70 g CHO/h runtime (Burke 2002, Hargreaves 2002, Jeukendrup 2002a) with derived values of 315 – 368 g CHO. On the other hand, total daily CHO intake during stage races lasting more than 4 – 5 hours of high intensity cycling is 12 – 13 g/kg reported for male cyclists (Burke 2001). The fact that the subject was a non–professional female is likely to explain the considerably lower amount of CHO consumed.

Post race. Following the experience gained by competing the TAC in 2003, sleeping time was strictly held from 10 p. m. to 6 a. m. in order to maximize recovery. Quick recovery is extremely important during stage races. The replenishment of muscle glycogen stores and fluid balance to pre race levels after daily competition is probably the most important factor

(Jeukendrup 2002a). To maximize glycogen storage, the ingestion of CHO rich fluids and easily digestible solid CHO rich foods such as bananas, is preferred (Jentjens 2002, Jeukendrup 2002a, Brouns et al. 1986). Even when CHO intake between successive days of racing is very high, the muscle glycogen levels might be suboptimal when the CHO need is critically high and when the next stage is started within 8 – 16 hours (Jentjens 2002, Jeukendrup 2002a). Since the female in the TAC 2004 was usually riding for 4 – 7 hours daily, there was barely enough time for eating large meals. However, the challenges posed be the practical constraints, both in terms of the limited time available for eating and the suppression of appetite after exhaustive exercise (Brouns et al. 1986, Burke 2001, Jeukendrup 2002a+b), appear to have been met by the subject. Relative daily post race ingestion from CHO nicely meets the recommendations for stage races with 5 – 6 h of extreme endurance effort of 1 – 1.2 g CHO/kg*h (Jentjens 2002, Jeukendrup 2002a). Derived ranges for the MTB athlete (490 – 590 g CHO/day) fits well with current results (529 g CHO). Contrary to road cycling, the most important occasions to eat were post exercise.

Energy Intake from Macronutrients

Compared to guidelines for endurance trained female athletes, fat intake (9.2 % of total EI) was found to be about half the recommended intake (Gabel 2002: 20 – 35 % of total EI) and relative protein intake was about twice the recommended levels (Lemon 1995: 1.2 – 1.4 g protein/kg*day). Protein requirements of endurance athletes are known to exceed those of recreational subjects (Gabel 2002). The mean daily intakes of protein and micronutrients are likely to meet or exceed advocated levels for the MTBer competing in TAC 2004, largely because of high EIs (Burke 2001, Saris et al. 1989).

Martin et al. (2002) studied the EI (self reported) and energy expenditure in eight elite female cyclists (members of the Australian national training squad: 25 years, 59 kg) during eight days of training and racing, including a five days stage race. They reported a mean EI of 14.87 MJ/day. During five days of racing, intake from fat and protein was reported to have been 59 g/day and 136 g/day, respectively. These values correspond with the current findings of fat (58 g/day) and protein (107 g/day).

Carbohydrate. The importance of CHO as a main source of fuel for performance during prolonged endurance exercise has been recognized since the 1930s (Jentjens 2002). Christensen and Hansen (1939) were among the first to demonstrate the influence of CHO on improving or maintaining exercise performance during exercise.

CHO replacement plays an essential role during prolonged intensive cycling races (Burke 2001). The oxidation of CHO can provide energy at a faster rate than fat oxidation. Therefore, CHO is the preferred fuel at exercise intensities higher than 80 % of maximum HR when large amounts of energy have to be generated over long periods of time (Jeukendrup 2002b, Burke 2001). Suitable food choices to attain such goals include concentrated sport drinks and portable CHO rich foods such as solid energy bars and gels (Jeukendrup 2002a, Brouns et al. 1986). CHO ingestion during exercise has been shown to improve race performance in events of more than 90 min of duration by maintaining both high levels of both plasma glucose and CHO oxidation. The increased availability of plasma glucose enables the athlete to postpone fatigue or to develop a higher PO in a final sprint following endurance exercise (Coggan and

Coyle 1987/1988/1989, Hargreaves et. al. 1984). A further mechanism to improve cycling performance by CHO ingestion might be also the resynthesis of muscle glycogen during periods of low intensity (Jeukendrup 2002a, Hargreaves et al. 1984).

In the current study, an intake of 1195 g/day came from CHO. Compared to Martin et al. (2002), who reported a CHO intake of 588 g/day during a race period of five days, the result of the MTBer is about twice the value of that for female road cyclists. Erp van–Baart et al. (1989), studying amateur cyclists in the Tour l`Avenir reported a daily intake of 873 g from CHO. Almost a decade later, Garcia–Roves et al. (1998) found a similar CHO intake during the Vuelta a Espana (841.4 g/day). Currently recommended energy from CHO for a more competitive woman participating in endurance and ultra endurance events had been given as 55 – 70 % of total intake (Gabel 2002). The total calories coming from CHO during TAC 2004 (83.3 %) exceed the advocated range by about 13.3 %. Relative CHO intake (24.4 g/kg*day) is twice as high as the recommendations of 8 – 12 g CHO/kg*day (Jentjens 2002, Jeukendrup 2002a) and more than twice the guidelines for female athletes of 6 – 10 g CHO/kg per day (Gabel 2002).

Dietary Intake in Vegan Athletes

The vegan diet is determined to be exclusively sourced from plant based nutrition, rejecting all products from animal sources (as one unit, ingredient or supplement) such as meat, fish, dairy products, egg and honey (see Figure 12).

The European Union currently has 1.73 % of its population (6.72 million people) following a vegetarian or vegan lifestyle (representative survey conducted by the European Commission: http://ec.europa.eu/food/animal/welfare/euro_barometer25_volA_en.pdf). *A* UK wide survey carried out by the Food Standards Agency (Consumer Attitudes to Food Standards *2007:* www.vegsoc.org/info/statveg.html*) in* 3513 adults found 2 % of respondents to be "completely vegetarian". The number of vegans in the UK is estimated to be at around 0.3 % of the population (180,000 people: www.imaner.net/panel/statistics). Further reliable information based on the available research (Dietary Habits of Adults 18 and Older in the United States) puts the figure ranging from 0.5 % – 1.4 % of the USA population to be vegan, with the possible exception of honey (2008: www.imaner.net/ panel/statistics.htm, 2006: www.vrg.org/journal/vj2006issue4/vj2006issue4poll.htm).

In general, vegetarians are known to be more "health conscious" than non–vegetarians (Bedford and Barr 2005). To date, the female MTB athlete has successfully followed a vegan lifestyle since 1999 and thus has gained previous experience.

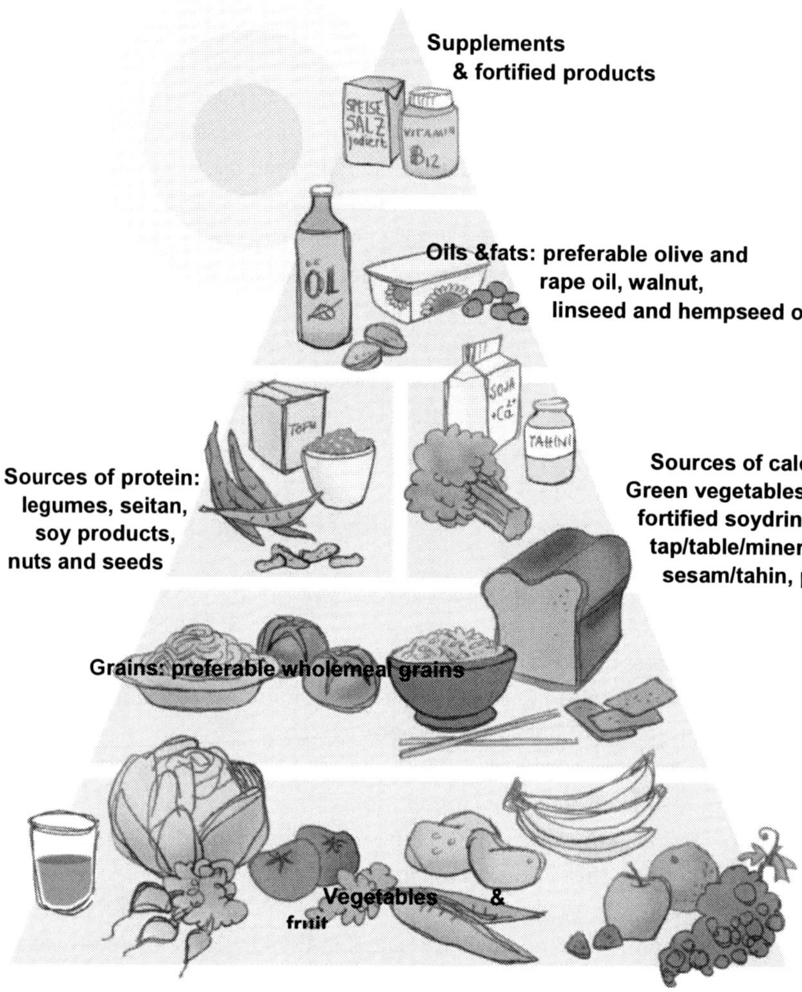
Supplements
& fortified products
SPEISE SALZ jodiert
VITAMIN B12
ÖL
Oils &fats: preferable olive and
rape oil, walnut,
linseed and hempseed oil
TOFU
SOJA +Ca
TAHINI
Sources of protein:
legumes, seitan,
soy products,
nuts and seeds
Sources of calcium:
Green vegetables,
fortified soydrinks,
tap/table/mineral water,
sesam/tahin, poppy...
Grains: preferable wholemeal grains
Vegetables &
fruit

Figure 12. Vegan nutrition pyramide after Petter and Pohlmann (2007: with permission).

According to the meta–analysis of the ADA (2003), a vegetarian – including vegan – diet can meet current recommendations for all nutrients. A well planned vegan and other type of vegetarian diet is appropriate for all stages of the life cycle, including during pregnancy, lactation, infancy, childhood and adolescence. Vegetarian diets offer a number of nutritional benefits as well as higher levels of CHOs.

"It is the position of the American Dietetic Association and Dietitians of Canada that appropriately planned vegetarian diets are healthful, nutritionally adequate, and provide health benefits in the prevention and treatment of certain diseases" (ADA 2003). Together, these advantages include lower risk for heart disease, blood cholesterol levels, blood pressure, hypertension, diabetes mellitus, obesity and some types of cancer (Kugler 2007, Campbell and Campbell 2006, Venderly and Campbell 2006, ADA 2003).

After many years of research, mainly focused on issues connected to health (nutritional adequacy and the implications for diseases of affluence) rather than on human performance issues, the effects of a plant based diet on athletic performance are still unclear. Little is know about the relationship between vegetarianism and athletic performance even today, in spite of the popular belief that these kinds of diet may be beneficial to some athletes. Thus, there is a certain lack of information relating to veganism and its relationship to endurance performance. All athletes at some time in their career look at alternative eating patterns in the effort to reach their full athletic potential. While some take pills and/or powders, others have changed their nutritional styles to a vegetarian diet to gain advantages in training and enhance performance (Berning 2002).

However, any athlete, regardless of whether omnivore or vegan, should plan his/her diet carefully to avoid the risk of nutritional deficiencies and adverse effects on performance (Venderly and Campbell 2006, Berning 2002). There is sufficient evidence from laboratory and field that a well planned vegetarian or vegan diet can meet the energy and nutrient requirements of a competitive athlete (Venderly and Campbell 2006, Barr and Rideout 2004, ADA 2003). The current findings confirm that this challenge can be met when the subject follows a well planned and monitored vegan diet.

As mentioned before, CHO is the vital fuel during prolonged intensive endurance exercise (Jeukendrup 2002a+b, Burke 2001). It is broadly accepted that endurance athletes involved in heavy endurance training and competition should ingest a higher amount of energy from CHO to maximize muscle glycogen synthesis. Niemann (1988) suggested that particularly those athletes training for more than 60 – 90 min/day should consume 60 – 70 % of their energy from CHO.

The main advantages of vegetarian diets are the higher amounts of CHO, including numerous higher CHOs, lower fat and adequate protein (Venderly and Campbell 2006, ADA 2003, Niemann 1988). Vegans in particular consume the majority of their energy from CHO (Venderly and Campbell 2006, Messina and Messina 1996). Messina and Messina (1996) summarizing dietary data from 63 studies, reported that among the general public, the CHO intake of vegans ranges from 50 – 65 % of total daily energy. Therefore, endurance athletes might adopt vegetarian diets as an optimum strategy in order to meet increased CHO needs and to assist in weight control (Cox 2000, Niemann 1988).

The formerly common opinion that a vegetarian diet is not advisable for athletes due to a small amount of high quality protein, cannot be hold nowadays. Appropriate protein provision is met by adopting a well–planned vegan diet (Williams 1997). With respect to the quality of animal protein repeatedly attested to in the literature as being "high", this level of quality has to be fundamentally questioned from a nutritional point of view. Meat, fish, egg and dairy products are produced by the commercial sector of livestock and animal farming industries. In order to maximize profits, processes aimed at the reaching of economic goals are often targeted at the practices within animal farming industries. Because the physiological units would not survive the conditions in life stocking, the production process has to be supported by the use of medical substances and supplements such as antibiotics, growth hormones, psychotropics and tranquillizers, which is commonly practice in animal farming industries. As a consequence, the excessive dose of medical treatment cannot be catabolized within very short lifetimes. Thus, a cocktail of residues from medical substances is contained within any kind of animal protein, as documented by numerous independent laboratories, widely known.

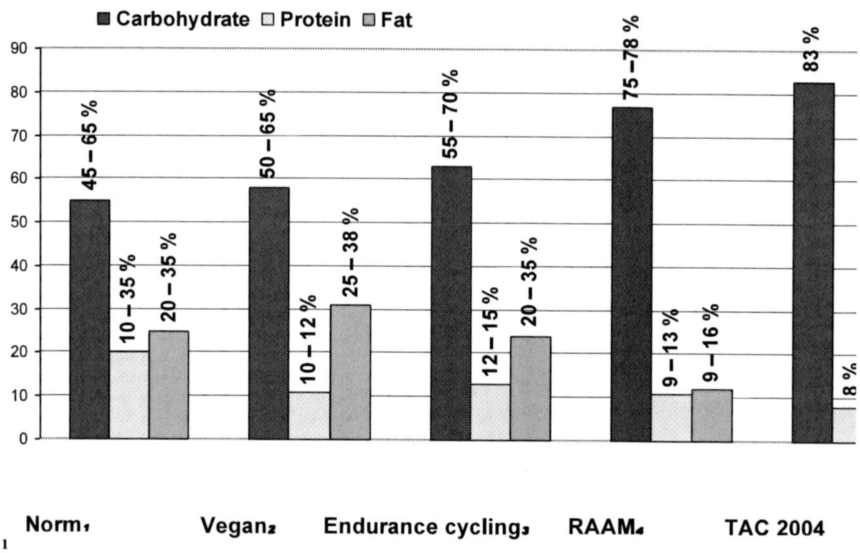

[1](Venderly and Campbell 2006), [2](Messina and Messina 1996), [3](Gabel 2002, Garcia–Roves et al.1998, Geiss and Hamm 1992, Saris et al. 1989, Niemann 1988), [4](Knechtle et al. 2005, Lindemann 1991)

Figure 13. Breakdown of macronutrients as a percentage of total energy intake according to type of activity or sports (derived from available literature). Norm = normal distribution of general population. Vegan = distribution of vegans (non-athletes). Endurance cycling = endurance cyclists (Tour de France, Vuelta a Espana, competitive endurance cyclists and athletes). RAAM = Race Across America. TAC 2004 = Transalp Challenge 2004.

Table 5. Distribution of macronutrients carbohydrate (CHO), protein and fat for each occasion. g = gram, kcal = kilocalorie, kJ = kilojoule, MJ = megajoule

	g	kcal	kJ	MJ	% Dish	% Total
Breakfast	1831	8180	34246	34.24		17.40 %
CHO	1501	6156	25774	25.77	75.30 %	
Protein	202	830	3474	3.47	10.10 %	
Fat	128	1194	4998	5	14.60 %	
Race	3980	16550	69293	69.30		35.20 %
CHO	3831	15706	65757	65.76	94.90 %	
Protein	104	426	1785	1.79	2.60 %	
Fat	45	418	1751	1.75	2.50 %	
Post Race	5069	22301	93370	93.37		47.40 %
CHO	4228	17334	72574	72.57	77.70 %	
Protein	548	2247	9407	9.41	10.10 %	
Fat	293	2720	11389	11.39	12.20 %	
Total TAC 2004	10880	47030	196909	196.91		
CHO	9560	39196	164105	164.11		83.30 %
Protein	854	3503	14666	14.67		7.50 %
Fat	466	4332	18138	18.14		9.20 %

Research indicates that vegan competitive athletes can meet protein requirements exclusively from plant based sources (which provide all essential amino acids and ensure adequate nitrogen retention) when a variety of plant foods is consumed and energy needs are met (ADA 2003). Due to the diminished digestibility of plant protein, the requirement of protein is classified to be 20 – 30 % higher than with an omnivore diet (Kugler 2007). However, typical protein intakes of vegans (10 – 12 % of EI) appear to meet and exceed requirements (Kugler 2007, Barr and Rideout 2004, Larson 2000, Messina and Messina 1996), without the use of specials foods or supplements (Larson 2000). Figure 13 depicts an overview of macronutrient intake reported and recommended in literature.

During the TAC 2004, the mean daily intakes of CHO and protein were found to meet or exceed recommended levels through a well planned vegan diet.

Iron status. Key nutrients for adolescent vegetarians include calcium, iron, zinc, vitamin D and B 12. A well planned vegan diet does not cause a deficiency in any of these nutrients when energy needs are met (Kugler 2007, ADA 2003).

Concerns about the iron status of vegetarian athletes are usually based on the bioavailability of iron from plant foods rather than the amount of total iron present in a vegetarian diet (Sabate et al. 1999/2001). Shaw et al. (1995) found in a comparative study that daily iron intake was similar in both vegetarian and non–vegetarian men, but iron intake was significantly higher in female vegetarians than non–vegetarians. It has been found that vegans can compensate for a diminished ingestion of calcium and iron by an adaptation of metabolism in both increased absorption and decreased losses (Kugler 2007, Hunt and Roughead 1999/2000). Saris et al. (1989) found high EI resulting in high calcium and iron intake during the Tour de France.

Since iron plays a critical role in oxidative energy metabolism, it is vital for endurance athletes to have adequate iron stores. It is used for the synthesis of hemoglobin and myoglobin, essential components in the transport and delivery of oxygen to muscles (Sabate et. al. 1999). Generally, endurance training and competition tend to reduce iron stores (ADA 2003). Messina and Messina (1996) reported that only 10 % of athletes have anaemia and thhat it is more commonly found among endurance athletes. In general, iron deficiency anaemia is rare in vegetarian athletes, but is commonly reported in female athletes (Venderly and Campbell 2006, Niemann 1999). Therefore, it is especially important to monitor iron status especially in endurance and female athletes.

However, iron deficiency is observed in 20 % of the world population, with a similar incidence of iron deficiency amongst vegetarians or vegans as amongst omnivores (Kugler 2007, ADA 2003). Vegan and omnivore athletes alike must consume sufficient iron to prevent deficiency, which will adversely affect performance. In general, vegetarian diets contain as much or more total iron than omnivore diets and is usually highest in vegans (ADA 2003, Messina and Messina 1996).

A late and severe period of training close to the TAC 2004 resulted in a trend of lower iron levels. Despite this, the pre race levels of iron, ferritin and vitamin B 12 were within a normal range in the female subject. In order to prevent an iron deficiency which might have resulted in a reduced aerobic capacity during the subsequent stage race, the female was treated by an intravenous application of iron supplement on 10 occasions including 100 mg of iron each (surgery). Sobal and Marquart (1994), reviewing 51 studies (10274 athletes), found a supplement use in female athletes of 57 %. Vitamin and mineral supplementation (orally or by intravenous injection) is common practice during professional tour races, especially after hard stages (Lucia et al. 2003, Saris et al. 1989), which ensures a daily micronutrient intake considerably higher than the recommended daily allowance, especially for iron and vitamin B 12 (Saris et al. 1989).

Despite the frequently proven benefits on health, sports scientists still doubt the advantageous effects of vegetarian diets on performance (ADA 2003), although an impressive number of high performance athletes (world record holders, national and international champions, attendants in World Championships, Olympic Games and World Cup, winners and multiple winners of major cycling tours etc.) from several disciplines such as marathon running, triathlon and ironman as well as cycling (including MTB sports) confirm the positive benefits for endurance performance.

Since professional cyclists like Adam Myerson (road–cycling), Christine Vardaros (cyclo–cross), Jason Sager (MTB), Sally Hibberd (British Women MTB Champion), Estelle Gray and Cheryl Marek (hold the world record for cross–country tandem cycling) and professional triathletes (ironman winners and finishers) like Brendan Brazier, Lucy Stephens and Ruth Heidrich have all adopted a vegan nutrition pattern (www.organicathlete.org/pro–activist, www.veganfitness.net/forum/viewtopic.php?t=723), the vegan diet has been demonstrated to be adequate for high performance events due to the advantageous effects on prolonged and high intensive endurance performance.

Limitations of this Case Report

The food diary is commonly used in most self–reported dietary surveys to monitor the intake during a specific event. Unfortunately, inaccuracies due to several factors (memory failure, frequency of consumption, estimating portion size by not weighing the mass of food) are a universal problem (Jeukendrup 2002b, Burke 2001). This might result in considerable errors, leading to underestimate or overestimate intake ranging from 20 – 50 % (Jeukendrup 2002b, Burke 2001).

However, the most accurate self–reports might be expected to be derived from athletes who are confident of their eating habits, aware of their body image and who are highly motivated to receive valuable feedback (Burke 2001). As mentioned before, the subject is highly self–aware, a very experienced vegan. Thus, the nutritional strategy during the TAC 2004 was carefully planned and accurately accomplished in order to minimize and control for the errors involved in the survey techniques described in the method section. Therefore, EI is probably not biased by either self report or race tactics (bunch building and/or drafting). Considering the former case reports on dietary pattern comparable to this case study (Knechtle et al. 2005, Lucia et al. 2003) the error of EI might be similar to those or perhaps of a considerably lesser magnitude. However, authors are absolutely aware that the use of self–reported dietary survey to determine the EI of a specific event is potentially limited.

Burke (2001) concluded in her review that dietary surveys during the racing practices of high level endurance cyclists provide a potential source of important information. Finally, since no indicators of dietary intake free from potential limitations exist, the use of self–reported dietary surveys can be acceptable for quantifying the EI in the present case report under authentic race burden of the TAC 2004.

Conclusion

This study was the first to report the dietary intake during the TAC 2004. It shows the vegan diet, when appropriately planned, to adequately meet the nutritional demands of one of the most difficult MTB stage races in the world. The current results might be useful to design specific training programs and to develop appropriate nutritional strategies for endurance athletes, particularly female and vegan, who need to sustain physical demands similar to this MTB race.

Well controlled long term studies assessing the effects of vegetarian diets on athletes have not yet been conducted. Therefore, prospective research should aim to focus on vegetarian and vegan dietary patterns and their influence on endurance performance, particularly on high performance cycling, stage racing and endurance trained female populations.

References

American Dietetic Association, Dietitians of Canada (ADA) (2003) Position of the American Dietetic Association and Dietitians of Canada. Vegetarian diets. *J Am Diet Assoc, 103(6)*, 748–765

Astrand, P. O. (1968). *Nutrition Today 3*: *no2*, 9-11

Barr SI and Rideout CA (2004). Nutritional Considerations for vegetarian athletes. *Nutrition* Jul-Aug, *20(7-8)*, 696-703.

Bedford, J. L. & Barr, S. I. (2005) Diets and selected lifestyle practices of self–defined adult vegetarians from a population–based sample suggest they are more 'health conscious'. *Int J Behav Nutr Phys Act*, Apr, *13*, 2(1), 4.

Below, P. R., Mora–Rodriguez, R., Gonzalez–Alonso, J. & Coyle, E. F. (1995). Fluid and carbohydrate ingestion independentely improve performance during 1 h of intense exercise. *Med Sci Sports Exerc.,* Feb, *27*, 200-210.

Berning, J. R. (2002) . The Vegetarian Athlete. In: Maughan RJ (ed) *Nutrition in Sport. Part 2: Special Considerations.,* Chapter 33, 442-456. Oxford: Blackwell Science

Borg, G. (1998) . The Borg RPE Scale. In: Borg G (ed) *Borg`s perceived exertion and pain scales.* Champaign: Human Kinetics.

Brouns, F. J., Saris, W. H. & ten Hoor, F. (1986) Dietary problems in the case of strenuous exertion. *J Sports Med Phys Fitness.,* Sep, *26(3)*, 306-319.

Burke, L. M. (2001) . Nutritional practices of male and female endurance cyclists. *Sports Med, 31(7)*, 521-532.

Burke, L. M. (2002) . Principles of Eating for Cycling. In: Jeukendrup AE (ed) *High–Performance Cycling. Part IV: Nutrition.* Chapter 16, 183-200. Champaign: Human Kinetics

Campbell, T. C. & Campbell, T. M. (2006) *The China Study. Startling implications for diet, weight loss and long–term health.,* Part I: 27-31, 43-67 and Part II: 109-225. Dallas, Texas: BenBella.

Chittenden, R. H. (1904). *Physiological economy in nutrition.,* New York: F. A. Stokes.

Chittenden, R. H. (1907). *The nutrition of man.* New York: F. A. Stokes.

Christensen, E. H. & Hansen, O. (1939). Arbeitsfähigkeit und Ernährung. *Scandinavian Archives of Physiology., 81*, 160-171.

Coggan, A. R. & Coyle, E. F. (1987) Reversal of fatigue during prolonged exercise by carbohydrate infusion or ingestion. *J Appl Physiol Dec., 63(6)*, 2388-2395.

Coggan, A. R. & Coyle, E. F. (1988) Effect of carbohydrate feeding during high–intensity exercise. *J Appl Physiol.,* Oct, *65(4)*, 1703-1709.

Coggan, A. R. & Coyle, E. F. (1989) Metabolism and performance following carbohydrate ingestion late in exercise. *Med Sci Sports Exerc.,* Feb, *21(1),* 59-65.

Cox, G. (2000). Special needs: the vegetarian athlete. In: Burke L, Deakin V (ed) *Clinical sports nutrition.*, Chapter, 20, 656-671. Sydney, NSW: McGraw-Hill.

Cramp, T., Broad, E., Martin, D. & Meyer, B. J. (2004). Effects of preexercise carbohydrate ingestion on mountain bike performance. *Med Sci Sports Exerc* Sept; *36(9)*, 1602–1609

Dietary Habits of Adults 18 and Older in the United States 2006: www.vrg.org/journal/vj 2006issue4/vj2006issue4poll.htm (15. 2. 2009).

Erp van-Baart, A. M., Saris, W. H., Binkhorst, R. A., Vos, J. A. & Elvers, J. W. H. (1989). Nationwide survey on nutritional habits in elite athletes. Part I, Energy carbohydrate, protein. *Int J Sports Med* May, *10(Suppl)1*, S3-S10.

Febbraio, M. A. (2002). Exercise in climatic extremes. In: Maughan RJ (ed) *Nutrition in Sport. Part 3: Practical Issues.,* Chapter, *38*, 497-509. Oxford: Blackwell Science.

Fisher, I. (1907). The Influence of Flesh Eating on Endurance. *Yale Medical Journal., 13(5)*, 205-211.

Food Standards Agency. Consumer Attitudes to Food Standards *2007:* www.vegsoc.org/ info/statveg.html (15. 2. 2009).

Gabel, K. A. (2002). The Female Athlete. In: Maughan RJ (ed) *Nutrition in Sport. Part 2: Special Considerations.,* Chapter., *31*, 417-428. Oxford: Blackwell Science.

Garcia–Roves, P. M., Terrados, N., Fernandez, S. F. & Patterson, A. M. (1998). Macronutrients intake of top level cyclists during continuous competition – change in the feeding pattern. *Int J Sports Med.,* Jan, *19(1)*, 61-67.

Geiss, K. R. & Hamm, M. (1992). *Handbuch Sportlerernährung.* Überarbeitete Neuausgabe. Kapitel, 2, 17-19 und Kapitel 4, 190-191. Reinbeck, Hamburg: Rowolth Taschenbuch Verlag, Sport rororo.

Gilman, M. B. & Wells, C. L. (1993) The use of heart rates to monitor exercise intensity in relation to metabolic variables. *Int J Sports Med.,* Aug, *14(6)*, 339-344.

Gilman, M. B. (1996) The use of heart rate to monitor the intensity of endurance training. *Sports Med.,* Feb, *21(2)*, 73-79.

Hargreaves, M. (2002). Carbohydrate Replacement during Exercise. In: Maughan RJ (ed) *Nutrition in Sport. Part 1: Nutrition and Exercise.,* Chapter, *8*, 112-118. Oxford: Blackwell Science

Hargreaves, M., Angus, D., Howlett, K., Conus, N. M. & Febbraio, M. (1996a). Effect of heat stress on glucose kinetics during exercise. *J Appl Physiol,* Oct, *81(4)*, 1594-1597

Hargreaves, M., Dillo, P., Angus, D., Howlett, K. & Febbraio, M. (1996b). Effect of fluid ingestion on muscle metabolism during prolonged exercise. *J Appl Physiol.,* Jan, *80(1)*, 363-366.

Hargreaves, M., Costill, D. L., Coggan, A., Fink, W. J. & Nishibata, I. (1984). Effect of carbohydrate feedings on muscle glycogen utilization and exercise performance. *Med Sci Sports Exerc.,* Jun, *16(3)*, 219-222.

Hunt, J. R. & Roughead, Z. K. (2000) Adaptation of iron absorption in men consuming diets with high or low iron bioavailability. *Am J Clin Nutr.,* Jan, *71(1)*, 94-102.

Hunt, J. R. & Roughead, Z. K. (1999). Nonheme–iron absorption, fecal ferritin excretion, and blood indexes of iron status in women consuming controlled loacto–ovovegetarian diets for 8 wk. *Am J Clin Nutr.,* May, *69(5)*, 944-952.

Hurst, H. T. & Atkins, S. (2006) Power output of field–based downhill mountain biking. *J Sports Sci.,* Oct, *24(10)*, 1047-1053.

Hurst, H. T. & Atkins, S. (2002). The physiological demands of downhill mountain biking as determined by heart rate monitoring. Communication to the 7th Annual Congress of the European College of Sports Sciences, Athens, Greece. http://ec.europa.eu/food (15. 2. 2009) http://ester (15. 2. 2009)

Impellizzeri, F. M., Rampinini, E., Sassi, A., Mognoni, P. & Marcora S (2005a). Physiological correlates to off–road cycling performance. *J Sports Sci.,* Jan, *23(1)*, 41-47

Impellizzeri, F. M., Marcora, S. M., Rampinini, E., Mognoni, P. & Sassi, A. (2005b). Correlations between physiological variables and performance in high level cross country off road cyclists. *Br J Sports Med.,* Oct; *39(10)*, 747-751.

Impellizzeri, F. M., Sassi, A., Rodriguez-Alonso, M., Mognoni, P. & Marcora. (2002). Exercise intensity during off–road cycling competitions. *Med Sci Sports Exerc* Nov, *34(11)*, 1808-1813.

Jentjens, R. (2002). Eating Strategies for Stage Races. In: Jeukendrup AE (ed). *High–Performance Cycling. Part IV: Nutrition.,* Chapter 15, 173-182. Champaign: Human Kinetics.

Jeukendrup, A. E. (2002a). Cycling. In: Maughan RJ (ed). *Nutrition in Sport. Part 4: Sport–specific Nutrition.,* Chapter 43, 562-573. Oxford: Blackwell Science.

Jeukendrup, A. E. (ed) (2002b). *High performance Cycling. Part IV: Nutrition.,* Chapter 12, 139-153. Champaign: Human Kinetics.

Knechtle, B., Enggist, A. & Jehle, T. (2005). Energy turnover at the Race Across America (RAAM) – a case report. *Int J Sports Med* Jul-Aug, *26(6)*, 499-503.

Kugler, H. G. (ed) (2007). *Vegetarisch essen – Fleisch vergessen. Ärztlicher Ratgeber für Vegetarier und Veganer.,* 17-19, 43, 57. Marktheidenfeld: Verlag DAS WORT GmbH.

Kuipers, H., Verstappen, F. T, Keizer, H. A., Geurten, P. & van Kranenburg, G. (1985). Variability of aerobic performance in the laboratory and its physiologic correlates. *Int J Sports Med.,* Aug, *6(4)*, 197-201.

Larson, D. E. (2000). Vegetarian athletes. In : Rosenblooom CA (ed) *Sports Nutrition. A Guide for the Professional Working with Active People.* 3rd edition: 405-425. Chicago, IL: American Dietetic Association, Sports, Cardiovascular, and Wellness Dietetic Practice Group.

Lemon, P. W. R. (1995). Do athletes need more dietary protein and amino acids? *Int J Sport Nutr.,* Jun; *5Suppl*, S39-S61.

Le Système International d'Unités: www.bipm.org, www.bipm.org/en/CGPM/db/11/12/ (15. 2. 2009).

Lindemann, A. K. (1991). Nutrient intake in an ultraendurance cyclist. *Int J Sport Nutr*., Mar, *1(1)*, 79-85.

Lucia, A., Hoyos, J., Santalla, A., Earnest, C. P. & Chicharro, J. L. (2003). Case Report. Giro, Tour and Vuelta in the same season. *Br J Sports Med., 37(5)*, 457-459.

Martin, M. K., Martin, D. T., Collier, G. R. & Burke, L. M. (2002) . Voluntary food intake by elite female cyclists during training and racing: influence of daily energy expenditure and body composition. *Int J Sport Nutr Exerc Metab.*, Sep, *12(3)*, 249-267.

Mastroianni, G. R., Zupan, M. F., Chuba, D. M., Berger, R. C. & Wile, A. L. (2000) . Voluntary pacing and energy cost of off–road cycling and running. *Appl Ergon.*, Oct, *31(5)*, 479-485.

Maughan, R. (2002) Fluid Balance. In: Jeukendrup AE (ed). *High–Performance Cycling. Part IV: Nutrition.* Chapter 13, 155-166. Champaign: Human Kinetics.

Messina, M. & Messina, V. (1996) Vegetarian diets for athletes. In: Messina M and Messina V (ed). *The dietitian`s guide to vegetarian diets: issues and applications.* p. 124–135, 354-367. Gaithersburg, MD: Aspen Publishers.

Niemann, D. C. (1999). Physical fitness and vegetarian diets: Is there a relation? *Am J Clin Nutr.,* Sep, *70(3Suppl)*, 570S-575S.

Niemann, D. C. (1988) Vegetarian dietary practices and endurance performance. *Am J Clin Nutr.,* Sep, *48(3Suppl)*, 754-761.

Padilla, S., Mujika, I., Orbananos, J., Santisteban, J., Angulo, F., Jose–Goiriena, J. (2001). Exercise intensity and load during mass–start stage races in professional road cycling. *Med Sci Sports Exerc.,* May, *33(5)*, 796-802.

Palmer, G. S., Hawley, J. A., Dennis, S. C. & Noakes, T. D. (1994) Heart rate responses during a 4–d cycle stage race. *Med Sci Sports Exerc.,* Oct, *26(10)*, 1278-1283.

Peters, E. M. (2003) Nutritional aspects in ultra–endurance exercise. *Curr Opin Clin Nutr Metab Care.,* Jul, *6(4)*, 427-434.

Petter, K. & Pohlmann, T. (2007). *Die große vegane Nährwerttabelle.* Wien: Eigenverlag. Available from URL: www.veganity.com/GVNWT/Naehrwerttabelle.pdf (15. 2. 2009).

Phillips, R. L., Lemon, F. R., Beeson, W. L. & Kzuma, J. W. (1978). Coronary heart disease mortality among Seventh–Day Adventists with differing dietary habits: a preliminary report. *Am J Clin Nutr.,* Oct, *31(10Suppl)*, S191-198.

Richardson, R. S., Verstraete, D., Johnson, S. C., Luetkemeier, M. J. & Stray–Gundersen, J. (1996). Evidence of a secondary hypervolemia in trained man following acute high intensity exercise. *Int J Sports Med.,* May, *17(4)*, 243-247.

Rose, S. C. & Peters, E. M. (2008) Ad libitum Adjustments to Fluid Intake in cool Environmental Conditions Maintain Hydration Status in a Three–Day Mountain bike Race. *Br J Sports Med.,* 2008, Jun; *6*(Epub ahead of print).

Sabate, J., Duk, A. & Lee, C. L. (1999). Publications trends of vegetarian nutrition articles in biomedical lieterature, 1966–1995. *Am J Clin Nutr.,* Sep, *70(3Suppl)*, 601S-607S.

Sabate, J., Ratzin-Turner, R. A. & Brown, J. E. (2001) Vegetarian diets: descriptions and trends. In: Sabate J (ed) *Vegetarian Nutrition.,* 3-17. Boca Raton, FL: CRC Press.

Saris, W. H. M., van Erp–Baart, M. A., Brouns, F., Westerterp, K. R. & ten Hoor, F. (1989). Study on food intake and energy expenditure during extreme sustained exercise: the Tour de France. *Int J Sports Med.,* May, *10(Suppl)* 1:S26-S31.

Seifert, J. G., Luetkemeier, M. J., Spencer, M. K., Miller, D. & Burke, E. R. (1997). The effects of mountain bike suspension systems on energy expenditure, physical exertion and time trial performance during mountain bicycling. *Int J Sports Med.,* Apr, *18(3)*, 197-200.

Shaw, N. S., Chin, C. J. & Pan, W. H. (1995). A vegetarian diet rich in soybean products compromises iron status in young students. *J of Nutr.,* Feb, *125(2)*, 212-219.

Sobal, J. & Marquart, L. F. (1994) Vitamin/mineral supplement use among athletes: a review of the literature. *Int J Sport Nutr.,* Dec, *4(4)*, 320-334.

Stapelfeldt, B., Schwirtz, A., Schumacher, Y. O. & Hillebrecht, M. (2004). Workload Demands in Mountain Bike Racing. *Int J Sports Med.,* May, *25(4)*, 294-300.

Takaishi, T., Yasuda, Y., Ono, T. & Moritani, T. (1996) Optimal pedalling rate estimated from neuromuscular fatigue for cyclists. *Med Sci Sports Exerc.,* Dec, *28(12)*, 1492-1497.

Union Cycliste Internationale. Available from URL: www.uci.ch (15. 2. 2009).

Venderly, A. M. & Campbell, W. W. (2006). Vegetarian Diets. Nutritional considerations for Athletes. *Sports Med 36(4)*, 293-305.

Whorton, J. C. (1982) *Crusaders for fitness.* Princeton, NJ: Princeton University Press.

Williams, M. H. (1997). *Ernährung, Fintness und Sport.* Berlin/Wiesbaden: Ullstein Mosby

Wingo, J. E., Casa, D. J., Berger, E. M., Dellis, W. O., Knight, J. C. & McClung, J. M. (2004). Influence of a Pre–Exercise Glycerol Hydration Beverage on Performance and Physiologic Function During Mountain–Bike Races in the Heat. *J Athl Train.,* Jun; *9(2)*, 169-175.

Wirnitzer, K. C. & Kornexl, E. (2008). Exercise intensity during an eight–day mountain bike marathon race. *Eur J Appl Physiol.,* Dec, *104(6)*, 999-1005. Epub 2008, Sep 6.

Wirnitzer, K. C. & Faulhaber, M. (2007). Hemoglobin and hematocrit during an 8 day mountainbike race: a field study. Letter to the Editor. *J Sports Sci Med* (serial online)6. Available from both URL (15. 2. 2009), www.jssm.org/vol6/n2/16/v6n2–16text.php, www.jssm.org/vol6/n2/16/v6n2–16pdf.pdf.

www.bleibfit.at/kalorientabelle–naehrwerte.phtml (15. 2. 2009).

www.dge.de/modules (15. 2. 2009).

www.imaner.net/panel/statistics (15. 2. 2009).

www.naehrwerttabelle.de (15. 2. 2009).

www.organicathlete.org/pro–activist (15. 2. 2009).

www.veganfitness.net/forum/viewtopic.php?t=723 (15. 2. 2009).

In: Encyclopedia of Sports and Athletics
Editors: Jack L. Murray and Emily O. Watson
ISBN: 978-1-61209-959-0

Chapter V

Substrates Mobilization and Utilization during Aerobic Exercise: Metabolic Health Benefits

Julien Aucouturier[1], Eric Doré[1], Sébastien Ratel[1], Craig A. Williams[2] and Pascale Duché[1*]

[1]Laboratory of Exercise Biology (BAPS EA 3533), Faculty of Sports Sciences, University of Blaise Pascal, Clermont-Ferrand, France

[2]Children's Health and Exercise Research Centre, School of Sport and Health Sciences, University of Exeter, Exeter, UK

Abstract

Over the last decade, there has been growing interest in the health benefits of exercise for the prevention and treatment of metabolic syndrome disorders.

Currently, the effectiveness of exercise to prevent fat mass gain or to improve the health status of obese people has mainly been assessed through the capacity of exercise to elicit the highest rate of whole body fat oxidation. Hence, low to moderate intensity exercise of duration between 30 to 45 minutes is widely recommended. However, numerous factors affect the mechanisms which control substrate mobilization and utilization. For example, maturation induces changes in substrate metabolism as children tend to oxidize more fat at the same relative submaximal intensity than do adults. Also, studies involving women participants have shown a larger contribution of lipids to energy expenditure. These differences are explained by the effects of ovarian hormones on lipids mobilization, muscle free fat and glucose uptake and oxidation. Acute carbohydrate (CHO) ingestion during exercise has been shown to promote increased CHO oxidation. Similarly, long term, diets rich in CHO and fat promote increased oxidation rates. Furthermore, metabolic alterations such as insulin resistance, abdominal obesity or decreased cardiorespiratory fitness are factors associated with alteration of the

* Corresponding author: Laboratory of Exercise Biology (BAPS), UFR STAPS, University of Blaise Pascal, BP. 104, 63172 Aubière, France, Tel: (33) 4-73-40-75-36, Mobile: (33) 6-19-98-73-81, Email: Pascale.DUCHE@univ-bpclermont.fr

mobilization and oxidation of lipids in fat depots. If exercise is to be used as a therapy, all these factors must be taken when establishing the intensity, duration and mode of exercise in children and adults.

However, other modes of aerobic exercise could be just as potent in the treatment of diseases associated with obesity. Indeed, results from a smaller number of investigations in trained individuals indicate that higher exercise intensities elicit a higher utilization of intramuscular triglycerides. Furthermore, it has been shown from the work of Essen in the 1970s that high intensity intermittent exercises, which also improve maximal aerobic capacity, can elicit rates of fat oxidation similar to those observed during moderate intensity continuous exercise. Therefore, it remains to be determined if this type of exercise is as effective as low intensity exercises in the treatment of metabolic diseases and to evaluate the relative importance of the fat oxidation rate as the best single criterion outcome.

This review will discuss the relationships between the substrates mobilization and utilization during aerobic exercise and the metabolic health benefits.

1. Physical Activity Recommendations

The health benefits of physical and sporting activities have been known since ancient times. Therefore, physical activity is in theory considered to be an important factor contributing to and maintaining health. However, how much exercise is necessary to improve public health for specific populations and outcomes - i.e. cardio-vascular risk, metabolic parameters or fitness -, is unknown. In fact, the evolution of international physical activity recommendations is interesting to consider because it reflects researchers' increasing understanding comprehension of the relationships between physical activity and health (Dunn et al. 1998; Blair et al. 2004; Haskell et al. 2007). Moreover, new recommendations have been established by health organizations in order to face the increased prevalence of obesity and associated diseases such as type 2 diabetes and metabolic syndrome.

The prevalence and severity of metabolic disorders is increasing with rising morbidity and mortality. For this reason there has been a growing interest over the last decade in the health benefits of exercise for the prevention of consequences associated with increased fat mass and the treatment of metabolic syndrome disorders. By increasing energy expenditure and substrates mobilization, muscle-skeletal activity plays an important role in the regulation of energy balance, fat balance, fat mass and glucose homeostasis. Furthermore, metabolic alterations such as insulin resistance, abdominal obesity or decreased cardio-respiratory fitness are factors associated with alteration of the mobilization and oxidation of lipids in fat depots. All these factors need to be taken into account when defining the intensity, duration and mode of exercise if it is to be used as a therapeutic agent for children and adults.

Adult public health recommendations to maintain and improve health are to accumulate 30 minutes or more of moderate intensity physical activity on most, preferably all, days of the week. These recommendations support the proposal that activity of continuous and moderate intensity can boost the contribution made by the lipids to energy expenditure and help improve body composition. Studies reported in the present review indicate that other modes of aerobic exercise could be just as potent in the treatment of diseases associated with obesity. Indeed, results from a smaller number of investigations in trained individuals indicate that higher exercise intensities elicit a higher utilization of intramuscular triglycerides.

Furthermore, high intensity intermittent exercises, which also improve maximal aerobic capacity, can elicit rates of fat oxidation similar to those observed during moderate intensity continuous exercise. Despite most physical activity guidelines recommending low intensity continuous exercise there is strong evidence that high intensity exercise may be as beneficial for many health outcomes, including energy metabolism. However, numerous factors affect the mechanisms which control substrate mobilization and utilization. Finally, although it is difficult to determine a healthy threshold of physical activity, this review will outline the components of exercise (i.e. intensity, frequency and duration) with regard to population characteristics.

1.1. Current Recommendations for Physical Activity Level and Public Health

The American College of Sports Medicine (ACSM) and the American Heart Association AHA) have recently updated their recommendations on physical health activities for maintaining good health for all adults aged from 18 to 65 years (Haskell et al. 2007). It is recommended to maintain and improve health by accumulating 30 minutes of physical activity of moderate intensity (such as continuous type aerobic exercise at an intensity comparable to walking at a brisk pace) at least 5 days a week, or performing physical activity of high intensity for 20 minutes 3 days per week (such as aerobic type exercise comparable to jogging). The presence of a dose-response relationship (intensity and health gain) confirms that additional health benefits may be obtained by exceeding the minimum recommended level. In addition, the scientific data obtained in the last decade showed that strength training also improves muscle quality and function. The specific recommendations are that these activities should be performed on at least 2, non-consecutive days each week, in the form of 8 to 10 exercises using the major muscle groups (with 8 to 12 repetitions of each exercise) (Franklin et al. 2000, Haskell et al. 2007).

A large prospective study comprising 250,000 participants and taking into account a very large number of adjustment factors compared inactive to active participants (Leitzmann et al. 2007). The recommendations for moderate intensity activity (at least 30 minutes on most days of the week) or for high intensity activity (at least 20 minutes 3 times per week) was associated with decreased mortality risk in the order of 30% (Leitzmann et al. 2007).

Thus, the public health recommendation is to have at least 150 minutes per week of moderate intensity physical activity. In energy calorific terms, this equates to between 1,000 and 1,700 kcal per week and could be associated with a significant reduction in mortality (Kesaniemi et al. 2001; Oguma et al. 2002). In terms of walking, to meet current guidelines, individuals are encouraged to walk a minimum of 3000 steps in 30 minutes on 5 days each week. Three bouts of 1000 steps in 10 minutes each day can also be used to meet the minimum recommended goal (Marshall et al. 2009).

2. Acute Effect of Exercise on Energy Metabolism

2.1. Effect of Exercise Intensity on Substrates Utilization

Free fatty acids (FFA) oxidized in skeletal muscle originate from adipose tissue which releases FFA in the circulation, intramuscular triglycerides and plasma triglycerides. Mobilization and utilization of FFA from these different adipose stores are influenced by factors such as the intensity of exercise, training level or body composition of participating subjects. When specifically focusing on obesity, factors other than whole body adiposity are linked with alterations of energy metabolism during exercise. Indeed, studies in obese subjects have led to conflicting results when investigating substrates utilization during exercise. For example, Pérez-Martin et al. (2001) have show that fat oxidation rates were lower in obese than in lean individuals during low intensity exercise. In contrast, Goodpaster et al. (2002) have reported that exercise at a higher intensity (50% of maximal oxygen consumption, VO_{2max}) in obese men relied more on lipid oxidation than it did in lean men. Factors that could explain discrepancies between studies may be specific to the population investigated in each study. Both Kanaley et al. (2001) in a population of obese women and Numao et al. (2006) have failed to show a difference in lipid oxidation rate between individual with an android or visceral localization of fat mass with those who had subcutaneous or gynoid adipose tissue localization. Hence, the severity of obesity, localization of abdominal adipose tissue, insulin resistance and lipid accumulation into muscle cells are all confounding variables which alter substrates utilization.

2.2. Assessment of Substrates Metabolism during Exercise

Based on results showing that adaptations of energy metabolism differ with exercise training programmes in the low or moderate intensity domains (Brandou et al. 2005; van Aggel-Leijssen et al. 2002), exercise testing procedures have been developed in order to assess the intensity of exercise which elicit the maximal fat oxidation rate. Several research teams have used incremental testing to measure the point of maximal fat oxidation (Achten and Jeukendrup 2003; Nordby et al. 2006; Perez-Martin et al. 2001). Exercises generally consist of exercise periods ranging between 3 and 6 minutes, VO_2 and VCO_2 measurements by indirect calorimetry are used to calculate rate of fat and carbohydrate (CHO) oxidation with stoechiometric equations. The maximal fat oxidation point is observed at intensities ranging between 50% and 70% of VO_{2max}. Romijn et al. (1993) observed that fat oxidation was maximal at 65% of VO_{2max} in trained individuals. Also in trained subjects, Van Loon et al. (2001) and Bergman et al. (1999) have reported intensities of 57% and 40% of VO_{2max} for the maximal fat oxidation point. However, in untrained individuals Bergman and Brooks (1999) have reported that fat oxidation was maximal at 59% VO_{2max}. Finally, in a population of more than 300 individuals heterogeneous in terms of physical activity level and physical fitness, the average fat oxidation was maximal at 48% VO_{2max} (Venables et al. 2005). However, there are some limitations to assess rate of fat oxidation through incremental exercises because significant differences of rate of substrates oxidation have been observed between values calculated during incremental exercises and those during square wave exercises matched for intensity (Steffan et al. 1999). Moreover, a study by Meyer et al. (2007) has shown similar rates of fat oxidation during square wave exercises performed at 55%, 65%, 75%, 85% and 95% of the intensity at the anaerobic threshold. Furthermore, when the values measured during the sixth minute of exercise were compared to those measured between the 30th and 40th minutes, significant differences were found. The implications from these findings are that exercise testing does not reflect accurately energy metabolism during long duration activity with low- compared to moderate-intensity exercises, which are typically recommended for exercise training in a health perspective. During exercise in the low- to moderate-intensity domain, a few studies have also failed to show a decline in fat oxidation with increases in exercise intensity in obese children (Maffeis et al. 2005) or in individuals with type 2 diabetes (Kang et al. 1999).

2.3. Plasma Free Fatty Acids Utilization

Utilization of FFA originating from the different lipid stores is also influenced by the intensity of exercise. The study by Romijn et al. (1993) using stable isotope tracers and indirect calorimetry showed that plasma FFA oxidation was maximal at 25% VO_{2max} whereas intramuscular triglycerides (IMTG) oxidation was maximal at higher intensity (65 % of VO_{2max}). A decrease in the contribution of plasma FFA to energy expenditure may partly be explained by a lower release of FFA into the circulation, a decrease in adipose tissue blood flow or an increased FFA re-esterification. However, FFA delivery cannot explain solely the decline in plasma FFA oxidation because an experimental rise in plasma FFA does not increase FFA oxidation during a 85% VO_{2max} exercise to the same level as during a 65% VO_{2max} exercise (Romijn et al. 1995). Hence, it is the increased predominance in CHO oxidation that explains the suppression of fat oxidation in skeletal muscle.

2.4. Intramuscular and Plasma Lipoprotein Derived Triglycerides Utilization

Given their role in fighting the aetiology of insulin resistance and type 2 diabetes, the utilization of intramuscular triglycerides during exercise is an important factor that must be taken into account. In mammals, according to Hoppeler and Weibel (1998) there is a structural limitation for CHO and lipid transport from the circulation to skeletal muscle which is maximal at approximately between 40 to 50% of VO_{2max}. This limitation is due to the sarcolemmal membrane and cannot be up-regulated. Hence, at higher intensities of exercise, energy is mainly provided by intramuscular glycogen and to a lesser extent by intramuscular triglycerides. Thus, in order to mobilize intramuscular triglycerides, intensities higher than 40 to 50% VO_{2max} should be recommended. This is consistent with data reported by Van Loon (2004) in a review that assessed the contribution of intramuscular triglycerides during exercise which showed that during exercise at intensities below 30% VO_{2max} there was only a minor contribution of intramuscular triglycerides to whole body fat oxidation whereas during exercise performed at moderate intensity (>40%VO_{2max}) between 30 to 50% of whole body fat oxidation was accounted for by non plasma FFA oxidation i.e. intramuscular triglycerides.

Lastly, because exercise improves skeletal muscle lipoprotein lipase activity (Nikkila et al. 1978; Seip et al. 1995) it is likely that when training improves non FFA plasma oxidation, a small part of the increase may be explained by an increase in lipoprotein-derived triglycerides (TG) oxidation.

2.5. Acute Regulation of Substrates Metabolism during High Intensity Intermittent Exercise

During a repetition of sprint exercise a progressive decline in power output occurs. The contributions of glycolysis to energy expenditure declines during repeated bouts of exercise even with recovery periods as long as an hour (Bangsbo et al., 1992a) and is not compensated for the increase in oxidative phosphorylation that occurs with the repetition of exercise bouts. Increased H^+, Ca^{2+}, ADP, AMP concentrations during a 30 s sprint and citrate produced by oxidative phosphorylation inhibit glycolytic enzymes, explaining that power output declines when a 30 s is repeated (Bangsbo et al. 1994). Moreover, the decline in power output appears to be dependent on the duration of the sprint performed. With short duration sprints peak power can be maintained during repeated bouts of exercise. Less than 5 minutes in men and 1 min in boys are necessary for creatine phosphate (PCr) re-synthesis (Ratel et al. 2002). Moreover, re-synthesis of PCr is faster in individuals with a high aerobic capacity (Yoshida and Watari 1994).

Several studies have shown that high intensity intermittent exercise can elicit a high rate of lipid oxidation. Studies by Essen et al. (1977 & 1978) have first shown that 15 s exercise periods at a work rate equal to power output at VO_{2max} interspersed with 15 s rest elicited a rate of fat oxidation that was similar to that measured during a continuous exercise at 50% VO_{2max}. Glycogen, ATP and PCr depletion and the increase in citrate concentration within muscle fibres were also similar in both types of exercise. However, there were also lactate differences between high intensity intermittent exercise and low intensity continuous exercise at 50% VO_{2max}. Thus, lipid oxidation during a continuous moderate intensity exercise contributes directly to the production of power output. But during a high intensity intermittent exercise it is a recovery mechanism that contributes to restore ATP and PCr, which are depleted during short and intense bouts of exercise. Moreover, according to Astrand et al. (1960) myoglobin is an O_2 store continuously depleted and reloaded during successive work and recovery periods. Hence, when the duration of work period increases during intermittent exercise, MbO_2 is depleted and glycolysis is activated in order to match the energy which is necessary to maintain the intensity of exercise. This has been confirmed in experiments using near infrared spectroscopy (NIRS) during intermittent exercise with 24 s work period which elicited a higher decline in HbO_2 than shorter exercise period of 6 s (Christmass et al. 1999b).

During exercise, for which power output exceeds maximal aerobic power, have also been shown to induce a significant lipid oxidation. For example, Balsom et al. (1999) have studied an exercise consisting of 6 s sprints interspersed with 30 s recovery performed until exhaustion, with mean power output during exercise period equal to 200% of maximal aerobic power. They showed that Respiratory Exchange Ratio (RER) was approximately 1.02 during exercise periods and ≈0.90 during recovery periods when subjects were fed with a high carbohydrate diet before exercise, and when fed a low CHO diet RER was ≈0.88 during exercise periods and ≈0.75 during recovery periods. By altering the diet composition, muscle glycogen content was increased or decreased and in addition to the intensity of exercise was a factor influencing the balance of substrates oxidation. Since the work by Essen et al., others have specified that both work period duration and the ratio between work period and recovery period duration affect substrate utilization. Increasing durations of work and rest periods, from 6 s work and 9 s recovery to 24 s work and 36 s recovery lead to an increased contribution of glycolysis to energy expenditure, an increase of RER and a decrease in mean VO_2, despite similar intensity of exercise and work/recovery ratio (Christmass et al. 1999a). Moreover, plasma lactate and pyruvate concentrations were higher during the work/recovery ratio 24/36 for all measurements. Glycerol concentration was lower during this ratio, but there was no difference for FFA.

Finally, besides its effects on skeletal muscle metabolism, high intensity exercise also stimulates lipolysis in adipose tissue. High intensity exercise can induce significant lipolysis stimulated by catecholamines, even if lipid oxidation is very low, perhaps as a consequence of catecholamine production which has been shown to rise exponentially with the intensity of exercise (Borsheim and Bahr, 2003). FFA released by lipolysis are then recycled in the triglycerides-fatty acids cycle, facilitating redistribution of endogenous triglycerides (Romijn et al. 1993).

2.6. Effects of Exercise on Energy Expenditure during Recovery

Exercise can increase energy expenditure more than 20 fold in skeletal muscle compared with resting conditions. Moreover, energy expenditure during the post exercise recovery is also increased compared to rest (Borsheim and Bahr 2003). Thus, when looking at the effects of exercise health practitioners should also take into account that the effects of exercise extend beyond the recovery period. The importance of this energy expenditure is generally investigated by the measurement of excess post-exercise oxygen consumption (EPOC) which can be increased for up to 24 hours. Hermansen et al. (1984) have observed an increase of 5.9 % in VO_2, compared with resting condition 24 hours after exercise but other studies have shown that after shorter exercise, EPOC did not exceed 40 minutes. Intensity is the main factor influencing EPOC despite some studies showing a more important effect of exercise duration (Chad and Quigley 1991). Intermittent exercise has been shown to increase EPOC significantly (Almuzaini et al. 1998; Kaminsky et al. 1990). The importance of EPOC is also dependent on the training status of subjects. A higher EPOC has been reported in trained women than sedentary women following exercise at the same submaximal relative intensity (Chad and Quigley 1991). This is explained by a higher VO_2 at the end of exercise in trained women whom VO_{2max} was higher than in sedentary women. Moreover, exercise increases oxygen consumption during a longer period after exercise in untrained subjects (Frey et al. 1993).

The physical activity level and physical fitness affect both the amplitude and duration of EPOC. Chad and Quigley (1991) have shown that trained women had a higher VO_2 after 30 min of exercise either at 50 or 70 % VO_{2max} which could be explained by a higher rate of fat oxidation during the recovery period. However, EPOC being shorter in trained women, because of faster declines of VO_2 and VE in trained individuals (Frey et al. 1993; Short and Sedlock 1997). Hence, these studies showed that highly fit subjects (high VO_{2max}) may exhibit greater amplitude of EPOC but shorter duration because of faster kinetics of ventilatory parameters during recovery. Logically, when exercise has a long duration with high intensity, EPOC remains over long periods of time. Hermansen et al. (1984) have observed that EPOC induced by a 80 min exercise at 75% VO_{2max} represented 48 L and that 24h after exercise VO_2 remained 6% higher than VO_2 during a control resting situation. However, the effect of intensity on the magnitude of EPOC predominates over the effect of exercise duration because according to Gore and Withers (1990a, b), the intensity explains 45% of the variation of EPOC, the duration only 9% and the interaction between duration and exercise 8%. Sedlock et al. (1989) have studied exercise matched for energy expenditure (300 kcal) performed at different intensities. EPOC after 30 minutes of exercise at 50% VO_{2max} was 2.5L whereas it was 6.0L after 20 minutes at 75% VO_{2max}. In comparison, the effect of exercise duration appears to be limited. Performing a 30 minute or a 60 minute exercise at 50% VO_{2max} does not significantly affect EPOC. Finally, the repetition of an exercise bout during a single day may also contribute to increase energy expenditure during post exercise recovery periods. Kaminsky et al. (1990) have shown that two 25 minute exercises at 70% VO_{2max} interspersed by 6.00 h induced a 3 L EPOC whereas it was only 1.4 L when the 50 minutes of exercise where performed in a single bout. Similarly Almuzaini et al. (1998) have measured a 7.4L EPOC during two 15 minute exercise bouts at 70% VO_{2max} whereas EPOC was equal to 5.3L during a 30 minute exercise at the same intensity.

Numerous hormonal responses are involved in increased energy metabolism, particularly when exercise bouts are repeated during the day (Ronsen et al. 2001). Blaak et al. (1993) have suggested that the increased sympathetic activity during post exercise recovery had a thermogenic effect. The importance of catecholamine action on energy metabolism could explain that the increase in EPOC is linearly related to the increase in exercise intensity because catecholamines level are exponentially related to exercise intensity, whereas increasing exercise duration results in a lower catecholamine increase (Borsheim and Bahr 2003). Moreover, even though to our knowledge no study has been conducted in order to assess an effect of protein synthesis on EPOC, it is an energetically costly process that could contribute to the increased energy expenditure.

In summary, the magnitude of EPOC, and subsequent energy expenditure and the balance of substrates utilization are influenced by factors such as physical activity level, physical fitness, exercise intensity and duration and nutritional status. Even though the differences in values are negligible when related to daily energy expenditure, these studies indicate that the intermittent or continuous characters of exercise affect energy expenditure. An exercise above 50 to 60% VO_{2max} seems to be necessary to induce a significant EPOC, and above 60% VO_{2max} a linear relation can be observed between EPOC and exercise intensity (Bahr et al. 1992). However, as far as we know no study has yet assessed EPOC after exercise in children and its effect on physical fitness and body composition.

2.7. Substrate Utilization during Post-Exercise Recovery

In addition to greater post-exercise energy expenditure, exercise induces a decrease in RER during the post-exercise recovery period, which is associated with exercise intensity (Bahr et al. 1991; Bahr et al. 1987). In comparison to lean individuals, obese individuals have been reported to have a lower EPOC and a higher RER during recovery (Wong and Harber 2006). This decrease in RER indicates that CHO oxidation is reduced and prevents a further depletion of glycogen stores after exercise. Insulin has an important role on both CHO and fat metabolism during the recovery period. An exercise bout induces increased fat oxidation during the recovery period even if food ingestion induces a rise in blood insulin. For example, it has been shown in healthy individuals that RER does not increase with an euglycemic hyperinsulinemic clamp during the 2.00 h following a 90 min exercise whereas RER increased significantly in the non-exercising control group (Perreault et al. 2004). In addition, exercise performed before energy intake can blunt the rise of post-prandial lipemia (Katsanos et al. 2004) which could be explained by increased muscle lipoprotein lipase activity in order to restore the IMTG pool depleted during exercise. Low RER is also explained by an in increase in the TG-FFA cycle because an important part of FFA released by lipolysis during exercise is not oxidized during exercise nor re-esterified during the recovery period (Bahr et al. 1990; Bahr et al. 1991). High intensity exercise results in an important release of FFA from adipose tissue but low lipid oxidation. The EPOC observed following this type of exercise could result from usage in the TG-FFA cycling (Borsheim and Bar, 2003). Catecholamines increase lipolysis through activation of hormone sensitive lipase (HSL) which could subsequently determine the activity of the TG-FFA cycle during recovery.

Finally, the increased contribution of fat utilization to energy expenditure during the post-exercise recovery period could induce an increase in VO_2 because of the higher oxygen cost to oxidize lipid than to oxidize CHO as fuel. Indeed, the oxidation of lipid is equivalent to ~4.7 mol per ATP/mol O_2 whereas CHO oxidation is equivalent to ~5.1 mol per ATP/mol O_2.

In summary, energy expenditure during the post-exercise period is mainly influenced by the intensity and mode (intermittent/continuous) of the preceding exercise bout. Whether this energy expenditure is important in terms of weight loss is debatable (Borsheim and Bahr, 2003). Intermittent exercise of a high intensity seems to be well adapted to obtain a maximal increase in energy expenditure during recovery. There is still a need for studies to investigate the effect of exercise on energy metabolism and its potential beneficial effects on lipemia, blood glucose or insulin, especially where exercise is performed before or soon after a meal.

3. Effects of Exercise Training on Energy Metabolism

Despite most physical activity guidelines recommending low intensity continuous exercise there is strong evidence that high intensity of exercise may be as beneficial for many health outcomes, including energy metabolism. Studies investigating the effects of exercise training on energy metabolism have focused attention on energy expenditure and the amount of lipid used during exercise and, in some cases, during recovery in order to improve energy and to balance lipid for fat mass reduction. More recently, researchers have rather focused on metabolic adaptations which may restore the action of insulin in tissues and, more generally, metabolic flux. Finally, other studies have rather focused on the signalling pathways involved in adaptations to exercise training. For example, training activates signalling cascades that induce expression of genes involved in muscle fibre type transformation, mitochondrial biogenesis and increase the content of substrates transporter such as GLUT-4 or FAT/CD36 across the sarcolemmal membrane of muscle cells (Perry et al. 2008).

Studies have shown that weight gain could be predicted from a low fat to CHO ratio during a 24 hour measurement of energy expenditure and substrates utilization. Moreover, obese individuals are considered to have a reduced ability for fat oxidation because of the low activity of oxidative enzymes,β-oxidation (Zurlo et al. 1994) and an altered lipid mobilization (Blaak et al. 1994). Hence, exercise training programmes in individuals with excess body weight and related metabolic disorders aim to restore muscle oxidative capacity and the utilization of fat as a substrate. For this purpose, low to moderate exercise intensities are widely recommended in training programmes in obese subjects because of the important contribution of lipids to the energy expended.

3.1. Adaptations of Muscle Oxidative Capacity with Training

Adherence to exercise may be better with low intensity exercise and reduces the risk of musculo-skeletal injuries. Van Aggel-Leijssen et al. (2002) have compared the effect of low and high intensity continuous exercise training on substrates oxidation in obese men. They showed a significant decrease of FFA plasma oxidation under resting conditions in the high intensity training group. The lipolytic rate was increased during exercise in the low intensity training group, concomitantly with an increase in the contribution of fat to energy expenditure from 35 % before training to 52 % after training. These findings were explained by an increased reliance on non plasma FFA oxidation, most likely IMTG. Nevertheless, the obese group who followed the high intensity training programme also exhibited adaptations of fat metabolism because the reliance on FFA plasma was decreased and non plasma FFA oxidation increased. Furthermore, studies using whole-room indirect calorimetry have failed to show any difference for 24 h energy expenditure and substrates utilization between days with low, high intensity exercises or resistance training (Melanson et al. 2002a; 2002b). Hence, according to Melanson et al. (2002a; 2002b) individuals wishing to experience maximal benefit in terms of energy expenditure and fat oxidation should exercise at the maximal intensity they can comfortably maintain for the time available. Finally, Van Aggel-Leijssen et al. (2002) also questioned that if the improvement of fat oxidation with exercise training was due to an increase of non plasma FFA (probably because of an increase in IMTG utilization), exercise training would not be effective to reduce fat mass and adipose tissue size.

High intensity of training seems to be a factor which is more important than the duration of training when the aim is to improve VO_{2max} and muscle oxidative capacity. Hence, it appears necessary to elicit high intensities of exercise to improve VO_{2max} (Baquet et al. 2003; Wenger and Bell 1986). High intensity intermittent training (HIIT) can be defined as brief periods of exercise at intensity near or above VO_{2max} alternating with periods of recovery. Several studies have indicated that this type of training may be as valuable as low intensity continuous exercise to induce improvements in CHO and lipid metabolism in untrained individuals. Sprint interval training or very high intermittent training differs from HIIT in that the elicited power output is exceedingly higher than the power output elicited at VO_{2max}. For example, Burgomaster et al. (2005) trained their volunteers with series of 4 to 7 Wingate tests (30 s maximal cycle sprint exercise) and investigators of other studies have used intensities ranging between 150 and 300% of power output elicited at VO_{2max}.

Spina et al. (1996) have shown that short-term endurance training induced an increase in activities of citrate synthase, beta-hydroxyacyl-CoA dehydrogenase (β-HAD), mitochondrial thiolase, and carnitine acetyltransferase. Short term HIIT has been shown to induce similar improvements at the skeletal muscle level; Perry et al. (2008) have observed that 6 weeks of training, 3 days a week consisting of 10 bouts of 4 min with 2 min recovery at 90% of VO_{2max} elicited similar increases in citrate synthase (CS), cytochrome c oxidase complex IV (COX IV), beta-hydroxyacyl-CoA dehydrogenase (β-HAD) and pyruvate dehydrogenase (PDH) activities. Also, the rate of fat oxidation at 60% VO_{2max} was significantly increased. In addition, fatty acids transport across sarcolemmal membrane or mitochondrial membrane was increased due to increases in fatty acids transport proteins (FAT/CD36 and FABPpm). MacDougall et al. (1998) have shown an improvement in both glycolytic and oxidative capacity with sprint training. In this study, young lean and healthy men performed 7 weeks of sprints training with 30s all-out exercise interspersed with 4min of recovery at the beginning of the program. Results showed increased phosphofructokinase (PFK) activity and glycolytic flux which are specific to sprint training, but VO_{2max} and activities of oxidative enzymes were also increased. An increased pyruvate flux to the mitochondria has been hypothesized to up-regulate the activities of oxidative enzymes such as CS, malate dehydrogenase, succinate dehydrogenase or β-HAD (MacDougall et al. 1998).

The time course of metabolic adaptations with exercise training occurs rapidly with endurance or high intensity intermittent training. With both types of training increases in oxidative enzymes activities occurred after six to seven training sessions (Gibala et al. 2006; Green et al. 1999; Spina et al. 1996). Gibala et al. (2006) compared endurance training and sprint training with programmes matched for the number of training sessions and recovery between sessions. The total amount of training was 15 minutes and 630 kJ during sprints training and 630 minutes and 6500 kJ during endurance training, and was thus considerably lower with sprint training. Both programmes were two weeks in duration with a total of 6 sessions. The results showed that both types of training induced improvements in short (≈2 min) and long duration (≈ 60 min) performance. In skeletal muscle, the two training programmes induced similar increases in the activity of cytochrome c oxidase (COX).

3.2. Adaptations of Muscle Substrates Stores

The different types of training induce adaptations of substrates storage and metabolism. Several recent studies have reported increased resting muscle glycogen content in response to a short-term training programme with high intensity intermittent exercise. Burgomaster et al. (2005) reported an increase in muscle glycogen content between 26% and 50% after sprint interval training and Perry et al. (2008) reported a 59% increase after a high intensity intermittent training with exercise bouts at 90% VO_{2max}. These values are slightly higher than those previously reported with short-term endurance training (Chesley et al. 1996; Green et al. 1995; Putman et al. 1998). However, in the study by Gibala et al. (2006) comparing the effects of endurance and sprint training, a similar increase in muscle glycogen content was observed with the two programmes. In addition, Talanian et al. (2007) did not observe any changes in resting muscle glycogen or in muscle lipid after seven training sessions of exercise over two weeks. Ross and Leveritt (2001) in a review about the effects of sprint training did not report a systematic increase in muscle glycogen stores after training. It seems that other factors than the intensity of exercise would affect metabolic adaptations. For example, a study by Parra et al. (2000) reported similar increase in glycolytic and oxidative enzyme activities during an interval sprint training performed every day for two weeks or one day every three days during six weeks. However, a reduced glycolytic capacity during a 30 second all out cycling sprint with the former training programme was found.

Lastly, amongst the studies that have investigated the effect of HIIT on energy metabolism, only Talanian et al. (2007) have measured IMTG utilization pre- and post-training as well as during exercise. However, these authors did not report any significant increases in IMTG utilization during 60 minutes endurance exercise, but whole body fat oxidation was improved. Hence, there is a need for future studies to investigate the effect of this type of exercise training on ectopic fat storage which more than body composition, are closely related to the development of metabolic disorders.

In summary, most of the studies showing comparable effects of HIIT and moderate intensity long-duration exercise on skeletal muscle oxidative capacities had durations ranging between 2 to 6 weeks. Such durations may however be too short to induce differences in metabolic adaptations and activate specific signalling pathways. In addition, subjects were generally untrained. Hence, one hypothesis is that when sedentary individuals undergo an exercise training programme, aerobic fitness and metabolic capacity are improved, even if exercises are performed in the anaerobic range of exercise intensity. The repetition of very intense bouts of exercise appears an interesting option compared to more traditional training generally recommended to improve aerobic fitness (VO_{2max}) or substrates metabolism during exercise.

4. Specificities of Exercise Training in Children

4.1. Current Guidelines for Young Populations

The data in children are insufficient to allow accurate recommendations. Recommendations similar to those for adults have been publicized, i.e. at least 30 minutes per day of moderate-intensity activity. One of the first recommendations was published by Simons-Morton et al. (1988) and recommended 20 minutes, 3 times per week with heart rate at ~70% of maximal heart rate. However, the conclusions of several recent publications all agreed that 30 minutes in young children are probably not enough to improve health (Andersen et al. 2006; Strong et al. 2005). A minimal daily amount of physical activity of 60 to 90 minutes at the moderate-to-heavy intensity appears necessary to reduce the risks of cardiovascular diseases. In addition, a 15-minute period of physical activity with vigorous intensity must be included each day (Ness et al. 2007). In adolescents, a daily physical activity of at least 30 minutes at moderate intensity is recommended. Three 20-minute sessions of physical activity at high intensity may be added. The type and form of activities should favour daily exercise and free play physical activity must be taken into account, with factors such as friendship and fun being paramount.

4.2. Energy Metabolism in Children during Exercise

Physical activity is widely recommended for the prevention of excessive weight gain and the treatment of obesity and associated diseases in children. As with to adults, studies investigating substrates metabolism during exercise in children from a health perspective have focused on long duration and low intensity exercise (Maffeis et al. 2005). Even though it has been known for more than 50 years that children do not spontaneously perform continuous and low intensity exercise (Astrand 1952). Paradoxically, the effect of this type of exercise on substrates metabolism is mostly studied for health purposes in children. Again as with adults, experimenters have focused on measuring the exercise intensity that elicits maximal fat oxidation in order to prescribe it during training programs. In obese children, Brandou et al. (2003) the maximal fat oxidation point occurred at 32% VO_{2max}. In obese children, Maffeis et al. (2005) have also observed that the maximal contribution of lipid utilization was obtained at low ambulatory speed (4 $km.h^{-1}$). However, no decline in the absolute rate of fat oxidation was observed for higher walking speeds and the increase in power output was explained by an increased CHO oxidation. In adolescents, Lazzer et al. (2007) reported a value of 41% of maximal aerobic power for the maximal fat oxidation point. Furthermore, in young obese subjects, maturation affects the rate of lipid oxidation. Indeed, the maximal fat oxidation point occurs at a higher intensity in pubertal obese subjects compared to pre-pubertal children (Brandou et al. 2006). However, others have only reported a minor decrease of the maximal fat oxidation point in pubertal compared to pre-pubertal obese subjects (46 *vs* 49% VO_{2max}) (Zunquin et al. 2006).

Healthy children compared to adults during exercise of similar intensities have a higher contribution of lipid oxidation to energy expenditure (Foricher et al. 2003; Martinez and Haymes 1992; Timmons et al. 2003). In addition, children may rely on oxidative metabolism during intense exercise more than adults. Several studies based on measurement of glycolytic enzymes activities in skeletal muscle have suggested that children have a reduced glycolytic capacity when compared to adults (Eriksson et al. 1971). However, other studies have shown by using ^{31}P Nuclear Magnetic Resonance that glycolytic capacity is not maturity dependent (Petersen et al. 1999) and that differences in glycogen utilization between children and adults could be explained by a low muscle glycogen content before puberty (Timmons et al. 2007).

Several studies have shown that when children engage in unstructured physical activity their activity pattern is characterized by short and repeated bursts of very intense exercise (Bailey et al. 1995; Duncan et al. 2008). When compared to adults, lower blood lactate, blood acidity and faster recovery between bouts of exercise may partly explain why high intensity exercise is perceived as less strenuous to children than adults. On the contrary, these advantages are less obvious during longer duration exercise. Indeed, in exercise lasting longer than 15 minutes the rise in RPE is faster than in adults (Bar-Or and Rowland, 2004).

From results of studies in adult populations, we can infer that high intensity intermittent training could increase the ability for fat oxidation during exercise. Exercise in the heavy intensity domain has already been shown to induce greater improvement in maximal aerobic capacity than training in the low- to moderate-intensity range. Baquet et al. (2003) who have specifically reviewed the studies reporting the effect of endurance training on VO_{2max} in children and adolescents have concluded that exercising at intensities above 80% VO_{2max} was necessary to obtain a significant improvement of VO_{2max}. Moreover, a high oxidative capacity could explain the fast recovery between sprints in children (Ratel et al., 2002a). Also, some studies have shown that muscle glycogen content may be reduced in children (Eriksson, 1980). Thus, as in adults with a low muscle glycogen level, the contribution of fat utilization to energy expenditure is increased and it is conceivable that prolonged high intensity intermittent exercise with children could result in improved lipid oxidation due to low glycogen availability.

In summary, there is some evidence that participation in exercise training programmes with high intensity intermittent exercise may be improved by reducing the perceived difficulty of the exercise. This is surprising since this type of exercise seems to be particularly well adapted to children's exercise preferences. Likewise, there is evidence in adult studies, that both maximal aerobic capacity and substrates metabolism can be improved with high intensity intermittent exercise. However, it remains to be determined whether this type of exercise is associated with higher rates of fat oxidation during acute exercise and metabolic adaptations with chronic training programmes.

5. Specificities of Exercise Training in the Elderly

5.1. Important Advance for Physical Activity in Elderly People

Recommendations on the types and amounts of physical activity for adults aged over 65 years and for patients suffering from chronic diseases over the age of 50 years have been published by the ACSM and AHA (Nelson et al. 2007a, b). These recommendations are essentially based on aerobic-type activities of moderate intensity for a minimum of 30 minutes per day, 5 days per week or of high intensive for 20 minutes per day, 3 days per week. However, special emphasis is placed on the individualisation of the intensity of the physical activity as advocated by using a visual analogue scale. The intensity level 5-6 on the scale is considered as moderate. Secondly, the diversification of activities is very important for this population. In addition to aerobic exercise, strength training should also be added to preserve and maintain muscular strength and balance. It is necessary to combine moderate and intense activities. In elderly people, physical activity for maintaining muscle and joint flexibility are recommended because of the association with balance exercises to prevent them from falling. People who wish to further improve their physical fitness, reduce their risk of chronic disease and disability or prevent excessive weight gain must follow at least the minimum physical activity recommended.

5.2. Effects of Acute Exercise on Substrates Utilization

Aging is associated with an increased risk of cardiovascular diseases and metabolic disorders such as type 2 diabetes. Alterations in muscle mitochondrial function in the elderly (Wallace 2005), and an increased prevalence of obesity with age are linked with the development of insulin resistance (Ryan 2000). In addition, aging is associated with a decrease in fat free mass and particularly muscle mass, which determines the largest component of energy expenditure and whole body fat oxidation. This can partially explain a decline in the rate of fat oxidation in absolute terms. At the whole body level, several studies have shown that aging is linked with a decline in fat oxidation (Nagy et al. 1996; Solomon et al. 2008) However, investigations at the muscle cell level indicate that CPT activity and muscle fat oxidative capacity are not reduced with aging (Rimbert et al. 2004). The latter study, which investigated the effects of age and physical inactivity on muscle fat oxidative capacity in young and old men who were sedentary or trained showed that the ability to use fat as a fuel was similar between young and old subjects with the same training status but was higher in groups of trained men compared to physically inactive men matched for age. However, it is of importance to note that muscle fat oxidative capacity was expressed as nanomoles of palmitate per gram of wet tissue per minute and thereby excludes the effect of muscle mass and aerobic fitness. Further to this, several other studies have compared young and older subjects for whole body rate of fat oxidation during exercise (Hagberg et al. 1988; Sial et al. 1998). Sial et al. (1998) and Hagberg et al. (1988) have report lower values of FFA oxidation in older subjects. Furthermore, lower FFA oxidation was observed in the former study in 66-79 year old men compared to 20-30 year old men whether subjects exercised at the same absolute or at relative intensity. Under resting conditions fat oxidation is reduced in the older subjects even when adjusted to fat free mass (Solomon et al. 2008). Moreover, the study by Solomon et al. (2008) showed that the rate of fat oxidation was positively correlated with VO_{2max} and negatively with age. As previously reported, these authors also observed the age-related physiological decline of VO_{2max}.

There is evidence that the contribution of fat oxidation to energy expenditure during submaximal exercise is higher in pre-menopausal women than in men (Ruby and Robergs 1994; Tarnopolsky 2000). In older individuals, this difference in fat oxidation is no longer apparent (Toth et al. 1998). Furthermore, this study also showed that under resting conditions fat oxidation is higher in men than in women. This study and others have shown that it is fat free mass reflecting metabolically active tissue rather than fat mass which is a determinant of basal lipolysis and FFA delivery and oxidation in individuals of normal weight (Calles-Escandon and Driscoll 1995; Toth et al. 1996; Toth et al. 1998).

5.3. Effects of Exercise Training

Studies investigating the effect of training on energy metabolism in the elderly have either focused on population with different training backgrounds alongside lifespan or the effect of short-term training programmes on energy metabolism in untrained men from baseline. Both types of studies generally show that training increases the reliance on fat as energy source during submaximal exercise (Boon et al. 2007; Schrauwen et al. 2002). However, these studies have also highlighted discrepancies between the time-course of metabolic adaptations with long-term or short-term training programmes. Boon et al. (2007) have for example hypothesized that short-term training induces an increase in fat oxidation through an early increase in muscle triglycerides and plasma triglycerides mobilization whereas long-term training adaptation occurs through a delayed rise in adipose tissue lipolysis and muscle FFA transport capacity. Indeed, Boon et al. (2007) have shown in 57-year old endurance-trained men that the contribution of muscle and plasma lipoprotein derived TG to energy expenditure was approximately 10% during an exercise set at 50% of maximal aerobic power. When compared to untrained age-matched men, greater FFA rate of appearance in the circulation, their uptake and oxidation in skeletal muscle explained the higher fat oxidation rate in older endurance trained-athletes. In contrast, Schrauwen et al. (2002) showed that after a 3-month endurance training programme in previously untrained subjects, the contribution of fatty acids derived from IMTG and/or plasma lipoprotein TG accounted for 40% compared to 20% before the beginning of training.

The reduction in aerobic capacity with age is explained, first, by a reduction in O_2 delivery because of a reduced cardiac output and peripheral oxygen uptake whereas the decreased fat free mass is an important factor to explain the decreased absolute value of VO_{2max} (Proctor and Joyner 1997). Endurance training in individuals above 60 years old has been shown to prevent the decline in muscle oxidative capacity linked with age. Short et al. (2004) also showed that endurance training 3 to 4 times per week could improve aerobic capacity and muscle protein synthesis. Moreover, this study also showed that aerobic exercise in older subjects induced an increase in muscle protein synthesis, possibly associated with an increased muscle protein turnover (Pikosky et al. 2006). The increased turnover may help to prevent the loss of fat free mass and may also improve mitochondrial biogenesis as suggested by increased mRNAs encoding mitochondrial proteins and transcription factors e.g. PGC1α. While many studies have focused on measurements of substrates oxidation at the whole body level or in skeletal muscle, others have also investigated the responses of hormones which regulate substrate mobilization during exercise (Manetta et al. 2005). For example, Manetta et al. (2005) have shown an increased epinephrine response in older trained cyclists, both in comparison to young trained men and to sedentary older men. This increased catecholamine response may help older trained subjects to maintain a high rate of CHO oxidation because the decline in CHO utilization that was associated with aging was lesser in trained cyclists than in sedentary men, especially for exercise intensities above the ventilator threshold.

In summary, oxidative capacity irrespective of the type of substrate which is used appears to be a major factor conditioning rate of fat oxidation. Some studies show that muscle fat oxidative capacity may not decrease with age but rather with physical activity. In addition, other factors condition are conditioning fat metabolism during exercise. These factors could be due to an age-related impairment of lipolytic responsiveness in adipose tissue and a reduced delivery of substrates to muscle cell because of a decline in capillary density in skeletal muscle or a decrease in fat free mass, which could explain the decline of rates of fat oxidation expressed in absolute values. It is not currently possible to provide exercise recommendations for a training programme specifically targeted to improve fat utilization in the elderly. However, given the strong link between aerobic fitness and fat oxidation which has been reported in the elderly, it may be of importance to slow down the physiological decline in VO_{2max} that occurs with age in order to prevent a reduction of substrates oxidation rate.

6. Summary and Conclusion

Exercise is an important part of therapeutic intervention for the treatment of obesity which has for its main purpose the improvement of body composition. However, health practitioners and physical activity instructors should also be aware that even moderate intensity activity can improve lipid mobilization and the contribution of fat oxidation to energy expenditure. Furthermore, regular physical activity of moderate intensity improves several abnormalities linked to the metabolic syndrome such as reducing the effects of insulin resistance, hyperglycemia, poor triglycerides and HDL cholesterol profiles and hypertension. It is very important to note that these beneficial modifications of sensitivity to insulin, tolerance to glucose and lipid profile under the effect of regular training can be observed. These changes are independent of modifications in weight or fat mass, and occur in the absence of major modifications of cardio-respiratory capacity (VO_{2max}). Indeed, there are also some findings indicating that the capacity for fat oxidation can be improved with low-intensity exercise in the absence of any changes in muscle oxidative capacity or VO_{2max}. Hence, in people with medical conditions that preclude high-intensity physical activity, low-intensity exercise may improve metabolic fitness without the positive effect of aerobic fitness. Finally, higher intensity of exercise and high-intensity intermittent exercise are also of interest because they induce rapid improvement in muscle oxidative capacity, enzymes involved in fat metabolism and aerobic fitness. These intensities could also elicit a higher mobilization of intramuscular triglycerides which are involved in the pathogenesis of insulin resistance and metabolic syndrome. Moreover, there is some evidence that this type of exercise appears to be perceived as less strenuous and may favour long-term adherence to physical activity programmes.

References

Achten, J. & Jeukendrup, A. E. (2003). Maximal fat oxidation during exercise in trained men. Int *J Sports Med.*, *24*, 603-608.

Almuzaini, K. S., Potteiger, J. A. & Green, S. B. (1998). Effects of split exercise sessions on excess postexercise oxygen consumption and resting metabolic rate. *Can J Appl Physiol.*, *23*, 433-443.

Andersen, L. B., Harro, M., Sardinha, L. B., Froberg, K., Ekelund, U., Brage, S. & Anderssen, S. A. (2006). Physical activity and clustered cardiovascular risk in children: a cross-sectional study (The European Youth Heart Study). *Lancet.*, *368*, 299-304.

Astrand, I., Astrand, P. O., Christensen, E. H. & Hedman, R. (1960). Myohemoglobin as an oxygen-store in man. *Acta Physiol Scand.*, *48*, 454-460.

Astrand, P. O. (1952). *Experimental studies of the physical working capacity in relation to sex and age*. Copenhagen: Munksgaard.

Bahr, R., Gronnerod, O. & Sejersted, O. M. (1992). Effect of supramaximal exercise on excess postexercise O2 consumption. *Med Sci Sports Exerc.*, *24*, 66-71.

Bahr, R., Hansson, P. & Sejersted, O. M. (1990). Triglyceride/fatty acid cycling is increased after exercise. *Metabolism.*, *39*, 993-999.

Bahr, R., Hostmark, A. T., Newsholme, E. A., Gronnerod, O. & Sejersted, O. M. (1991). Effect of exercise on recovery changes in plasma levels of FFA, glycerol, glucose and catecholamines. *Acta Physiol Scand.*, *143*, 105-115.

Bahr, R., Ingnes, I., Vaage, O., Sejersted, O. M. & Newsholme, E. A. (1987). Effect of duration of exercise on excess postexercise O2 consumption. *J Appl Physiol.*, *62*, 485-490.

Bailey, R. C., Olson, J., Pepper, S. L., Porszasz, J., Barstow, T. J. & Cooper, D. M. (1995). The level and tempo of children's physical activities: an observational study. Med Sci Sports Exerc., *27*, 1033-1041.

Balsom, P. D., Gaitanos, G. C., Soderlund, K. & Ekblom, B. (1999). High-intensity exercise and glycogen availability in humans. *Acta Physiol Scand.*, *165*, 337-345.

Bangsbo, J., Graham, T., Johansen, L. & Saltin, B. (1994). Muscle lactate metabolism in recovery from intense exhaustive exercise: impact of light exercise. *J Appl Physiol.*, *77*, 1890-1895.

Baquet, G., van Praagh, E. & Berthoin, S. (2003). Endurance training and aerobic fitness in young people. *Sports Med.*, *33*, 1127-1143.

Bergman, B. C. & Brooks, G. A. (1999). Respiratory gas-exchange ratios during graded exercise in fed and fasted trained and untrained men. *J Appl Physiol.*, *86*, 479-487.

Blaak, E. E., van Baak, M. A., Kemerink, G. J., Pakbiers, M. T., Heidendal, G. A. & Saris, W. H. (1994). Total forearm blood flow as an indicator of skeletal muscle blood flow: effect of subcutaneous adipose tissue blood flow. *Clin Sci (Lond).*, *87*, 559-566.

Blaak, E. E., van Baak, M. A., Kempen, K. P. & Saris, W. H. (1993). Role of alpha- and beta-adrenoceptors in sympathetically mediated thermogenesis. *Am J Physiol.*, *264*, E11-17.

Boon, H., Jonkers, R. A., Koopman, R., Blaak, E. E., Saris, W. H., Wagenmakers, A. J. & L. J. VANL. (2007). Substrate source use in older, trained males after decades of endurance training. *Med Sci Sports Exerc.*, *39*, 2160-2170

Borsheim, E. & Bahr, R. (2003). Effect of exercise intensity, duration and mode on post-exercise oxygen consumption. *Sports Med.*, *33*, 1037-1060.

Brandou, F., Savy-Pacaux, A. M., Marie, J., Bauloz, M., Maret-Fleuret, I., Borrocoso, S., Mercier, J. & Brun, J. F. (2005). Impact of high- and low-intensity targeted exercise training on the type of substrate utilization in obese boys submitted to a hypocaloric diet. *Diabetes Metab.*, *31*, 327-335.

Brandou, F., Savy-Pacaux, A. M., Marie, J., Brun, J. F. & Mercier, J. (2006). Comparison of the type of substrate oxidation during exercise between pre and post pubertal markedly obese boys. Int J Sports Med *27*, 407-414.

Burgomaster, K. A., Hughes, S. C., Heigenhauser, G. J., Bradwell, S. N. & Gibala, M. J. (2005). Six sessions of sprint interval training increases muscle oxidative potential and cycle endurance capacity in humans. *J Appl Physiol.*, *98*, 1985-1990.

Calles-Escandon, J. & Driscoll, P. (1995). Diet and body composition as determinants of basal lipolysis in humans. *Am J Clin Nutr.*, *61*, 543-548.

Chad, K. E. & Quigley, B. M. (1991). Exercise intensity: effect on postexercise O2 uptake in trained and untrained women. *J Appl Physiol.*, *70*, 1713-1719.

Chesley, A., Heigenhauser, G. J. & Spriet, L. L. (1996). Regulation of muscle glycogen phosphorylase activity following short-term endurance training. *Am J Physiol.*, *270*, E328-335.

Christmass, M. A., Dawson, B. & Arthur, P. G. (1999a). Effect of work and recovery duration on skeletal muscle oxygenation and fuel use during sustained intermittent exercise. *Eur J Appl Physiol Occup Physiol.*, *80*, 436-447.

Christmass, M. A., Dawson, B., Passeretto, P. & Arthur, P. G. (1999b). A comparison of skeletal muscle oxygenation and fuel use in sustained continuous and intermittent exercise. *Eur J Appl Physiol Occup Physiol.*, *80*, 423-435.

Duncan, J. S., Badland, H. M. & Schofield, G. (2008). Combining GPS with heart rate monitoring to measure physical activity in children: A feasibility study. *J Sci Med Sport.*

Eriksson, B. O., Karlsson, J. & Saltin, B. (1971). Muscle metabolites during exercise in pubertal boys. *Acta Paediatr Scand Suppl.*, *217*, 154-157.

Essen, B. (1978). Studies on the regulation of metabolism in human skeletal muscle using intermittent exercise as an experimental model. *Acta Physiol Scand Suppl.*, *454*, 1-32.

Essen, B., Hagenfeldt, L. & Kaijser, L. (1977). Utilization of blood-borne and intramuscular substrates during continuous and intermittent exercise in man. *J Physiol.*, *265*, 489-506.

Franklin, B., Whaley, M. & Howley, E. (2000). ACSM 's Guidelines for Exercise Testing and Prescription. 6th Edition. 137-164.

Foricher, J. M., Ville, N., Gratas-Delamarche, A. & Delamarche, P. (2003). Effects of submaximal intensity cycle ergometry for one hour on substrate utilisation in trained prepubertal boys versus trained adults. *J Sports Med Phys Fitness.*, *43*, 36-43.

Frey, G. C., Byrnes, W. C. & Mazzeo, R. S. (1993). Factors influencing excess postexercise oxygen consumption in trained and untrained women. *Metabolism.*, *42*, 822-828.

Gibala, M. J., Little, J. P., van Essen, M., Wilkin, G. P., Burgomaster, K. A., Safdar, A., Raha, S. & Tarnopolsky, M. A. (2006). Short-term sprint interval versus traditional endurance training: similar initial adaptations in human skeletal muscle and exercise performance. *J Physiol.*, *575*, 901-911.

Goodpaster, B. H., Wolfe, R. R. & Kelley, D. E. (2002). Effects of obesity on substrate utilization during exercise. *Obes Res.*, *10*, 575-584.

Gore, C. J. & Withers, R. T. (1990a). Effect of exercise intensity and duration on postexercise metabolism. *J Appl Physiol.*, *68*, 2362-2368.

Gore, C. J. & Withers, R. T. (1990b). The effect of exercise intensity and duration on the oxygen deficit and excess post-exercise oxygen consumption. *Eur J Appl Physiol Occup Physiol 60*, 169-174.

Green, H., Grant, S., Bombardier, E. & Ranney, D. (1999). Initial aerobic power does not alter muscle metabolic adaptations to short-term training. *Am J Physiol.*, *277*, E39-48.

Green, H. J., Cadefau, J., Cusso, R., Ball-Burnett, M. & Jamieson, G. (1995). Metabolic adaptations to short-term training are expressed early in submaximal exercise. *Can J Physiol Pharmacol.*, *73*, 474-482.

Hagberg, J. M., Seals, D. R., Yerg, J. E., Gavin, J., Gingerich, R., Premachandra, B. & Holloszy, J. O. (1988). Metabolic responses to exercise in young and older athletes and sedentary men. *J Appl Physiol.*, *65*, 900-908.

Haskell, W. L., Lee, I. M., Pate, R. R., Powell, K. E., Blair, S. N., Franklin, B. A., Macera, C. A., Heath, G. W., Thompson, P. D. & Bauman, A. (2007). Physical activity and public health: updated recommendation for adults from the American College of Sports Medicine and the American Heart Association. *Circulation.*, *116*, 1081-1093

Hermansen, L., Grandmontagne, M. & Mæhlum, S. (1984). Post exercise elevation of resting oxygen uptake - possible mechanisms and physiological significance from intense intermittent running and prolonged walking. In: Marconnet P., Poortmans J, Hermansen L., editors Medicine and sport Science Basel: *Karger.*, *17*, 119-129

Hoppeler, H. & Weibel, E. R. (1998). Limits for oxygen and substrate transport in mammals. *J Exp Biol.*, *201*, 1051-1064.

Kaminsky, L. A., Padjen, S. & LaHam-Saeger, J. (1990). Effect of split exercise sessions on excess post-exercise oxygen consumption. *Br J Sports Med.*, *24*, 95-98.

Kanaley, J. A., Weatherup-Dentes, M. M., Alvarado, C. R. & Whitehead, G. (2001). Substrate oxidation during acute exercise and with exercise training in lean and obese women. *Eur J Appl Physiol.*, *85*, 68-73.

Kang, J., Kelley, D. E., Robertson, R. J., Goss, F. L., Suminski, R. R., Utter, A. C. & Dasilva, S. G. (1999). Substrate utilization and glucose turnover during exercise of varying intensities in individuals with NIDDM. *Med Sci Sports Exerc.*, *31*, 82-89.

Katsanos, C. S., Grandjean, P. W. & Moffatt, R. J. (2004). Effects of low and moderate exercise intensity on postprandial lipemia and postheparin plasma lipoprotein lipase activity in physically active men. *J Appl Physiol.*, *96*, 181-188.

Kesaniemi, Y. K., Danforth, E., Jr., Jensen, M. D., Kopelman, P. G., Lefebvre, P. & Reeder, B. A. (2001). Dose-response issues concerning physical activity and health: an evidence-based symposium. *Med Sci Sports Exerc.*, *33*, S351-358.

Lazzer, S., Busti, C., Agosti, F., De Col, A., Pozzo, R. & Sartorio, A. (2007). Optimizing fat oxidation through exercise in severely obese Caucasian adolescents. *Clin Endocrinol (Oxf).*, *67*, 582-588.

Leitzmann, M. F., Park, Y., Blair, A., Ballard-Barbash, R., Mouw, T., Hollenbeck, A. R. & Schatzkin, A. (2007). Physical activity recommendations and decreased risk of mortality. *Arch Intern Med.*, *167*, 2453-2460.

MacDougall, J. D., Hicks, A. L., MacDonald, J. R., McKelvie, R. S., Green, H. J. & Smith, K. M. (1998). Muscle performance and enzymatic adaptations to sprint interval training. *J Appl Physiol.*, *84*, 2138-2142.

Maffeis, C., Zaffanello, M., Pellegrino, M., Banzato, C., Bogoni, G., Viviani, E., Ferrari, M. & Tato, L. (2005). Nutrient oxidation during moderately intense exercise in obese prepubertal boys. *J Clin Endocrinol Metab.*, *90*, 231-236.

Manetta, J., Brun, J. F., Prefaut, C. & Mercier, J. (2005). Substrate oxidation during exercise at moderate and hard intensity in middle-aged and young athletes vs sedentary men. *Metabolism.*, *54*, 1411-1419.

Marshall, S. J., Levy, S. S., Tudor-Locke, C. E., Kolkhorst, F. W., Wooten, K. M., Ji, M., Macera, C. A. & Ainsworth, B. E. (2009). Translating physical activity recommendations into a pedometer-based step goal: 3000 steps in 30 minutes. *Am J Prev Med.*, *36*, 410-415.

Martinez, L. R. & Haymes, E. M. (1992). Substrate utilization during treadmill running in prepubertal girls and women. *Med Sci Sports Exerc.*, *24*, 975-983.

Melanson, E. L., Sharp, T. A., Seagle, H. M., Donahoo, W. T., Grunwald, G. K., Peters, J. C., Hamilton, J. T. & Hill, J. O. (2002a). Resistance and aerobic exercise have similar effects on 24-h nutrient oxidation. *Med Sci Sports Exerc.*, *34*, 1793-1800.

Melanson, E. L., Sharp, T. A., Seagle, H. M., Horton, T. J., Donahoo, W. T., Grunwald, G. K., Hamilton, J. T. & Hill, J. O. (2002b). Effect of exercise intensity on 24-h energy expenditure and nutrient oxidation. *J Appl Physiol.*, *92*, 1045-1052.

Meyer, T., Gassler, N. & Kindermann, W. (2007). Determination of "Fatmax"with 1 h cycling protocols of constant load. *Appl Physiol Nutr Metab.*, *32*, 249-256.

Nagy, T. R., Goran, M. I., Weinsier, R. L., Toth, M. J., Schutz, Y. & Poehlman, E. T. (1996). Determinants of basal fat oxidation in healthy Caucasians. *J Appl Physiol.*, *80*, 1743-1748.

Nelson, M. E., Rejeski W. J., Blair SN., Duncan PW., Judge JO., King AC., Macera CA. & Castaneda-Sceppa C. (2007a). Physical activity and public health in older adults: recommendation from the American College of Sports Medicine and the American Heart Association. *Med Sci Sports Exerc.*, *39*, 1435-1445.

Nelson, M. E., Rejeski, W. J., Blair, S. N., Duncan, P. W., Judge, J. O., King, A. C., Macera, C. A. & Castaneda-Sceppa, C. (2007b). Physical activity and public health in older adults: recommendation from the American College of Sports Medicine and the American Heart Association. *Circulation.*, *116*, 1094-1105.

Ness, A. R., Leary, S. D., Mattocks, C., Blair, S. N., Reilly, J. J., Wells, J., Ingle, S., Tilling, K., Smith, G. D. & Riddoch, C. (2007). Objectively measured physical activity and fat mass in a large cohort of children. *PLoS Med 4*, e97.

Nikkila, E. A., Taskinen, M. R., Rehunen, S. & Harkonen, M. (1978). Lipoprotein lipase activity in adipose tissue and skeletal muscle of runners: relation to serum lipoproteins. *Metabolism.*, *27*, 1661-1667.

Nordby, P., Saltin, B. & Helge, J. W. (2006). Whole-body fat oxidation determined by graded exercise and indirect calorimetry: a role for muscle oxidative capacity? *Scand J Med Sci Sports 16*, 209-214.

Numao, S., Hayashi, Y., Katayama, Y., Matsuo, T., Tomita, T., Ohkawara, K., Nakata, Y. & Tanaka, K. (2006). Effects of obesity phenotype on fat metabolism in obese men during endurance exercise. *Int J Obes (Lond).*, *30*, 1189-1196.

Oguma, Y., Sesso, H. D., Paffenbarger, R. S. & Jr., Lee, I. M. (2002). Physical activity and all cause mortality in women: a review of the evidence. *Br J Sports Med.*, *36*, 162-172.

Parra, J., Cadefau, J. A., Rodas, G., Amigo, N. & Cusso, R. (2000). The distribution of rest periods affects performance and adaptations of energy metabolism induced by high-intensity training in human muscle. *Acta Physiol Scand 169*, 157-165.

Perez-Martin, A., Dumortier, M., Raynaud, E., Brun, JF., Fedou, C., Bringer, J. & Mercier, J. (2001). Balance of substrate oxidation during submaximal exercise in lean and obese people. *Diabetes Metab.*, *27*, 466-474.

Perreault, L., Lavely, J. M., Bergman, B. C. & Horton, T. J. (2004). Gender differences in insulin action after a single bout of exercise. *J Appl Physiol 97*, 1013-1021.

Perry, C. G., Heigenhauser, G. J., Bonen, A. & Spriet, L. L. (2008). High-intensity aerobic interval training increases fat and carbohydrate metabolic capacities in human skeletal muscle. *Appl Physiol Nutr Metab 33*, 1112-1123.

Petersen, S. R., Gaul, C. A., Stanton, M. M. & Hanstock, C. C. (1999). Skeletal muscle metabolism during short-term., high-intensity exercise in prepubertal and pubertal girls. *J Appl Physiol.*, *87*, 2151-2156.

Pikosky, M. A., Gaine, P. C., Martin, W. F., Grabarz, K. C., Ferrando, A. A., Wolfe, R. R. & Rodriguez, N. R. (2006). Aerobic exercise training increases skeletal muscle protein turnover in healthy adults at rest. *J Nutr.*, *136*, 379-383.

Proctor, D. N. & Joyner, M. J. (1997). Skeletal muscle mass and the reduction of VO2max in trained older subjects. *J Appl Physiol.*, *82*, 1411-1415.

Putman CT., Jones NL., Hultman E., Hollidge-Horvat MG., Bonen A., McConachie DR. & Heigenhauser, G. J. (1998). Effects of short-term submaximal training in humans on muscle metabolism in exercise. *Am J Physiol 275*, E132-139

Ratel S., Bedu M., Hennegrave A., Dore E. & Duche P. (2002). Effects of age and recovery duration on peak power output during repeated cycling sprints. *Int J Sports Med 23*, 397-402

Rimbert V., Boirie Y., Bedu M., Hocquette JF., Ritz P. & Morio B. (2004). Muscle fat oxidative capacity is not impaired by age but by physical inactivity: association with insulin sensitivity. *FASEB J 18*, 737-739

Romijn JA., Coyle EF., Sidossis LS., Gastaldelli A., Horowitz JF., Endert E. & Wolfe RR. (1993). Regulation of endogenous fat and carbohydrate metabolism in relation to exercise intensity and duration. *Am J Physiol 265*, E380-391

Romijn JA., Coyle EF., Sidossis LS., Zhang XJ. & Wolfe RR. (1995). Relationship between fatty acid delivery and fatty acid oxidation during strenuous exercise. *J Appl Physiol 79*, 1939-1945

Ronsen O., Haug E., Pedersen BK. & Bahr R. (2001). Increased neuroendocrine response to a repeated bout of endurance exercise. *Med Sci Sports Exerc 33*, 568-575

Ross A. & Leveritt M. (2001). Long-term metabolic and skeletal muscle adaptations to short-sprint training: implications for sprint training and tapering. Sports Med *31*, 1063-1082

Ruby BC. & Robergs RA. (1994). Gender differences in substrate utilisation during exercise. *Sports Med 17*, 393-410

Ryan AS. (2000). Insulin resistance with aging: effects of diet and exercise. *Sports Med 30*, 327-346

Schrauwen P., van Aggel-Leijssen DP., Hul G., Wagenmakers AJ., Vidal H., Saris WH. & van Baak MA. (2002). The effect of a 3-month low-intensity endurance training program on fat oxidation and acetyl-CoA carboxylase-2 expression. *Diabetes 51*, 2220-2226

Sedlock DA., Fissinger JA. & Melby CL. (1989). Effect of exercise intensity and duration on postexercise energy expenditure. *Med Sci Sports Exerc 21*, 662-666

Seip RL., Angelopoulos TJ. & Semenkovich CF. (1995). Exercise induces human lipoprotein lipase gene expression in skeletal muscle but not adipose tissue. *Am J Physiol 268*, E229-236

Short KR. & Sedlock DA. (1997). Excess postexercise oxygen consumption and recovery rate in trained and untrained subjects. *J Appl Physiol 83*, 153-159

Short KR., Vittone JL., Bigelow ML., Proctor DN. & Nair KS. (2004). Age and aerobic exercise training effects on whole body and muscle protein metabolism. *Am J Physiol Endocrinol Metab 286*, E92-101

Sial S., Coggan AR., Hickner RC. & Klein S. (1998). Training-induced alterations in fat and carbohydrate metabolism during exercise in elderly subjects. *Am J Physiol 274*, E785-790

Simons-Morton BG., Parcel GS., O'Hara NM., Blair SN. & Pate RR. (1988). Health-related physical fitness in childhood: status and recommendations. *Annu Rev Public Health 9*, 403-425

Solomon TP., Marchetti CM., Krishnan RK., Gonzalez F. & Kirwan JP. (2008). Effects of aging on basal fat oxidation in obese humans. *Metabolism 57*, 1141-1147

Spina RJ., Chi MM., Hopkins MG., Nemeth PM., Lowry OH. & Holloszy JO. (1996). Mitochondrial enzymes increase in muscle in response to 7-10 days of cycle exercise. *J Appl Physiol 80*, 2250-2254

Steffan HG., Elliott W., Miller WC. & Fernhall B. (1999). Substrate utilization during submaximal exercise in obese and normal-weight women. *Eur J Appl Physiol Occup Physiol 80*, 233-239

Strong WB., Malina RM., Blimkie CJ., Daniels SR., Dishman RK., Gutin B., Hergenroeder AC., Must A., Nixon PA., Pivarnik JM., Rowland T., Trost S. & Trudeau F. (2005). Evidence based physical activity for school-age youth. *J Pediatr 146*, 732-737

Talanian JL., Galloway SD., Heigenhauser GJ., Bonen A. & Spriet LL. (2007). Two weeks of high-intensity aerobic interval training increases the capacity for fat oxidation during exercise in women. *J Appl Physiol 102*, 1439-1447

Tarnopolsky MA. (2000). Gender differences in substrate metabolism during endurance exercise. *Can J Appl Physiol 25*, 312-327

Timmons BW., Bar-Or O. & Riddell MC. (2003). Oxidation rate of exogenous carbohydrate during exercise is higher in boys than in men. *J Appl Physiol 94*, 278-284

Timmons BW., Bar-Or O. & Riddell MC. (2007). Influence of age and pubertal status on substrate utilization during exercise with and without carbohydrate intake in healthy boys. *Appl Physiol Nutr Metab 32*, 416-425

Toth MJ., Arciero PJ., Gardner AW., Calles-Escandon J. & Poehlman ET. (1996). Rates of free fatty acid appearance and fat oxidation in healthy younger and older men. *J Appl Physiol 80*, 506-511

Toth MJ., Gardner AW., Arciero PJ., Calles-Escandon J. & Poehlman ET. (1998). Gender differences in fat oxidation and sympathetic nervous system activity at rest and during submaximal exercise in older individuals. Clin Sci (Lond) *95*, 59-66

van Aggel-Leijssen DP., Saris WH., Wagenmakers AJ., Senden JM. & van Baak MA. (2002). Effect of exercise training at different intensities on fat metabolism of obese men. J Appl Physiol *92*, 1300-1309

van Loon LJ. (2004). Use of intramuscular triacylglycerol as a substrate source during exercise in humans. J Appl Physiol *97*, 1170-1187

van Loon LJ., Greenhaff PL., Constantin-Teodosiu D., Saris WH. & Wagenmakers AJ. (2001). The effects of increasing exercise intensity on muscle fuel utilisation in humans. *J Physiol 536*, 295-304

Venables MC., Achten J. & Jeukendrup AE. (2005). Determinants of fat oxidation during exercise in healthy men and women: a cross-sectional study. *J Appl Physiol 98*, 160-167

Wallace DC. (2005). A mitochondrial paradigm of metabolic and degenerative diseases., aging., and cancer: a dawn for evolutionary medicine. *Annu Rev Genet 39*, 359-407

Wenger HA. & Bell GJ. (1986). The interactions of intensity., frequency and duration of exercise training in altering cardiorespiratory fitness. *Sports Med 3*, 346-356

Wong T. & Harber V. (2006). Lower excess postexercise oxygen consumption and altered growth hormone and cortisol responses to exercise in obese men. *J Clin Endocrinol Metab 91*, 678-686

Yoshida T. & Watari H. (1994). Exercise-induced splitting of the inorganic phosphate peak: investigation by time-resolved 31P-nuclear magnetic resonance spectroscopy. *Eur J Appl Physiol Occup Physiol 69*, 465-473

Zunquin, G., Theunynck, D., Sesboue, B., Arhan, P. & Bougle D. (2006). [Effects of puberty on glucose-lipid balance during exercise in the obese child]. *Appl Physiol Nutr Metab 31*, 442-448.

Zurlo, F., Nemeth, P. M., Choksi, R. M, Sesodia, S. & Ravussin, E. (1994). Whole-body energy metabolism and skeletal muscle biochemical characteristics. *Metabolism., 43*, 481-486.

In: Encyclopedia of Sports and Athletics
Editors: Jack L. Murray and Emily O. Watson
ISBN: 978-1-61209-959-0

Chapter VI

Cardiovascular Adaptation to Aerobic Training in Prepubertal Children

Stephane Mandigout[1,2*], Jonathan Kim[3,4] and Aaron Baggish[3,4]
[1]Faculty of Sciences, University of Limoges, France
[2]Laboratory of Exercise Biology (BAPS, EA 3533), University of Blaise Pascal, UFR STAPS, 63172 Aubière, France
[3]Department of Medicine, Massachusetts General Hospital, Boston, MA, US
[4]Division of Cardiology, Massachusetts General Hospital, Boston, MA, US

Summary

This chapter presents the effects of aerobic training on the adaptation of the cardiovascular system to exercise in prepubertal boys and girls. The major results of the scientific literature showed that the training program led to a rise in maximal O_2 uptake (VO_{2max}), brought about however only by an increase in SVmax in both sexes. Moreover, boys increased their VO_{2max} to a greater extent than girls only because of a higher SVmax improvement. No alterations were noticed in the SV pattern from rest to maximal exercise, indicating that the increase in SVrest was a key factor in the improvement of SVmax and thus VO_{2max}. Regarding resting echocardiographic data, an increase in left ventricular end-diastolic diameter, concomitant with an improvement in diastolic function, were observed after training and constituted an essential element in the rise in VO_{2max} after training in these children. Also, during maximal exercise, a decrease in systemic vascular resistances, probably indicating peripheral cardiovascular alterations, could have also play an important role in the increase in VO_{2max}.

I. Introduction

The primary goal of the cardiovascular system is to supply the visceral organs, central nervous system, and peripheral skeletal musculature with energy-rich substrates and

* Corresponding author : Faculté des Sciences et Techniques, 123 Avenue Albert Thomas, 87060 LIMOGES, Tel : (0 33)5 55 45 73 91, Email : stephane.mandigout@unilim.fr

oxygenated blood. During vigorous physical exercise, metabolic demands of the body increase dramatically. Successful performance of intense exercise relies on the cardiovascular system's ability to increase supply of substrate to match this demand.

The cardiovascular system is comprised of the 4 major cardiac chambers and heart valves, the large central capacitance arteries, the medium caliber resistance vessels, the micro-vascular capillary network, and the venous circulation. In conjunction with the autonomic nervous system, precisely controlled changes at all levels of the cardiovascular system ensure that exercising skeletal muscles are provided with the necessary fuel to perform the desired tasks. The ability of the cardiovascular system to augment and sustain cardiac output by more than 5 times resting levels is truly one of the most amazing phenomena in all of human physiology.

During vigorous physical exercise, dramatic increases in blood pressure, heart rate, and both intra-cardiac volume and pressure represent a stress for the cardiovascular system. If encountered with sufficient frequency and intensity, these stressors stimulate structural and functional cardiovascular adaptation. Such adaptations are thought to improve the overall efficiency thereby allowing an individual maximize exercise performance while minimizing further stress to the cardiovascular system.

Cardiovascular adaptations to exercise training including cardiac remodeling, changes in vascular function, and altered autonomic nervous system function have been well characterized in adults. Copious cross-sectional and more recently longitudinal data have led to a firm understanding of how the adult human cardiovascular system responds to repeated exercise training. Further, the importance of these adaptations with respect to human performance and health has been well documented. To date, far less is known about how the youthful body responds to exercise training.

This paper will provide a thorough review of prior work examining the response of the childhood cardiovascular system to exercise training. This discussion will be limited to studies of pre-pubertal children and an attempt will be made to provide information about the exact ages and gender of children included in all relevant studies. Unless otherwise specified, the term exercise training will refer to programs utilizing aerobic or endurance type training characterized by sustained high cardiac output and every effort will be made to provide detailed description of the exact exercise stimuli. It is our hope that this review of prior work will clarify what is known and what major areas of uncertainty are in need of future work.

II. Measuring the Impact of Exercise on Cardiac Structure and Function

Scientific examination of the interplay between exercise and cardiovascular function in children is a challenging task. Meaningful data is best generated through studies that utilize precisely characterized exercise stimuli and a measurement technique that provides accurate and reproducible cardiovascular data. Prescribing exercise as an effective research intervention requires the creation of an exercise program that is of sufficient duration and intensity to stimulate significant cardiovascular adaptation. Because the dose-response relationship between exercise and cardiac adaptation has yet to be established in either adults or children, there has been no uniform approach to this task. In fact, the vast majority of "exercise" studies have been cross-sectional analyses in which single time point measurements have been made in trained or athletic children and compared with those derived from untrained or sedentary controls. Although such observational data are hypothesis generating, they do not permit the establishment of causality and thus only set the stage for longitudinal studies in which serial data are prospectively collected and individuals serve as their own controls. Recently, such studies have begun to become available and the causal data they afford continues to mount.

Measurement of cardiac parameters among individuals participating in exercise training has long been an area interest. The first report of an association between vigorous physical exercise and changes in cardiac parameters came from the Swedish clinician Henschen in 1899.[1] Using the rudimentary yet elegant physical examination technique of cardiac percussion, he documented enlarged cardiac silhouettes in elite Nordic skiers. Since the time, advances in our understanding of the relationship between exercise training and cardiovascular adaptation have paralleled the development of cardiovascular diagnostic technologies. Initially, the use of plain radiographs was used to confirm and more accurately quantify cardiac enlargement in physically trained individuals. The development and subsequent widespread application of 12-lead electrocardiography led further understanding of heart structure and function in athletic individuals. Though plain film radiography and ECG led to important advances in our understanding of how training affects the heart, these measurements techniques provided indirect surrogates of underlying cardiac parameters.

The advent of transthoracic echocardiography and its application in the field of sports cardiovascular research led to an explosion of data with respect to the cardiac parameters in athletes. Early echocardiographic investigation relied on M-mode imaging, 2-dimensional, and acoustic Doppler imaging. For example, Morganroth et al used M-mode echocardiography to document cardiac enlargement in trained athletes and were the first to suggest the concept of sport specific or physiology specific cardiac remodeling. Morganroth's [2] work paved the way for a number of landmark echocardiography-based studies examining the prevalence and patterns of cardiac structural enlargement in trained athletes. Recent imaging advances including harmonic imaging, tissue-Doppler imaging, and 3-dimensional imaging and novel post-processing techniques such as gray scale speckle-tracking which allow for direct measurement of myocardial function have led to further important studies of cardiovascular function and exercise.

There are several reasons why echocardiography has been and continues to be the most widely used investigative modality for the characterization of cardiac parameters in exercise-trained individuals. First, it has the capacity to provide precise, reproducible measurements of cardiac chamber sizes and wall thickness. Second, it has the capacity to quantify cardiac function with respect to myocardial mechanics, intracardiac pressures, and blood transit. Third, it is a non-radiating method of anatomic imaging and thus serves as a minimal risk technique for assessing young, healthy individuals. Finally, it is the imaging modality best suited to assessment of cardiac behavior during vigorous exercise. Much of the subsequent text will review the role of echocardiography in the study of exercise training and cardiac function in children.

III. Effect of Exercise Training on VO_{2max} in Children

Peak exercise oxygen consumption (VO_{2max}) is the most widely used metric to define cardiorespiratory fitness and exercise capacity. Numerous studies have examined the impact of exercise training on VO_{2max} in children [3, 4] The majority of pediatric VO_{2max} work has utilized observational, cross sectional study designs which impart significant limitations as previously delineated. As such, this review will focus on prior data that has been derived from longitudinal study.

A. Controversial Results from Prior Work

A detailed review of the literature reveals the existence of very controversial results regarding the impact of exercise training on VO_{2max} in children. Specifically, some studies suggest that endurance training has no effect on VO_{2max} (particularly among the youngest children) beyond that attributable to normal growth and development [5,6,7] while others suggest that exercise training can increase VO_{2max} significantly [4, 8-11]. Key factors with respect to study design and study participants likely explain these seemingly discrepant findings. First, it is noteworthy that the vast majority of exercise training studies in children have been conducted using only male participants. Second, there has been marked heterogeneity with respect the training type, training frequency, training duration, and training intensity. Third, there has been considerable disparity with respect to age among representative studies. Finally, there has been important heterogeneity with respect to baseline cardiorespiratory fitness in both the exercise-trained and "sedentary" control groups in prior studies. The fact that most children engage in a significant, though difficult to quantify, amount of physical activity during recreational sports, school-sponsored physical education programs, and casual play introduces considerable potential confounding bias in the study of the effects of exercise training. Despite the above summarized issues, the bulk of evidence supports the notion that children can increase their VO_{2max} when exercise training sessions are of sufficient intensity, frequency and duration [3, 4].

B.) The Magnitude of VO_2max Increase in Children

An intriguing and relatively consistent finding is that the magnitude of VO_{2max} response appears limited when compared to adults [12]. In fact, when the training stimuli are similar between adults and children, most of the longitudinal studies demonstrate that the changes in VO_{2max} are considerably less in children (↑ 5-15 %) than those observed in adults (↑15-30%). Although it appears that children demonstrate less VO_{2max} augmentation after exercise training than adult counterparts, there has been marked heterogeneity in the magnitude of VO_{2max} response even among children as a group. Factors that appear to contribute to the magnitude of VO_{2max} increase resulting from exercise training include the specifics of the training program and attributes of the study population.

Training programs are generally designed with consideration of several important variables including training type (i.e. running, cycling, rowing, etc.), intensity (based on subjective measures such as perceived exertion or objective measures such as heart rate /power output), duration (minutes or hours per training session), and frequency (i.e. number of training sessions per unit time). Interpretation of VO_{2max} data within any given study must be considered following careful scrutiny of these factors. Study participant attributes including age/maturity status, gender, group constitution, initial VO_{2max} and pre-study physical activity level will have important effects on the observed response to exercise training. In aggregate, these factors appear to account for the wide range of previously reported VO_{2max} responses to exercise training.

At the present time, available data support several logical conclusions. First, it appears that a minimum of 2 sessions / week is necessary for significant VO_{2max} gains. Second, it appears that these session need to involve relatively high intensity exercise as defined by maximum heart rate of > 80% age-predicted maximum[3] With regards to specifics of the of exercise sessions, it appears that continuous, relatively low intensity exercise is a less potent VO_{2max} stimulus than interval-based training that includes repetitive periods of intense activity [3].

C.) The Impact of Gender on the Vo2max Response to Training

There are very sparse direct data comparing VO_{2max} responses among male and female children exposed to the same exercise stimuli. Mandigout et al [13]. found a non-significant trend toward higher increases in VO_{2max} among girls than among boys in a study examining the response to 13 weeks of running training (1 hour, 3 times weekly). The authors speculated that this observation was a function of differences in the pre-training fitness levels between girls and boys (VO_{2max} pre-test: 38.59±4.45 vs 47.27±7.88 $ml.min^{-1}.kg^{-1}$, $p<0,001$). Indeed, a significant relationship ($p<0,001$) was observed between pre-test VO_{2max} and the VO_{2max} percentage increase after 13 weeks of training (Figure 1). This finding led to the conclusion initial fitness level is a key determinant of VO_{2max} response to training. At present time, there are insufficient data to draw conclusions about the importance the actual type of aerobic exercise with respect to VO_{2max} changes in children.

In conclusion, it appears VO_{2max} does increase in response to exercise training in children though to a lesser degree than what would be expected in adults. The absolute magnitude of VO_{2max} increase depends upon several key factors including exercise duration and intensity. At present, there are no compelling data to support an important contribution from gender.

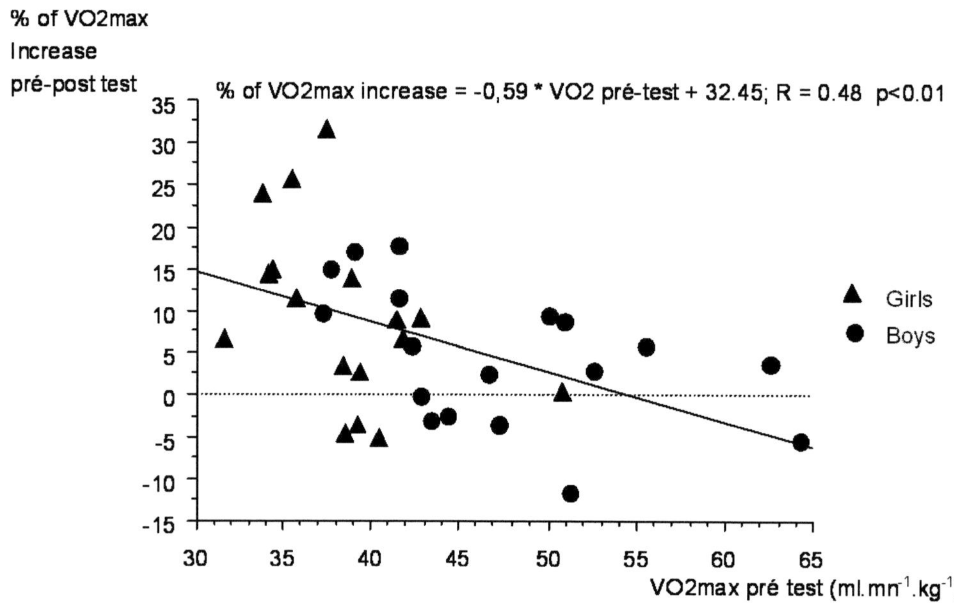

Figure 1. Relation between the VO2max percentage change post-training and VO2max pre-training in thirty five prepubertal children (Mandigout et al. [13]).

IV. Effect of Exercise Training on Left Ventricular Parameters

Left ventricular remodeling in response to exercise training is well documented in adults [14, 15]. At the present time, the cardiac structural and functional responses to exercise training are not as well documented in children as in the adult population. Among studies that have been conducted, results have been inconsistent [9,16-21] but the majority of evidence suggests that the hearts of children do remodel when exposed to significant exercise training. Further, the observed magnitude of left ventricular physiologic remodeling in children has been highly variable but overall appears to be less than that observed in older individuals [8, 16]. A review of relevant studies and discussion of the observed heterogeneity will now be further discussed.

Left Ventricular Structure

Several investigators have reported cross-sectional data from small case-control studies examining left ventricular chamber size in childhood athletes. In a small cohort of 10 to 11 year old swimmers (n=9), Obert et al [18]. reported increased left ventricular internal diameter and mass compared to less active controls. In this comparative study, there were no significant differences in left ventricular wall thickness between the two groups [18]. Similar findings have been reported by Ozer *et al.* in a larger cohort of young swimmers[19]. In contrast, Rowland and colleagues studied slightly older swimmers (11 to 13-year-old males, n=10), and found that although maximal oxygen uptake (VO_{2max}) was higher than controls, there was no difference in left ventricular chamber size or wall thickness.

Several longitudinal studies examining LV chamber size have also been conducted. For example, Geenen *et al.* observed no changes in left ventricular internal dimensions in 6 to 7-year-old children after an 8 month training program consisting of aerobic games and dance (4 days per week for 20 minutes at a heart rate of 150-160 beats/minute) [22]. In contrast, a study of 6-10 year-old children involved in an intense swimming program (2 years) demonstrated significant increases in left ventricular size when compared to non-training controls [23]. In similar fashion, Hayashi *et al.* also found a significant enlargement in left ventricular internal dimensions in 10 to 11-year-old obese children after an intense 1 year running program[24]. Most recently, Obert *et al* found data in accordance to the latter 2 studies, namely an increase in left ventricular internal dimensions by +4.6% in a group of 10-11 year-old children involved in a 13 week running program (3 days per week for 1 hour sessions at a heart rate of greater than 80% max predicted)[13]. It seems most likely that the lack of change observed in the Geenen study[22] was attributable to the relatively low intensity / low duration of the exercise stimuli examined.

The impact of exercise training on left ventricular wall thickness has also been examined. Maingourd *et al.* reported increases in left ventricular wall thickness in national-level youth ice hockey players over a 5 year follow-up period [25]. It is noteworthy that between the ages of 10-12 years, no changes in left ventricular wall thickness occurred but between ages 12-14, significant LV hypertrophy developed. Maturation related changes in testosterone levels and age related changes in age systolic blood pressure response to exercise may underlie these observation [16,26]. However, LV wall thickening was subsequently reported by Hollman et al [23]. after 2 years of intensive swimming in 6-10 year old children. This finding suggests that younger individuals have the capacity to mount a left ventricular hypertrophic response to training [23]. An intriguing yet difficult to reconcile observation was made by Obert et al [27], who reported thinning of the interventricular septum and posterior left ventricular wall after 13 weeks of running training. As similar observations have not been made in other studies of either children or adults exposed to exercise training and as such, the explanation and importance of this finding remains unclear [13].

Left Ventricular Systolic Function

Structural left ventricular adaptations to exercise training in pre-pubertal children do not appear to affect resting left ventricular systolic function [13, 16, 18, 22]. Further, there are data which suggest that the exercise training induced left ventricular chamber enlargement coupled with preserved contractile function may be an important mechanism for the documented increases in exercise capacity following training. In a study by Obert *et al,* increases in VO_{2max} following training were accounted for by increases in both resting and exercise stroke volume [28].

Left Ventricular Diastolic Function

Augmentation of diastolic function has been consistently observed among adults exposed to exercise training [29]. Studies examining the affects of endurance exercise training on diastolic function in children are limited. Several cross-sectional studies have failed to show any differences in left ventricular diastolic filling characteristics between highly trained pre-pubertal athletes and controls. To date, the only longitudinal study examining diastolic properties was done by Obert *et al*, and did show enhancement of early diastolic left ventricular (LV) filling with a concomitant reduction in the late diastolic active LV filling after training [13, 27, 30-32]. Using complementary indices of diastolic filling including time velocity integral of early diastolic rapid inflow (TVI-E) and the rapid filling fraction (RFF), the authors showed enhanced early diastolic filling after training and subsequent regression to baseline following detraining. As the authors appropriately acknowledge, the use of trans-mitral Doppler-derived flow parameters has important limitations. However this valuable data is the best evidence to support the ability of exercise to improve diastolic function in pre-pubertal children.

There are a number of potential factors that contribute to the variability in the magnitude of left ventricular remodeling that has been observed in children. Study population differences including gender, level of maturation, and training program variability (type, intensity, and frequency) are likely contributory. In addition, differences in genetic factors are also of importance[33]. Further work using longitudinal studies designed to control for these confounding variables are needed.

V. Effect of Exercise Training on the Hemodynamic Response to Exercise

As previously detailed, numerous studies have shown that exercise training of sufficient intensity, frequency, and duration leads to increases in maximal oxygen uptake (VO_{2max}) in children [3-5, 28]. Because VO_{2max} is determined by a number of factors including cardiovascular function, pulmonary gas exchange, and peripheral muscle metabolism, mechanisms responsible for changes in VO_{2max} may be challenging to define. Consequently, physiological factors responsible for the higher VO_{2max} in athletes compared to non-athletes and for the observed increases in VO_{2max} after exercise training have areas of great interest.

Despite increasing interest in paediatric exercise physiology, little information is available on the cardiovascular changes in exercising children that may account for observed increases in VO_{2max}. A simplistic yet useful method of parsing out the major physiologic determinants of VO_{2max} is consideration of the Fick relationship which states that oxygen consumption (both at maximal and submaximal exercise) is the product of heart rate (HR), stroke volume (SV) and the arterial-venous oxygen content difference (a-vO_2). In this section, the impact of exercise training on each component of the Fick relationship will be examined in an effort to elucidate mechanisms for the observed increases in VO_{2max}.

Heart Rate during Exercise

Although exercise training has been shown to reduce resting heart rates in children, there does not appear to be any difference in maximal heart rate between trained and untrained children [28, 33]. The observation suggests that maximal heart rate is not responsible for differences in VO_{2max} between trained and untrained children. As has been shown for adults, it appears that exercise training does not influence the mechanisms responsible for defining the upper limits of the sinoatrial node's response to exhaustive exercise.

Arterial –Venous Oxygen Difference (a-v O_2)

In similar fashion, the majority of prior studies suggest that a-v O_2 is not an important determinant of VO_{2max} in trained children [28, 33]. It is important to note that in these study, a-v O_2 was assessed by the indirect method of calculating the ration of systemic oxygen uptake to cardiac output. Both at rest and at maximal exercise intensity, a-v O_2 was similar between exercise trained and non-trained children. As such, it appears that a-v O_2 does not appear to contribute to variation in VO_{2max} in children with aerobic training.

Stroke Volume

Having shown that neither maximal heart rate nor a-v O_2 at peak exercise explains variability in VO_{2max} among children, attention must be focused on stroke volume. Stroke volume is the amount of blood ejected from the heart with each cardiac cycle. Stroke volume and heart rate (number of beats per minute) determine cardiac output. It has been shown that trained children have similar resting cardiac outputs to sedentary children [9, 34, 35], However, trained children demonstrate higher cardiac output at maximal exercise than non-trained children. Because there is no explanatory difference in maximal heart rate, the observed difference in maximal cardiac must be explained by stroke volume. Indeed, there are some primary data which suggest that maximal stroke volume is the principle physiological factor responsible for the higher VO_{2max} in exercise trained children[9].

Three studies have investigated stroke volume kinetics during progressive exercise performed until exhaustion in children and have produced inconsistent results [36-38]. Rowland et al. [35] and Nottin et al. [36] showed a similar pattern of stroke volume characterized by initial increase followed by plateau among trained child cyclists and sedentary controls. In contrast, a progressive rise in stroke volume from rest to maximal exercise was observed in a group of child runners [38]. Further studies are required to better understand whether sports or testing modality specificities can explain these different results. In adults, some questions arise regarding the effect of endurance training on the pattern of SV during exercise as different patterns have also been reported in endurance trained subjects [39,40]. It is possible that the method used to measure Q could explain these differences. In fact, all the studies demonstrating an increase in SV during exercise have used indirect methods [40], whereas most of the studies using dye dilution, thermodilution and the Fick technique have shown that SV is constant during exercise [41, 42].

The physiologic determinants of stroke volume are numerous. Nottin et al [36] examined some of the physiological factors underlying stroke volume during exercise in children. In this study, similar increases in stroke volume during exercise were observed between trained and untrained children. Further, the patterns of left ventricular end systolic diameter and fractional shortening (indices of contractility) and systemic vascular resistance (index of afterload) were similar in trained and untrained children when examined at rest and during exercise. Because trained children had higher end-diastolic left ventricular chamber dimensions and preserved systolic function at rest and during exercise, absolute stroke volumes were larger in all conditions. As such, the authors concluded that the higher values of SV at submaximal and maximal exercise in trained children result mainly from larger left ventricular chambers sizes. These results suggest that exercise training-induced left ventricular remodelling, specifically increases in left ventricular end-diastolic chamber size and thus stroke volume, is the primary cardiovascular factor leading to improvements in VO_{2max} in exercise trained children.

Data regarding determinants of VO_{2max} in children have largely been derived from cross-sectional studies. As such, causality has been difficult to establish. Specifically, it has been difficult to definitively separate the effects of exercise training from other determinants of performance such as underlying genetic endowment. To our knowledge, only two longitudinal studies have investigated the effect of aerobic training on hemodynamic parameters during submaximal and maximal exercise in children with similar results were reported in these two studies [28, 33]. VO_{2max} enhancement was observed after 16 weeks [33] and 13 weeks [28, 33], of exercise training. In these two studies, training programs were similar (1h session, 3 times per week under the supervision of an experienced physical education instructor). The training was predominantly aerobic and consisted of interval training and continuous long distance running. The training intensities were designed to induce a HR's higher than 90 and 80 percent of each child's HRmax for the interval and continuous running, respectively. In Eriksson et al [33] study, VO_{2max} demonstrated a 19% rise whereas in Obert et al [28] study 10% increased were found in experimental group. Key findings from the study by Obert et al [28] are presented in Table 1 and Figure 2 and 3. In this study, participants were assessed at rest and during exercise before and after exercise training. Following training, individuals all demonstrated lower resting heart rate and higher in stroke volume at rest. During submaximal exercise, there were no differences in stroke volume patterns when compared with those observed prior to training. Specifically, there was an initial rise in stroke volume at the onset of exercise (i.e. from rest to SM-1, Figure 1) and then a plateau which persisted from moderate workloads until exhaustion. Although this rise and plateau phenomenon was not changed by training, absolute SV was significantly higher at rest, during submaximal exercise, and during maximal exercise after the training period. Also, the increase in VO_{2max} in these two study [28, 33] induced by aerobic training program in children was explained only by an increase in SV_{max}, since no changes in HR_{max} and $AVO\text{-}D_{max}$ were reported.

Table 1. Rest and maximal metabolic and cardiovascular data before and after 13 weeks endurance training program in prepubertal children. (Obert et al .[28])

	Experimental Group				Control Group			
	Rest		Maximal exercise		Rest		Maximal exercise	
	Before	After	Before	After	Before	After	Before	After
VO_2 *(ml.min^{-1}.kg^{-1})*								
Boys	7.0±0.7	7.0±0.6	44.1±6.1	50.9±6.7***	8.0±1.9	7.5±1.9	51.5±6.3	50.3±6.1
Girls	6.9±1.3	6.7±1.1	40.9±8.9	44.2±8.4†*	8.8±1.8	8.8±2.4	42.4±5.6‡	42.6±5.7‡
HR *(beat.min^{-1})*								
Boys	86±10	76±11*	202±7	201±6	83±17	81±18	199±9	197±11
Girls	95±8	86±6*	202±7	200±5	84±7	84±9	204±5	204±6
Q-I *(L.min^{-1}.BSA^{-1})*								
Boys	3.3±0.6	3.2±0.6	10.5±1.8	12.1±1.5**	2.8±0.5	2.7±0.4	9.7±0.8	9.8±1.0
Girls	3.1±0.5	3.1±0.5	9.4±1.4†	10.4±1.0†**	2.9±0.5	2.8±0.6	9.4±1.2†	9.4±1.7†
SV-I *(ml.BSA^{-1})*								
Boys	38.6±7.4	43.1±5.5*	52.2±8.2	60.2±7.2**	35.2±6.3	34.8±5.9	49.1±4.8	49.6±5.4
Girls	33.3±6.2	36.1±4.9*	46.5±6.8†	51.9±4.3‡**	34.1±6.1	32.9±6.3	46.1±6.0†	46.0±8.7†
a-vO_2 *(ml.100ml^{-1})*								
Boys	6.7±1.8	6.8±1.5	13.0±2.1	13.1±1.9	8.8±2.1	8.5±2.0	15.6±1.5	15.2±1.3
Girls	6.7±0.9	6.7±1.4	13.2±1.6	13.0±1.9	9.0±2.8	9.5±3.4	13.1±2.8†	13.3±1.9†
SVR *(U.I.)*								
Boys	20.8±5.0	19.4±3.5	7.1±1.5	5.8±0.9***	22.1±5.5	21.2±4.2	7.1±0.9	6.7±0.8
Girls	20.3±4.2	18.7±2.8	7.5±1.2	6.6±0.8†***	23.6±5.0	23.7±7.6	7.5±0.7	7.5±1.2

VO_2: oxygen uptake; HR : heart rate; Q-I : cardiac output indexed to body surface area ; SV-I : stoke volume indexed to body surface area ; a-vO_2 : arterio-venous oxygen difference ; SVR: systemic vascular resistances. * p<0.05; ** p<0.01; *** p<0.001: significant difference between before and after the study period in the same group; † p<0.05; ‡ p<0.01: significant difference between boys and girls in the same group.

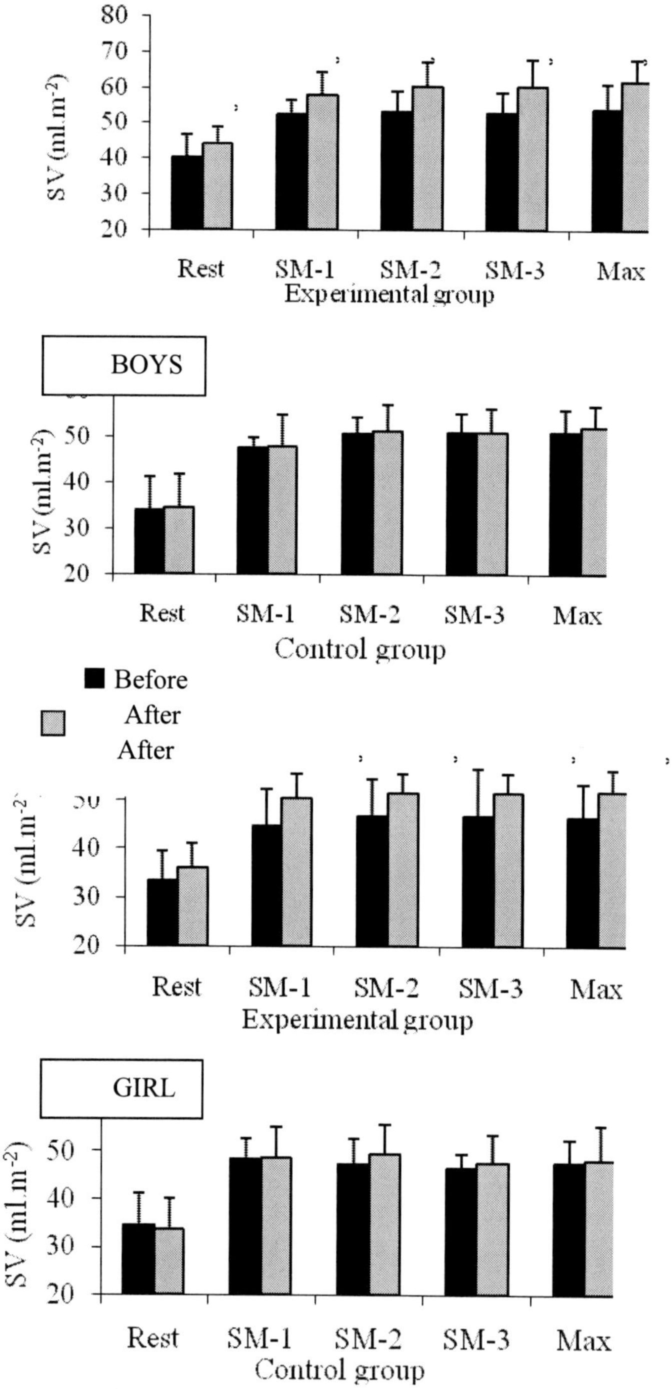

Figure 2. Stroke volume kinetics from rest to maximal exercise in the boys and the girls of experimental group which realised 13 weeks endurance training program (Obert et al [28]), before ■ and after□ the study period. * $p<0.05$, ** $p<0.01$: significant difference between before and after study period.

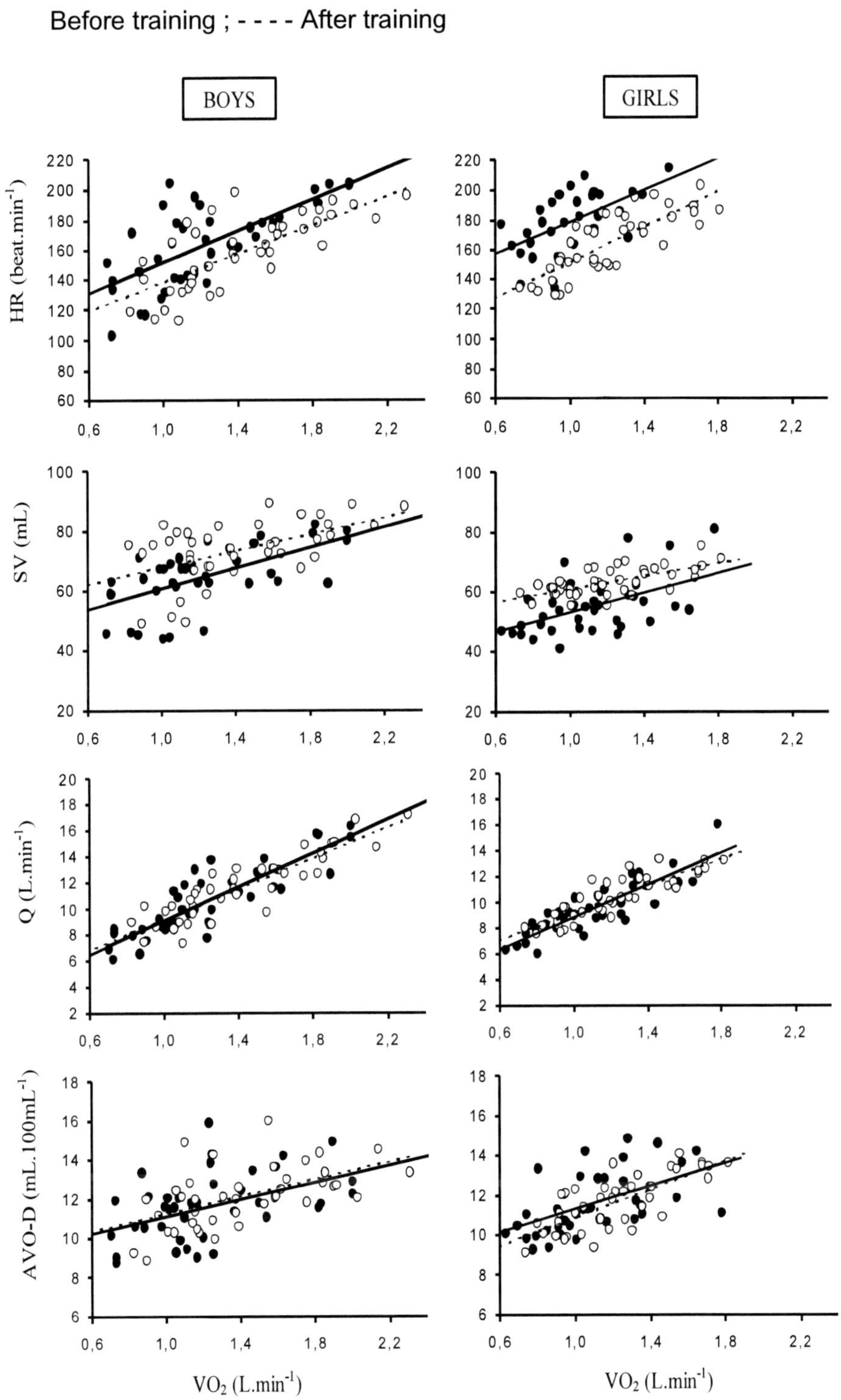

Figure 3. Submaximal cardiovascular responses at a given VO_2 in the boys and the girls of experimental group which realised 13 weeks endurance training program (Obert et al [28]), before (●) and after (○) training. HR : heart rate ; SV : stroke volume ; Q : cardiac output ; AVO-D : arterio-venous oxygen difference.

In aggregate, it appears that exercise training-induced increases in VO_2max in children can, at least in part, be attributed to increases in stroke volume. Both cross-sectional and longitudinal data suggest that increases in left ventricular end-diastolic volume coupled with preserved systolic function lead to high stroke volume and thus improved oxygen delivery.

VI. Effect of Exercise Training on Autonomic Nervous System Function as Reflected by Heart Rate Variability (HRV)

The term heart rate variability (HRV) refers to the beat-to-beat fluctuations in heart rate. The measurement of the heart rate variability (HRV) is a useful tool for the quantification of autonomic nervous system control on cardiovascular function in adults as well as in children [43]. Specifically, indices of HRV have been shown to correlates strongly with activity in both the sympathetic and parasympathetic arms of the autonomic nervous system. The use of HRV as a research tool and a clinical prognostic markers has been demonstrated [44, 45].

Measurement of HRV

Traditionally, HRV has been used exclusively in research settings given the expertise required for measurement and interpretation. More recently, commercially available devices have been developed which provide accurate automated HRV measurements. However, interpretation of HRV data remains a formidable task. To address this challenge, a joint European Society of Cardiology / North American Society of Pacing and Electrophysiology Task Force have developed standards for interpretation [46]. The specific goals of this effort were to (1) standardize nomenclature and develop definitions of terms, (2) specify standard methods of measurement, (3) define physiological and pathophysiological correlates, (4) describe currently appropriate clinical applications, and (5) identify areas for future research.

HRV may be evaluated by a number of methods. The most common approach involves measurements of the time domain and the frequency domain. The more simple of these two metrics is the time domain. Time domain measure is the calculation of the standard deviation of beat-to-beat intervals (Table 2). In other words, the duration of time intervals across successive heart beats can be statistically analyzed to obtain information about the autonomic nervous system. In contrast, the frequency domain method is the application of discrete Fourier transformation to the beat-to-beat interval time series. Assessment of variation across different frequency spectra provides information about different physiologic controls of heart rate. Several frequency bands of interest have been defined in humans including the high, low, very low, and ultra-low bands (Table 2).

Effects of Exercise Training on HRV

It has been well established that exercise training can alter the autonomic balance in adults[47,48]. Specifically, exercise trained individuals generally demonstrate increased parasympathetic tone relative to sympathetic tone [47]. Although many questions regarding the precise relationship between exercise and nervous system function remain unanswered, it appears that moderate to high intensity is necessary to produces significant alterations in autonomic nervous system function [49].

There are relatively few data examining the HRV and autonomic nervous system response to exercise training in children [50, 51, 52, 53, 54, 55]. Among prior work, there are inconsistant conclusions.

In a cross sectional study by Triposkiadis et al. [51] HRV in the time and frequency domain was assessed in 25 highly trained preadolescent swimmers and in 20 non trained children. The results showed that the response to intensive training includes vagal predominance in prepubertal swimmers (RR, SDNN, PNN50 and HF power were greater in swimmers than in controls). However, a similar study by Vinet et al [50], led to conflicting results. Specifically, data examining the impact of an intensive training program (8-10h/week) suggested that it did not induce changes in HRV indices in prepubertal boys. The difference between the results of these two studies may lie in the differences in the population studied as well as methodological factors.

Table 2. Selected time-domain and frequency domain measures of HRV

Variables	Unit	description	
Time domain measures			
SDNN	ms	Standard deviation of all NN intervals	reflects all the cyclic components responsible for variability
SDANN	ms	Standard deviation of the averages of NN intervals in all 5 min segments of the entire recording	measures the variability due to cycles shorter than 5 min
RMSSD	ms	The square root of the mean of the sum of the squares of differences between adjacent NN intervals	estimate of short-term components of HRV
PNN50	%	NN50 count divided by the total number of all NN intervals.	estimate high frequency variations
Frequency domain measures			
VLF	ms^2	Very low frequency	Not well known, but it had been attributed to thermal regulation
LF	ms^2	Low frequency	derives from parasympathetic and sympathetic activity
HF	ms^2	High frequency,	Reflects vagal activity or the parasympathetic system
LF/HF			Index of sympathetic to parasympathetic balance of heart rate fluctuation

Results from the above mentioned cross-sectional studies have been difficult to reconcile. Fortunately, longitudinal studies examining the impact of exercise training on HRV have been conducted (Table 3). Despite important differences in study design, these efforts consistently demonstrate the fact that exercise training has the potential to profoundly affect autonomic nervous system function.

Nagai et al [53] reported that all the frequency components of the HRV were significantly increased after the submaximal exercise training period in children with normal HRV. Gutin et al [54] showed that training significantly increased RMSSD (+9.8%, $p<0.05$), decreased LF power expressed as a percentage of total power (-7.6%, $p<0.03$) as well as LF/HF ratio (-0.7%, $p<0.01$), and tended to decrease resting heart rate.

In Mandigout et al. [52] study, endurance training induced alteration in HRV, characterized by an increase in the majority of spectral (VLF, LF, HF) and time (SDNN, RMSSD, PNN50) HRV components. However, when the frequency components (i.e. VLF, LF, HF) were expressed as a percentage of TP, it appeared that sympathetic, parasympathetic activities as well as and sympatho-vagal balance were not altered by training in prepubertal children. Finally in Gamelin et al. [55] study, the major finding was the non significant effect of high intensity intermittent exercise training on the autonomic cardiovascular control of prepubescent children, despite a large increase in aerobic fitness. The single difference between these two last studies which could explain the training response on the HRV was the training duration (13weeks vs 7 weeks respectively). Some studies, in adults, reported an increase in vagal modulation of HR after 2 or 12 weeks of moderate training. Nevertheless, in children autonomic nervous activity is dependant of the maturation state with in particular a greater vagal tone than adults [43]. This relation allowed to conclude that for the greater vagal tone is, the less important the increase of HRV will be for the same training characteristics between children and adults.

Although the majority of data support the fact exercise training alters autonomic nervous system function, it remains uncertain what physiological factors are responsible for the observed changes. One hypothesis is that increased HRV may result from enhanced blood flow in the microcirculation of the autonomic nervous system, as previously suspected in trained adults [56]. Alternatively, chronic strenuous exercise may trigger non-neural adaptation [57]. Further work will be required to determine the mechanisms by which exercise leads to alterations in HRV. Further questions about the impact of age, gender, and training type are important areas of future work.

VII. Physiological Factors Responsible for Training-Induced Increases in VO_{2max}

Previous studies have shown the favorable effects of chronic exercise on maximal oxygen uptake ($VO_{2\,max}$) in children with various pathologies, such as obesity and cardio-respiratory disease [58-62]. This has also been shown in healthy pre-pubertal children [4, 5, 63], but the degree of improvement appears limited when compared with adults [64]. Data supporting the mechanism in adults which accounts for this increase in VO_{2max} explains that it is related to both central and peripheral cardiovascular adaptations, as shown by an increase in cardiac output and maximal a-v O_2 [65, 66]. The data in pediatrics is far more limited, and most of the studies have been cross-sectional.

Table 3. Effects of training on HRV in prepubertal children. Cross- sectional an longitudinal studies are presented in chronological order

Study	Sex	Age	Exercise	n	Training	Results
Cross-sectional studies						
Triposkiadis et al. [51]	F/M	10/12	Swimmer Control	25 20	10-12h/wk	Vagal predominance in swimmer
Vinet et al. [50]	M	11-12	Swimmer Control	11 9	8-10h/wk	No changes in HRV indices

Longitudinal studies

Study	Sex	Age (year)	Exercise	N	Length (week)	Intensity	Frequency (n/wk)	Duration	Results
Gutin et al. [54]		7-11	 Control	17 18	17	>150 BPM	4-5	40min	RMSSD ↗ , resting HR↘ and LF/HF↘
Mandigout et al .[52]	F/M	10-11	School training Control	12 7	12	>80%HRmax	3	1h	HRV↗ in absolute values but not in percentage of total power
Nagai et al. [53]	F/M		School exercise control	24 24	52	HR:130-140BPM	5	20min	HRV↗
Gamelin et al. [55]	F/M	9-10	School training Control	22 16	7	100-190% maximal aerobic velocity	3	30min	No modification on the autonomic cardiovascular control

Cross-sectional studies suggest that a higher VO_{2max} in endurance-trained children is secondary only to higher maximal stroke volume [37, 38, 61, 67-69]. Rowland *et al.* used Doppler echocardiography to assess cardiac function in 8 trained runners and 14 controls [37, 67]. When assessed during progressive upright cycle exercises, it was noted that the trained children had higher indexed stroke volumes at all workloads when compared to controls. Additionally, it was found that values for maximal indexed stroke volumes were less in the child runners than those typically seen in trained adults. A second study by Rowland *et al.* compared the hemodynamic response of progressive cycle exercise in 7 child cyclists and in 39 age matched controls [38, 61, 68, 69]. Higher mean VO_{2max} was found in the athletes (60 mL/kg·min vs 47 mL/kg·min), as well as a higher indexed stroke volume at rest (59 mL/m^2 vs 44 mL/m^2) and at maximal exercise (76 mL/m^2 vs 60 mL/m^2). The ratio of maximal to rest stroke volume index, however, was similar in both groups. In both groups, there was a plateau in stroke volume beyond low intensity work with no difference in maximal a-v O_2. It was concluded that maximum stroke volume was critical in determination of VO_{2max}, and that factors influencing resting stroke volume are important in defining differences between child athletes and non-athletes. Given the nature of such cross-sectional studies, however, it could not be determined if the differences noted were a function of exercise training or other factors.

Two longitudinal studies have examined the effect of exercise training on the cardiovascular function and exercise capacity [28, 33, 70]. Eriksson *et al.* studied boys, and found that there was an increase in VO_{2max} after training and that this was attributed to an increase in SV_{max} [33]. The training program consisted of 3 sessions per week at 1h per session under the supervision of an experienced physical education instructor. Training was predominantly aerobic and consisted of intervals and continuous long distance running. The training intensities were defined so as to induce a HR higher than 80-90 percent of each child's HR_{max} for the interval and continuous running, respectively. Unfortunately, mechanisms looking into improvement of SV_{max} were not studied, and females were not investigated. Studies that have looked into gender differences in VO_{2max}, have found that girls have a lower VO_{2max} boys [38]. The most recent study by Obert *et al.* was designed to determine the effect of an endurance program on cardiac function, and also to determine whether gender affects the training induced cardiovascular response [28]. Nineteen (19) children (10 girls, 9 boys) participated in a 13 week training program (3hrs/wk, >80% HR max) compared to 16 controls (7 girls, 9 boys). The training was predominantly aerobic and was described as consisting of short distance interval training as well as continuous long distance running. Echocardiograms and a maximal upright cycle test were performed in all participants before and after the study period. The results confirmed a rise in VO_{2max} brought about by an increase in SV_{max}. Moreover, boys increased their VO_{2max} to a greater extent than girls (+15% compared to +8%) because of a higher SV_{max} (+15% compared to +11%). Regardless of gender, increases in VO_{2max} after training was the result of an increase in SV_{max} only, as HR_{max} and a-vO_s were not altered after training in boys or girls.

Obert *et al.* provided the first data examining the potential contributing factors involved with SV enhancement in children [28]. Though not all factors affecting SV were evaluated at maximal exercise, several mechanisms were proposed by the authors to explain this phenomenon. The most important finding from this study was the increase in E-wave (early diastolic trans-mitral filling velocity) after training. As acknowledged by the authors, E-wave velocity is the result of numerous factors including left ventricular preload and ventricular compliance [71-73]. The results of a study by Koch *et al.*, which examined endurance trained 13-15 year old boys, found higher blood volumes than in untrained controls, and substantiated a role for preload [74].

Left ventricular enlargement is a second mechanism by which SV could be enhanced. As mentioned previously, Obert[28] performed trans-thoracic echocardiograms on all subjects in this study at rest, before and after the study period. Significant increases in LV internal chamber size and mass were found after training, as well as a highly significant correlation between LVEDd (LV end diastolic dimension) and SV_{max} or VO_{2max}, suggesting that LVEDd may play a significant role in improved VO_{2max} and SV_{max}. There was no gender difference with regard to an improvement in LV internal dimensions[28]. Previous cross-sectional data has also reported similar results in terms of increased left ventricular internal chamber dimensions[9, 18]. Whether the increased LV dimensions is a result of repetitive overload on the ventricle after training or from an increase in preload secondary to blood volume enhancement remains unclear. Previous animal studies by Moore and Palmer showed that endurance training leading to repetitive overload on the LV, did induce a longitudinal growth of cardiac myocytes, leading to LV chamber enlargement and SV enhancement[75].

Improved diastolic function leading to higher left ventricular end-diastolic volume could also contribute to an improved SV_{max}. Obert *et al.* did show improvement in peak E, as mentioned earlier, as well as an improved E/A ratio in boys and girls[28]. Further, in a previous longitudinal study from Obert *et al.*, improved diastolic filling in pre-pubertal children after an intense training regimen was described, although no change in stroke volume index was found [27]. The most recent data from Obert *et al.* looked at LV wall motion velocities by tissue Doppler imaging in 25 children vs 25 controls. Subjects were enrolled in a 2 month, high intensity aerobic training program. Interestingly, there was no improvement in trans-mitral inflow velocities or early and late wall motion [76].

Finally, systemic vascular resistance, a surrogate for measure of afterload, was also evaluated by Obert[28]. Longitudinal studies in adults have shown a decrease in SVR_{max} (maximum systemic vascular resistance) after training [77, 78]. Similar results were found in Obert *et al.* as well as a highly significant relationship between stroke volume and SVR_{max}, suggesting a decrease in afterload contributing to the measured improvement in SV_{max} [28]. The boys exhibited a greater decrease than the girls, which could be one explanation for better stroke volume augmentation in boys. This data was the first to demonstrate this, and was in contrast to previous data by Eriksson *et al.* [33]. Nottin *et al.* published another cross-sectional study that assessed SVR_{max} in child cyclists and found no difference between the trained cyclists and the controls [36]. Though studies exist in the adult population looking at arterial compliance and vasodilatation, there are no such studies in the pediatric literature.

Data regarding mechanisms of improved VO_{2max} in pre-pubertal children are limited when compared to the same topic in adults. Both cross-sectional as well as longitudinal studies, however, have shown that SV_{max} is the primary cause of improved VO_{2max} after aerobic exercise. Only one study examined gender effects on the cardiovascular response to training in pre-pubertal children, and showed that boys increase their VO_{2max} to a greater extent than girls, mostly due to a higher SV_{max} improvement. The physiological factors responsible for the rise in VO_{2max} and SV_{max} are likely multi-factorial, and could be due to increases in preload, LV internal dimensions/improved diastolic function, and reduced afterload. Further work is needed to examine each of these individual parameters.

VIII. Conclusions

Exercise training has long been known to be a potent stimulus for physiologic cardiac remodeling and disease prevention in adults. Recently, similar advances in our understanding of how exercise affects the cardiovascular system in children have been made. Important heterogeneity in study design and the cross-sectional nature of most data have led ambiguity with respect to important issues. Fortunately, recent longitudinal studies have begun to clarify the confusion. It is now clear that exercise training can lead to objective improvements in exercise capacity in children. Further, it appears that physiologic cardiac remodeling with resultant augmentation of stroke volume is the primary cardiovascular adaptation that facilitates improvements in exercise performance. Building on these findings, there is much future work to be done to understand the complex interplay between physical activity and cardiovascular health and disease in children.

References

[1] Henschen, S. Skidlauf und Skidwettlauf. Eine medizinische Sportstudie. *Mitt Med Klin Upsala.,* 1899, 2(15).

[2] Morganroth, J; Maron, BJ; Henry, WL; Epstein, SE. Comparative left ventricular dimensions in trained athletes. *Ann Intern Med.,* 1975, 82(4), 521-524.

[3] Baquet, G; van Praagh, E; Berthoin, S. Endurance training and aerobic fitness in young people. *Sports Med.,* 2003, 33(15), 1127-1143.

[4] Shephard, RJ. Effectiveness of training programmes for prepubescent children. *Sports Med.,* 1992, 13(3), 194-213.

[5] Rowland, TW. Aerobic response to endurance training in prepubescent children: a critical analysis. *Med Sci Sports Exerc.,* 1985, 17(5), 493-497.

[6] Turcotte, RA; Belcastro, AN. Time dependent response of cardiac myofibrillar ATPase activity to exercise. *Int J Biochem.,* 1989, 21(12), 1329-1335.

[7] Vaccaro, P; Mahon, A. Cardiorespiratory responses to endurance training in children. *Sports Med.,* 1987, 4(5), 352-363.

[8] Rowland, TW. Trainability of the cardiorespiratory system during childhood. *Can J Sport Sci.* 1992, 17(4), 259-263.

[9] Rowland, TW; Delaney, BC; Siconolfi, SF. 'Athlete's heart' in prepubertal children. *Pediatrics.* 1987, 79(5), 800-804.

[10] Krahenbuhl, GS; Skinner, JS; Kohrt, WM. Developmental aspects of maximal aerobic power in children. *Exerc Sport Sci Rev.,* 1985, 13, 503-538.

[11] Brown, CH; Harrower, JR; Deeter, MF. The effects of cross-country running on pre-adolescent girls. *Med Sci Sports.,* 1972, 4(1), 1-5.

[12] Howard, A; Wenge; HA; Gordon, JB. The interaction of intensity, frequency and duration of exercise training in altering cardiorespiratory fitness. *Sports Med.* 1986, 3(1), 346-356.

[13] Mandigout, S; Lecoq, AM; Courteix, D; Guenon, P; Obert, P. Effect of gender in response to an aerobic training programme in prepubertal children. *Acta Paediatr.* 2001, 90(1), 9-15.

[14] Rawlins, J; Bhan, A; Sharma, S. Left ventricular hypertrophy in athletes. *Eur J Echocardiogr.,* 2009, 10(3), 350-356.
[15] Pelliccia, A. Athlete"s heart and hypertrophic cardiomyopathy. *Current cardiology reports.,* 2000, 2(2), 166-171.
[16] Rowland, TW. Effect of prolonged inactivity on aerobic fitness of children. *J Sports Med Phys Fitness.* 1994, 34(2), 147-155.
[17] Gutin, B; Mayers, N; Levy, JA; Herman, MV. Physiologic and echocardiographic studiers of age-group runners. *Competitive Sport for Children and Youth.,* 1988, 117-128.
[18] Obert, P; Stecken, F; Courteix, D; Lecoq, AM; Guenon, P. Effect of long-term intensive endurance training on left ventricular structure and diastolic function in prepubertal children. *Int J Sports Med.* 1998, 19(2), 149-154.
[19] Ozer, S; Cil, E; Baltaci, G; Ergun, N; Ozme, S. Left ventricular structure and function by echocardiography in childhood swimmers. *Japanese heart journal.,* 1994, 35(3), 295-300.
[20] Telford, RD; McDonald, IG; Ellis, LB; Chennells, MH; Sandstrom, ER; Fuller, PJ. Echocardiographic dimensions in trained and untrained 12-year-old boys and girls. *Journal of sports sciences.,* 1988, 6(1), 49-57.
[21] Thoren, CAR; Asano, K. Functional capacity and cardiac function in 10-year-old boys and girls with high and low running performance. *Children and Sport.,* 1984, 183-188.
[22] Geenen, DL; Gilliam, TB; Crowley, D; Moorehead-Steffens, C; Rosenthal, A. Echocardiographic measures in 6 to 7 year old children after an 8 month exercise program. *Am J Cardiol.* 1982, 49(8), 1990-1995.
[23] Hollmann, W; Rost, R; De Meirleir, K; Liesen, H; Heck, H; Mader, A. Cardiovascular effects of extreme physical training. *Acta medica Scandinavica.,* 1986, 711, 193-203.
[24] Hayashi, T; Fujino, M; Shindo, M; Hiroki, T; Arakawa, K. Echocardiographic and electrocardiographic measures in obese children after an exercise program. *Int J Obes.* 1987, 11(5), 465-472.
[25] Maingourd, Y; Bourges-Petit, E; Tanguy, C; Quintard, JM; Medelli, J; Freville, M. [Peripubertal longitudinal study by echocardiography of left heart development in a group of ice hockey players]. *Arch Mal Coeur Vaiss.,* 1990, 83(3), 371-375.
[26] Wanne, OPS; Haapoja, E. Blood pressure during exercise in healthy children. *Eur J Appl Physiol.* 1986, 11, 66-79.
[27] Obert, P; Mandigout, S; Vinet, A; N'Guyen, LD; Stecken, F; Courteix, D. Effect of aerobic training and detraining on left ventricular dimensions and diastolic function in prepubertal boys and girls. *Int J Sports Med.* 2001, 22(2), 90-96.
[28] Obert, P; Mandigouts, S; Nottin, S; Vinet, A; N'Guyen, LD; Lecoq, AM. Cardiovascular responses to endurance training in children: effect of gender. *Eur J Clin Invest.,* 2003, 33(3), 199-208.
[29] Fagard, RH. Impact of different sports and training on cardiac structure and function. *Cardiol Clin.* 1997, 15(3), 397-412.
[30] Nottin, S; Vinet, A; Lecoq, AM; Guenon, P; Obert, P. [Study of the reproducibility of cardiac output measurement during exercise in pre-pubertal children by doppler echocardiography and CO2 inhalation]. *Arch Mal Coeur Vaiss.* 2000, 93(11), 1297-1303.

[31] Obert, P; Mandigout, M; Vinet, A; Courteix, D. Effect of a 13-week aerobic training programme on the maximal power developed during a force-velocity test in prepubertal boys and girls. *Int J Sports Med.* 2001, 22(6), 442-446.
[32] Vinet, A; Nottin, S; Lecoq, AM; Guenon, P; Obert, P. Reproducibility of cardiac output measurements by Doppler echocardiography in prepubertal children and adults. *Int J Sports Med.* 2001, 22(6), 437-441.
[33] Eriksson, BO; Koch, G. Effect of physical training on hemodynamic response during submaximal and maximal exercise in 11-13-year old boys. *Acta Physiol Scand.* 1973, 87(1), 27-39.
[34] Rowland, TW. Evolution of maximal oxygen uptake in children. *Med Sport Sci.* 2007, 50, 200-209.
[35] Rowland, TW; Cunningham, LN. Oxygen uptake plateau during maximal treadmill exercise in children. *Chest.,* 1992, 101(2), 485-489.
[36] Nottin, S; Vinet, A; Stecken, F; Nguyen, LD; Ounissi, F; Lecoq, AM; Obert, P. Central and peripheral cardiovascular adaptations during a maximal cycle exercise in boys and men. *Med Sci Sports Exerc.* 2002, 34(3), 456-463.
[37] Rowland, T; Goff, D; Popowski, B; DeLuca, P; Ferrone, L. Cardiac responses to exercise in child distance runners. *Int J Sports Med.,* 1998, 19(6), 385-390.
[38] Rowland, T; Wehnert, M; Miller, K. Cardiac responses to exercise in competitive child cyclists. *Med Sci Sports Exerc.,* 2000, 32(4), 747-752.
[39] Crawford, MH; Petru, MA; Rabinowitz, C. Effect of isotonic exercise training on left ventricular volume during upright exercise. *Circulation.,* 1985, 72(6), 1237-1243.
[40] Gledhill, N; Cox, D; Jamnik, R. Endurance athletes' stroke volume does not plateau: major advantage is diastolic function. *Med Sci Sports Exerc.,* 1994, 26(9), 1116-1121.
[41] Ginzton, LE; Conant, R; Brizendine, M; Laks, MM. Effect of long-term high intensity aerobic training on left ventricular volume during maximal upright exercise. *J Am Coll Cardiol.* 1989, 14(2), 364-371.
[42] Jensen-Urstadt, M; Bouvier, F.; Nejat, M; Saltin, B; Brodin, LA. Left ventricular function in endurance runners during exercise. *Acta Physiol Scand.* 1998, 164, 167-172.
[43] Lenard, Z; Studinger, P; Mersich, B; Kocsis, L; Kollai, M. Maturation of cardiovagal autonomic function from childhood to young adult age. *Circulation.* 2004, 110(16), 2307-2312.
[44] Molgaard, H; Sorensen, KE; Bjerregaard, P. Circadian variation and influence of risk factors on heart rate variability in healthy subjects. *Am J Cardiol.* 1991, 68(8), 777-784.
[45] Hayano, J; Sakakibara, Y; Yamada, A; Yamada, M; Mukai, S; Fujinami, T; Yokoyama, K; Watanabe, Y; Takata, K. Accuracy of assessment of cardiac vagal tone by heart rate variability in normal subjects. *Am J Cardiol.,* 1991, 67(2), 199-204.
[46] Heart rate variability. Standards of measurement, physiological interpretation, and clinical use. Task Force of the European Society of Cardiology and the North American Society of Pacing and Electrophysiology. *Eur Heart J.,* 1996, 17(3), 354-381.
[47] Shin, K; Minamitani, H; Onishi, S; Yamazaki, H; Lee, M. Autonomic differences between athletes and nonathletes: spectral analysis approach. *Med Sci Sports Exerc.* 1997, 29(11), 1482-1490.
[48] Stein, PK; Ehsani, AA; Domitrovich, PP; Kleiger, RE; Rottman, JN. Effect of exercise training on heart rate variability in healthy older adults. *Am Heart J.* 1999, 138(3 Pt 1), 567-576.

[49] Aubert, AE; Seps, B; Beckers, F. Heart rate variability in athletes. *Sports Med.* 2003, 33(12), 889-919.
[50] Vinet, A; Beck, L; Nottin, S; Obert, P. Effect of intensive training on heart rate variability in prepubertal swimmers. *Eur J Clin Invest.,* 2005, 35(10), 610-614.
[51] Triposkiadis, F; Ghiokas, S; Skoularigis, I; Kotsakis, A; Giannakoulis, I; Thanopoulos, V. Cardiac adaptation to intensive training in prepubertal swimmers. *Eur J Clin Invest.* 2002, 32(1), 16-23.
[52] Mandigout, S; Melin, A; Fauchier, L; N'Guyen, LD; Courteix, D; Obert, P. Physical training increases heart rate variability in healthy prepubertal children. *Eur J Clin Invest.* 2002, 32(7), 479-487.
[53] Nagai, N; Moritani, T. Effect of physical activity on autonomic nervous system function in lean and obese children. *Int J Obes Relat Metab Disord.* 2004, 28(1), 27-33.
[54] Gutin, B; Barbeau, P; Litaker, MS; Ferguson, M; Owens, S. Heart rate variability in obese children: relations to total body and visceral adiposity, and changes with physical training and detraining. *Obes Res.* 2000, 8(1), 12-19.
[55] Gamelin, FX; Baquet, G; Berthoin, S; Thevenet, D; Nourry, C; Nottin, S; Bosquet, L. Effect of high intensity intermittent training on heart rate variability in prepubescent children. *Eur J Appl Physiol.* 2009, 105(5), 731-738.
[56] Loimaala, A; Huikuri, H; Oja, P; Pasanen, M; Vuori, I. Controlled 5-mo aerobic training improves heart rate but not heart rate variability or baroreflex sensitivity. *J Appl Physiol.* 2000, 89(5), 1825-1829.
[57] Casadei, B; Cochrane, S; Johnston, J; Conway, J; Sleight, P. Pitfalls in the interpretation of spectral analysis of the heart rate variability during exercise in humans. *Acta Physiol Scand.* 1995, 153(2), 125-131.
[58] Huttunen, NP; Knip, M; Paavilainen, T. Physical activity and fitness in obese children. *Int J Obes.* 1995, 10, 519-525.
[59] LeMura, LM; Maziekas, MT. Factors that alter body fat, body mass, and fat-free mass in pediatric obesity. *Med Sci Sports Exerc.* 2002, 34, 487-496.
[60] Ram, FS; Robinson, SM; Black, PN. Effects of physical training in asthma: a systematic review. *Br J Sports Med.* 2000, 34(3), 162-167.
[61] Rowland, T; Whatley Blum, J. Cardiac dynamics during upright cycle exercise in boys. *Am J Hum Biol.* 2000, 12(6), 749-757.
[62] Williams, CA; Armstrong, N; Powell, J. Aerobic responses of prepubertal boys to two modes of training. *Br J Sports Med.* 2000, 34(3), 168-173.
[63] Mahon, AD; Vaccaro, P. Cardiovascular adaptations in 8- to 12-year-old boys following a 14-week running program. *Can J Appl Physiol.,* 1994, 19(2), 139-150.
[64] Rowland, TW; Boyajian, A. Aerobic response to endurance exercise training in children. *Pediatrics.,* 1995, 96(4 Pt 1), 654-658.
[65] Wilmore, JH; Stanforth, PR; Gagnon, J; Rice, T; Mandel, S; Leon, AS; Rao, DC; Skinner, JS; Bouchard, C. Cardiac output and stroke volume changes with endurance training: the HERITAGE Family Study. *Med Sci Sports Exerc.,* 2001, 33(1), 99-106.
[66] Saltin, B; Blomqvist, G; Mitchell, JH; Johnson, RL. Jr., Wildenthal K; Chapman CB. Response to exercise after bed rest and after training. *Circulation.* 1968, 38(5 Suppl):VII1-78.

[67] Rowland, TW; Melanson, EL; Popowski, BE; Ferrone, LC. Test-retest reproducibility of maximum cardiac output by Doppler echocardiography. *Am J Cardiol.* 1998, 81(10), 1228-1230.

[68] Rowland, T; Goff, D; Martel, L; Ferrone, L. Influence of cardiac functional capacity on gender differences in maximal oxygen uptake in children. *Chest.,* 2000, 117(3), 629-635.

[69] Rowland, T; Potts, J; Potts, T; Sandor, G; Goff, D; Ferrone, L. Cardiac responses to progressive exercise in normal children: a synthesis. *Med Sci Sports Exerc.* 2000, 32(2), 253-259.

[70] Vinet, A; Mandigout, S; Nottin, S; Nguyen, L; Lecoq, AM; Courteix, D; Obert, P. Influence of body composition, hemoglobin concentration, and cardiac size and function of gender differences in maximal oxygen uptake in prepubertal children. *Chest.* 2003, 124(4), 1494-1499.

[71] Pathe, M; Laurenceau, JL; Baron, B; Marchand, X; Rocha, P; Zannier, D; Kahn, JC. [Influence of preload changes on the filling function of the left heart ventricle studied by Doppler echocardiography]. *Arch Mal Coeur Vaiss.* 1990, 83(14), 2061-2066.

[72] Krip, B; Gledhill, N; Jamnik, V; Warburton, D. Effect of alterations in blood volume on cardiac function during maximal exercise. *Med Sci Sports Exerc.* 1997, 29(11), 1469-1476.

[73] Vlahovic, A; Popovic, AD. [Evaluation of left ventricular diastolic function using Doppler echocardiography]. *Medicinski pregled.* 1999, 52(1-2), 13-18.

[74] Koch, G. Muscle blood flow in pre-pubertal boys. *Med Sport.,* 1978, 1978, 39-46.

[75] Moore, RL; Palmer, BM. Exercise training and cellular adaptations of normal and diseased hearts. *Exerc Sport Sci Rev.* 1999, 27, 285-315.

[76] Obert, P; Nottin, S; Baquet, G; Thevenet, D; Gamelin, FX; Berthoin, S. Two months of endurance training does not alter diastolic function evaluated by TDI in 9-11-year-old boys and girls. *Br J Sports Med.* 2009, 43(2), 132-135.

[77] Ogawa, T; Spina, RJ; Martin, WH; 3rd; Kohrt, WM; Schechtman, KB; Holloszy, JO; Ehsani, AA. Effects of aging, sex, and physical training on cardiovascular responses to exercise. *Circulation.,* 1992, 86(2), 494-503.

[78] Ferguson, S; Gledhill, N; Jamnik, VK; Wiebe, C; Payne, N. Cardiac performance in endurance-trained and moderately active young women. *Med Sci Sports Exerc.,* 2001, 33(7), 1114-1119.

In: Encyclopedia of Sports and Athletics
Editors: Jack L. Murray and Emily O. Watson
ISBN: 978-1-61209-959-0

Chapter VII

The Health Benefits of Aerobic Activity and Physical Fitness in Young People

Craig A. Williams[1], Julien Aucouturier[2], Eric Doré[2], Pascale Duché[2] and Sébastien Ratel[2*]

[1]Children's Health and Exercise Research Centre, School of Sport and Health Sciences, University of Exeter, Exeter, UK

[2]Laboratory of Exercise Biology (BAPS EA 3533), Faculty of Sports Sciences, University of Blaise Pascal, Clermont-Ferrand, France

Abstract

Results from studies involving adult participants have definitively established that physical activity and cardiorespiratory fitness are inversely correlated to morbidity and mortality. The evidence of the health benefits for physically active and fit adults is well known. There is a wealth of data which has shown that physically active and fit adults can help attenuate the effects of hypertension, insulin resistance, hyperlipidemia, obesity and cancer. However, the relationship between activity, fitness and the health benefits during childhood are less well established. Although it is intuitive to propose that an active child will become an active adult, the research evidence is weak. Similarly, the extent to which children's fitness and activity must decrease to seriously compromise their current or future health is also unknown. There is however growing concern for the future health status of children due to the increased levels of overweight and obese children and increased reporting of cardiovascular risk factors. Prospective data is needed to elucidate the complexity of these relationships. This complexity is partially due to problems related to 1) methodology i.e. how do we measure activity and health outcomes precisely; 2) biology i.e. children are growing and maturing at different rates and 3) sociology i.e. the effects of the environment. These problems therefore pose real challenges for policy makers as to whether they should concentrate resources on those child individuals who are deemed 'at risk' i.e. low fitness and low physical activity

* Corresponding author: Laboratory of Exercise Biology (BAPS), UFR STAPS, University of Blaise Pascal, BP. 104, 63172 Aubière, France., Tel: (33) 04-73-40-54-86, Mobile: (33) 06-82-13-62-73, Email: Sebastien.RATEL@univ-bpclermont.fr

patterns or to focus across the whole child population. This review will explore the relationships between physical fitness, activity and health in young people as well as describing the evidence for health benefits in this age group. The review will also discuss the implications for strategies of health related physical activity promotion at local and national levels.

I. The Relationship between Activity, Health and Fitness in Young People

Over the last twenty years there have been comprehensive reviews about the measurement and assessment procedures used to define the physical activity patterns of young people and adults (Corder and Ekelund, 2008). Although there is no one gold standard for the measurement of physical activity, the various pedometers, accelerometers, heart rate monitors, indirect calorimetry, double labelled water, direct observation and questionnaire methods have broadly found similar results. That is, boys are more active than girls, activity declines with age and the relationship between fitness and activity becomes stronger the older the participant. The latter finding is important because it has yet to be conclusively shown that physical activity is a strong predictor for fitness in young people as it is in adults. When the two measureable outcomes of activity and fitness in adults are linked to morbidity and mortality, the link is even stronger. In young people, there is as yet no consensus. The associations between health, activity and fitness are important to understand in order for them to be translated into policy, thus ensuring meaningful enhancements in health throughout childhood, adolescence and adulthood. The declining levels of physical activity, not only in adults but also young people, are a major concern world wide. The increasing incidence of life-style related chronic diseases (previously called hypokinetic diseases) once associated only with adults are now being observed in young people e.g. the increasing incidences of overweight and obesity. Researchers had considered that children have not yet lived long enough before major health problems occurred due to a lack of activity, but now there is empirical evidence that children and adolescents' health is suffering (Viner and Barker, 2005).

I.1. Definitions of Physical Activity, Health and Fitness

There is common agreement that physical activity is a behaviour and therefore subject to a multitude of extraneous factors (Casperson *et al.*, 1985). Although physical activity can be described as any bodily movement produced by the skeletal muscles resulting in energy expenditure, knowing the context for how and when young people move is important. It is likely that researchers have underestimated how complex activity is. Activity is both context and task specific e.g. type, duration and frequency of activity, as well as, whether the activity is performed habitually as part of one's work or recreationally. In children, the activity behaviour is confounded by the growth, maturation and development of the young person. Participation in activity is influenced by peer group behaviour, the increasing levels of independence with age and/or the increasing availability of monies to engage in different activities.

Physical fitness is defined as an attribute and has usually been referred to in the context of physical work. This is largely as a consequence of research work in the 19th and 20th century which quantified how much physical work labourers could perform during set jobs. Therefore, fitness was related to performance, although within the last 30 years there has been a broader move to incorporate fitness to health outcomes. Fitness is generally sub-divided into endurance or cardiovascular fitness (often described as aerobic), strength, speed, power and flexibility. From a performance perspective and depending on the relative importance of these sub-divisions to a particular sport, they can be easily measured. From an adult health perspective, there is more empirical evidence for cardiovascular fitness, strength and flexibility compared to speed and power. However, in young people, there is still too little information to describe the associations between fitness and health. This is mainly because fitness has a large genetic component to it and although it can be improved through training; there are too few training studies which have focused on health outcomes in children and adolescents.

Fitness training for health has not been extensively studied in young people possibly due to the fact that mortality rates in developed countries have shown a downward trend and therefore, the emphasis on this attribute is not a priority. However, in terms of morbidity many countries are showing adverse trends or maintenance of high levels related to obesity, smoking, asthma, diabetes, sexually transmitted diseases and pregnancy (Newacheck and Taylor, 1992). Particularly in the case of overweightness and obesity the gradual process of the disease has, until now, distracted professionals' attention away from the problem. Now most countries around the world have developed strategies to combat the spread of these lifestyle diseases (WHO, 1995; Health Education Authority, 1996; Dept of Health, 2004).

I.2. Physical Activity Guidelines and Young People

The first set of recommendations for physical activity guidelines were produced by the American College of Sports Medicine in 1988. Although the recommendations were based on adult guidelines, it was proposed that children should engage in at least 20 minutes of vigorous physical activity each day. A more considered approach was taken by an International Conference on Physical Activity Guidelines for Adolescents who in 1993 also attempted to base guidelines on empirical evidence (Sallis and Patrick, 1994). The consensus of the panel was that adolescents should;

1. be active on a daily basis, whether it be through work, play, physical education, sport, or active transport.
2. engage in at least 20 min of sustained moderate to vigorous activity at least three times a week.

In 1997, the Health Education Authority (England) convened a meeting to produce guidelines for activity in children (Biddle *et al.*, 1998). Again systematic reviews were conducted and attempts to base the recommendations on empirical evidence were conducted. The recommendations proposed that;

1. currently active children should achieve a minimum of 60 min of moderate activity per day, whereas less active children should strive for at least 30 min of moderate activity
2. children should also engage at least twice per week in activities designed to promote bone growth, flexibility, and strength.

One of the differences between the first two sets of American recommendations to those from England was that the Health Education Authority panel attempted to take into account individual differences (Pate *et al.*, 1998). A distinction was made between those children who were already active and those who were least active. In 2004, these recommendations were re-affirmed by the Chief Medical Officer's report on physical activity and health (Department of Health, 2004). These guidelines have since been further reviewed by researchers in the United States who concluded that school children should engage in at least 1 hour of moderate to vigorous activity per day and that activities should be enjoyable and developmentally suitable.

Recent evidence from the European Youth Heart Study has however questioned the evidence base for these guidelines and suggested these are not robust enough (Bo Andersen *et al.*, 2006). They randomly selected 1732 children aged between 9 and 15 years old across Denmark, Estonia and Portugal, risk factors such as systolic blood pressure, triglyceride, insulin resistance, skinfolds amongst others were collected. Their study found a graded negative relationship between clustering of the risk factors and physical activity. This risk was raised in the first three quintiles compared to the most active quintile. It was proposed that the current guidelines of at least 1 hour could be an underestimation of the activity necessary to prevent clustering. Their conclusion was that achieving 90 minutes of daily physical activity might be necessary to prevent insulin resistance and the clustering within cardiovascular disease risk factors. As to which guidelines are the most appropriate is debatable. It is important to emphasise, as it is often mis-quoted in the media that all the recommendations are only *guidelines*. All the members of the panels have struggled to interpret the data on activity and fitness of children and the impact on health, as well as predicting the impact on future adult health. All the panels have, in order to produce recommendations that can be understood by the general public, had to over simplify and treat physical activity as a one dimensional phenomenon. It is therefore unsurprising, given the social, physiological, psychological, environmental and temporal factors which influence activity, that researchers are no closer to precisely defining physical activity recommendations. Whether there are *optimal* levels of physical activity is debatable and might result in a search by future investigators for the "holy grail" of recommendations. Currently, the physical activity guidelines in both America and the United Kingdom are being revised.

I 3. The Adult-Child Relationships between Physical Activity, Health and Fitness

Blair *et al.* (1989) produced a flow diagram which highlighted the inter-links between:

1. childhood activity and childhood,
2. childhood activity to adult health,
3. childhood activity to adult activity,
4. adult activity and adult health,
5. childhood health to adult health.

Whilst this diagram simplistically represents the proposed relationships between activity, health and age, it has provided a model to investigate and rationalise why childhood activity is beneficial. The rationale for ensuring a physically active childhood includes sociological, psychological and physiological enhancement from activity which has a direct impact on childhood health. Secondly, a strategy of reducing the impact of health risks e.g. avoiding becoming overweight as a child and the direct impact on a healthy lifestyle as an adult. And thirdly, the intuitive proposition that an active child is more likely to develop into an active adult.

From the bullet points 1-3 in the above list by Blair and colleagues, it is still yet to be conclusively established that positive associations in childhood activity will impact either on child or adult health. By far the strongest evidence is for the relationship between adult activity and adult fitness (see point #4 above). Both fitness and activity are strongly and independently associated with health in adults, whilst the relationships are weaker in children. The strong and inverse relationship between activity and fitness, particularly cardiovascular, in adults is such that inactivity (sedentary activity) is prevalent and carries a risk as high as other risk factors e.g., smoking (Leon *et al.*, 1987). Therefore, one of the strategies that organisations and Governments must focus on is to decrease the amount of sedentary behaviour.

So far in this review, the focus has been on increasing physical activity but the reverse of this scenario is decreasing the amount of sedentary behaviour. It is important to note that they are not one and the same. The reasons for being active or being sedentary will of course be complex, but they are very different concepts. Therefore, many researchers over the last 10 years have focused their attention on decreasing the amount of sedentary behaviour exhibited by children. Research has invariably focused on television watching and computer playing and although this subject is beyond the scope of this review, readers are referred to a review by Marshall *et al.* (2006).

I 4. Physical Activity, Health and Fitness of Children

Activity is important for the development of children's physical and mental well being, and this fact is well accepted. As previously discussed the problem is how much activity is best for the growing child. Although this might be difficult to ascertain for a child who is healthy, who engages in sport or other leisure activities, the answers might be more forthcoming if we examine children who are not active. This inactivity could be either through choice or because they have a medical condition which prevents them being active. Researchers are therefore concerned about declining activity levels particularly in the adolescent years and the potential impact on future health. Early work by the Children's Health and Exercise Research at the University of Exeter examining activity, fitness and health and found that children did possess a range of cardiovascular risk factors e.g. high blood pressure, cigarette smoking or were overweight (Armstrong *et al.*, 1991). However, they concluded that the relationships between activity and fitness were weak and that there was not enough longitudinal evidence to show a connection between child health and future adult health. However, there have now been a number of publications which suggest stronger associations between being active and possessing a more favourable weight status or healthier cardiovascular disease profile (Brage et al., 2004; Andersen *et al.*, 2006; Ness *et al.*, 2007).

One of the main difficulties is that the common measure of health is 'mortality' which cannot be appropriately used in child studies. The other measure of health, 'morbidity' can be used with such outcomes as raised blood pressure, lipid profiles or fatness being recorded. But even these factors will only account for a certain percentage of the eventual cardiovascular mortality. A more immediate problem is the issue of increasing fatness in children and where there is a very strong relationship between cardiovascular fitness and fatness (Boreham *et al.*, 1997; Winsley *et al.*, 2006). It is important to highlight that the cardiovascular fitness of the overweight or obese child is compromised by the amount of fatness *per se*, not because the cardiovascular fitness of the child is deficient. When appropriately scaled for body fatness, overweight and normal weight children have similar aerobic fitness.

Therefore, whilst relationships between activity, fitness and health in adults are stronger than children and adolescents, it is intuitive to try to instil an active lifestyle in our young people. Data which tracks activity in childhood through to adolescence and into adulthood has shown a weak to moderate relationship (Malina, 2001). However, just because it is a weak relationship does not make it unimportant. Given the complexity of the relationships and confounding variables such as the environment, impact of work and family, times when ill, the relationship might only ever be weak or moderate. This observation should not detract from practitioners advocating physical activity as a preventative strategy to ill health throughout the life cycle.

I.5. Hypoactivity/Deconditioning Due to Illness - Asthma and Obesity

Hypoactivity is defined as an activity level which is lower than that of healthy peers of similar age, gender, cultural and socioeconomic background. Childhood diseases can both be a direct and indirect cause of hypoactivity. For example, a child with severe arthritis or muscular dystrophy is very limited in their movement patterns because of the disease. Conversely, a child with mild asthma can be active but often is not, but the hypoactivity might be co-incidental to the disease. There are many reasons why the disease might lead to a state of hypoactivity other than the actual disease restricting movement. These include over protection by parents or carers, fear of the consequence of performing activity, social isolation and ignorance about the effects of activity. All these factors including the progression of the diseases lead to a 'detraining effect' and functional deterioration. In particular functions which decline include; the maximal oxygen uptake (a measure of aerobic fitness), the elevation of the metabolic cost of submaximal tasks and the increased perception of effort in performing the tasks, and the reduction in strength, anaerobic power, and flexibility.

Physical activity recommendations for children with chronic diseases are uncommon, for some some of the reasons outlined above in healthy children, i.e. the complexity of the relationships between fitness, activity and how the processes evolve over time. In the case of children with chronic diseases there is the added issue of understanding the pathology of the disease and how physical activity may or may not affect the condition of the disease. In very few cases activity will affect the pathology of the disease, an exception is obesity or perhaps type 2 diabetes when insulin resistance is decreased. In other cases, activity may only be used to retard the disease process. For example, in cystic fibrosis it has been shown that the higher the aerobic fitness of the child, the longer the survival rate of the individual will be. Therefore, exercise is used as one therapy to increase length of life. In Duchenne muscular dystrophy, the use of exercise is controversial with some advocates suggesting exercise can do more damage to the muscle proteins, whilst others argue if strength can be improved, the increased mobility can have a significant impact on quality of life. Two particular diseases for which there is a growing amount of information about the relationship between fitness and activity is asthma and obesity and these will be reviewed in the next section.

II. Fitness and Physical Activity in Children with Diseases

II.1. Children with Asthma

II.1.1. Background

Asthma is a very common chronic disease involving the respiratory system in which the airways constrict and become inflamed. Airway obstruction is reversible either spontaneously or with treatment. One characteristic of asthma is that the bronchial system is hyper-responsive to a variety of triggers. These stimuli include airway infections, exposure to allergens or air pollutants, inhalation of dry and cold air, and exercise if it is of a sufficient intensity and duration. A considerable proportion of asthmatic children are affected by exercise-induced asthma (EIA), with the prevalence believed to be around 90 % (Wilkerson, 1998). In most patients, EIA leads to coughing, wheezing and shortness of breath in a short period after exercise (Storms 1999). Some patients complain about chest discomfort, nausea and stomach ache after exercise. In children, symptoms usually resolve within 10-90 min after the cessation of exercise. The purpose of the following sections will be to discuss the relationship between asthma and exercise when dealing with an active paediatric population to establish whether significant differences exist in the levels of habitual physical activity and aerobic fitness.

II.1.2. Asthma and physical activity

Although having a diagnosis of asthma or EIA does not necessarily prevent participation in sporting activities, there is a common perception that asthmatic children have a reduced capacity for exercise. In other words, it is perceived that asthmatic children, particularly those with EIA are not as physically active as their non-asthmatic counterparts. Despite the amount of speculation, only a limited number of studies have assessed the physical activity levels of asthmatic children and the results of these were highly controversial. These discrepancies are mostly associated with the difficulty of measuring with a high reliability, the habitual levels of physical activity by questionnaire, particularly in children (Kowalski *et al.*, 1997). For instance, Nystad (1997) administered the ISAAC (International Study of Asthma and Allergies in Childhood) questionnaire (Asher *et al.*, 1995) to 4021 school children living in three different areas of Norway and showed no difference in the physical activity levels between asthmatic and non-asthmatic children. Furthermore, the authors showed no difference in the exercise frequency and the number of hours spent exercising per week between the two groups. In the same way, using the 7-day recall Physical Activity Questionnaire for Children (PAQ-C) (Crocker *et al.*, 1997), Welsh *et al.* (2002) reported no differences in the physical activity levels of 28 asthmatic children and 200 non-asthmatic children. Conversely, Weston *et al.* (1989) found that asthmatic children were more frequently active than their non-asthmatic counterparts as measured by a self-administered questionnaire. Although asthmatic children were found to experience higher degrees of anxiety prior to exercise, they were characterized by higher school and daily physical activity levels.

In summary, these data suggest that asthmatic children have comparable physical activity levels compared to their non-asthmatic counterparts. However, in order to make definitive conclusions about this issue, further studies need to be carried out using more accurate recording systems of habitual physical activity and daily energy expenditure (e.g. accelerometry associated with or without heart rate recordings) rather than questionnaires.

II.1.3. Asthma and Aerobic Fitness

It also remains unclear whether significant differences exist in the aerobic fitness between asthmatic children and their non-asthmatic counterparts. Whilst some studies reported no difference in the aerobic fitness levels between asthmatic and non-asthmatic children and adolescents (Hedlin *et al.*, 1986; Fink *et al.*, 1993; Santuz *et al.*, 1997; Boas *et al.*, 1998), others demonstrated reduced aerobic fitness in asthmatic children. For instance, Boas et al. (1998) found similar values of VO_2max in 22 asthmatic children and adolescents and 22 age-matched non-asthmatic controls. Likewise, Fink *et al.* (1993) found no differences in VO_2max values between active and inactive groups of stable asthmatic and non-asthmatic children. On the contrary, Varray *et al.* (1989) found that 11 asthmatic children had significantly lower VO_2max values when compared with 11 non-asthmatic children matched for age, sex, height and weight. Similarly, Counil *et al.* (1997) reported reduced VO_2max values of around 10 % in 19 asthmatic boys when compared to 14 non-asthmatic boys of the same age. Despite these controversies, it has been suggested that the reduced aerobic fitness of any asthmatic child is associated with their sedentary lifestyle and that endurance training can enhance their aerobic fitness to be comparable to that found in non-asthmatic children (Fink *et al.*, 1993). According to some authors, asthmatic children are able to achieve similar levels of aerobic fitness as long as their physical activity levels are comparable with those of normal children (Santuz *et al.*, 1997). However, it is worth noting that in general, the benefits of increased physical activity are more pronounced in children and adolescents with severe disease compared to those with only moderately severe asthma (Hebestreit, 2008).

II.1.4. Recommendations

Children with asthma can exercise safely. Additionally, they can successfully participate in competitive sports at a very high level. However, a number of principles need to be adopted to minimize exercise-related risks (Hebestreit, 2008). Firstly, children with asthma should select the least asthmogenic activities. For instance, asthmatic children should be encouraged to practise swimming rather than land-based activities since EIA is less common. However, this recommendation does not apply to those few patients who experience bronchial constriction when swimming in chlorinated water. Also, it is well known that inhaling cold and dry air whilst exercising increases the risk of a severe bronchial obstruction. Therefore, asthmatic children are sometimes advised not to participate in winter sport activities. If children with asthma are led to practise skiing in dry air and cold temperature conditions, it is advised to wear a face mask to prevent the loss of heat and water from the bronchial system (Silvers *et al.*, 1994). Asthmatic children also have to be especially careful if exercise is performed in an environment with a high level of dust or ozone and a high concentration of allergens in the air (Mussaffi *et al.*, 1986). Furthermore, children should not exercise during a period of severely reduced airway patency. It is also worth noting that the warm-up is crucial before exercise to lower the risk for EIA during the subsequent 2 hours (Reiff *et al.*, 1989). However, the optimal pattern of the warm-up should be determined individually. Finally, children with asthma should inhale anti-inflammatory drugs (e.g. β_2-adrenergic agonists as salbutamol) 10-20 min before exercise and even during exercise in case of EIA (Hebestreit, 2008).

II.2. Obese Children

II.2.1. Background

Since the 1970s, the childhood obesity rate in the United States has more than doubled for children aged 2-5 years and adolescents aged 12-19 years, and it has more than tripled for children aged 6-11 years (Institute of US Medicine Web site, 2004). As a result, children are at increased risk of acute and chronic medical problems, which are associated with increased morbidity and mortality. These associated problems include insulin resistance, type 2 diabetes mellitus, coronary artery disease, hypertension, stroke and heart failure (Eckel and Krauss, 1998). The evidence of the increasing prevalence of obesity during childhood is particularly alarming since it has been assessed that 80 % of obese adolescents become obese adults (Schonfeld-Warden and Warden, 1997). The causes of obesity in children and adolescents are multiple and are continuously being debated. However, the increase of body fatness during childhood and adolescence has been associated with a decline in reported time for exercise (Watts *et al.*, 2005). The purpose of the following sections will be to discuss whether body fatness and aerobic fitness are associated or considered as independent risk factors for health. The aim is to ascertain whether significant differences exist in the aerobic fitness between obese and normal-weight children. Furthermore, it is also considered as to whether aerobic exercise training alone has a beneficial effect on body composition, blood profile and aerobic fitness in overweight and obese children.

II.2.2. Obesity and Aerobic Fitness

Confusion exists on the proper expression of VO_2max data when comparing obese and normal weight individuals. According to Goran *et al.* (2000), VO_2max should be expressed per unit of fat-free mass ($mL \cdot kg\ FFM^{-1} \cdot min^{-1}$) when comparing the physiological ability of the tissue to maximally consume oxygen, since FFM is more metabolically active than fat mass (FM). Conversely, when looking at endurance performance or the ability to perform a submaximal aerobic exercise, oxygen consumption relative to body mass should be used. Comparisons in VO_2max values relative to body mass appear to be clear, with numerous studies reporting a significantly reduced VO_2max in obese children compared with normal-weight children (Epstein *et al.*, 1983; DeMeersman *et al.*, 1985; Zanconato *et al.*, 1989; Rowland TW, 1991; Maffeis *et al.*, 1994; Goran *et al.*, 2000). This is certainly attributed to the overcorrection related to the excess of body fatness in obese individuals. However, when scaling for FFM, VO_2max data were found to be similar between obese and normal-weight children (Cooper *et al.*, 1990; Maffeis *et al.*, 1993; Maffeis *et al.*, 1994; Treuth *et al.*, 1998; Goran *et al.*, 2000). These findings support the proposition that the maximal oxygen consumption of fat-free tissue is independent of the body fatness rate and the limiting factor in aerobic-type activities for the obese individual is not the cardio-respiratory system. Some studies showed that it was physiologically more difficult for the obese individuals to do the same amount of work as normal weight individuals, at least in weight-bearing activities (Mattsson *et al.*, 1997; Goran *et al.*, 2000). For instance, Mattsson *et al.* (1997) reported that obese women used 57 % of VO_2max during normal walking, whereas their normal weight counterparts used only 36 % of VO_2max. In the same way, Goran *et al.* (2000) found that heavier individuals required a greater percentage of VO_2max than normal weight subjects to complete the same running task (44 vs 37 % in children, respectively; 44 vs 36 % in adults, respectively). Their finding was associated with a higher submaximal heart rate, a higher respiratory exchange ratio and shorter time to exhaustion in obese individuals. Therefore, obese individuals were found to be limited in their ability to perform sub-maximal aerobic exercises.

In summary, obese children do not have lower maximal aerobic power of their fat-free mass compared with their lean counterparts or impaired cardio-respiratory and pulmonary responses to exercise. On the contrary, the overweight and obese children require a greater proportion of their aerobic capacity to perform weight-bearing physical activities. Therefore, children with obesity are likely to fatigue more quickly during submaximal exercise, which requires the mobilisation of their increased body mass.

II.2.3. Exercise training, body composition, blood profile and aerobic fitness

The majority of studies that controlled exercise training independently of dietary modification on body composition, blood profile and aerobic fitness showed beneficial effects in childhood and adolescent obesity. For instance, after a 1-year exercise intervention, Hayashi *et al.* (1987) demonstrated a decrease in bodyweight and resting heart rate and an increase in left ventricular end-diastolic dimension in obese children aged 10-11 years. Conversely, the normal-weight control group who participated in their regular physical education classes gained weight and no changes in their cardiac dimensions over the year. Furthermore, Gutin *et al.* (1997) found in 35 obese children aged 7-11 years that a 4-month programme involving 40 min of aerobic exercise 5 days per week resulted in decreased levels of body fat (-4.1 %) and an enhanced cardiac autonomic function by a decreased ratio of sympathetic to parasympathetic activity. The same intervention programme also resulted in a decreased subcutaneous abdominal tissue (-16.1 %) and less accumulation of visceral adipose tissue in 74 obese children compared with a non-exercise control group (Owens *et al.*, 1999). It is also worth noting that the 4 months of aerobic exercise training in the absence of changes in diet, decreased the levels of fasting plasma insulin and leptin in association with decreased plasma triglyceride levels (-0.24 $mmol \cdot L^{-1}$), suggesting that exercise training may improve glycaemic control and decrease the insulin resistance syndrome in obese children (Ferguson *et al.*, 1999; Gutin *et al.*, 1999). However, those benefits were lost when obese children became less active (Ferguson *et al.*, 1999; Gutin *et al.*, 1999).

In summary, the well controlled studies that examined the effects of exercise training alone on body composition and the detrimental metabolic consequences of childhood and adolescent obesity were small. However, the studies discussed above suggest that exercise training beneficially modifies body composition without changes in bodyweight and body mass index. Furthermore, exercise training is associated with increases in cardiovascular fitness in obese children. However, whilst exercise training is not always associated with large changes on blood lipid profile and glycaemic control, diet may be a more important determinant in obese young people (Watts *et al.*, 2005).

II.2.4. Recommendations

Many studies have failed to provide adequate information regarding important elements of the exercise prescription such as intensity. On the basis of the studies cited above, children should regularly participate 5 days per week in 40 min or more of moderate to vigorous physical activity. Furthermore, it is advised obese children practise low intensity non-weight bearing activities like bike riding and swimming, as these may result in greater ease of performing the physical tasks, resulting in greater energy expenditure and weight loss. Also, the physical activity sessions should be supervised by a qualified exercise leader.

III. Promotion of Health, Physical Activity and Fitness Schemes – Policy and Practice

III.1. Environmental factors

In 2008, NICE (National Institute for Health and Clinical Excellence) a National Health Service organisation (NHS) in the U.K. issued guidelines on promoting and creating built or natural environments to promote physical activity. A specific guideline was the need for environmental factors to be implemented thus making it as easy as possible for people to be habitually active. The guidelines which could be applied to children and adolescents included:

- Ensuring planning applications for new developments always prioritise the need for people to be physically active as a routine part of their daily lives.
- Ensuring pedestrians, cyclists and other modes of physically active transport are given the highest priority when developing or maintaining streets and roads.
- Ensuring new workplaces are linked to walking and cycling networks.

Whilst past environmental interventions such as legislating for treating waste products and enhancing and maintaining food and water quality have been success stories, this cannot be stated for cases of environmental interventions and physical activity (Sallis *et al.*, 1998). This lack of success may be due to the difficulty of not being able to separate the different social, personal and cultural factors from the environmental impact thereby showing a direct effect due to the environmental changes. Models of ecological theory of physical activity such as the one proposed by Sallis and Owen (1996) accounts not only for the specific environment in which the physical activity takes place, but the social and cultural context, as well as, the "behaviour setting". For example, sports fields and gymnasia in schools have both a physical and social setting that are designed to promote physical activity in schools. This example is also the consequence of a public policy because the various school laws, in different countries, specify the amount of physical education and curriculum time children should engage in physical activity. In the context of the behaviour setting, some children will engage more actively in the lesson than others and therefore might benefit to a greater extent. The above scenario is a very direct example, mainly because the activity i.e. the P.E. lesson is enshrined in law, but there are also other environmental examples that can affect physical activity. For example, in many westernised countries, one strategy has been to try to increase the number of children that walk or bike to school. This has meant important co-operation is needed between parents, the school and the local authority to ensure such resources as a safe route maps to school, organising bike and walk days to school and/or walking bus schemes, as well as having available better road signage and cycle paths to schools.

More recently, another theoretical model known as the Environmental Research framework for weight gain prevention (EnRG) has been proposed (Kremers *et al.*, 2006). This framework encompasses social, psychological and ecological models of health behaviour to investigate obesogenic (low physical activity and excessive energy intake) environments. A range of mediating factors such as personality, sedentary behaviour, active transport, attitude, self-efficacy and intentions are all considered in an attempt to explain the outcomes on physical activity and energy intake. Clearly, the more detailed the models become, the more complex are the data sets and therefore, the more difficult is the interpretation. However, it is vitally important that investigators develop and adapt these models theoretically from the empirical evidence, in order to prioritise what are the key determinants.

Environmental interventions to increase physical activity in children need to be based on empirical findings, a theoretical framework and as important, be practical. Unfortunately, research literature is sparse and cannot at present evaluate the influence and impact of the environment. Past health promotions have focused on altering attitudes to activity, the determinants of activity e.g. accessibility or cost and the environment e.g. open spaces to promote activity or decrease sedentary behaviour. However, more research is needed in this area.

III.2. School Factors

The promotion of enhanced physical activity through additional physical education has been a favoured intervention strategy in many countries. The opportunity for a 'captive' audience in which to deliver the physical activity message is clearly an opportunity that cannot be missed. Coupled with the fact that children attend school from an early age provides a setting that affects positive behaviours. Although rigorously controlled studies of physical activity intervention studies are sparse, results have been positive. Most outcomes have tended to focus on knowledge of health, physical fitness tests and attitudes to activity. However, it should be noted that studies tend to be short in duration, with little opportunity for follow up evaluations. Not all researchers are convinced that better facilities or increased time allocated to PE will improve activity levels in children and will impact on the rising epidemic of obesity (Metcalf *et al.*, 2004).

However, given the multi-dimensional aspects of health, promoting early life experiences through physical activity is considered an important strategy to foster good habits. Primary school age (typically 5-11 years) is often a time when movement skills, co-operative games are emphasised rather than competitive games and the intensity of these activities has been criticised as being too low to enhance health (Mota, 1994). But, the development of foundational skills and competencies and making the first experiences of activity to be fun and inclusive probably takes precedence. Perhaps the impact of the enhancement of health via the intensity of activity becomes more important during their secondary school years (typically 11-16 years). However, it is also a time when it is known that physical activity patterns decline dramatically, particularly in girls (Armstrong and Van Mechelen, 1998). Therefore, we would advocate a strong focus of research attention on the adolescent years to understand why these patterns change and how the declining patterns can be reversed or slowed. The adolescent period is also a period, particularly in the U.K. when physical activity through the national curriculum of P.E and games varies considerably between schools. The national recommended amount is 8-10 % of total curriculum time but few schools meet this target. Although the U.K. Government has targeted fours hours of PE for the future, it is unclear if this target will be met. Interestingly, those studies which have examined academic performance and increased physical activity have not found a negative impact on academic performance. Although the empirical evidence is limited and definitive conclusions incomplete, there is scope in this area to show school head teachers that increased physical activity can have additional benefits besides health ones e.g., improvement in cognition, academic test scores, attention in class, absenteeism and behaviour (Dwyer *et al.*, 1983; Sallis *et al.*, 1999; Coe *et al.*, 2006; Ahamed *et al.*, 2007).

Strategies to either objectively measure or enhance the frequency of physical activity in schools are common across the developed world. These include the 'JUMP-in' programme in Amsterdam, Holland (Jurg *et al.*, 2006), the National Health and Nutrition Examination Survey (2003-04) in the U.S., the health-related fitness and later health-related physical activity P.E. curriculum in England during the late 1980s and early 1990s and project SHAPE in Australia (Dwyer *et al.*, 1983). Despite these resources and considerable attention from programmes world wide, there is still an urgent need for action on children's health within a school setting. However, schools must not be considered as a panacea to society's problems of worsening health issues for children and adolescents. As much as physical activity is multi-dimensional, so too must the problem be tackled from numerous other organisations. This includes political intervention.

III.3. Local and National Government Policies

In their review Sallis and colleagues (1998) emphasised the importance of inter-agency advocacy, coordination and planning. Using a model developed through the New South Wales (Australia) Physical Activity Task Force (1997), agencies from the police, criminal justice, community organisations were identified to work together. Transportation departments were also involved to assist in urban planning, public transport and cycling paths. In the U.K. the guidance by NICE encourages local authorities, transport, planning and development professionals to work together on making towns and cities more liveable by advocating a healthy lifestyle through increased physical activity. Other groups including the media and education services were also identified as important agents in affecting change. It is clear that this level of co-ordination is needed to have the maximum effect of increasing physical activity levels not just in children, but also adults.

In the U.S. a National Coalition to Promote Physical Activity (NCPPA) was formed in 1995. Bringing together many of the key medical, sports and educational organisations to promote physical activity, NCPPA models itself on the coalition that has had such success on combating tobacco use in the U.S. One of the key strategies of the NCPPA has been to work with legislative bodies at both national and state levels. These types of strategies are being replicated from country to country such that levels of involvement and co-operation between the different organisations have increased. For a review see the work of Blair and colleagues (1996). As yet however, there appears to be little evaluation from which to conclude their effectiveness (Kremers *et al.*, 2008).

IV. Summary and Conclusion

There is a logical rationale for promoting physical activity in children and adolescents, despite the current evidence being weak to moderate with regards to its influence on adult health. However, more studies are being conducted to elucidate the complex relationships between health, activity and fitness during childhood, adolescence and into adulthood. Physical activity has been shown to be important for improving the health of the overweight, obese or Type 2 diabetic child and adolescent. Strategies to enhance physical activity have often been focused within schools, although the amount of PE and games within schools is often a legislative matter in many countries and therefore prone to political changes. Wider strategies beyond the school gate have highlighted the importance of trying to engage with as many organisations as possible to maximise effectiveness. To this end a clear lead by Government departments and world agencies e.g. the World Health Organisation must be sought to promote physical activity as a cornerstone to good health.

References

Ahamed, Y., MacDonald, H., Reed, K., Naylor, P. J., Liu-Ambrose, T. & McKay, H. (2007). School-based physical activity does to compromise children's academic performance. *Med Sci Sports Exerc.*, *39*, 371-376.

Andersen, L. B., Harro, M., Sardinha, L. B., Froberg, K., Ekelund, U., Brage, S. & Andersen, S. A. (2006). Physical activity and clustered cardiovascular risk in children: A cross-sectional study (The European Youth heart Study). *The Lancet.*, *368*, 299-304.

Armstrong, N., Williams, J., Balding, J., Gentle, P. & Kirby, B. (1991). Cardiopulmonary fitness, physical activity patterns, and selected coronary risk factor variables in 11 to 16 years olds. *Ped Exerc Sci.*, *3*, 219-228.

Armstrong, N. & Van Mechelen, W. (1998). Are young people fit and active? In: *Young and Active?* (Editors: Biddle S, Sallis J and Cavill N). London, Health Education Authority, 69-97.

Asher, M. I., Keil, U., Anderson, H. R., Beasley, R., Crane, J., Martinez, F., Mitchell, E. A., Pearce, N., Sibbald, B., Stewart, A. W., et al. (1995). International Study of Asthma and Allergies in Childhood (ISAAC): rationale and methods. *Eur Respir J., 8,* 483-491.

Biddle, S. J. H., Sallis, J. F. & Cavill, N. A. (1998). Young and active? Young People and Health Enhancing Physical Activity. *Evidence and Implications*. London, Health Education Authority.

Blair, S. N., Clark, D. G., Cureton, K. J. & Powell, K. E. (1989). Exercise and fitness in childhood: Implications for a lifetime of health (Editors: Gisolfi CV and Lamb DR) In: *Perspectives in exercise science and sports medicine*, Benchmark press, Indianapolis, IN, pp. 401-430.

Blair, S. N. & Booth, M., Gyarfas I., et al. (1996). Development of public policy and physical activity initiatives internationally. *Sports Med., 21,* 157-163.

Boas, S. R., Danduran, M. J. & Saini, S. K. (1998). Anaerobic exercise testing in children with asthma. *J Asthma., 35,* 481-487.

Boreham, C. A. G., Strain, J. J., Twisk, J. W. R., Van Mechelen, W., Savage, J. M. & Cran, G. W. (1997). Aerobic fitness, physical activity and body fatness in adolescents. (Editors : Armstrong N, Welsman J and Kirby B) In: *Children and exercise*, E&FN Spon, London., 69-75.

Brage, S., Wedderkopp, N., Ekelund, U., Franks, P. W., Wareham, N. J., Andersen, L. B. & Froberg, K. (2004). Objectively measured physical activity correlates with indices of insulin resistance in Danish children. The European Youth Heart Study (EYHS). *Int J Obes., 28*, 1503-1508.

Casperson, C. J., Powell, K. E. & Christenson, G. M. (1985). Physical activity, exercise, and physical fitness : definitions and distinctions for health-related research. *Pub Health Reports., 100,* 126-131.

Childhood obesity in the United States: facts and figures. Institute of Medicine Web site. September 2004. Available at: http://www.iom.edu/Object.File/Master/22/606/FINALfactsandfigures2.pdf. *Accessed March., 19,* 2009.

Coe, D. P., Pivarnik, J. M., Womack, C. J., Reeves, M. J. & Malina, R. M. (2006). Effect of physical education and activity levels on academic achievement in children. *Med Sci Sports Exerc., 38,* 1515-1519.

Corder, K. & Ekelund, U. (2008). Physical activity. In *Paediatric Exercise Science and Medicine, 2nd Edition* (Editors: Armstrong N and Van Mechelen W), Oxford University Press, Oxford, pp.128-143.

Cooper, D. M., Poage, J., Barstow, T. J. & Springer, C. (1990). Are obese children truly unfit? Minimizing the confounding effect of body size on the exercise response. *J Pediatr., 116,* 223-230.

Counil, F. P., Varray, A., Karila, C., Hayot, M., Voisin, M. & Préfaut, C. (1997). Wingate test performance in children with asthma: aerobic or anaerobic limitation? *Med Sci Sports Exerc., 29,*430-435.

Crocker, P. R., Bailey, D. A., Faulkner, R. A., Kowalski, K. C. & McGrath, R. (1997). Measuring general levels of physical activity: preliminary evidence for the Physical Activity Questionnaire for Older Children. *Med Sci Sports Exerc., 29,* 1344-1349.

DeMeersman, R. E., Stone, S., Schaefer, D. C. & Miller, W. W. (1985). Maximal work capacity in prepubescent obese and nonobese females. *Clin Pediatr., 24,* 199-200.

Department of Health Physical Activity Health Improvement and Prevention. (2004). *At least five a week: Evidence of the impact of physical activity and its relationship to health.* Department of Helath, London.

Dwyer, T., Blizzard, L. & Dean, K. (1996). Physical activity and performance in children. *Nutr Rev., 54,* S27-31.

Eckel, R. H. & Krauss, R. M. (1998). American Heart Association call to action: obesity as a major risk factor for coronary heart disease. AHA Nutrition Committee. *Circulation, 97,* 2099-2100.

Epstein, L. H., Koeske, R., Zidansek, J. & Wing, R. R. (1983). Effects of weight loss on fitness in obese children. *Am J Dis Child., 137,* 654-657.

Ferguson, M. A., Gutin, B., Le, N. A., Karp, W., Litaker, M., Humphries, M., Okuyama, T., Riggs, S. & Owens, S. (1999). Effects of exercise training and its cessation on components of the insulin resistance syndrome in obese children. *Int J Obes Relat Metab Disord, 23,* 889-895.

Fink, G., Kaye, C., Blau, H. & Spitzer, S. A. (1993). Assessment of exercise capacity in asthmatic children with various degrees of activity. *Pediatr Pulmonol., 15,* 41-43.

Goran, M., Fields, D. A., Hunter, G. R., Herd, S. L. & Weinsier, R. L. (2000). Total body fat does not influence maximal aerobic capacity. *Int J Obes Relat Metab Disord., 24,* 841-848.

Gutin, B., Owens, S., Slavens, G., Riggs, S. & Treiber, F. (1997). Effect of physical training on heart-period variability in obese children. *J Pediatr., 130,* 938-943.

Gutin, B., Ramsey, L., Barbeau, P., Cannady, W., Ferguson, M., Litaker, M. & Owens, S. (1999). Plasma leptin concentrations in obese children: changes during 4-mo periods with and without physical training. *Am J Clin Nutr., 69,* 388-394.

Hayashi T., Fujino M., Shindo M., Hiroki T. & Arakawa K. (1987). Echocardiographic and electrocardiographic measures in obese children after an exercise program. *Int J Obes., 11,* 465-472.

Health Education Authority. (1996). Active for Life Campaign. London, *Health Education Authority.*

Hebestreit, H. (2008). Exercise, physical activity, and asthma. In: Paediatric Exercise Science and Medicine, 2nd Edition (Editors: Armstrong N and Van Mechelen W). Oxford University press, 431-439,

Hedlin, G., Graff-Lonnevig, V. & Freyschuss, U. (1986). Working capacity and pulmonary gas exchange in children with exercise-induced asthma. *Acta Paediatr Scand., 75,* 947-954.

Jurge, M. E., Kremers, S. P. J., Candel, M. J. J. M., Van der Wal, M. & De Meij, J. (2006). A controlled trial of a school-based environmental intervention to improve physical activity in children: JUMP-in, kids in motion. *Health Promot Int., 21,* 320-330.

Kowalski, K. C., Crocker, P. R. E. & Faulkner, R. A. (1997). Validation of the physical activity questionnaire for older children. *Pediatr Exerc Sci., 9,* 174-186.

Kremers, S. P. J., De Bruijn, G. J., Vissher, T. L. S., Van Mechelen, W., De Vries, N. K., Brug, J. (2006). Environmental influences on energy balance-related behaviors: A dual-process view. *Int J Behav Nutr Phys Act., 3,* 9.

Kremers, S. P. J., Schaalma, H., Meertens, R. M., Van Mechelen, W. & Kok, G. J. (2008). Systematic promotion of physical activity. In *Paediatric Exercise Science and Medicine*, 2nd Edition (Editors: Armstrong N and Van Mechelen W), Oxford University Press, *Oxford.*, 409-417.

Leon, A. S., Connett, J., Jacobs, D. R. & Rauramaa, R. (1987). Leisure-time physical-activity levels and risk of coronary heart-disease and death-The multiple risk factor intervention trial. *JAMA.*, *258,* 2388-2395.

Maffeis, C., Schutz, Y., Schena, F., Zaffanello, M. & Pinelli, L. (1993). Energy expenditure during walking and running in obese and nonobese prepubertal children. *J Pediatr.*, *123,* 193-199.

Maffeis, C., Schena, F., Zaffanello, M., Zoccante, L., Schutz, Y. & Pinelli, L. (1994). Maximal aerobic power during running and cycling in obese and non-obese children. *Acta Paediatr.*, *83,* 113-116.

Malina, R. M. (2001). Tracking of physical activity across the lifespan. *Res Digest*, *3,* 1-7.

Marshall, S. J., Gorely, T. & Biddle, S. J. (2006). A descriptive epidemiology of screen-based media use in youth. A review and critique. *J Adolesc.*, *29,* 333-349.

Mato, J. (1994). Children's physical education activity, assessed by telemetry. *J Hum Mov Stud.*, *27,* 245-250.

Mattsson, E., Larsson, U. E. & Rössner, S. (1997). Is walking for exercise too exhausting for obese women? *Int J Obes Relat Metab Disord*, *21,* 380-386.

Metcalf, B., Mallam, K., Voss, L., Jeffrey, A., Snaith, R., Alba, S. & Wilkin, T. (2004). The regulation of physical activity in young children. *Educ Health.*, *61,* 61-64.

Mussaffi, H., Springer, C. & Godfrey, S. (1986). Increased bronchial responsiveness to exercise and histamine after allergen challenge in children with asthma. *J Allergy Clin Immunol.*, *77,* 48-52.

Ness, A. R., Leary, S. D., Mattocks, C., Blair, S. N., Reilly, J. J., Wells, J., Ingle, S., Tilling, K., Smoth, G. D. & Riddoch, C. (2007). Objectively measured physical activity and fat mass in a large cohort of children. *Plos Med*, *4,* 476-484.

New South Wales Physical Activity Task Force. Simply active every day: a discussion document from the NSW Physical Activity Task Force on proposals to promote physical activity in NSW., 1997-2002. *Summary report.* Sydney, Australia: New South Wales Health Department, 1997.

Newacheck, P. & Taylor, W. (1992). Childhood chronic illness: prevalence, severity and impact. *Am J Public Health.*, *82,* 364-371.

NICE (National Institute for Health and Clinical Excellence). (2008). *Physical activity and the environment.* Accessed April 2009 at http://www.nice.org.uk

Owens, S., Gutin, B., Allison, J., Riggs, S., Ferguson, M., Litaker, M. & Thompson, W. (1999). Effect of physical training on total and visceral fat in obese children. *Med Sci Sports Exerc.*, *31,* 143-148.

Pate, R., Trost, S. & Williams, C. (1998). Critique of existing guidelines for physical activity in young people. In: Young and active? Young People and Health Enhancing Physical Activity. *Evidence and Implications* (Editors: Biddle SJH, Sallis JF, Cavill NA) London, Health Education Authority, 162-175.

Reiff, D. B., Choudry, N. B., Pride, N. B. & Ind, P. W. (1989). The effect of prolonged submaximal warm-up exercise on exercise-induced asthma. *Am Rev Respir Dis.*, *139,* 479-84.

Rowland, T. W. (1991). Effects of obesity on aerobic fitness in adolescent females. *Am J Dis Child, 145,* 764-768.

Sallis, J. F. & Patrick, K. (1994). Physical activity guidelines for adolescents: consensus statement. *Pediatr Exerc Sci., 20,* 422-423.

Sallis, J. F. & Owen, N. (1996). Ecological models. In: Health behaviour and health education. Theory, research, and practice, 2nd Edition (Editors: Glanz K., Lewis FM., and Rimer BK) Jossey-Bass, *San Fransico.*, 403-424.

Sallis, J. F., Bauman, A. & Pratt, M. (1998). Environmental and policy interventions to promote physical activity. *Am J Prev Med., 15,* 379-397.

Sallis, J. F., McKenzie, T. L., Boldan, K., Lewis, M., Marshall, S. & Rosengard, P. (1999). Effects of health related physical education on academic achievement: Project SPARK. *Res Q Exerc Sport., 70,* 127-134.

Santuz, P., Baraldi, E., Filippone, M. & Zacchello, F. (1997). Exercise performance in children with asthma: is it different from that of healthy controls? *Eur Respir J., 10,* 1254-1260.

Schonfeld-Warden, N., Warden, C. H. (1997). Pediatric obesity. An overview of etiology and treatment. *Pediatr Clin North Am., 44,* 339-61.

Silvers, W., Morrison, M. & Wiener, M. (1994). Asthma ski day: cold air sports safe with peak flow monitoring. *Ann Allergy., 73,* 105-108.

Storms, W. W. (1999). Exercise-induced asthma: Diagnosis and treatment for the recreational or elite athletes. *Med Sci Sports Exerc.*, 31 (Suppl. 1), S33-S38.

Treuth, M. S., Figueroa-Colon, R., Hunter, G. R., Weinsier, R. L., Butte, N. F. & Goran, M. I. (1998). Energy expenditure and physical fitness in overweight vs non-overweight prepubertal girls. *Int J Obes Relat Metab Disord., 22,* 440-447.

Varray, A., Mercier, J., Ramonatxo, M., et al. (1989). Maximal exercise in asthmatic children: aerobic limitation or anaerobic compensation? *Sci Sports., 4,* 199-207.

Viner, R. M. & Barker, M. (2005). Young people's health: the need for action. *BMJ., 330,* 901-903.

Watts, K., Jones, T. W., Davies, E. A. & Green, D. (2005). Exercise training in obese children and adolescents. *Sports Med., 35,* 375-392.

Welsh, L., Roberts, R. G. D. & Kemp, J. G. (2002). Aerobic fitness, physical acitvity and asthma in Australian school children [abstract]. *Am J Respir Crit Care Med.*, 165(8), A740.

Weston, A. R., Macfarlane, D. J. & Hopkins, W. G.. (1989). Physical activity of asthmatic and nonasthmatic children. *J Asthma., 26(5)*, 279-286.

Wilkerson, L. A. (1998). Exercise-induced asthma. *J Am Osteopath Assoc, 11(4)*, 322-331.

Winsley, R. J., Middlebrooke, A. R., Armstrong, N. & Williams, C. A. (2006). Aerobic fitness and visceral adipose tissue in children. *Acta Paediatrica., 95(11)*, 1435 - 1438.

World Health Organisation. (1995). Exercise for health. *WHO/FIMS Committee on Physical Activity for Health.* Bulletin of the WHO, *73*, 135-136.

Zanconato, S., Baraldi, E., Santuz, P., Rigon, F., Vido, L., Da Dalt, L. & Zacchello, F. (1989). Gas exchange during exercise in obese children, *Eur J Pediatr., 148*, 614-7.

In: Encyclopedia of Sports and Athletics
Editors: Jack L. Murray and Emily O. Watson

ISBN: 978-1-61209-959-0

Chapter VIII

Physical Activity and Women: Unique Issues

Linda May, Sarah Pyle and Richard Suminski
Kansas City University of Medicine and Biosciences, Kansas City, MO, US

Abstract

Physical activity is vital for overall health maintenance, particularly cardiovascular health. Additionally, physical activity is important for decreasing the risk of cancer and osteoporosis in women. Physical fitness, a benefit of physical activity, is important during pregnancy and postpartum periods for both women and their babies. As women became more aware of this issue, their participation in physical activity increased. Upon becoming pregnant, many women posed their Ob/Gyn physicians with the question, "is physical activity during pregnancy safe?" Initially, little was known about the effects physical activity had on the expectant mother or fetal development. Research has led to a better understanding of maternal and fetal physiology and findings highlight the importance of physical activity during this time. This chapter provides an overview, which examines aspects of physical activity in regard to pregnant and lactating women. Based on the available literature, physicians have shifted their focus from assuring patients that physical activity during gestation is safe to encouraging physical activity during pregnancy because of the potential benefits to both the fetus and mother. Ultimately, these benefits are realized at labor and delivery and during the mother's recovery period. Current research into the fetal and neonatal benefits of maternal physical activity is explored. Lactation represents a continuation of the pregnancy, as the mother continues to supply nourishment for her infant. The effects of physical activity during lactation are viewed from the maternal and infant perspective. As research advances, American College of Obstetricians and Gynecologists (ACOG) guidelines continue to reflect these gains in information. An overview of the current ACOG guidelines is considered. Lastly, the chapter expresses what has been done, and what is currently being done to encourage women to stay physically active during their pregnancy.

Introduction

Since the 1930's, women's attitudes about physical activity have gone through a dramatic, intellectual transformation. Over the last half century, women have started to take a more intentional approach in respect to their physical activities. For instance, many women participate in competitive sports. Large numbers of females engage in club sports and recreational activities. These increases in opportunities for women to be physically activity have generated a dramatic and positive shift in the health consciousness of women.

Many of the women engaging in physical activity pursuits are of reproductive age and plan to bear children at some point in their lives. The question often arises about the safety and benefit of engaging in physical activity during pregnancy. Additionally, women wonder what effects physical activity has on lactation. Consequently, there is a growing field of interest in the scientific literature focusing on physical activity during periods of pregnancy and lactation. Furthermore, researchers in this area are examining the benefits of physical activity during pregnancy to the fetus and the newborn child.

Physical Activity during Pregnancy

Starting in the 1960s, researchers around the globe began to investigate the relationship between physical activity and pregnancy (Sazontov et al 1952, Von Rutte et al. 1951, Bader et al. 1955, Hart et al. 1956). Initial research focused on examining the effects of physical activity prior to pregnancy and focusing on changes that were teratogenic, or harmful, to the fetus. Physical activity results in acute cardiovascular, hormonal, nutritional, thermoregulatory, and biomechanical responses. There was concern these acute responses could have an impact on the developing fetus. The acute responses with exercise may apply to females who were physically active or sedentary prior to their pregnancy. Long term, consistent exercise leads to biochemical, physiological, and metabolic changes. These changes apply to exercise trained pregnant women.

Initial studies in the 1950s focused on the critical issue of hemodynamic responses of uterine blood flow during aerobic exercise in pregnant mothers. In the non-pregnant state moderate aerobic exercise causes vasoconstriction of splanchnic blood supply, which supplies the uterus, and vasodilation of vessels supplying working muscle. This causes a decrease in blood flow to the uterus of about 50% which could affect the developing fetus (Clapp 1978). Therefore, physical activity during pregnancy was thought to be detrimental to fetal health and development. Although research studies have differing results depending on exercise regime and measuring techniques, the current consensus is that blood flow to the utero-placental bed decreases during a pregnant mother's exercise. However, this decrease is not as great as in the non-pregnant state and is accompanied by other adaptations. For example, oxygen transport capacity is enhanced by increases in cardiac output (Clapp 2003, Weissgerber). Additionally, maternal blood volume increases to maintain an adequate nutrient supply to the developing fetus (Clapp 2003, Hart et al. 1956, Morrow et al. 1969). Exercise training during pregnancy increases resting maternal plasma volume, intervillous space blood volume, and red cell mass (Clapp 2003, Hytten and Chamberlain 1991). Other adaptations specific to the placenta occur and will be discussed later.

Typically, catecholamine levels decrease during pregnancy (Metcalfe et al. 1988). However, an exercise bout leads to a release of norepinephrine. Physicians were concerned that this change in hormonal milieu may affect the smooth muscle contractility of the uterus. Research has shown that the hormonal changes during exercise do not alter the endocrine milieu greatly during pregnancy. In the last trimester of pregnancy, levels or norepinephrine are diminished compared to the 1st and 2nd trimesters and to non-pregnant controls (Bonen et al. 1995). Upon the completion of exercise, hormone concentrations rapidly return to normal as in the non-pregnant state. (Bonen et al. 1995). None of the studies noted any increased incidence of uterine contractions or pre-term labor indicating the catecholamines do not have a stimulatory effect on the quiescent pregnant uterus. Therefore, catecholamine levels are similar in pregnant and non-pregnant exercisers and have little affect on the pregnancy in general even though norepinephrine can cross the placental barrier (ref). Thus, hormonal changes due to exercise do not compromise the developing fetus. The potential direct effects of catecholamines on the fetus will be discussed later.

Other exercise hormones, insulin and glucagon, are important for maintaining cells' metabolic demands for energy. Exercise promotes increases in glucagon and decreases in insulin (Gollnick 1985). This effect causes an intensity-dependent, hyperglycemic response to supply glucose to working muscle (Clapp and Capeless 1991). During pregnancy, though, insulin levels are elevated in order to maintain glucose delivery to the developing fetus (Metcalfe 1988). When exercise is combined with pregnancy the release of insulin becomes progressively decreased as gestation continues (Clapp and Capeless 1991). As the pregnancy progresses, a women normally becomes more insulin resistant in order to shunt blood glucose to the fetus, thus leaving maternal cells to use free fatty acids for fuel (Hytten and chamberlain 1991). Eventually the response of the pregnant mother to exercise becomes hypoglycemic instead of hyperglycemic and is no longer related to intensity (Clapp and Capeless 1991). A mother's glycemic response to exercise is influenced by whether she has ingested a high-glycemic or low-glycemic carbohydrate diet (Clapp 1998). Since there are so many factors that influence maternal glucose response (frequency, intensity, time, type of exercise, glycemic load of carbohydrates, women training status, etc.) there is not a defined response for blood glucose during pregnancy and exercise. Nonetheless, there is no evidence suggesting growth restriction of the fetus when exposed to maternal exercise (Clapp and Capeless 1990, Lokey et al. 1991). This is due to increases in dietary intake of food to maintain or increase availability of substrates and precursors for fetal-placental metabolism (Weissgerber TL and Wolfe LA) Hence, there are compensatory mechanisms to maintain fetal substrates for proper growth and development.

Another area of concern relates to the known physiological effect of hyperthermia during exercise and the potential teratogenic effect on the fetus. Depending on the intensity and environmental conditions, exercise can cause an increase of 1 to 3 degrees Celsius while 1.5 to 2.5 degrees Celsius is a known teratogen in some animal models (Clapp 1988, Metcalfe et al. 1988, Rowell 1974, Rowell 1983). The concern was that similar mechanisms would lead to harm for the fetus during maternal exercise. A normal compensatory mechanism of pregnancy is a lower body temperature (Clapp 1993). This lower temperature maintains a heat gradient away from the developing fetus. Additionally, the mother has increased blood flow to the skin during exercise (Clapp 1993). These adaptations are coupled with a lower sweating threshold to improve heat dissipation (Clapp 1993). Throughout the pregnancy, increased heat from exercise will be efficiently removed from the fetus.

During exercise there can be increases in stresses on joints and other portions of the body. Little was known about the effect of these forces on the growing uterus. Furthermore, as the pregnancy progresses, the expanding uterus changes a woman's body mass distribution, center of gravity, and increases joint laxity. The two questions raised concern whether these stresses from exercise during pregnancy could jeopardize the pregnancy (i.e. rupture membranes, preterm labor, injure the fetus) and whether it increases the mother's chances of injury. However, research has found no increase in spontaneous abortions or placental abnormalities. Studies looking at various exercises, including high impact activities, have demonstrated no differences in spontaneous abortion, malformations, placental complications (i.e. placenta previa), or pregnancy induced hypertension between exercising and non-exercising mothers (Clapp 1989, Clapp 1993-ch.2). As far as maternal injury, studies have not been able to find maternal injuries associated with exercise (McNitt-Gray 1991, Karzel et al. 1991, Work 1989). Many of the initial concerns with exercise during pregnancy were found to have no merit.

Outside of the acute affects of exercise on pregnant women, question has been raised about the chronic adaptations to exercise such as: cardiovascular, biochemical, and metabolic alterations. Exercise adaptations of the cardiovascular system include increased stroke volume and cardiac output at a given heart rate, increased plasma volume, and resting venous capacitance (Clapp 1988, Hytten and Chamberlain 1980, Rowell 1974). These adaptations are beneficial during pregnancy and allow for an increased heart rate reserve during exercise and may be a reason for the attenuated decrease of exercise induced uterine blood flow (Clapp 1990). Whether these known positive changes, such as improved maternal heart and vascular function, can improve pregnancy complications such as gestational hypertension is a current area of research. Various biochemical parameters change in response to regular physical activity such as: alteration of phospholipids composition, antioxidant status, and immune responses. Exercise changes the phospholipids fatty acid composition, which allows for improved insulin sensitivity (Borkman et al. 1993). Although the exact role this plays in maternal glucose metabolism is unknown, the fetal supply of glucose is maintained (ref). None of these biochemical changes has been shown to detrimentally affect the health and well-being of the developing fetus. Lastly, question has been raised about how gross anatomical changes that result from regular maternal exercise affect the pregnancy. In general, women who exercise regularly have decreased fat deposition. A decrease in the thickness of the panniculus adiposus may seem to put the fetus at increased risk of blunt damage by removing this cushioning layer, but this is not the case. As mentioned previously, the mother adjusts her eating to maintain her body weight and the energy requirements of the pregnancy. Exercise helps mothers use insulin to shuttle glucose into cells while still maintaining the level of glucose available for the baby. In this respect, exercise does not put the fetus at increased risk for trauma from blunt damage or for energy deprivation.

Early research demonstrated that the maternal body compensates well to acute bouts of exercise. Additionally, many physiological adaptations of exercise are beneficial to the pregnant women as well. Finally after many years of research, physicians can feel confident telling patients that exercise during pregnancy is safe.

Outcomes of Pregnancy Exposed to Exercise

Various studies have looked at pregnancy outcomes from mothers who exercised during pregnancy. Some parameters which have been measured are neonatal morbidity, APGAR scores, and fetal measurements. To date, no differences have been noted in neonatal morbidity from maternal exercise (Collings et al.1983, Hall and Kaufmann 1987, Kulpa et al. 1987, Sibley et al.1981). Even if exercise training was initiated during the pregnancy there is no increase in neonatal morbidity. Another important indicator of neonatal health is the Apgar score. The APGAR test rates five components of neonatal health: Appearance (skin color), Pulse (heart rate), Grimace (reflex irritability), Activity (muscle tone), and Respiration (breathing rate). Studies have shown no differences at birth in neonates exposed to exercise versus those who were not exposed to exercise in utero.

Ob/Gyn physicians tracked common fetal measurements (head circumference, body length, birth weight, etc.) in order to determine if exercise during pregnancy affected fetal growth and development. Head circumference and crown-heel length show no variation in infants whether exposed or not to exercise (Clapp 1990). The measures that show great variation are birth weight, percent body fat, and ponderal index. The ponderal index, similar to the body mass index concept, is a way of expressing the relationship of height to body mass. Therefore the main differences of infants exposed to exercise relative to their non-exposed counterparts are their birth weight and percent body fat. In general, a woman who continues exercise throughout the duration of her pregnancy will have a lighter infant. The decreased weight of the infant is due solely to decreased body fat (Clapp 1990). However, if a pregnant mother exercises during the first and second trimesters only and discontinues her regimen in the last trimester then the birth weight is similar to non-exercise exposed infants (Clapp 1990). Again these differences in birth weight are due to the change in fat deposition. Exercise studies show that pregnant women who eat more refined carbohydrates and sugars had fatter babies relative to pregnant mothers who ate whole grains and vegetables. Additionally, if the exercise regime is maintained in the third trimester, when the energy requirements are greatest for the fetus, the baby is often born lighter as a result of decreased fat storage. While maternal glucose is used for working muscle and this glucose is also the fetuses' first source of energy, research has shown that, with a relative maintenance of blood supply, the baby's increased ability to extract glucose is maintained. The last trimester of pregnancy is the critical period for fetal fat deposition and exercise, as well as different food intake, both of which can affect the amount of fat tissue the infant has at birth. For example, Clapp et al found that if a mother maintained exercise in the third trimester, the infant had a decreased body weight at birth due to decreased fat deposition relative to other baby's not exposed to exercise. When mothers decreased or stopped exercise during the last trimester, the baby's body weight was the same or increased due to a change in fat deposition relative to same age counterparts. Other factors can affect pregnancy outcomes, such as on the frequency, intensity, time, and type of exercise, and level of training prior to pregnancy.

Based on the findings that exercising mothers tended to have lighter babies, research was done into whether leaner or fatter babies were healthier. Clapp et al (1998) has demonstrated that children exposed to exercise in utero are morphometrically similar to counterparts at one year. Parameters compared among the two groups included weight, length (height), percent body fat, head circumference, chest circumference, and abdominal circumference (Clapp et al. 1998). However, in a different population of women, Clapp found children exposed to exercise in utero were leaner at five years of age compared to their counterparts who had not been exposed to exercise in utero (Clapp et al. 1996). However, past one year of age, it is difficult to determine if the effects are from nature (in utero exercise exposure) versus nurture (raised in a health conscious household) or a product of both. While the relationship between long-term leanness and maternal exercise while pregnant is still being elucidated, research has consistently found no negative impact of exercise exposure in utero on fetal development. In light of the childhood obesity pandemic, the decreased fat deposition may be a potential benefit to the children in the future.

Maternal Benefits

During the course of the research with pregnant women, some researchers noticed that many of the healthy pregnant volunteers had fewer complaints during pregnancy, which lead to investigation of the potential benefits received by the mother from exercise during pregnancy. Common ailments of pregnancy include back discomfort, difficulty with some movements, swelling, and anxiety. Researchers found that women who exercised during pregnancy had less pregnancy related complaints relative to their counterparts. There are varying hypotheses for what accounts for this relationship. It could be that exercising mothers actually had less aches and pains of pregnancy or that they had a higher pain threshold based on their exercise. Research has not determined which hypothesis is a more accurate reflection of pregnant women's experiences. Nonetheless, it is clear that exercising women report feeling better during their pregnancy than their non-exercising peers. Concern has been raised that, with the increase in physical activity, women whom exercise during pregnancy would be more likely to fall or have some trauma to the abdomen which could seriously harm the baby. Research has shown women who exercise are less likely to fall during their pregnancy due to increased flexibility and kinesthetic awareness. Even though fewer falls and abdominal trauma occur with exercise, the American College of Obstetrics and Gynecologists (ACOG) discourages some physical activities due to increased likelihood of abdominal trauma such as skiing, soccer, and skydiving. In general, exercise is known to alleviate stress and this effect remains true also during pregnancy. In addition to reporting less anxiety, women who exercise during pregnancy are more likely to feel less pains and more "in control" of the process of pregnancy.

One aspect of pregnancy that produces anxiety, especially for first time mothers, is the unknown experience of labor and delivery. Some of the potential benefits gained from maternal exercise are seen at labor and delivery. Many mothers who exercise deliver closer to their estimated due date than non-exercisers (Clapp) which can lead to decreases in anxiety of the mothers. Additionally, maternal exercise tends to decrease the total time of labor and delivery, which is often one of the most exciting benefits of maternal exercise, at least to mothers. Maintaining muscle tone logically leads to the ability of mothers to "perform" better during the energy intensive time of delivery. The decrease in time is even more prevalent for multiparous females than first time mothers.

Placental Adaptations

Once it was determined that exercise was not a teratogen to the fetus and the maternal benefits were recognized, many physicians and researchers began to explore what other benefits may occur, such as at the placenta. The placenta is the interface between mother and fetus where oxygen, nutrients, and hormones are transferred to the fetus while waste products are eliminated from the fetus without an intermixing of fetal and maternal blood. The placenta is a unique transient organ that begins developing around day 12 after fertilization, which translates to day 24-26 of the menstrual cycle. This process often begins before the woman knows she is pregnant. Additionally, the placenta is a combination of fetal and uterine (mother's) tissues. The fetal tissue invades the maternal uterus until it encounters the maternal decidual vessels. Once these vessels are penetrated villi begin to form; these are the functional extension of the fetal portion of the placenta to increase surface area for exchange between fetus and mother. Investigation of the effects of exercise on the placental structure has resulted in several findings. First, the jarring and impact from high intensity aerobic activity was not found to have a detrimental affect on fetal growth and development or the placenta. Numerous studies have shown that exercise does not increase spontaneous abortions or placenta complications (placenta previa, PROM, pre-term labor, etc.). Second, if the mother exercises during the period of placentation, or forming of the placenta, there are an increased number of villi which means increased surface area for exchange of nutrients between fetus and mother. Therefore, the infants of exercising mothers receive increased oxygen and nutrients during exercise. This is evidenced in umbilical cord erythropoietin levels, a marker of fetal oxygenation levels, at birth.

Fetal Benefits

Measuring fetal stress

Of particular focus for researchers in this area is the benefit of maternal exercise to the fetus. Trying to determine if the fetus was stressed in any way during pregnancy proves to be challenging, at best. Some measurements used to determine fetal well-being include fetal heart rate (FHR), fetal breathing, fetal movements, and fetal activity states. The most obvious measure of fetal well-being and health is the fetal heart rate (FHR). FHR is the most common and straightforward measure and is a standard measure during pregnancy. So far, research in this area has not found a consistent link between maternal exercise and fetal heart rate. Numerous studies show exercise increases, some show a decrease, some show both affects, and others show no change. It has been hypothesized that some of these differences are due to methodology employed by the studies with FHR being measured before exercise, during exercise, or after exercise in different studies. While the most accurate picture of resting FHR should be before an exercise bout, additional factors need to be considered: time of day, time of mother's last meal, baby's gender, and fetal activity state. The process of measuring FHR during exercise is problematic considering the maternal abdomen moves during an exercise bout there is too much artifact to get accurate EKG or ultrasound recording, at least with the current technology available.

Another common measure used to determine if fetal well being has been affected by maternal exercise has been fetal breathing movements (FBM). Again, the findings are variable including increased FBM, decreased FBM, and no changes in FBM. The differences again can be attributed to different techniques used. However, a major reason for differences, only more recently being investigated, is the effect of fetal state on the previous measurements. Fetal activity states are based on activity state patterns recognized in neonates and adapted to the fetus. Often the classification into the different activity states (1F, 2F, 3F, 4F) are based on heart rate, body movement, breathing movements, and even eye movements with more activity being higher numbers. For instance, comparing fetuses in different activity states is similar to comparing one subject's resting heart rate (HR) to another subject's exercising HR. Therefore, current research regarding fetal HR, breathing, or body movements must make sure the fetuses are in the same activity state In order to draw any valid conclusions.

Post birth measurements also have been examined to determine the relationship between maternal exercise and neonatal outcomes. Some common measurements used to substantiate this claim are Apgar scores, birth weight, and body fat. No differences have been found in Apgar scores between neonates exposed to exercise in utero and those not exposed to exercise. As previously mentioned, neonates exposed to exercise during pregnancy may have lower birth weights due to decreased fat deposition, but they may be of normal weight as well depending on the maternal exercise regime in the last trimester as well as the type of carbohydrates consumed during the pregnancy.

Physiological changes to the neonate: fetal benefits

Besides the physiological adaptations that occur with the female's body, such as improved heat dissipation, increased villous surface area, and improved cardiac function (Clapp 1993, Clapp 1994, Clapp 1990), some researchers believe adaptations to exercise also take place in the growing fetus. Rodent studies demonstrate that the hearts from offspring of exercised pregnant rats have increased cardiac capillary and muscle fiber density, increased number and viability of cardiac myocytes, decreased diffusion distances, and a slower beating rate (Blake and Hazelwood 1971, Bonner et al. 1978, Parizkova 1975, Parizkova 1979). Additionally, research in humans demonstrates that fetal heart rate rises during maternal exercise suggesting maternal exercise stimulates the developing autonomic nervous system (Clapp 1990, Clapp 1985, Collings and Curet 1996, Cooper 1984, Gorski 1985, McMurray et al 1995, McMurray 1993, Parizkova 1975, Steegers 1988). Furthermore, baseline fetal heart rate during rest is lower in the fetus of an exercising mother (Clapp 1985).

The autonomic nervous system (ANS) is the primary regulator of neural homeostasis. Early in gestation, fetal HR is primarily under control of the sympathetic nervous system. (Renou, Newman et al. 1969). As the parasympathetic nervous system matures (vagal stimulation), fetal HR decreases while fetal heart rate variability (HRV) steadily increases. (Pillai and James 1990) As HR increases and decreases over time, the interval between each consecutive beat (R-R interval) varies within a few milliseconds. This beat-to-beat variability is an index of cardiac autonomic control and is a sign of proper functioning of CNS regulatory pathways that decrease vagal activity with a short time delay. HRV increases with gestational age due in part to maturation of the ANS, but also in response to changes in fetal state, increased activity and respiratory movements. (Gagnon, Campbell et al. 1987; Hirsch, Karin et al. 1995) It has been shown that inter-individual differences in HR and HRV persist from prenatal to postnatal life. (Thomas, Haslum et al. 1989; DiPietro, Costigan et al. 2000) Trends in heart rate (HR) and heart rate variability (HRV) are influenced by non-neural and neural components to meet the changing cardiovascular needs and function over time (DiPietro 2005). In adults, children, and pregnant females, the decreased HR and increased HRV are characteristic of improved vagal tone. For the fetus, similar changes represent maturation of the neural components, such as the autonomics and changes within the medulla oblongata (DiPietro 2005).

Research studies have recently investigated the model of prenatal programming (Barker 2004a, Barker 2004b, Barker 2002, Barker 1994) which focuses on the effects of intrauterine events on fetal development and the relationship to long-term outcomes (DiPietro et al. 2000, Wintour et al. 2003). Currently, this hypothesis is being tested in relation to harmful stimuli in utero and its negative consequences in the future; however, this hypothesis can apply to positive stimuli. For example, research by DiPietro et al (2000) demonstrates significant associations between maternal physiologic function, fetal heart rate and heart rate at one year. This study is the first to directly associate maternal physiology and its effect on fetal autonomic function. Increased HRV (higher vagal tone) has been associated with higher Bayley scores (DeGangi, DiPietro et al. 1991) shorter visual fixation duration, (Richards 1985) more advanced language and play, (Seuss and Bornstein 2000) and temperament (Calkins 1997; Huffman, Bryan et al. 1998) in children. With this in mind, infants born of mothers who exercised during pregnancy had less body fat, improved psychomotor scores and percentiles, and a trend toward earlier ambulation at one year follow-up compared to infants from non-exercising mothers (Clapp 1998). One study looking at five year old children from exercising mothers did better in the areas of general intelligence and oral language, and had better overall score of neurodevelopmental skills than children from non-exercising mothers (Clapp 1996). If there is a fetal programming from maternal exercise during pregnancy, then it should be readily identified by measurements of autonomic tone and reflected in lower heart rate and higher heart rate variability (DiPietro et al. 2000). To date, research is currently being done to test this hypothesis. Preliminary results suggest that after taking gender, age, and activity state into consideration, fetuses exposed to exercise in utero have a lower heart rate compared to fetuses not exposed to exercise (May et al. unpublished data). The results suggest that maternal exercise influences the development of the fetus's nervous system.

Exercise during Lactation

Since it is now known that exercise during pregnancy is not harmful and there are maternal and placental adaptations as well as potential benefits to the infant, the question has been raised about whether, without further stimulus post birth, the infant will have decreased effects similar to a detraining period of an athlete. However, the mother still has an important influence on the neonate's health via breastfeeding. Breastfeeding represents an extension of the in utero environment. Usually up to about 3 to 6 months the mother is the sole supplier of the baby's nutritional and immunological needs. Again, the question arises how the mother's exercise affects the baby who is now a neonate. Before studying what molecular concentrations within breast milk change in response to exercise, it is imperative to understand what components are normally present in milk and what factors affect their presence and concentration.

There are numerous proteins besides the major and minor whey proteins and alpha-casein and lactalbumin (Koch et al. 1991) such as: galanin, neurotensin (Chen et al. 1999), pro-gamma-melanocortin (Werner et al. 1985 sites Ekman et al. 1985), Leptin (Donnet-Hughes 2000), bombesin and bombesin-like peptides (Koch 1991, Koldovsky et al. 1989, Werner et al. 1985 sites Ekman et al. 1985), delta-sleep-inducing peptide (Koch 1991, Koldovsky et al. 1989- sites Banks, Kastin, and Coy 1983, Horne et al. 2004), motilin (DeClercq et al. 1998), and fibronectin (Fukushima et al 1994). It is known that exercise increases galanin and fibronectin levels in the mother's plasma, while other proteins decrease, For some of the proteins, there is no conclusive evidence about the effects of exercise. For elevated proteins such as galanin and fibronectin, though, it is not known if the breast milk concentration also increases or if is remains unchanged in response to the exercise. It is well established that the GI tract of neonatal mammals is permeable and therefore peptides and proteins can be transported across the intestinal epithelium (Koch et al. 1991 sites Koldovsky 1980; West 1989). How exercise affects protein levels within breast milk is unknown but an area of potentially exciting research.

Breast milk normally includes various hormones such as hypothalamic releasing factors (GHRH, GnRH, TRH), most pituitary hormones (prolactin, oxytocin, melatonin, somatostatin, TSH), thyroid hormones (T3 and T4), some steroid hormones (estrogen, progesterone, corticosteroids) and others (insulin, Calcitonin, and erythropoietin). Many hormones within breast milk are present in concentrations that exceed those in plasma (Polk 1992). Although exercise affects the concentration of these hormones in the maternal plasma, it is not known how these changes affect the concentration within the mother's milk. For example, thyroid hormone levels within the breast milk are primarily determined by maternal circulating triiodothyronine (T3) levels (Oberkotter 1989). Therefore, if maternal thyroid hormones increase, due to exercise, then there will be an increase of this hormone in the breast milk (Amarant et al1982); Koldovsky et al. 1980). Although no research on the affect of these increases to the infant has specifically been done in humans, rodent research has shown that T3 to lactating rats caused increased T3 in serum and milk of mom (Strbak 1984, Michalickova). The increased thyroid hormone in milk caused decreased iodine uptake of thyroid, deceased thyroid hormone secretion, suppressed plasma TSH, causing high plasma T4 which led to accelerated eye opening. These effects caused increased sucrase and maltase activity, and increased activity of liver enzymes (i.e. beta-glycosidases) of the rat pups (Strbak 1984). The low plasma TSH which led to high plasma T4 caused higher growth rate and accelerated overall maturation in rat pups. Since we know that the hypothalamic-pituitary-thyroid axis is mature in the newborn and is activated immediately after birth (Strbak and Michalickova 1984), the infant thyroid gland can respond as an adult thyroid to the presence or absence of hormones in milk.

Some hormones will maintain the same concentration between mother's milk and plasma. Other hormones will be diluted in the milk, and still others will be concentrated in the breast milk. Many growth factors are made de novo at the mammary gland regardless of the maternal plasma concentration of these factors (Polk 1992). It is known that insulin decreases during exercise while glucagon, epinephrine, NE, growth hormones, and cortisol increase. The concentration of growth hormone (GH), or growth related factor (GRF) in breast milk exceed plasma values by several fold. Hence, it has been found in animal research to be concentrated from blood to milk by the mammary gland and was found to reach the stomach of the pups in an intact form (Werner 1986). Purified milk extracts induced the secretion of

GH from rat pituitary cells in culture and centrally administered GRF has a stimulatory effect on food intake in rats and a stimulatory effect on digestive enzyme secretion from an exocrine pancreatic preparation. Milk GRF may be involved in regulation of GH secretion from the pituitary of the neonate (Werner et al. 1986) and therefore may benefit the growth of the neonate. Some of the growth factors known to be present in breast milk are: EGF, NGF, TGF, and MGF. Although maternal exercise may increase the presence of growth factors, this may not translate into increased concentration in the breast milk. However, it is not known how exercise affects mammary gland production of these growth factors.

It is known that milk contains cytokines and other immunomodulatory agents and living cells (Savilahti 2005). Breast milk also contains a number of nonspecific anti-infectious substances such as iron-binding lactoferrin, bacteriocide, lysozyme, and the oligosaccharide inhibiting microbial attachment to epithelial cells (Savilahti 2005). Current research has shown that a mother's moderate exercise has no effect on the concentrations of IgA, lactoferrin, or lysozyme in her milk (Lovelady et al. 2003). The affects of exercise on the immune system status of lactating mothers was also determined by measuring: complete blood cell counts, differential leukocyte counts; percentages and absolute counts of peripheral lymphocyte cells (CD3+, CD3+CD8+, CD3+CD4+, CD19+, CD56+); neutrophil killing and oxidative burst activity; and in vitro mitogenic responsiveness of lymphocytes. The exercise during lactation had no affect on immune status compared to matched sedentary lactating mothers (Lovelady et al. 2004).

Since lactation is a continuation of the female body supplying the needs of a new quickly growing infant, it is important to understand the effects of exercise on breast milk composition. The presence of biologically active peptides, hormones, growth and immune factors in milk is evident. The notion that these factors have a physiological role in the development of the newborn is strongly supported by research. However, there is still much that needs to be learned. This is an area of where more research needs to be done.

Exercise in the lactation period offers benefits to the mother as well. Of course, breastfeeding allows for bonding between mother and child as well as nutrient exchange, but breastfeeding is a selfless act by the new mother that requires physical, mental, nutritional, and energy stores focused on her new baby. Especially for first time mothers, this bonding experience is a blend of bliss and anxiety. Exercise during this period allows a new mother a sense of taking care of herself and improves recovery to pre-pregnancy weight, and helps to balance the emotions during this difficult time of transition.

Types of Physical Activities

Since women have their own preferences and dislikes, there are a variety of physical activities that they like to participate in during pregnancy. Thus far, research has been done on most of these types of physical activities ranging from aerobic to weight lifting types. In general, most types of aerobic activity are safe to perform during an uncomplicated healthy pregnancy. From low impact aerobic walking to high impact aerobic running, all of these physical activities are safe IF there are not complications or symptoms during the pregnancy. Some activities will need to be modified to keep both the mother and fetus safe. For example, instead of bicycling outside on a trail, a pregnant mother can exercise on a stationary bicycle to avoid an accident. Even weight training and abdominal exercises are acceptable during pregnancy. Again, some physical activities should be modified to keep the pregnancy safe. For example, instead of free weights for resistance, a pregnant female can use weight machines, which control the range of motion and the weights. Abdominal exercises are important since these muscles will be necessary during delivery, but after six months a pregnant mother cannot lay on her back. During pregnancy, a mother needs to do crunches either upright or at an angle rather than flat on her back, to prevent compression of the vessels. All contact types of physical activities or physical activities that have the potential for abdominal trauma are to be avoided during pregnancy, such as soccer, football, racquetball, skydiving, etc. For a complete list of acceptable activities and when to discontinue safe activities please see the American College of Obstetrics and Gynecologists (ACOG) website.

Application

What does this mean for pregnant women? If a woman was active prior to becoming pregnant then she can continue activity during the pregnancy, as long as the pregnancy progresses normally and without complications. If there are complications that arise during the pregnancy, then a woman should discuss with her OB/Gyn physician the possibility of maintaining physical activity throughout the pregnancy. If a woman was not active prior to becoming pregnant then she can still exercise during pregnancy. However, she must start out slowly and lightly and should do so under the supervision of a trained professional. Regardless, of whether a woman was active prior to pregnancy or not the exercise should be self limiting and pain free.

What does this mean for people working with pregnant women? Let the woman set her own limitations and boundaries, with reason. For the most, the pregnant mother knows what her limitations are from her exercise regime, therefore, she should know what she can and cannot do. Although, woman do like for people to dote on them during this wonderful time of their life, it is important to remember to treat her as a fully capable individual. The pregnancy does not make her incapable of doing everyday tasks; so people should treat her as they always have.

The Following Lists are Guidelines Based on ACOG Recommendations

Absolute Contraindications to Aerobic Exercise during Pregnancy (with Permission from ACOG)

- Haemodynamically significant heart disease
- Restrictive lung disease
- Incompetent cervix/cerclage
- Multiple gestation at risk for premature labour
- Persistent second or third trimester bleeding
- Placenta praevia after 26 weeks gestation
- Premature labour during the current pregnancy
- Ruptured membranes
- Pregnancy induced hypertension

Relative Contraindications to Aerobic Exercise during Pregnancy (with Permission from ACOG)

- Severe anaemia
- Unevaluated maternal cardiac arrhythmia
- Chronic bronchitis
- Poorly controlled type I diabetes
- Extreme morbid obesity
- Extreme underweight (body mass index <12)
- History of extremely sedentary lifestyle
- Intrauterine growth restriction in current pregnancy
- Poorly controlled hypertension/pre-eclampsia
- Orthopaedic limitations
- Poorly controlled seizure disorder
- Poorly controlled thyroid disease
- Heavy smoker

Warning Signs to Terminate Exercise While Pregnant

- Vaginal bleeding
- Dyspnoea before exertion
- Dizziness
- Headache
- Chest pain
- Muscle weakness
- Calf pain or swelling (need to rule out thrombophlebitis)
- Preterm labour
- Decreased fetal movement
- Amniotic fluid leakage

Women are strongly encouraged to discuss exercise during pregnancy with their Ob/Gyn physicians.

Conclusion

Myriad research studies have reiterated that exercise during pregnancy is not harmful to the fetus or its development. Additionally, this exercise has various positive adaptations for the mother, such as less weight gain. If exercise occurs early enough to influence placentation, then beneficial changes occur to increase villous surface area. The potential benefits a fetus receives from exercise exposure in utero is a growing area of research, especially as it relates to programming later in life. Although lactation represents a continuation of the in utero environment, as far as the mother supplying all of the neonate's needs, there is relatively little research looking at the affects of exercise on breast milk composition. Overall, exercise is beneficial at any age and stage of a female's life and can offer many benefits to the baby as well.

References

Bader, RAME; Rose, DFE. Hemodynamics at rest and during exercise in normal pregnancy as studies by cardiac catheterization. *J Clin Invest.*, 1955, Oct, 34(10), 1524-36.

Barker, DJP. Maternal and fetal origins of coronary heart disease. *J Royal Coll Phys London.*, 1994, 28(6), 544-551.

Barker, DJ. The developmental origins of adult disease. *J Am Coll Nutri.*, 2004a, 23 (6 Suppl): 588S-595S.

Barker, DJ. The developmental origins of well-being. *Phil Trans R Soc B Biol Sci.,* 2004b, 359, 1449 1359-1366.

Barker, DJ. Fetal Programming of coronary heart disease. *Trends Endocrinol Metab.,* 2002, 13(9), 364-368.

Blake, CA; Hazelwood, RL. Effect of pregnancy and exercise on actomyosin, nucleic acid, and glycogen content of the rat heart. *Proc Soc Exp Biol Med*, 1971, 136(2), 632-636.

Bonen, A; Campagna, PD; Gilchrist, L; Beresford, P. Substrate and hormonal responses during exercise classes at selected stages of pregnancy. *Can J Appl Physiol.*, 1995, Dec; 20(4), 440-51.

Bonner, HW; Buffington, CK; et al. Contractile activity of neonatal heart cells in culture derived from offspring of exercised pregnant rats. Eur *J Appl Physiol Occup Physiol.*, 39(1), 1-6. (1978).

Calkins, SD Cardiac vagal tone indices of temperamental reactivity and behavioral regulation in young children. *Dev Psychobiol.*, 1997 Sep; 31(2), 125-35.

Clapp, JF. A Clinical Approach to Exercise. *The Athletic Woman.*, 13(2), 443-448. (1994).

Clapp, JF. Exercise in pregnancy: Brief Clinical Review. *Fet Med Rev.,* 1990, 2, 89-101.

Clapp, JF. Exercise in pregnancy: Good, Bad, or Indifferent? *Current Obstetr Med.,* 1993, vol 2, 25-49. Mosby.

Clapp, JF 3rd. Effect of dietary carbohydrate on the glucose and insulin response to mixed caloric intake and exercise in both nonpregnant and pregnant women. *Diabetes Care.*, 1998, Aug; 21 Suppl 2:B107-12.

Clapp, JF. Fetal heart rate response to running in mid-pregnancy and late pregnancy. *Am J Ob/Gyn* 1985, 153, 251-252.

Clapp, JF 3rd. The effects of maternal exercise on fetal oxygenation and feto-placental growth. Eur *J Obstet Gynecol Reprod Biol.*, 2003, Sep 22, 110 Suppl 1, S80-5.

Clapp, JF. 3rd. The relationship between blood flow and oxygen uptake in the uterine and umbilical circulations. Am *J Obstet Gynecol.*, 1978, Oct 15, 132(4):410-3.

Clapp, JF. Maternal physiological adaptations to early human pregnancy. *Am J Obstet Gynecol,* 1988, 159, 1456-60.

Clapp, JF. 3rd. Morphometric and neurodevelopmental outcome at age five years of the offspring of women who continued to exercise regularly throughout pregnancy. *J Pediatr* 1996, 129, 856-863.

Clapp, JF. 3rd, Capeless EL The changing glycemic response to exercise during pregnancy. *Am J Obstet Gynecol.*, 1991, Dec, 165(6 Pt 1), 1678-83.

Clapp, JF; Capeless, EL. Neonatal morphometrics following endurance exercise during pregnancy: *Am J Obstet Gynecol.*, 1990, 163, 1805-1811.

Clapp, JF; 3rd, Simonian, S; Lopez, B; Appleby-Wineberg, S; Harcar-Sevcik, R. The one-year morphometric and neurodevelopmental outcome of the offspring of women who continued to exercise regularly throughout pregnancy. *Am J Obstet Gynecol.*, 1998, 178, 594-599.

Collings, CA; Curet, LB; Bullin, JP. Maternal and fetal responses to a maternal aerobic exercise program. *Am J Obstet Gynecol.*, 1983, 145, 702-707.

Cooper, KA; Hunyor, SN; Boyce, ES; O'Neill, ME; Frewin, DB. Fetal heart rate and maternal cardiovascular and catecholamine responses to dynamic exercise. *Am J Ob/Gyn* 1984, 149, 560-568.

DiPietro, JA. Neurobehavioral Assessment before Birth. *Mental retardation and Developmental Disabilities Research Reviews.*, 2005, 11, 4-13.

DiPietro, JA; Costigan, KA; Pressman, EK; et al. Antenatal origins of individual differences in heart rate. *Dev Psychogiol.*, 2000, 37, 221-228.

Gagnon, R; Campbell, K. et al. Patterns of human fetal heart rate accelerations from 26 weeks to term. *Am J Obstet Gynecol.*, 157(3), 743-8. (1987).

Gollnick, PD Metabolism of substrates: energy substrate metabolism during exercise and as modified by training. *Fed Proc.*, 1985 Feb, 44(2), 353-7.

Gorski, J. Exercise during pregnancy: maternal and fetal response: A brief review. *Med Sci Sports Exer.*, 17(4), 407-416. (1985).

Hall, DC; Kaufmann, DA. Effect of aerobic and strength conditioning on pregnancy outcomes. *Am J Obstet Gynecol.*, 1987, 157, 1199-1203.

Hart, A; Morris, N; Osborn, SB; Wright, HP. Effective uterine blood flow during exercise in normal and pre-eclamptic pregnancies. *Lancet.*, 1956 Sep 8, 271(6941), 481-4.

Hirsch, M; Karin, J. et al. Heart Rate Variability in the Fetus. *Heart Rate Variability.* M. Malik and A. Camm. New York, Futura Publishing., 1995, 517-531.

Huffman, LC Infant temperament and cardiac vagal tone: assessments at twelve weeks of age. *Child Dev.*, 1998, Jun, 69(3), 624-35.

Hytten, F; Chamberlain, G. *Clinical Physiology in Obstetrics*, 3rd ed. London, Blackwell Scientific, 1991.

Karzel, RP; Friedman, MJ. Orthopedic injuries in pregnancy, in Mittlemark RA, Wiswell RA, Drinkwater, FL (eds): *Exercise in Pregnancy, 2nd ed* Baltimore, Williams & Wilkins, 1991. 123-132.

Kulpa, PJ; White, BM; Visscher, R. Aerobic exercise in pregnancy. *Am J Obstet Gynecol.* 1987, 156, 1395-1403.

Lokey, EA; Tran, ZV; Wells, CL; et al: Effects of physical exercise on pregnancy outcomes: A meta-analytic review. *Med Sci Sports Exerc.,* 1991, 23, 1234-1239.

Lovelady, CA; Fuller, CJ; Geigerman, CM; Hunter; Kinsella, TC. Immune status of physically active women during lactation. *Med Sci Sports Exerc.,* 2004, Jun, 36(6), 1001-7.

Lovelady, CA; Hunter; Geigerman, C. Effect of exercise on immunologic factors in breast milk. *Pediatrics.,* 2003, Feb, 111(2), E148-52.

McMurray, RG; Katz, VL; Poe, MP; Hackney, AC. Maternal and fetal response to low-impact aerobic dance. *Am J Perinatol.*, 1995, 12 (4): 282-285.

McMurray, RG; Mottola, MF; Wolfe, LA; Artal, R; Millar, L; Pivarnik, JM. Recent advances in understanding maternal and fetal response to exercise. *Med Sci Sports Exer.*, 1993, 25 (12), 1305-1321.

McNitt-Gray, JL. Biomechanics related to exercise in pregnancy, , in Mittlemark RA; Wiswell RA; Drinkwater, FL (eds): *Exercise in Pregnancy, 2nd ed* Baltimore, Williams & Wilkins, 1991, 133-140.

Metcalfe, J; Stock, MK; Barron, DH. Maternal physiology during gestation. In: Knobil E; Neil J eds. *The physiology of reproduction,* New York: Raven Press., 1988, 1995-2021.

Morrow, RJ; Ritchie, JW<, Bull, SB. Fetal and maternal hemodynamic responses to exercise in pregnancy assessed by Doppler ultrasonography. *Am J Obstet Gynecol.*, 1969, 160, 138-40.

Parizkova, J. *Cardiac microstructure in female and male offspring of exercised rat mothers.* Acta Anat (Basel)., 1979, 104(4), 382-387.

Parizkova, J. Impact of daily work-load during pregnancy on the microstructure of the rat heart in male offspring. *European Journal of Applied Physiology*, 1975, 34, 323-326..

Pillai, M; James. D. The development of fetal heart rate patterns during normal pregnancy. *Obstet Gynecol,* 1990, 76(5 Pt 1), 812-6.

Renou, P; Newman, W. et al. Autonomic control of fetal heart rate. Am *J Obstet Gynecol.*, 1969, 105(6), 949-53.

Richards, JE. Respiratory sinus arrhythmia predicts heart rate and visual responses during visual attention in 14 and 20 week old infants. *Psychophysiology.*, 1985, Jan, 22(1), 101-9.

Rowell, LE. Cardiovascular aspects of human thermoregulation. *Circ Res.,* 1983, 52, 367-379.

Rowell, LE. Human cardiovascular adjustments to exercise and thermal stress. *Physiol Rev.,* 1974, 54, 75-159.

Sazontov, NV; Gambarjan, L. Exercise in pregnancy and puerperium. *Prakt Lek.*, 1952, Feb 5, 32(3), 51-5.

Seuss, PE; Bornstein, MH. Task-to-task vagal regulation: Relations with play and language in 20-month-old children. *Infancy,* 2000, 1, 303-322.

Sibley, L; Ruhling, RO; Cameron-Foster, J; Christensen, C; Bolen, T. Swimming and physical fitness during pregnancy. *J Nurse Midwif*., 1981, 26, 3-12.

Steegers, EAP; Buunk, G; Binkhorst, RA; Jongsma, HW; Wijn, PFF; Hein, PR. The influence of maternal exercise on the uteroplacental vascular bed resistance and the fetal heart rate during normal pregnancy. *Euro J Ob/Gyn Repro Bio.*, 27, 21-26. (1988).

Thomas, PW; Haslum, MN; MacGillivray, I; Golding, MJ. Does fetal heart rate predict subsequent heart rate in childhood? *Early Hum Dev.* 1989, May; 19(2), 147-52.

Von Rutte, U. Effect of exercise during pregnancy on labor. *Gynaecologia.,* 1951, Nov, 132(5), 274-6.

Weissgerber, TL; Wolfe, LA. Physiological adaptation in early human pregnancy: adaptation to balance maternal-fetal demands. *Appl Physiol Nutr Metab.*, 2006, Feb, 31(1), 1-11.

Wintour, EM; Johson, K; Koukoulas, I; Moritz, K; Tersteeg, M; Dodic, M. *Programming the Cardiovascular System, Kidney, and the Brain—a Review.* Placenta 24 (Supp. A, Trophoblast Research 17), S65-S71. 2003.

Work, JA. Is weight training safe during pregnancy? *Physician Sports Med.*, 1989, 17, 257-259.

In: Encyclopedia of Sports and Athletics
Editors: Jack L. Murray and Emily O. Watson
ISBN: 978-1-61209-959-0

Chapter IX

Biomechanics of Martial Arts and Combative Sports: A Review

Osmar Pinto Neto
Laboratory of Applied Biomechanics – Institute of Research and Development (IP&D)
University of Vale do Paraiba (UNIVAP), Sao Paulo, Brazil

Abstract

The pioneer studies on the biomechanics of martial arts were published in the nineteen sixties and seventies. After these articles were published, several other biomechanical studies have been conducted about martial arts and other related punching sports using a variety of different measures and methods, especially in the last decade. In general, these studies were concerned with the enhancement of performance and extending the understanding of injury risk. This paper presents a comprehensive review on this subject. It is divided in two major topics: the first topic covers articles about the kinetics, kinematics and electromyography of specific hand strikes, kicks, throws and fall techniques; the second topic focus on some aspects of motor behaviors and perceptual abilities fundamental for efficient and successful performances in martial arts and combative sports (i.e. repeatability of movement, reaction times).

1. Introduction

In the past 15 to 20 years the participation of athletes in martial arts and combative sports has increased dramatically (Oler et al., 1991; Pieter and Lufting, 1994). Along with the increase in participation an increase in the number of scientific papers published about martial arts and combative sports has also increased. These manuscript reviews the advancements made on the biomechanics of martial arts and combative sports.

Fights among unarmed men are probably as old as men themselves, in contrast scientific studies of fighting are very recent. The pioneer studies on this subject were published in the 1960s and 1970s. Vos and Binkhorst (1966) were fundamental to set start the scientific investigations of martial arts with their article entitled "Velocity and force of some karate arm-movements" published at "Nature". During the 1960s, other important article was published, entitled "Karate strikes", by J.D. Walker (1975) in the American Journal of Physics. Finally, in 1978 an article entitled "The physics of karate" by Feld, McNair and Wilk published in the Scientific American, would contribute largely to the popularization of the studies on the biomechanics of martial arts.

After these articles were published, several other biomechanical studies have been conducted about martial arts and other related punching sports using a variety of different measures and methods, especially in the last decade. In general, these studies were concerned with the enhancement of performance and extending the understanding of injury risk. This paper presents the first review on this subject. It is divided in two major topics: the first topic covers articles about the kinetics, kinematics and electromyography of specific hand strikes, kicks, throws and fall techniques; the second topic focus on some aspects of motor behaviors and perceptual abilities fundamental for efficient and successful performances in martial arts and combative sports (i.e. repeatability of movement, reaction times).

1.1. Different Styles of Martial Arts and Combative Sports

The articles cited in this review are based on results coming from five different modalities: Kung Fu, Karate, Taekwondo, Judo and Boxing. This section gives a brief description of these styles.

1.1.1. Kung Fu

Kung fu is a popular term that expresses Chinese martial arts in general. Colloquially, the term "kung fu" in Chinese alludes to any individual accomplishment or cultivated skill obtained by long and hard work. The origins of Kung Fu can be traced over 6,000 years ago to self-defense needs, hunting activities and military training in ancient China. From this beginning, Chinese martial arts proceeded to incorporate different philosophies and ideas into its practice expanding its purpose from self-defense to health maintenance and finally as method of self-cultivation. Through Chinese kung fu history, various warriors developed different techniques (styles) of self-defense with particular sets of movements and ideas (Despeux, 1981). Most of these styles were developed as progressions and offshoots of the styles created in two main ancient schools of martial arts in China (Reid & Croucher, 1983). These schools were located at two philosophical and religious centers, the Shaolin Temple (Buddhist) and the Wudang Mount (Taoist) (Despeux, 1981). Today there are more hundreds of Kung Fu styles. Although its popularity, the great number of styles and its ancient history, studies on the biomechanics of Kung Fu are still rare.

1.1.2. Karate

Karate is one of the most widespread martial art and combative sport; it involves primarily the use of punches, kicks and blocking techniques (Halabchi et al., 2007). There are not nearly as much styles of Karate as there is of Kung Fu; the main differences among Karate styles are in the way they compute, since their strikes, punches and kicks are similar. Due to its early wide popularity in the United States Karate was the first martial art to be investigated scientifically (Vos and Binkhorst, 1966).

Karate began as a common fighting system known as "te" among the samurai class of the Ryukyu Islands. Riukyu Islands are located west of China between Japan and Taiwan; Okinawa is its largest island. Still in its early history, two main factors furthered the development of karate in Okinawa. The first, in 1372, was the establishment of trade relationships between Okinawa and the Ming dynasty of China, which caused many forms of Chinese martial arts to be introduced to Okinawa. The second was the 'Policy of Banning Weapons,' enforced in Okinawa during the late 1400's. (Reid and Croucher, 1983)

Because of the Chinese influence, the word karate was originally a way of expressing "Chinese hand." In 1933, the Okinawan art of karate was recognized as a Japanese martial art and karate started to be written in Japanese characters now as "empty hand". (Higaonna, 1985)

1.1.3. Taekwondo

Taekwondo is a Korean martial art very popular worldwide and the national sport of South Korea. In Korean, tae means "foot"; kwon means "fist"; and do means "way". Traditional Taekwondo is typically not competition-oriented and stems from military roots. Modern Taekwondo, which is much more popular, on the other hand, tends to emphasize competition. Formally, there are two main styles of Taekwondo. Although there are doctrinal and technical differences between the two main styles and among the various organizations, the art in general emphasizes kicks. The roots of Taekwondo go back thousands of years. In 1955, a number of similar schools of martial arts were merged, and the resulting style was named Taekwondo. An important figure in this effort was Choi Hong Hi, a Korean general who worked to combine a traditional Korean foot-fighting technique called "tae kyon" with Japanese Karate. In 1966, General Choi established the International Taekwondo Federation (ITF) (Tae Kwon Do, 2008). As for Kung Fu, studies on the biomechanics of Taekwondo are also rare.

1.1.4. Judo

Judo is a modern Japanese martial art and combat sport that originated in Japan in the late nineteenth century. Unlike Kung-fu, Karate and Taekwondo there is only one style of Judo. Its most prominent feature is its competitive element, where the ultimate goal is to either throw one's opponent to the ground at his back, or immobilize or force one's opponent to quit with grappling maneuvers. Judo was developed by Jigoro Kano (1860–1938). In 1880, Kano reformed an ancient Japanese martial art called jujutsu with a new set of rules for competition and with focus on development of the body, mind and character of the practitioners. The word "judo" is formed by two characters: "ju", which means soft method and "do", which means, as in Taekwondo, way, road or path. (Group, 1977)

1.1.5. Boxing

Boxing, also known as Western boxing or pugilism, is a combat sport in which two participants, generally of similar weight, fight each other with their fists wearing padded gloves. Boxing is supervised by a referee and is typically engaged in during a series of one to three-minute rounds. Victory in boxing can be achieved in three different ways: by points at the end of the bout, given by judges' scorecards; by Knockout, when a fighter is knocked down and unable to get up before the referee counts to ten seconds; or by Technical Knockout, when a fighter is considered too injured to continue. (Group, 1977)

Boxing first appeared as a formal Olympic event in the 23rd Olympiad (688 BC), but fist-fighting contests must certainly have had their origin in mankind's prehistory. The earliest visual evidence for boxing appears in Sumerian relief carvings from the 3rd millennium BC (boxing, 2008). Modern boxing evolved in Europe, particularly Great Britain. During the early 18th century, in Great Britain, boxing was done bare-knuckle and referred to as prizefighting. The first documented account of a bare-knuckle fight in England appeared in 1681 in the London Protestant Mercury. This is also the time when the word "boxing" first came to be used (Roberts and Skutt, 1999). Pugilism is a much older word, it indicates the ancient origins of the sport in its derivation from the Latin "pugil", which mean a boxer, related to the Latin "pugnus", which means fist, and derived in turn from the Greek "pyx", which means with clenched fist (boxing, 2008).

2. Kinetics, Kinematics and Electromyography of Martial Arts and Combative Sports

Since the beginning of martial arts biomechanics research, scientists were intrigued in quantifying the forces involved in strikes performed by highly trained subjects. Recently, although still in a discrete manner, a few articles have been published trying to understand how trained subjects can achieve such performances. Along with that, there have been a few attempts to compare trained and untrained subjects' performances. These studies are important not only for the enhancement of performance but the understanding of injury risk. Recently, advancements have been made in the quantification of the forces that are exerted on the human body, when hit by a martial arts or combative sport strike during a real fight or competition. Other advancement recently made in the biomechanics of martial arts relates to the quantification of ground reaction forces during fall. Research indicates that martial arts techniques present ways to reduce forces exerted in the human body during falls. This topic covers articles about the kinetics, kinematics and electromyography of specific hand strikes, kicks, throws and fall techniques.

2.1. Biomechanics of Hand Strikes and Kicks

2.1.1. Kinetics and Kinematics

Joch et al. (1981) measured average punch impact forces of 3453 N for elite and 2932 N for intermediate boxers. Wilk et al. (1983) reported that adept karate practitioners could obtain maximum speeds values in the range of 5.7-9.8 m/s when performing straight punches, and impact forces in the range of 2400-2800 N when hitting a concrete patio block. Voigt (1989) built a dynamometer to analyze punches of 10 well trained karate students. He found peak impact force of 3334 N (2345 - 4866 N), and maximal speed of the hand before impact of 9.5 m/sec (8.2 - 10.7 m/s). Smith et al. (2000) measured average impact forces, using a sport-specific designed dynamometer, of 4800 N (SD = 601) for elite and 3722 N (SD = 375) for intermediate boxers. Gulledge (2008) compared mechanical factors in the reverse and three-inch power punches performed by twelve expert male Karate martial artists. They used a force plate to measure horizontal peak forces, and subsequently impulses. The power punch produced smaller fist velocities immediately before impact than the reverse punch, 4.09 vs. 6.43 m/s. The peak force exerted by the fist was much smaller in the power punch than in the reverse punch 790 vs. 1450N. However, they found that the linear impulse exerted by the fist during the first 0.20s of contact was slightly larger in the power punch than in the reverse punch (43.2 vs. 37.7N.s). They concluded that the power punch is less powerful than the reverse punch, but slightly more effective for throwing the opponent off balance.

The values of force shown above were not estimated considering impacts to objects comparable in mass and biofidelity to segments of the human body, thus the risk of injury cannot be reliably estimated from these forces. In an effort to better understand the relationship between forces delivered to human body and the risk of injury, a few studies have been conducted. Schwartz et al (1986) investigated the relative force of kicks and punches thrown at a dummy head, which was mounted 175 cm above the floor, their mechanism was contrived to provide constant rotational stiffness, and springs provided constant restorative moments about the three axes. They asked fourteen karate experts to punch and kick the dummy and measured accelerations ranging from 90 to 120 g. Walilko et al. (2005) submitted Olympic class boxers to perform straight punches thrown at an instrumented Hybrid III headform that simulated a human head. They calculated impact force and impact power values for seven boxers' punches and obtained an average impact force of 3427 N (SD = 811) and an average impact power of 6574 W (SD = 3453); they reported an average hand speed of 9.14 m/s (SD = 2.06). Pierce et al., (2006) obtained the first direct measurement of punch force in professional boxing matches through boxing gloves incorporating the *bestshot* System ™, a proprietary system created by SensorPad Systems, Inc. (SPS; Norristown, PA). They obtained force data across all rounds of six professional boxing matches across five different weight classes. Mean punch forces delivered ranged from 866.6 N to 1149.2 N. These measurements are considerably less than those reported above found in laboratory demonstrations, and may better reflect the actual forces exchanged in the ring. More studies should be done in order to verify if these forces do represent better the forces exchanged during actual boxing matches.

Several articles have made contribution in the attempt to understand how martial artists could obtain such values of force and power as described above, and why and how they perform different than untrained subjects. Wilk et al. (1983) suggested that the hand speed right before the impact was the primary factor contributing for the greater impact force of a karate martial artist strike compared to a non-martial artist. However, they did not verify this suggestion in their study. Walker (1975) suggested that another important variable, the effective mass of impact, could vary in different forms of karate strikes and affect the impact force; however, he did not report values of this variable.

The effective mass of impact is a measure of a body's inertial contribution to the transfer of momentum during a collision. In the case of a martial art strike, the effective mass can be seen as the mass of an imaginary rigid body that could replace the striker and with the same speed as the hand speed before the impact produce the same effect on the collision as the striker would. Blum (1977) suggested that an adept Karate practitioner achieves a "high mass" by tightening all the appropriate arm and upper body muscles at the moment of impact, but further insight into this theory was not provided.

Smith and Hamill (1986) were the first authors to investigate this suggestion. They measured the fist velocities from karate athletes of different skill levels and the relative momentum of a 33 kg punching bag. The bag momentum was greatest for the highest skilled subjects compared to the lower skilled punchers even though their respective fist velocities were approximately the same (11.03 (standard deviation (SD) 1.96) m/s for all subjects). Smith and Hamill (1986) suggested that the increase in bag momentum was due to the skilled boxer's ability to generate a greater effective mass during the impact than the lower skilled boxers. The estimated average effective mass for the highest skilled boxers was approximately 4.1 kg. Since this value is greater than the mass of the hand, the authors believed it reflected the ability of the athletes to link the mass of the arm into the punch. Voigt (1989) found the effective mass of karate punches calculated from calibrated punching dynamometer to be 1.4 kg (1.0 - 2.2 kg) and calculated from stroboscopic recordings to be 4.0 kg (2.5 - 4.5 kg). Walilko et al. (2005) reported a mean effective punch mass of 2.9 (SD 2.0) kg and a slight linear association of the effective mass with the weight of the boxer.

Neto et al. (2007c) was the first study that calculated values of effective mass from both trained and untrained subjects. In their study, the subjects were asked to strike a basketball at rest on a table five times with maximum force using a palm strike. Kung Fu athletes presented significantly higher averages of effective mass, hand speed and performance (ball speed after collision) than control group. The average effective mass for the Kung Fu group was 2.62 (SD 0.33) kg and for the control group was 1.33 (SD 0.19) kg. The average hand speed was 6.67 (SD 1.42) m/s for the Kung Fu group and 5.04 (SD 0.57) m/s for the control group. The average ball speed was 9.00 (1.89) m/s and 5.72 (SD 0.44) m/s for the Kung Fu group and control group, respectively. Comparing the values obtained for the average effective mass and hand and forearm mass estimated using regression equations, the authors found that for the control group the effective mass was statistically equivalent to the mass of the hand and forearm, while for the Kung Fu group the effective mass was significant greater than the mass of the hand and forearm. Contrary to what was found by Walilko et al. (2005), for both groups and all subjects no significant correlation was found between the values of effective mass and body mass. The authors concluded that because of the higher effective masses of the KF athletes, the KF group performance increases approximately twice as much with the increase of hand speed than the performance of the control group and that the effective mass is the main factor that distinguish a trained from a non-trained subject. Accordingly, Neto et al. (2008b) found a significant linear relationship between the values of average muscle and impact power for experienced Kung Fu Yau-Man practitioners, but not for the non-experienced participants. In other words, for the experienced participants an increase in muscle power was directly reflected in an increase in impact power, while for the non-experienced participants a higher muscle power did not necessarily corresponded to a higher impact power.

There are not as many studies on the biomechanics of kicks as there is of hand strikes. All articles reviewed are based on kicks performed by taekwondo athletes. Pieter and Pieter (1995) measured forces up to 620 N for the round kick against a water-filled bag with a built-in force sensor unit. Conkel, et al. (1988) used piezoelectric film, similar to that used to measure pressure distribution on the foot during gait, and attached it to a heavy bag to measure the impact force of front, side, back and roundhouse kicks. Impact forces of up to 470 N were recorded for the roundhouse kicks. Pieter and Pieter (1995), Conkel, et al. (1988) and Serina and Lieu (1991) have measured linear velocity of the foot immediately before impact during the execution of the round kick ranging from 14 to 16 m/s. Boey et al. (2002) reported kinematical results of turning kick performance of 4 athletes, two men and two women, in the Singapore National Taekwondo squad. Kicks speeds ranged from 11.53 to

15.04 m/s for the women and 17.12 to 22.7 m/s for the men. Pedzich et al. (2006) investigated the side-kick and spinning back kick performed by 5 competitors with mastery class of taekwondo. They reported average maximal stroke force values of 9015±2382 N (right leg) and 8294±2308 N (left leg) for the side-kick and 8569±2381 N (right leg) and 7751±2570 N (left leg) for the spinning back kick. Tsai et al. (2007) reported values of ankle speed of 9.55±1.65 m/s for the spin-whip kick performed by eight elite Taekwondo male college students.

2.1.2. Electromyography

As far as I know only three articles on the electromyography of hand strikes were published. Neto et al. (2007a) compared the electromyographic activity of the triceps brachii, biceps brachii and brachioradialis muscles during palm strikes with and without impacts. Electromyography analyses were done in the time and wavelet domains. Morlet wavelet power spectra were obtained and an original method was used to quantify statistically significant regions on the power spectra. The results both in the time and frequency domains indicated higher triceps brachii and brachioradialis muscle activity for the strikes with impacts. No significant difference was found for the biceps brachii in the two different scenarios. Neto et al. (2008a) reported a kinematical and electromyographic analysis of Kung Fu Yau-Man Palm strikes without impact. An empirical model applied to data obtained by a high-speed camera (1000 Hz) described the kinematical characteristics of the movement. Similar to Neto et al. (2007a), the authors analyzed the electromyographic patterns of the biceps brachii, brachioradialis and triceps brachii muscles during the strike in the time and frequency domains. The electromyography results showed a well developed muscle coordination of the practitioners in agreement with kinematical results. In an attempt to further understand the difference between highly trained martial arts athletes and untrained subjects, Neto et al. (2007b) evaluated the coordination between agonists and antagonists muscles of the arm in a movement of Kung Fu performed by trained and untrained subjects. The authors demonstrated, using wavelet transforms to analyze the data in the frequency domain through time, that the untrained subjects presented much higher undesired co-contractions during the strikes.

Electromyographic studies of kicks are also very rare. Sorensen et al. (1996) examined whether proximal segment deceleration during kicks is performed actively by antagonist muscles or is a passive consequence of distal segment movement, and whether distal segment acceleration is enhanced by proximal segment deceleration. Their results were based on data collected from seventeen skilled taekwondo practitioners were filmed using a high-speed camera while performing a high front kick, and electromyography recordings from five major lower extremity muscles. Their results indicated that thigh deceleration was caused by motion-dependent moments arising from lower leg motion and not by active deceleration.

Aggeloussis et al. (2007) conducted a research to study the repeatability of electromyography waveforms of major lower limb muscles during the axe kick in taekwondo. They recorded data from the rectus femoris, biceps femoris, gastrocnemius lateralis and tibialis anterior during 10 successive kicks performed to a fixed target by each participant. The electromyographic activity during the kicks presented coefficient of variation greater than 80%. The authors concluded that only ensemble averages of electromyography waveforms obtained from more than ten kicks may be considered representatives of the muscle function in this type of kicks.

2.2. Throws and Falls

To date, only a handful of studies have investigated judo from a biomechanical perspective. Harter and Bates (1985) studied the ground reaction forces associated with the harai-goshi throw. A tri-modal peak anteroposterior ground reaction forces pattern indicating a pull-push-pull effort by thrower was found during the throw. Tezuka et al. (1983) also measured the ground reaction forces of haraigoshi and found similar results.

Pucsok et al., (2001) analyzed and compared the kinetic and kinematic characteristics of the throwing technique Harai-goshi (hip throw), of novice and advanced judo competitors. Kinetic and kinematic data were collected by utilizing the Kistler Instrument Corporation Multicomponent Force Measuring Platform System and the Peak Technologies Motion Video Analysis System. This article revealed a significant difference in horizontal force application, between novice and advanced judo competitors. Numerous significant relationships among mean horizontal ground reaction force application and horizontal leg sweep velocity in was found in 19 of the 28 participants of the study. They suggested that leg sweep velocity is a function of ground reaction force application and horizontal leg sweep velocity plays a primary role in good technical execution of the Harai-goshi throw.

Imamura and Johnson (2003) recorded twenty male judo players, 10 black belts and 10 novices, executing the major outer leg reap with maximal effort. Statistical analysis found that peak angular velocity of the trunk and peak angular velocity of the ankle differed significantly from the performance of the experienced and novice participants. These differences were attributed to good upper body to upper body contact or impact, and stressed the importance of executing plantar flexion near sweep contact. Their results emphasized the importance of using the sweeping leg in a sequential kinetic link motion rather than as a single rigid segment.

Imamura et al. (2006) filmed and analyzed four black belt throwers in three dimensions using two video cameras (JVC 60 Hz) and motion analysis software. They investigated three different throwing techniques: Harai-goshi (hip throw), Seoi-nage (hand throw), and Osoto-gari (leg throw). Each throw was broken down into three main phases; balance breaking, fit-in and actual throw. Their results showed that for the Harai-goshi and Osoto-gari throws, impulse measurements were the largest within the first two phases of the movement. The Seoi-nage throw demonstrated the lowest impulse and maintained forward momentum on the body of faller throughout the entire throw.

Imamura et al. (2007) was the first article to consider the biomechanics of judo throwing out of isolated laboratory conditions. They compared the kinematics of throwing under competitive and non-competitive conditions under a real-life competitive condition and a simulated laboratory condition. Their results were based on data collected from a third degree black belt subject served as the thrower for both conditions, and two black belt participants ranked as first degree and fourth degree that served as the faller. They found that the directional velocity patterns of the peak velocity for the center of mass of the thrower and faller were similar in both conditions. They did find differences in timing and magnitude of peak center of mass directional velocity and peak angular velocity of the thrower's trunk. During competition, thrower created larger peak center of mass directional velocities onto the faller, which indicated greater throwing power. Peak velocities for thrower center of mass were larger during the noncompetitive condition since faller resistance was minimal.

As much as martial arts practitioners train to throw opponents to the ground, they must train to fall to the ground without getting hurt. For that, martial artists train specific fall techniques. For almost a decade, it has been suggested that that martial arts fall techniques can reduce hip impact forces (Sabick et al., 1999). Groen et al. (2007) quantified the role of hand impact, impact velocity, and trunk orientation in the reduction of hip impact force in martial arts techniques. In their study six experienced judokas performed sideways falls from kneeling height using three fall techniques: using the arm to break the fall, martial art rolling technique with use of the arm to break the fall, and martial art technique without use of the arm. Their results showed that the martial art technique can reduced the impact force by approximately 30%. Impact velocity was also significantly reduced in the falls done with the rolling technique. They found no significant differences between the rolling techniques using and without using the hands. The fact martial arts fall technique can contribute to the reduction of impact forces without using the arm to break the fall provided support for the incorporation of these techniques in fall prevention programs for elderly. Weerdesteyn et al. (2008) took one step further and investigated whether hip impact forces and velocities in martial arts falls would be smaller than simply using the arm to break the fall in ten young adults without any prior experience after a thirty minutes training session in sideways martial arts fall techniques. They found that martial arts falls had significantly smaller hip impact forces (17%) and velocities (7%). They concluded that training in martial arts techniques is very promising with respect to their use in interventions to prevent fall injuries.

3. Motor Behaviors and Perceptual Ability

Successful performance in martial arts and combative sports requires efficient execution of motor behavior and a high level of perceptual ability. This topic reviews articles about a couple of fundamental aspects of motor behavior and perceptual ability, repeatability of movement and reaction time.

3.1. Repeatability of Movement

The quantitative analysis of the repeatability of martial arts strikes and combative sports can help the better understanding of practitioners' motor control, as well as serve as a valuable tool for training. Ravier and Millot (1999) analyzed links between decision-making and motor control through karate techniques. In their study six karate practitioners had to perform two movements previously automatized in three experimental situations. The first was a simple situation in which the subject had no opponent and had to perform the parries (only one possibility). The second was a situation with choice, in which the subject still had no opponent and had to perform one of the parries at the trainer's request (two possibilities). In the third situation the subjects had to choose between the two movements to lock the attack of an opponent. They measured angular variations of elbow and knee joints as well as their duration were measured, using goniometry and showed a significant decrease in the precision of technical skills in the third situation compared with the simple situation.

Sforza et al. (2000) quantified the repeatability of the displacement of thirteen body landmarks of seven karate practitioners while performing two different basic karate hand strikes. Subjects were filmed with an optoelectronic computerized instrument (100 Hz) while performing 10 repetitions of straight punches and lunge punches. From the data of each subject, they calculated the average time of execution and the standard deviations of each of the three spatial coordinates x, y, z were computed for each landmark. The results showed that for all subjects, the execution of lunge punch took longer. For both punches and almost all landmarks, the largest repeatability (smallest standard deviation) was found in the vertical direction, while the smallest was found in the anteroposterior direction (direction of movement). Considering all karate practitioners, they showed that the lunge punch had a total standard deviation about 3 to 6 times larger than that measured during the performance of straight punches. In a similar study, Sforza et al. (2002) studied the repeatability of the karate front kick when performed by 13 black belt karate practitioners. The results showed that two experienced athletes presented the lower variability. The best repeatability was found in the horizontal plane, and in general for the hips and head movements.

Roosen and Pain (2007) examined the execution of a popular kicking combination during training in two level of intensity. 3D movement data were captured at 250Hz using a VICON motion analysis system from five taekwondo practitioners. They found that execution in two different intensity levels cause changes in angle data. Their data suggested that the first kick in the sequence showed the most differences in general. For all kicks, most differences are seen in the central segments. Angles related to the head and to the pelvis show most variability.

3.2. Reaction Time

In sport science, two types of perceptual abilities have been considered relevant to player's successful performance. One is primitive, basic sensory functions which are not specific to particular types of sport expertise. The other type of perceptual processing is sport-specific perceptual skills (Mori, 2002). Research on the perceptual abilities of martial artists and combative sports athletes is scarce. Layton (1993), citing one of his previous studies (Layton, 1991), reported that reaction time for hitting a punch bag in response to a sound stimulus were faster for karate black belts, although the reaction times of the advanced athletes did not differ in proportion to their grades. Kim and Petrakis (1998) the administered Identical Pictures Test, a time-constrained multiple-item test of perceptual judgments, to 50 male and 45 female volunteer karate practitioners who were classified by skill and belt-rank into three groups. Their results showed that black belts and the women had faster visual-perceptual speed.

Lee et al., (1999) reported that the reaction time to perform a ballistic finger extension movement in was significantly shorter in kendo (143 +/- 12 ms) and karate (146 +/- 11 ms) athletes compared to sedentary subjects (176 +/- 12 ms). They suggested that the RT is shortened through motor learning in the kendo and karate athletes who trained for momentary movements. Williams and Elliott (1999) have used more realistic stimuli and tasks to examine expertise anticipation of karate athletes, which is one important aspect of perceptual skill. In their study, the stimuli were dynamic film displays of karate athletes performing offensive attacks against the viewer. The film was presented on a large screen to give a real-size view of the performing athletes. The participant's task was a choice reaction time task, where the participants had to respond differently, as soon and accurately as possible, to the attacking positions. In this scenario, anticipating the attacking position from an early part of the video sequence would lead to faster reaction times and/or higher accuracy. The results showed that expert karate athletes were no faster but more accurate than the novices. In a similar study Mori et al. (2002) investigated simple reaction times, choice reaction times and anticipation of karate athletes. Their results showed significant differences between the karate athletes and the novices in the choice reaction time task, but not in the simple reaction time. O'Donovan et al. (2006) examined simple reaction times, choice reaction times and movement times of thirteen Taekwondo and Kung Fu practitioners and a control group. The experiment consisted of the subjects releasing an initiation button and depressing a stop button 25 cm away. Results indicated that during the simple and choice reaction time tasks the martial artists were no quicker in lifting their hand off a button in response to a sound stimulus, but were significantly faster in moving to press another button. Fontani et al. (2006) examined 18 karate practitioners, 9 of High Experience and 9 of Low Experience and showed that experience Karate practitioners reacted faster than those of low experience on the simple RT test (204 vs. 237 ms, $p< .01$).

Perez (2006) presented an extensive study on reaction time of karate athletes. In his study, 169 adults practitioners of karate, and 32 non-practitioners performed a choice reaction time test created using a computer software called SuperLab Pro version 2.0 (Cedrus Corporation, USA). Reaction time task consisted on pushing a button of a computer keyboard as quickly as possible, when a black square appeared on the screen. The black square could be in four different positions, and the subject had to press a different key according with the position. Each subject performed the test one hundred times and the authors calculated their efficiency in the task considering the reaction time and the number of mistakes made. They also collected personal and sport data using a questionnaire, tapping test in 10, 20 and 30 seconds data and hand grip strength data. Comparisons were made considering the subjects' competition specialty (fighting or forms), sport rank (regional, national without medal, national with medal and international) and sex. No significant differences were found in any of the comparisons. They also found that karate athletes were no different than the general population in the choice reaction time task. They found that reaction time was correlated to tapping and hand grip strength. They also found differences in reaction time depending on gender, concluding that men were faster than women.

4. Final Remark

This manuscript has presented a comprehensive review on the biomechanics of martial arts and combative sports. It has described the advancements made in this area, especially in the topics of kinetics, kinematics, electromyography and perceptual and motor skills. Most of the studies available in the literature are related to hand strikes, kicks, throws and fall techniques from five different modalities: Kung Fu, Karate, Taekwondo, Judo and Boxing.

References

Aggeloussis, N., Vassilis, G., Sertsou, M., Giannakou, E. & Mavromatis, G. (2007). Repeatability of electromyographic waveforms during the Naeryo Chagi in taekwondo. *Journal of Sports Science and Medicine, 6(CSSI-2),* 6-9.

Blum, H. (1977). Physics and the art of kicking and punching. *American Journal of Physics, 45*, 61-64.

Boey, L. W. & Xie, W. (2002). Experimental investigation of turning kick performance of Singapore national Taekwondo players. *Proceeding of ISBS*, Caceres–Spain, 302-305.

boxing. (2008). In *Encyclopaedia Britannica*, 2008/12/12, Available from: Encyclopædia Britannica Online: http://www.britannica.com/EBchecked/topic/76377/boxing

Chow, D. & Spangler, R. (1982). *Kung Fu, History, Philosophy and Technique.* North Hollywood, CA: Unique Publications.

Conkel, B. S., Braucht, J., Wilson, W., Pieter, W., Taaffe, D. & Fleck, S.J. (1988). Isokinetic torque, kick velocity and force in taekwondo. *Medicine and Science in Sports and Exercise, 20(2),* S5.

Despeux, C. (1981). *Tai-Chi Chuan: Arte Marcial Técnica de Longa Vida* (5th edition). São Paulo, SP: Círculo do Livro S.A. (in Portuguese).

Feld, M. S., McNair, R. E. & Wilk, S. R. (1979). The physics of karate. *Scientific American, 240(4),* 150-158.

Fontani, G., Lodi, L., Felici, A., Migliorini, S. & Corradeschi, F. (2006). Attention in athletes of high and low experience engaged in different open skill sports. *Perceptual & Motor Skills. 102(3),* 791-805.

Groen, B. E., Weerdesteyn, V. & Duysensa, J. (2007). Martial arts fall techniques decrease the impact forces at the hip during sideways falling. *Journal of Biomechanics, 40,* 458-462.

Group, D. (1977). *Enjoying Combat Sports.* (1st edition) New York, NY, Paddington Press.

Gulledge, J. K. & Dapena, J. (2008). A comparison of the reverse and power punches in oriental martial arts more options. *Journal of Sports Sciences, 26(2),* 189-196

Halabchi, F., Ziaee, V. & Lotfian, S. Injury profile in women Shotokan Karate Championships in Iran (2004-2005) (2007). *Journal of Sports Science and Medicine 6(CSSI-2),* 52-57.

Harter, R. A. & Bates, B. T. (1985). Kinematic and temporal characteristics of selected judo hip throws. *Proceedings of ISBS*, Del Mar, CA, 141-150.

Higaonna, M. (1985). *Traditional Karatedo-1 Fundamental Techniques.* Tokyo: Minato Research and Publishing Co. Ltd.

Imamura. R. & Johnson, B. (2003). A kinematic analysis of a judo leg sweep: major outer leg reap-osoto-gari. *Sports Biomechanics, 2(2),* 191-201.

Imamura, R. T., Hreljac, A., Escamilla, R. F. & Edwards, W. B. (2006). A three-dimensional analysis of the center of mass for three different judo throwing techniques. *Journal of Sports Science and Medicine, 5* (CSSI), 122-131.

Imamura, R. T., Iteya, M., Hreljac, A. & Escamilla, R. F. (2007). A kinematic comparison of the judo throw Harai-goshi during competitive and non-competitive conditions. *Journal of Sports Science and Medicine.*, *6*(CSSI-2), 15-22.

Joch, W., Fritche, P. & Krause, I. (1981). Biomechanical analysis of boxing. In K. Morecki, K. Fidelius, K. Kdzior & A. Wit (Eds.), *Biomechanics VII-A* (343-349). Baltimore, MD: University Park Press.

Kim, H. S. & Petrakis, E. (1998). Visuoperceptual speed of karate practitioners at three levels of skill. *Perceptual & Motor Skills, 87(1),* 96-98.

Layton, C. (1991). How fast are the punches and kicks of traditional Shotokan karateka? *Traditional Karate, 4,* 29-31.

Layton, C. (1993). Reaction time + movement-time and sidedness in Shotokan karate students. *Perceptual & Motor Skills, 76,* 765-766.

Lee, J. B., Matsumoto, T., Othman, T., Yamauchi, M., Taimura, A., Kaneda, E., Ohwatari, N. & Kosaka, M. (1999). Coactivation of the flexor muscles as a synergist with the extensors during ballistic finger extension movement in trained kendo and karate athletes. *International Journal of Sports Medicine 20,* 7-11.

Mori, S., Ohtani, Y. & Imanaka, K. (2002). Reaction times and anticipatory skills of karate athletes. *Human Movement Science* 21, 213-230.

Neto, O. P., Magini, M. & Pacheco, M. T. T. (2007a). Electromyographic study of a sequence of Yau-Man Kung Fu palm strikes with and without impact. *Journal of Sports Science and Medicine, 6, 23-27.*

Neto, O.P., Magini, M., Marzullo, A. C. M. & Pacheco, M. T. T. (2007b). Estudo Eletromiográfico da coordenação entre músculos agonistas e antagonistas do braço durante um golpe de Kung Fu Yau-Man. *Terapia Manual, 4,* 303-306. (In Portuguese)

Neto, O. P., Magini, M. & Saba, M. M. F. (2007c). The role of effective mass and hand speed in the performance of kung fu athletes compared to non-practitioners. *Journal of Applied Biomechanics, 23,* 139-148.

Neto, O. P. & Magini, M. (2008a). Electromyography and kinematic characteristics of Kung Fu Yau-Man palm strike. *Journal of Electromyography and Kinesiology, 18,* 1047-1052.

Neto, O. P., Magini, M., Saba, M. M. F. & Pacheco, M. T. T. (2008b). Comparison of Force, Power, and Striking Efficiency for a Kung Fu Strike Performed by Novice and Experienced Practitioners: Preliminary Analysis. *Perceptual and Motor Skills, 106,* 188-196.

O'Donovan, O., Cheung, J., Catley, M., McGregor, A. H. & Strutton, P. H. (2006). An investigation of leg and trunk strength and reaction times of hard-style martial arts practitioners. *Journal of Sports Science and Medicine, CSSI,* 5-12.

Oler, M., Tomson, W., Pepe, H., Yoon, D., Branoff, R. & Branch, J. (1991) Morbidity and mortality in the martial arts: a warning. *The Journal of Trauma, 31,* 251-253.

Pedzich, W., Mastalerz, A. & Urbanik, C. (2006). The comparison of the dynamics of selected leg strokes in taekwondo WTF. *ACTA of Bioengineering and Biomechanics, 8,* 63-81.

Pérez, O. M. Q. (2003). El tiempo de reacción visual en el Karate. PhD. thesis -Universidad Politécnica de Madrid. (In Spanish).

Pierce, J. D. Jr., Reinbold, K. A. Lyngard, B. C., Goldman, R. J. & Pastore, C. M. (2006). Direct Measurement of Punch Force During Six Professional Boxing Matches, *Journal of Quantitative Analysis in Sports* [http://www.bepress.com/jqas/vol2/iss2/3] 2(2).

Pieter, F. & Pieter, W. (1995). Speed and force in selected taekwondo techniques. *Biology of Sport, 12(4),* 257-266.

Pieter, W. & Lufting, R. (1994). Injuries at the 1991 taekwondo world championships. *Journal of Sports Traumatology and Related Research, 16,* 49-57.

Pucsok, J. M., Nelson, K. & Ng E. D. (2001). A kinetic and kinematic analysis of the Harai-goshi judo technique. *ACTA Physiologica Hungarica, 88 (3-4),* 271-280.

Rasch, P. J. & Pierson, W. R. (1963). Reaction and movement time of experienced karateka. *The Research Quarterly, 34*, 242-243.

Ravier, G. & Millot, J. L. (1999). Etude des ajustements moteurs mis en oeuvredans des situations d'apprentissage (kihon) et appliqués en karate. *Science & Sports*, *14*, 130-136 (in French).

Reid, H. & Croucher, M. (1983). *The way of the warrior: the paradox of the martial arts.* (2nd edition) London: Century Pub.

Roberts, J. B. & Skutt, A. G. (2002). *The Boxing Register (3rd edition)* Ithaca, NY McBooks Press.

Roosen, A. & Pain, M. T. G. (2007). Kinematic changes in the reproduction of a taekwondo kicking combination. *Journal of Biomechanics, 40*, 455-455.

Sabick, M. B., Hay, J. G., Goel, V. K. & Banks, S. A. (1999). Active responses decrease impact forces at the hip and shoulder in falls to the side. *Journal of Biomechanics*., *32,* 993-998.

Schwartz, M. L., Hudson, A. R., Fernie, G. R., Hayashi, K. & Coleclough, A. A. (1986).Biomechanical study of full-contact karate contrasted with boxing. *Journal of Neurosurgery, 64(2),* 248-252.

Serina, E. R. & Lieu, D. K. (1992). Thoracic injury potential of basic competition taekwondo kicks. *Journal of Biomechanics, 25(10),* 1247-8.

Sforza, C., Turci, M., Grassi, G., Fragnito, N., Pizzini, G. & Ferrario, V. F. (2000). The repeatability of choku-tsuki and oi-tsuki in traditional Shotokan karate: a morphological three-dimensional analysis. *Perceptual & Motor Skills, 90(3 Pt 1),* 947-60.

Sforza, C., Turci, M., Grassi, G. P., Shiray, Y. F., Pizzini, G. & Ferrario, V. F. (2002). Repeteability of Mae-Geri_Keage in tradiotional Karate: A three-dimensional analysis with black-belt karateka. *Perceptual & Motor Skills, 95,* 433-444.

Smith, M. S., Dyson, R. J., Hale, T. & Janaway, L. (2000). Development of a boxing dynamometer and its punch force discrimination efficacy. *Journal of Sports Sciences, 18*, 445-450.

Smith, P. K. & Hamill, J. (1986). The effect of punching glove type and skill level on momentum transfer. *Journal of Human Movement Studies*., *112,* 153-161.

Sorensen, H., Zacho, M., Simonsen, E., Dyhre-Poulsen, P. & Klausen, K. (1996). Dynamics of the martial arts high front kick. *Journal of Sports Sciences, 14*, 483-495.

Tae Kwon Do. (2008). In *Microsoft Encarta Online Encyclopedia*, 2008/12/12, Available from: http://encarta.msn.com/encyclopedia_761585873/Tae_Kwon_Do.html.

Takahashi, R. (1992). The application of biomechanics to judo technique "OKURI-ASHI-BARAI" (Sweeping Ankle Throw). *Sports coach, 15*, 30-33.

Tezuka, M., Funk, S., Purcell, M. & Adrian, M. (1983). Kinetic Analysis of judo technique. In: *Biomechanics, VIII-B*. Eds: Matsui, H. & Kobayashi, K. Champaign, IL: *Human Kinetics*. 869-875.

Voigt, M. (1989). A telescoping effect of the human hand and forearm during high energy impacts t. *Journal of Biomechanics, 22(10),* 1065.

Vos, J. A. & Binkhorst, R. A. (1966). Velocity and force of some Karate arm-movements. *Nature, 211*, 89-90.

Walilko, T. J., Viano, D. C. & Bir, C. A. (2005). Biomechanics of the head for Olympic boxer punches to the face. *British Journal of Sports Medicine*., *39,* 710-719.

Walker, J. D. (1975). Karate Strikes. *American Journal of Physics*., *43*, 845-849.

Weerdesteyn, V., Groen, B. E., Van Swigchem, R. & Duysens, J. (2008). Martial arts fall techniques reduce hip impact forces in naïve subjects after a brief period of training. *Journal of Electromyography and Kinesiology., 18,* 235-242.

Wilk, S. R., McNair, R. E. & Feld, M. S. (1983). The Physics of Karate. *American Journal of Physics., 51,* 783-790.

Williams, A. M. & Elliott, D. (1999). Anxiety, expertise, and visual search strategy in karate. *Journal of Sport & Exercise Psychology., 21,* 362-375.

Reviewed by Prof. Marcio Magini, PhD. Laboratory of Applied Mathematics - Institute of Research and Development, University of Vale do Paraiba, Sao Paulo - Brazil

In: Encyclopedia of Sports and Athletics
Editors: Jack L. Murray and Emily O. Watson
ISBN: 978-1-61209-959-0

Chapter X

Assessment of Cyclic Sports Performance

Ricardo Fernandes**, *Eduardo Oliveira and Paulo Colaço
Faculty of Sport, CIFI^{2}D, University of Porto, Portugal

Abstract

Training control and evaluation of athletes is, nowadays, seen as a fundamental tool to increase the efficiency of the training process. Thus, coaches and their collaborators often implement a set of tasks that allow evaluating the level of development of the athletes' performance determinant factors as well as the result and adequacy of the training exercises and programs.

Sport modalities like running, swimming, cycling and rowing, due to their characteristics (individual, cyclic, closed and combined modalities) are more easily measurable. From the several determinants of the specific performance of these athletes, the bioenergetical and biomechanical factors seem to be the most important and, consequently, the most studied.

The purpose of the present chapter is to present recent data obtained in protocols implemented in cyclic sports, giving more emphasis in running and swimming. The bioenergetical studies presented focus on the characterization of the capacity and power of the two larger body energy systems (the aerobic and the anaerobic ones) through the assessment of well-known physiological parameters like the anaerobic threshold, the maximal oxygen uptake (and the corresponding velocities) and the maximal blood lactate concentrations. Complementarily, recently proposed tests are also presented (e.g. critical velocity).

We hope that the presented protocols could be well accepted and applied by athletes, coaches and scientists in their training control programs, helping them to increase the training efficiency and even contributing to predict performance.

Keywords: Training control, athletes evaluation, advice, physiology

* Corresponding author: Email: ricfer@fade.up.pt

1. Conceptualization

Some of the main tasks of coaches and sport scientists are the training control and evaluation of athletes, which are seen as fundamental tools to increase the efficiency of the training process and to predict performance. By training control and evaluation of athletes is considered a set of tasks that allow the evaluation of the results and adequacy of the training exercises and programs as well as the level of development of the athletes' performance determinant factors.

Sport modalities like running, swimming, cycling and rowing, being individual, continuous, cyclic, closed and combined modalities, are more easily measurable than collective sports. Running and swimming have been along the years the primary areas of research in Sport Sciences, being published technical and scientific experimental studies since the 1930s (Billat, 1998). Scientific studies of rowing and cycling have more constantly appeared since the 1970s. Due to the high influence of external factors (e.g. wind, water conditions and temperature) that may influence the rowing and cycling tests results when conducted in normal competition conditions, experimental protocols have been conducted manly in laboratory conditions (Lucía et al., 2001; Maestu et al., 2005).

Since the enhancing of athletes' performance can no longer be obtained only by the increasing of training volume and by the use of non specific methodologies (Olbrecht, 2000) more objective and specific training sets are required to improve the quality of the training process. Therefore, the importance of the knowledge on performance determinant factors, performance diagnosis methods, and training control and evaluation, is rising in the last two decades.

Following Cazorla (1984), the main aim of the specialists in sports testing is to develop, for each athlete (independently of age or proficiency level), methods to assess his/her motor capacities in order to better understand and develop his/her motor background. Moreover, sports testing should be divided in two complementary activities - the control of training loads and the evaluation of the athletes' evolution - keeping in mind that these two items only have meaning when related to each other.

There are several reasons why sport testing is vital for increasing athletes' performance (Pyke, 2000): (i) it establish the individual's strengths and weaknesses; (ii) it allows to monitor progress, controlling the effectiveness of the prescribed training program; (iii) it permits to provide feedback of specific test scores, being an incentive for an athlete to improve in a particular area; (iv) it can educate coaches and athletes by providing them with a better understanding of the demands of the sport and the attributes required to be successful; (v) it allows prediction of the performance potential through the identification of individuals more suitable for a specific sport modality. We include the illness, injury and overtraining prevention in the period leading up to the competition, which is often seen as a fundamental aspect of the training process.

The first task to accomplish when constructing a testing program is to analyze the sport modality and define which are its performance influencing factors (Cazorla, 1984). Figure 1 illustrates a number of requirements for competitive running, swimming, cycling and rowing. As it is possible to observe, bioenergetical, biomechanical and psychological factors assume a direct influence and genetic and contextual factors an indirect influence in athletes' performance. The fact that this diagram is referring to individual, cyclic and closed sport modalities somehow reduces the number of variables to consider and therefore the internal variability spectrum. Complementarily, it is important to notice that each group of parameters is closed related with the others, having a strong reciprocal influence.

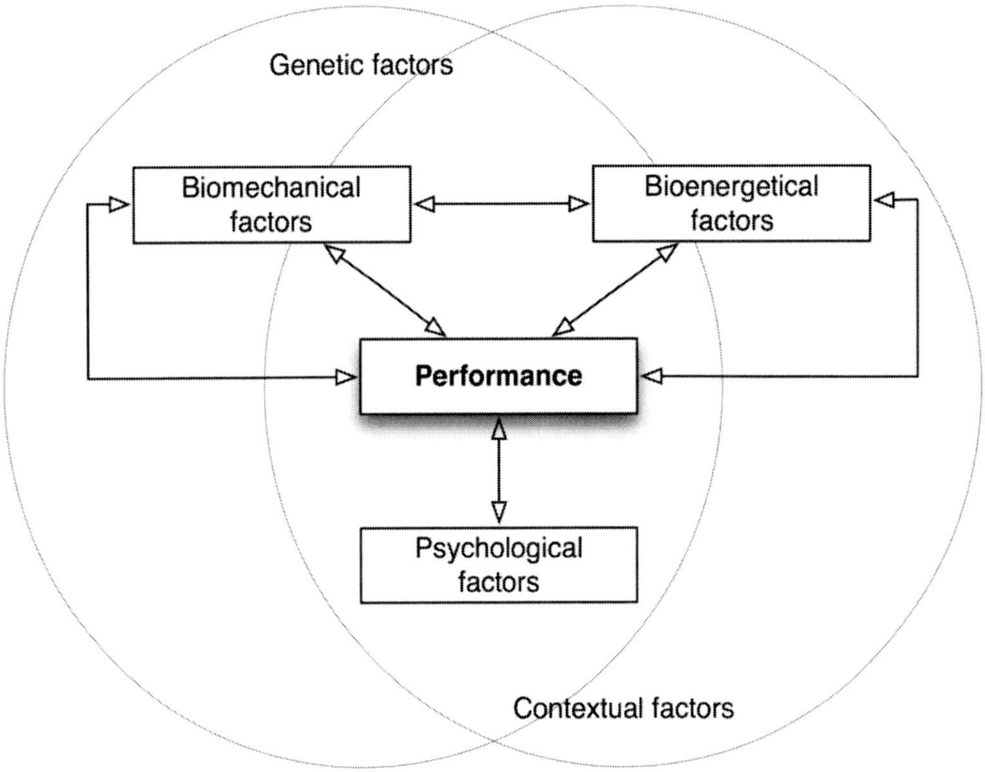

Figure 1. Determinant performance factors in cyclic sports (adapted from Fernandes et al., 2008a).

From the several performance determinants presented in Figure 1, although no attempt was made to quantify the importance of each factor, it seems logical that bioenergetical parameters are among the principal determinants. To evaluate the above-referred parameters there are a number of criteria that need to be considered, namely that the fact that tests should be relevant (for the athlete's sport), specific (simulating the competition conditions), practical (concerning the location and the availability of subjects), valid (measuring what it claims to measure) and accurate (when compared to a criterion method).

Considering that running, swimming, cycling and rowing are modalities in which bioenergetical factors assume a fundamental performance influencing role, the main propose of the present chapter is to present recent data obtained in experimental protocols. It is expected that it could be well accepted and applied by coaches and scientists in their training control programs, helping them to increase the training efficiency and even to explain future performance. In the following sections it will be presented some studies more centered in running and swimming sport modalities, focusing in the characterization of the capacity and power of the aerobic and the anaerobic energy systems through the assessment of well known physiological parameters. In a future paper, some biomechanical studies will be also shown, centering the attention on movement analysis through bi/three-dimensional kinematics, electromyography and dynamometry.

2. Bioenergetical Studies

2.1. Introduction

Nowadays, being the bioenegetical factors some of the most important and consequently frequently studied, its main purpose is to determine the athlete's bioenergetical profile and to observe the corresponding physiological changes due to the training process. Inclusively, it is well accepted that the increasing development of a series of bioenergetical tests is due in some part to the great interest in the correct establishment of training volumes and intensities and in the selection of the ideal work/rest ratios (Troup, 1995). Thus, it will be shown some valid and well accepted tests conducted by our group that allow coaches and scientists to dispose objective and pertinent data related to the aerobic and anaerobic body energy systems. Due to the characteristics of the majority of the events in running, swimming, cycling and rowing, the energetic contribution of high-energy phosphates was considered less important and therefore was not evaluated.

2.2. Aerobic System

Our studies have been supported in the proposals of Mader et al. (1976) and Heck et al. (1985), namely when we estimate the maximal lactate steady-state (Maxlass), trying to achieve an objective indicator to be used in the training field. However, the Maxlass concept is dificult to operate in the training process due to the high number of sessions needed to assess it. In this sense, to determine the correct training intensities in order to develop the aerobic capacity, the anaerobic threshold (AnT) seems to be an accurately way to achieve the Maxlass (Heck et al., 1985; Jones and Doust, 1998). A widely known procedure to assess AnT is to use the blood lactate concentration ([La^-]) values specific of an exercise intensity corresponding to a balance between its production and removal (Heck et al., 1985; Svedhal & MacIntosh, 2003).

The AnT can be determined using several protocols (cf. Svedhal & MacIntosh, 2003). Bearing in mind some specific limitations such as the athlete's age (Santos e Ascenção, 1999), accumulated training and training characteristics (Esteve-Lanao et al., 2005), we have been using the step test (Heck et al., 1985) to assess the running velocity corresponding to 4 mmol/l of [La^-] (v4), a well-accepted valid indicator of AnT. This test is composed by 4 x 2000 m (velocity of 4.2-5.8 m/s according with the athlete's level), increments of 0.4 m/s between each step and 1 min of interval (used to capillary blood collection). Our experience with the use of AnT has been very useful considering the feedbacks reported by coaches and athletes during the training advice. One of the most relevant results obtained was the high correlation values between AnT and performance for different running events (Table 1).

The results from this table suggest that the AnT can be a valid performance predictor particularly in long distances, which is in accordance with several authors (e.g. Roecker et al.,

1998; Papadopoulos et al., 2003). The data obtained also confirm that the determination of AnT can be extremely useful even in middle distances, following the proposals of Duffield et al. (2005) and Spencer & Gastin (2001), respectively for the 800 m and 1500 m events. This fact is more relevant when velocity at AnT is similar to the velocity obtained in competition, as it happens in Half Marathon runners (Figure 2).

Table 1. Correlation values obtained between different middle and long distance running events and anaerobic threshold (adapted from Colaço, 2007)

Event (m)	Subjects (gender/age in years)	Velocity (m/s)	Correlation ($p < 0.05$)
800	12 males (18.6±0.5)	6.76±0.20	r=0.77
1500	20 males (25.9±2.5)	6.32±0.25	r=0.87
5000	20 males (29.0±4.5)	5.79±0.44	r=0.89
Half Marathon (21097)	20 males (28.6±3.7)	5.17±0.46	r=0.95

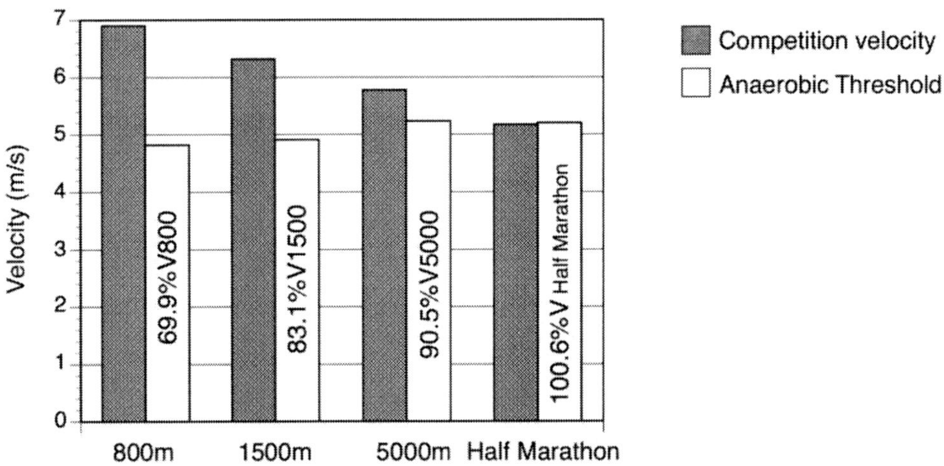

Figure 2. Percentage of v4 values relatively to competition velocity for each middle and long distance event (n = 80; 20 athletes/event). Adapted from Colaço (2007).

In swimming, due to the mechanical constraints imposed by the aquatic environment, it is common to assess AnT through simple non-invasive tests. From those, we would like to stand out the 30 min continuous test - T30 (Olbrecht et al., 1985) and the critical velocity test (Wakayoshi et al., 1992), which are valid and well accepted by coaches and scientists. Fernandes and Vilas-Boas (1999) observed high relationships between T30 and v4 ($r = 0.86$, $p < 0.01$), as well as between critical velocity and v4 ($r = 0.82$, $p < 0.01$), being v4 assessed by Mader's two-speed test (Mader et al., 1976). Other works of our group highlighted the relevance of the critical velocity test to training control and evaluation of swimmers of several ages, being easily conducted in a training session (cf. Vilas-Boas et al., 1997; Fernandes et al., 2000; Soares et al., 2003). Examples of critical velocities in age-group to senior swimmers are given in Table 2 (all values were different between genders).

However, when it is required a more "physiological" approach of the AnT phenomena, swimming coaches and scientists conduct a 7 x 200 m intermittent incremental protocol (Pyne et al., 2000; Cardoso et al., 2003), in which it is possible to identify the moment from which the rising of [La$^-$] starts to be non-linear (Figure 3). This methodology allows us to dispose higher number of [La$^-$]/velocity points which help us to better determine the [La$^-$] correspondent to the AnT. Thus, we obtain a better individualization of the AnT (IndAnT) value when comparing to the Mader's two-speed test.

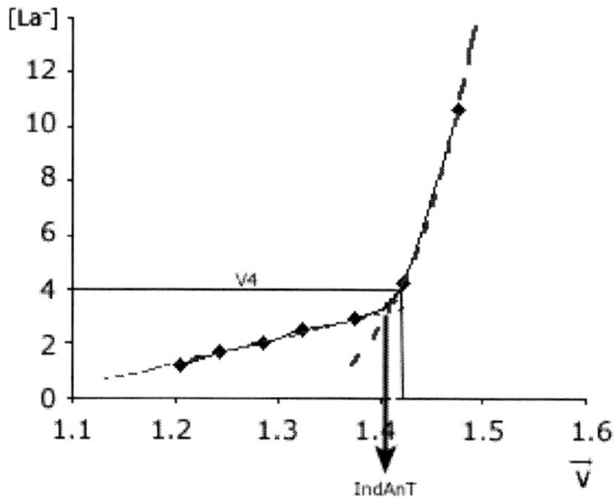

Figure 3. Individual blood lactate concentrations/velocity curve in the incremental test for VO_2max determination. Individual AnT (IndAnT) assessment is represented by the interception of a rectilinear and an exponential line (v4 is also marked). Adapted from Fernandes et al. (2005).

In this figure, it can be observed that the individual [La$^-$] values corresponding to AnT is approximately 3 mmol/l, lower than the 4 mmol/l value traditionally used. As observed in Santos and Ascensão (1999), in running, this individual value might also achieve higher values than 4 mmol/l. This reality seems to be explained by the high inter-subject variability of the [La$^-$] corresponding to AnT in swimming (Urhausen et al., 1993), as well as by the fact that the [La$^-$] values corresponding to AnT being specific for every sport (Beneke and Duvillard, 1996). Other studies of our group corroborate the example of Figure 3, referring a mean value of 2.99 ± 0.80 mmol/l (Morais et al., 2006) and 2.59 ± 0.97 mmol/l (Fernandes et al., 2008b) for the [La$^-$] at AnT.

The blood lactate concentration of 4 mmol/l is also a common reference in rowing, being described that the oxygen consumption, power (W) and velocity at that [La$^-$] is closely related to the 2000 m ergometer performance time (Ingham et al., 2002; Womack et al., 1996). However, Beneke (1995) and Jurimae et al. (2001) found values lower than 4 mmol/l for AnT: 3.0 ± 0.6 and 3.7 ± 0.6, respectively. Complementarily, Boiirgois and Vrijens (1998), stated that using fixed or individual lactate threshold values measured on a rowing ergometer as guidelines for training intensity must be viewed with caution because they do not exactly mirror the blood lactate at steady-state for rowers, which emerge the necessity of higher specificity of testing protocols.

Being cycling a long-duration and high intensity sport, it requires participants to possess high AnT (Lucía et al., 2001). Regarding the metabolic methods that can be used to determine the AnT, some authors chosen protocols (4 min increments) to determine the exercise intensity eliciting a blood level of 4 mmol/L (Padilla et al., 1999) or the IndAnT (Fernández-García et al., 2000). Our group has some experience in determining AnT in professional cyclists, namely by conducting an open road intermittent incremental protocol (4 steps of 5 min, with increments of 1.39 m/s) to assess the AnT. In Table 3 it is possible to observe the mean and SD values for the heart rate and [La$^-$] for each step of the protocol (n = 14). The mean and SD value for the v4 was 11.32 ± 1.05 m/s.

The [La$^-$]/velocity values referred in the above paragraphs also allow to monitor the exercise increase after the AnT intensity. Data show that, for intensities above the AnT, the increase [La$^-$] rate can be exponential, changing the former linear raising. This fact is more evident in middle distance efforts, in which the exercise intensity is higher. As we can see in Figure 4, the increase [La$^-$] rate is individualized, being different between athletes. This phenomena needs to be regarded as an important factor to be considered (and improved) during the practice. In this sense, the athlete needs a well developed AnT, but also a lower increase [La$^-$] rate for higher exercise intensities.

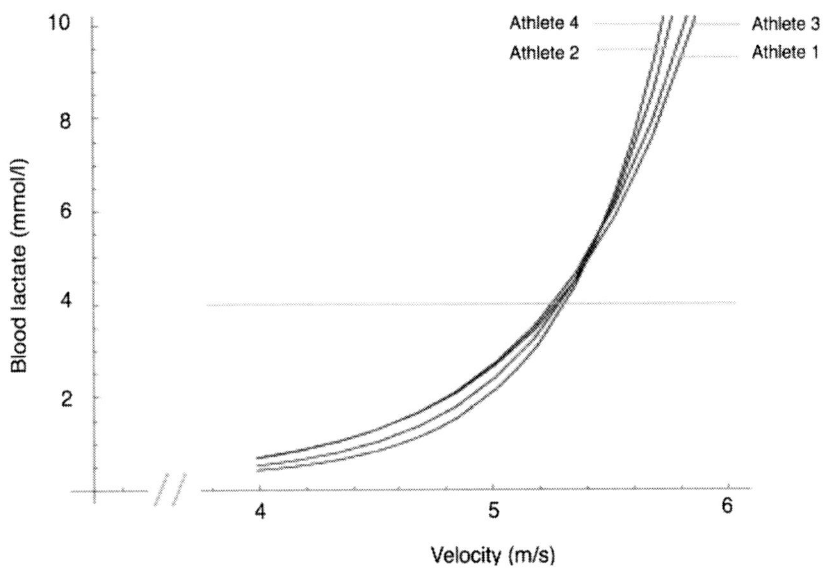

Figure 4. Increase of blood lactate concentration rate in four runners (adapted from Pedro, 2006).

It is possible to observe that the athletes with a better running AnT have a higher increase [La$^-$] rate after v4, which is a finding not commonly expected (Pedro, 2006).

In this sense, choosing the correct training volumes for certain specific intensities, it is possible and advisable to adapt the training process in order to combine a well developed AnT and a lower increase [La$^-$] rate for higher running velocity. This procedure has been carried out by some of the best coaches (e.g. Canova, 2004), accepting that a well-established physiological adaptation to higher intensities (e.g. 7 mmol/L) lead to a more easily and stable running.

In swimming the increase [La$^-$] rate is also studied by us, represented as the slope of the line obtained between 2 steps. In Figure 5, it is possible to observe an example of two [La]/velocity curves (conducted in different moments of the training season) for the same swimmer. We can observe a significant development in the anaerobic component, probably due to the use of more specific training methods recruiting other energy pathways.

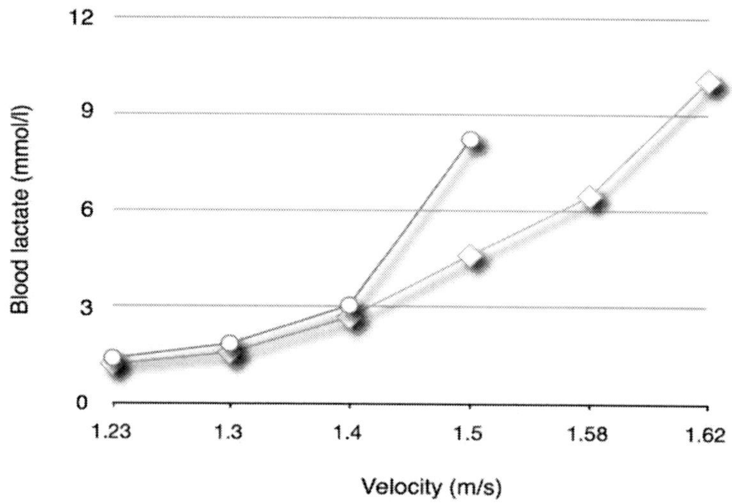

Figure 5. Example of two blood lactate concentrations/velocity curves for the same swimmer conducted in the different moments of the season (Fernandes et al, unpublished data).

Table 2. Mean plus SD of critical velocity (m/s) for male and female age-group swimmers (adapted from Soares et al., 2003)

	Infant (50 and 400 m)	Juvenile (100 and 800/1500 m)	Junior (100 and 800/1500 m)	Senior (50 and 800/1500 m)
Female	1.10±0.07	1.23±0.05	1.29±0.05	1.34±0.05
Male	1.18±0.08	1.32±0.06	1.36±0.04	1.38±0.07

Our experiments have been showing the importance of the "increase [La$^-$] rate" concept and can justify the reason why some athletes with a lower developed AnT can achieve best results in comparison with others. Thus, in Figure 6, it is possible to observe that the athlete #1, presenting a not so well developed AnT, has a lower increase [La$^-$] rate (defined by a lower slope), which allows him to achieve a better result in Half Marathon compared with other runners (the higher increase [La$^-$] rate after the AnT can make them less competitive).

Table 3. Mean plus SD of heart rate and (beats/min) and blood lactate concentrations in a cycling incremental intermittent protocol (Colaço et al., unpublished data)

	1st step (9.72 m/s)	2nd step (11.11 m/s)	3rd step (12.50 m/s)	4th step (13.88 m/s)
Heart rate (beats/min)	141.2±14.2	158.6±14.3	172.7±8.0	179.4±8.7
Blood lactate concentrations (mmol/l)	1.9±0.6	4.1±2.2	6.0±2.5	7.6±2.6

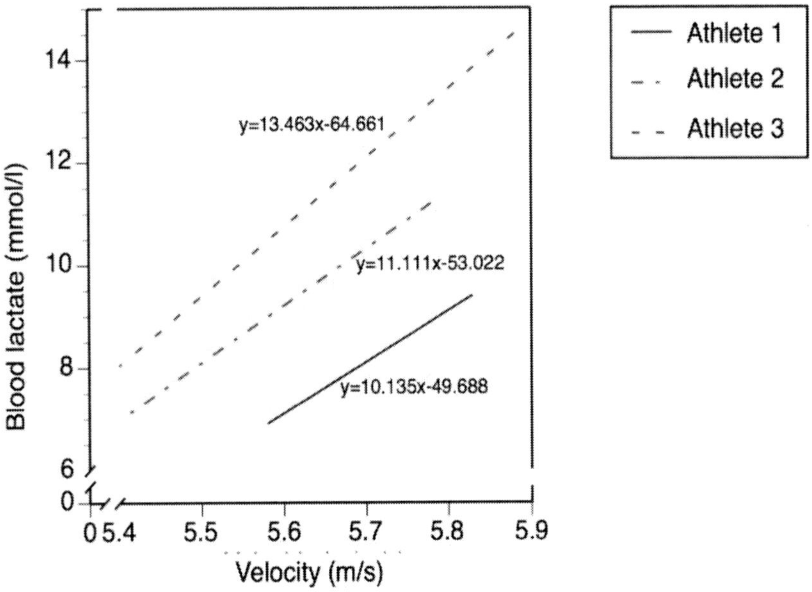

Figure 6. Lines and equations illustrating the increase of blood lactate concentrations rate obtained for three runners in the two last steps of an anaerobic threshold test (adapted from Colaço, 2007).

Additionally, according with other study of our group (Pedro, 2006), it is possible to find higher correlation between the 5000 m distance and the velocity corresponding to 6 mmol/L and 7 mmol/L ($r = 0.91$, $p < 0.01$) than for v4, which reinforces the importance of increase [La$^-$] rate after the AnT for middle distance runners. Following the same testing procedure, increase [La$^-$] rate was also evaluated in different moments of the season, which can be fundamental to understand the athlete's progression and to find some eventual evolution problems. It is important to underline that the training adaptations should be conducted in order to improve the AnT, or, in some moments of the season (e.g. the pre-competitive period), to maintain its level of development but also to promote the increase [La$^-$] rate for higher exercise intensities (Figure 7).

From Figure 7 it is possible to state that, during a season, the athlete should improve the AnT but the improvements corresponding to higher [La$^-$] values can be superior. These results suggest that the employ of more specific training (as intensive interval training), conducted at higher exercise intensities (e.g. near or at VO2max), can be responsible for the reported improvements. Monitoring these changes can be very useful to readjust the training prescription in a more accurately way. In this sense, we suggest organizing the training process through different bioenergetical training zones and control possible changes during the season (cf. Olbrecht, 2000).

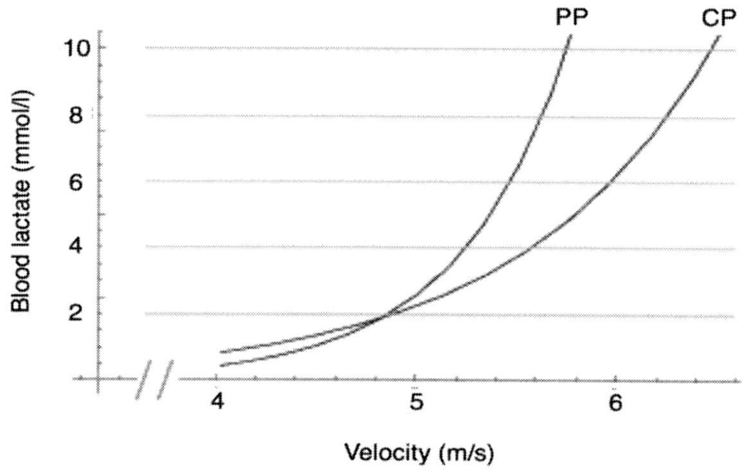

Figure 7. Blood lactate concentration curves corresponded to the preparatory period (PP) and Competitive Period (CP) of a runner (adapted from Pedro, 2006).

Considering the establishment of different training zones, we have been studying changes associated to [La⁻]/velocity curves during the season, determining adjacent areas in different [La⁻] intervals and corresponding running velocity, which allow comparing changes for each athlete during the season (Figure 8). Notice that the higher the area between two [La] values most prepared the athlete is to perform at those intensities.

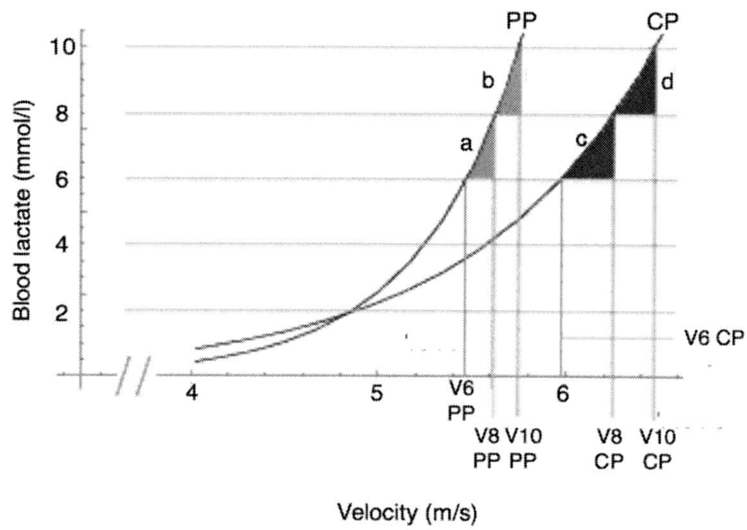

Figure 8. Representation of adjacent areas of blood lactate concentration curves in function of the running velocity, for Preparatory Period (PP - a and b areas) and Competitive Period (CP - c and d areas). Adapted from Pedro (2006).

The oxygen uptake kinetics should also be taken into consideration when evaluating the athletes. Although it is well-known that the methodological procedures to assess VO_2 during exercise are easier to implement in ergometers, some studies of our group were conducted in specific competition conditions. Using the above-referred 7 x 200 m incremental protocol, the

VO_2max values for front crawl swimming and its corresponding velocities were assessed in a 25 m swimming pool. The results were 52.1 ± 6.5 ml/kg/min and 1.16 ± 0.10 m/s, 69.9 ± 9.3 ml/kg/min and 1.40 ± 0.06 m/s, and 71.7 ± 6.1 ml/kg/min and 1.45 ± 0.05 m/s, respectively for recreational, competitive and elite male level swimmers (Fernandes et al., 2006a; Fernandes et al., 2008b). At the minimum intensity of VO2max (vVO_2max), the [La^-] were situated between 8-9 mmol/l and heart rate values between 180-190 b/min, which is in accordance with the specialized literature.

In continuation, we find very interesting to study the swimmer's ability to sustain the vVO_2max intensities, i.e., the swimming intensities that elicit their maximal aerobic power. So, recently, we started focusing in the determination of the time of exercise to exhaustion at vVO_2max (TLim-vVO_2max). This concept has arisen in the last years, seeming to be a very interesting matter for assessing various aspects of performance and training of endurance athletes (Billat et al., 1994). The first studies (e.g. Billat et al., 1996) that assessed TLim-vVO_2max in swimming were conducted using front crawl in swimming flume, not in specific training and competition conditions. As it is accepted that performing in a flume could bring some mechanical constraints, our TLim-vVO_2max related studies were always conducted in a swimming pool. We find a low inter-individual variability in TLim-vVO_2max values, ranging from 215 s in elite swimmers (Fernandes et al., 2008b) to 325 s in low level swimmers (Fernandes et al., 2003a), which are in accordance with the data obtained by Billat et al. (1996) and Demarie et al. (2001) for flume swimming. Those results suggest a lower variation of this parameter in swimming, compared with the results presented for other sports by Billat et al. (1994), namely treadmill running (range 4-11 min). This fact advocate coaches and swimmers to use lower duration of training sets when aiming to develop aerobic power: approximately 5 min in a continuous effort or until 10 min if intermittent training series are used. Moreover, no differences were observed in front crawl TLim-vVO_2max values between genders (Fernandes et al., 2005b), as well as between swimming strokes (Fernandes et al., 2006b), pointing out that the phenomenon is similar in male and female swimmers as well as in all four strokes. In Figure 9 it is represented a typical example of the VO_2 pattern during the TLim-vVO_2max test.

It is possible to see, after the fast rise of the VO_2 in the beginning of exercise (just following the cardiodinamic component in the first seconds of exercise), a secondary slower phase of VO_2 kinetics. This phenomenon, denominated oxygen slow component (O_2SC), seems to contradict the traditional idea of a systematic appearance of a VO_2 plateau after the fast VO_2 kinetics phase in heavy exercise. This fact corroborates the previous studies performed in cycling and running that stated that exercise at metabolic rates above the AnT, i. e., in the heavy or severe intensity domains, evidences a slowly-developing component of the VO_2 kinetics that is superimposed upon the rapid increase of $\dot{V}O_2$ initiated at exercise onset (Bearden and Moffatt, 2000).

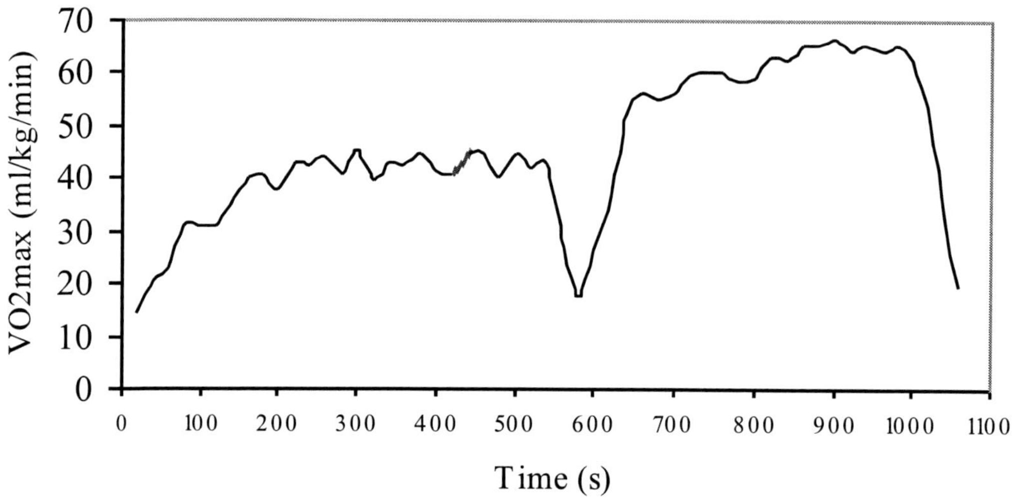

Figure 9. A typical example of the VO_2 pattern during the swimming TLim-vVO_2max test. (i) warm-up; (ii) 20 s rest for capillary blood collection and (iii) maintenance of swimming vVO_2max until exhaustion. The arrows delimit the period where the O_2 slow component was calculated (Fernandes et al., unpublished data).

In our studies, O_2SC was assessed as the difference between the last VO_2 measurement of the TLim-vVO_2max test and the one measured during the second min (Koppo and Bouckaert, 2001) or the third min of exercise (Demarie et al., 2001), being observed amplitudes of 279.0±195.2 ml/min in recreational swimmers (Fernandes et al., 2003a) and 274.1±152.8 in competitive swimmers (Fernandes et al., 2003b) that are in agreement with the Demarie et al. (2001) reports for pentathletes performing in swimming flume. These values seem to be lower than those for running and cycling (Billat et al., 1998), which could be justified by the chosen high exercise intensity and the specificity of this modality. Additionally, in the swimming studies above referred, it were obtained positive relationships between TLim-vVO_2max and O_2SC, which appear to express that the higher the TLim-vVO_2max was, the higher the O_2SC amplitude was expected to be, being in accordance with other groups (e.g. Gaesser and Poole, 1996). The cause of the O_2SC appearance is still a matter of debate, seeming to be explained by the increased number of recruited motor units in heavy efforts. In this sense, this concept is still difficult to use in training prescription.

2.3. Anaerobic System

Nonetheless the importance of aerobic capacity in running, swimming, cycling and rowing performance, the anaerobic energy system is a significant contributor during short distances, namely the ones lasting less than 2 min (Gastin, 2001). However, quantitative assessments of anaerobic metabolism are difficult to achieve, since invasive measures (e.g. muscle biopsies, blood samples and magnetic resonance) are costly and unavailable in a field test setting, once it demands knowledgeable technicians and require a considerable amount of sophisticated equipment.

In middle and long distance running events, anaerobic performance is expressed in differently accordingly to the dependence of each event from its energetic supporting system: it is clear that an 800 m runner will recruit much more energy from anaerobic pathways than a Marathon runner. However, it is not easy to identify the exact contribution of each body energy systems. In Table 4, it is possible to observe some literature proposals about this topic in running.

The observed differences for each event can be justified by different methodological and instrumental procedures, as well as by the subjects' level.

Table 4. Percentage values attributed by different authors to the contribution of different energetic systems, in different running events

Authors	Anaerobic	Aerobic
800m		
Spencer e Gastin (2001)	34%	66%
Duffield et al. (2005a)	40%	60%
1500m		
Spencer e Gastin (2001)	16%	84%
Duffield et al. (2005b)	23%	77%
5000m		
Newsholme et al. (1992)	12.5%	87.5%
Marajo et al. (1994)	20%	80%
Half Marathon		
Newsholme et al. (1992)	0-3%	97-100%
Péronnet et Thibault (1989)	5-10%	90-95%

Considering this topic, we have been using a two-speed test (Mader et al., 1980) based in a distance in accordance with the competition event (600, 1200 or 2000 m respectively for 800, 1500 and 5000 m, and Half Marathon runners). The selected distance is performed at different intensities (80% for the first and higher than 95% for the second repetition), using a complete interval between them. Lactate blood samples are taken in each min after each repetition until the maximum lactate value is obtained. With this test is possible to understand the increase of $[La^-]$ with velocity, compare the slopes, balance results of velocity associated to certain $[La^-]$ values and understand how an athlete is progressing in the $[La^-]$ /velocity relationship (Figure 10).

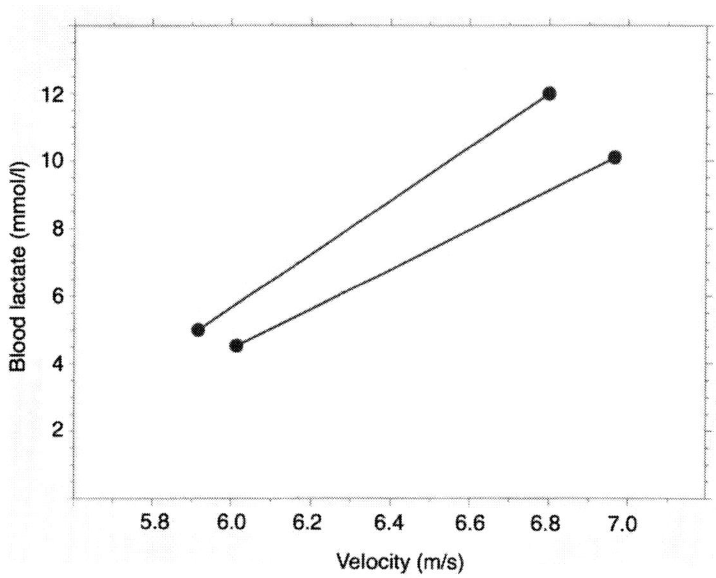

Figure 10. Graphical representation of two lines obtained from the two speed test, applied to a female runner (adapted from Colaço, 2007).

Thus, by using this test it is possible to compare the behavior of different lines obtained in different moments of the season, better explain diverse competitive performance levels and understand if the training process is promoting the expected levels of anaerobic adaptation. Simultaneously to the monitoring of the anaerobic changes, it should be observed the aerobic variations (through an AnT test) and have a better understanding of the connection between the test results and the specific performance changes for each event.

The purpose of our studies has been two-fold: (i) observing different performance levels between athletes (Colaço, 2007) and (ii) comparing the same athlete in different moments (Pedro, 2006). So, using the two-speed test, it was used the slope and area values trying to find the athlete with less increase [La$^-$] rate with velocity increment, especially for intensities that are connected with the athlete's event. In this perspective, we can notice that, for events with a significant anaerobic contribution, the lines behavior in higher intensities can be more performance discriminative, particularly when aerobic level seems to be similar between athletes with different performance levels (Figure 11).

When this test is applied in middle distance runners (Colaço, 2007), it is possible to observe different performance levels. However, when we are working with 5000 m and Half Marathon runners, it seems that this test lose relevance. However, considering that some athletes can achieve similar aerobic levels, the specific use of some anaerobic contribution can determine different final results and also need to be taken in consideration in the training control and evaluation of these athletes. As an example, it is important to refer that the values obtained using the 2 x 2000 m test can be particularly discriminating of performance (Colaço, 2007), which happens particularly when the athletes with similar AnT have their performance level distinguished by the anaerobic energy contribution (Figure 12).

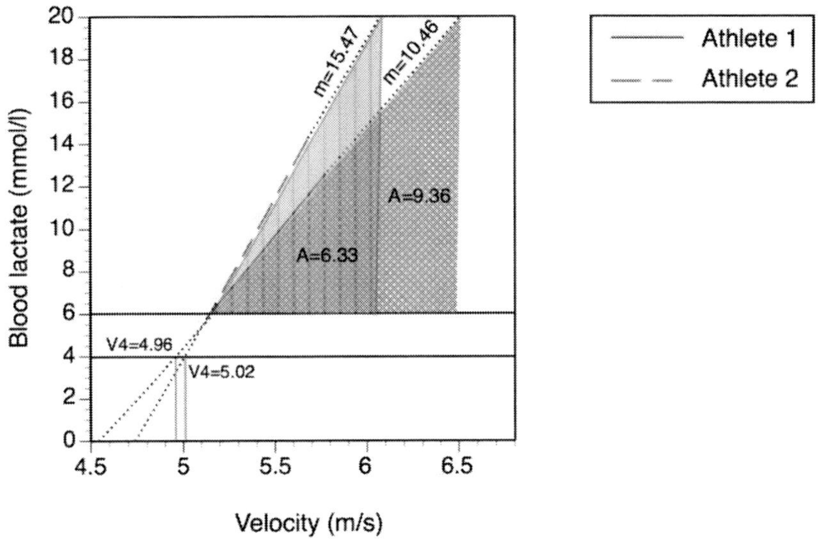

Figure 11. Representation of the two speed test of two 1500 m runners, with the slope (m) area obtained by the lines extrapolation until 20 mmol/l value and 6 m/s of running velocity (adapted from Colaço, 2007).

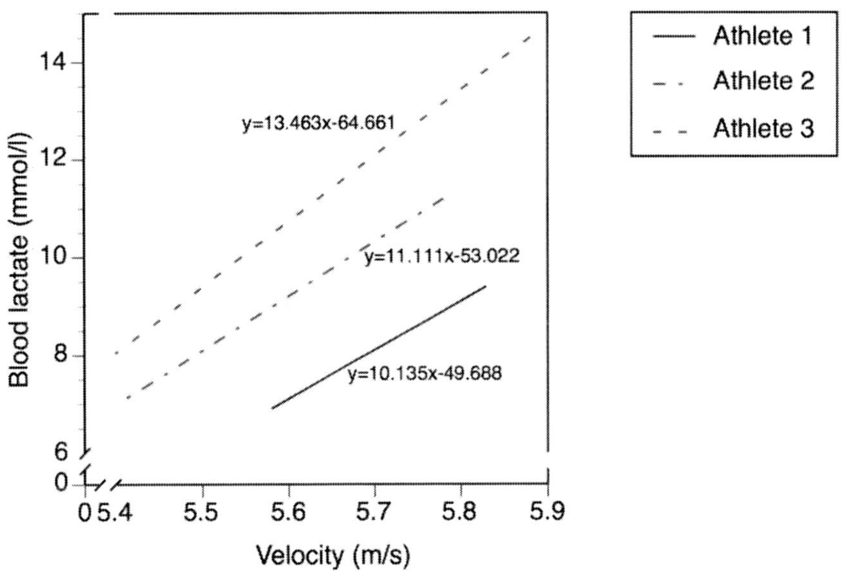

Figure 12. Lines and equations obtained throughout the two speed test for three 5000 m runners. Notice that the athlete 1 had the lower competitive level, although his higher anaerobic threshold (adapted from Colaço, 2007).

In swimming, knowing that the majority of the competitive events last less than 2 min, the importance of the anaerobic energy system is clearly stated. Holmér (1983) referred that for the 50 and 100 m events the anaerobic contribution is about 80%, or even more. Thus, a large anaerobic capacity, with high rates of glycogen breakdown and glycolytic enzyme activities in the muscles, seems to be a prerequisite for fast swimming (Trappe, 1996). In this sense, complementarily to the traditionally used maximal [La⁻] values obtained in the final steps of incremental progressive tests or even in the end of short duration events, we have implemented some protocols to control and evaluate the anaerobic system contribution in swimming.

In a recent publication, Fernandes et al. (2008a) proposed the anaerobic critical velocity test, assessed in front crawl, as a simple and non-invasive methodology that could allow coaches and scientists to have a new tool for swimmers training advice. This test was based upon the concept of the (aerobic) critical velocity method, using the regression line equation obtained by the relationship between sprint distances and the respective time durations, to provide a hypothetical measure of the functional anaerobic capacity of swimmers. In Figure 13 it is possible to observe that anaerobic critical velocity was assessed through the slope of the regression equation established between the 12.5, 25 and 50 m test distances and the corresponding test times. Anaerobic critical velocity (represented as a and expressed in m/s) was calculated from the slope of the distance (y) versus time (x) relationship, and b is y-interception value, according to this equation:

$$y = ax + b \tag{1}$$

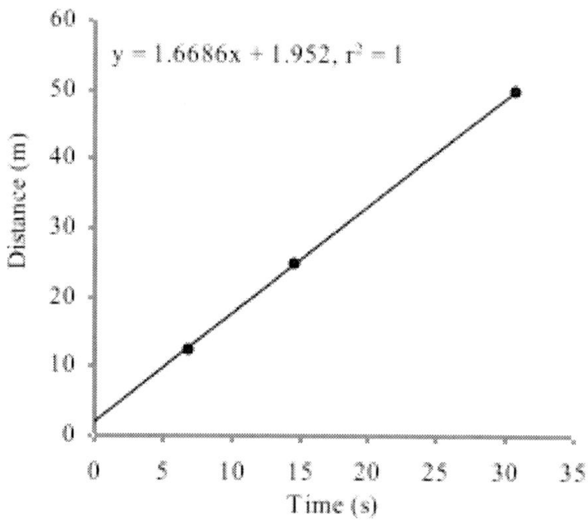

Figure 13. Example of a swimming anaerobic critical velocity assessment (Fernandes et al., unpublished data).

In the study of Fernandes et al. (2008a) it was found a strong inverse relationship between the anaerobic critical velocity and the 100 m front crawl time ($r = -0.84$), the first 50 m partial ($r = -0.87$) and the second 50 m partial ($r = -0.79$), all for a $p < 0.001$. Complementarily, the value of the anaerobic critical velocity converted in 100 m time was not different of the 100 m front crawl event duration. Even more recently, our group (unpublished data) observed moderate to high correlation values between the anaerobic critical velocity and the specific velocities obtained in the 100 m butterfly, backstroke, breaststroke and freestyle events ($r > 0.60$, $p < 0.05$). These authors also referred the non-existence of differences between anaerobic critical velocity and the velocity of the last 50 m of the above-referred events. Although future studies in larger samples should be implemented, the results obtained suggest that anaerobic critical velocity can be used as measure of the anaerobic swimming potential.

Other area of interest, when referring to evaluating anaerobic swimming potential, is the assessment of fatigue thresholds. Nonetheless the study of fatigue thresholds is more evident at aerobic intensities, namely studying the AnT, we were able to observe the existence of velocity, force and power time-curves with one or two fatigue thresholds during 30 s tests (Soares et al., 2006 and Soares et al., 2008). Conducting five different tests with the same effort duration, being three general (cycloergometer Wingate test, crank ergometer Wingate test and simulated swimming on a biokinetic swim bench) and two specific (free swimming with connection to a cable velocimetric system and tethered swimming), these authors observed that in curves with one threshold, fatigue appears around 13 s from the beginning of the effort and, in curves with two fatigue thresholds, they become visible around 8 s and 18 s of exercise. In Figure 14, it is possible to observe a velocity-time trace of a swimmer in which the determined fatigue thresholds were plotted in (vertical lines).

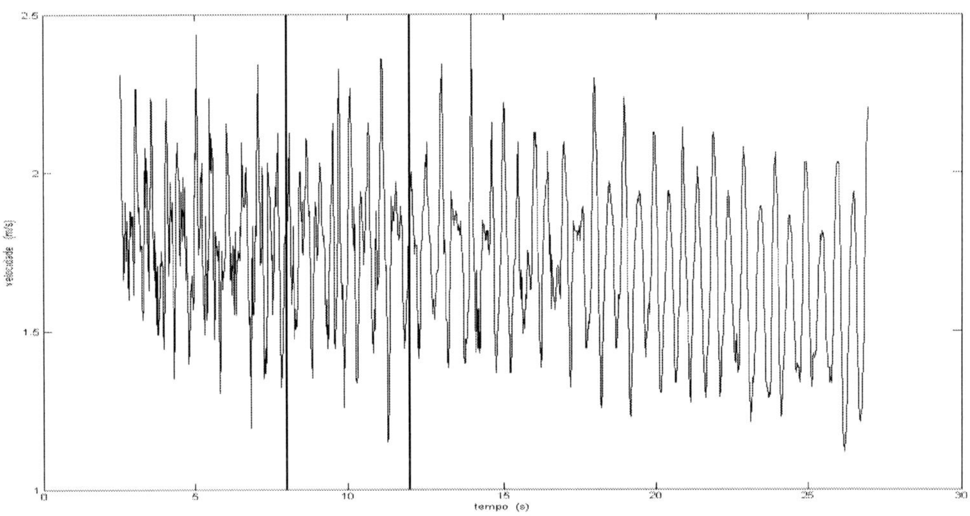

Figure 14. Velocimetric trace (with start, glide and arrival removed) of a swimmer with fatigue thresholds identified with vertical lines (Soares et al., unpublished data).

The above-referred authors concluded that fatigue thresholds appearance seem to be independent of the kind of effort performed by swimmers and speculate about the possibility of using velocity curves to determine an individual alactic-lactic threshold and better plan and control the anaerobic training. In this domain, the same authors have conducted a simple test for metabolic fatigue thresholds determination through $[La^-]$ kinetics during an incremental 30 s protocol. Results showed differences in $[La^-]$ near to 15 s swimming effort. Metabolic thresholds were close to velocimetric thresholds of v(t) curves.

3. Conclusion

We expect that the presented protocols, conducted in the bioenergetical area of expertise, could be well accepted and applied by athletes, coaches and scientists in their training control and athletes' evaluation programs. We keep on saying that reliable and systematic control and evaluation is a precious tool to increase the training efficiency and even contributing to predict performance.

As observed during the text, there is a large number of protocols to evaluate athletes and control the training process. Considering the different possibilities, we have been choosing those that allow getting the more applied results to training. Complementarily, we also have being trying to select tests with a good prediction capacity to help coaches and athletes to know the exact moments of the season to schedule their competitions.

One of our most important concerns has been to indirectly estimate some of the most used bioenergetical parameters and to state them in a comprehensible way to coaches and athletes. Finally, we expect to work in the future with as large number of athletes in longitudinal studies trying to perfect and individualize these methodologies.

References

Bearden, S. E. & Moffatt, R. J. (2001). VO2 slow component: to model or not to model? *Med. Sci. Sports Exerc., 33(4)*, 677-680.

Beneke, R. (1995). Anaeroboc threshold, individual threshold, and maximal steady state in rowing. *Med Sci Sports Exerc., 27(6)*, 863-867.

Beneke, R. & von Duvillard, S. (1996). Determination of maximal lactate steady state response in selected sports events. *Med Sci Sports Exerc., 28*, 241-246.

Billat, V. (1998). Physiologie et méthodologie de l'entraînement. *De la théorie à la pratique*. De Boeck Université, Paris, France.

Billat, V., Renoux, J. C., Pinoteau, J., Petit, B. & Koralsztein, J. P. (1994). Reproducibility of running time to exhaustion at VO2max in subelite runners. *Med. Sci. Sports Exerc., 2*, 254-257.

Billat, V., Faina, M., Sardella, F., Marini, C., Fanton, F., Lupo, S., Faccini, P., De Angelis, M., Koralsztein, J. P. & Dal Monte, A. (1996). A comparison of time to exhaustion at VO2max in elite cyclists, kayac paddlers, swimmers and runners. *Ergonomics., 39(2)*, 267-277.

Billat, V., Richard, R., Binsse, V. M., Koralsztein, J. P. & Haouzi, P. (1998). The VO2 slow component for severe exercise depends on type of exercise and is not correlated with time to fatigue. *J. Appl. Physiol., 85*, 2118-2124.

Boiirgois J. and Vrijens J. (1998). Metabolic and cardiorespiratory responses in young oarsmen during prolonged exerci.se tests on a rowing ergometer at power outputs corresponding to two concepls of anaerobic threshold. *Eur J Appl. Physiol., 77*: 164-9.

Canova R (2004). *Development of strenght endurance: the key to improve in middle and long distance events*. EACA Coaching Congress. Abano Terme. Italy.

Cardoso, C., Fernandes, R., Magalhães, J., Santos, P., Colaço, P., Soares, S., Carmo, C., Barbosa, T., Vilas-Boas, J.P. (2003). Comparison of a continuous and intermittent triangular protocols for direct VO2max assessment in swimming. In: J.-C. Chatard (edt.), *Proceedings of the IXth World Symposium on Biomechanics and Medicine in Swimming,* pp. 313-318. Saint-Etienne, France.

Cazorla, G. (1984). De l'evaluation en activité physique et sportive. Travaux et recherches en E.P.S. n° 7, *Evaluation de la valeur physique.*, 7-35. INSEP, Paris.

Colaço, P. (2007). Aerobic and anaerobic evaluation of middle distance and long distance runners (in Portuguese). *Doctoral Thesis.* Faculty of Sport, Porto University. Portugal.

Demarie, S., Sardella, F., Billat, V., Magini, W. & Faina, M. (2001). The VO2 slow component in swimming. *Eur. J. Appl. Physiol., 84,* 95-99.

Duffield, R., Dawson, B. & Goodman, C. (2005). Energy contribution to 400-metre and 800-metre track running. *J. Sports Sci.,* 23 (3), 299-307.

Esteve-Lanao, J., Juan, A., Earnest, C., Foster, C. & Lucia, A. (2005). How do endurance runners actually trains? Relationship with competition performance. *Med. Sci. Sports Exerc., 37,* 3, 496-504.

Fernandes, R. & Vilas-Boas, J. P. (1999). Critical velocity as a criterion for estimating aerobic training pace in juvenile swimmers. In: K. Keskinen, P. Komi, P. Hollander (eds.), *Proceedings of the VIII International Symposium of Biomechanics and Medicine in Swimming,* 233-238. University of Jyvaskyla, Finland.

Fernandes, R., Guerra, S., Lamares, J. P. & Vilas-Boas, J. P. (2000). Critical velocity in swimming: three different methodologies for its determination. In: J., Avela, P., Komi, & J., Komulainen (eds.), *Proceedings of the 5th Annual Congress of the European College of Sport Science,* pg 260. University of Jyvaskyla, Finland.

Fernandes, R., Billat, V., Cardoso, C., Barbosa, T., Soares, S., Ascensão, A., Colaço, P., Demarle, A. & Vilas-Boas, J. P. (2003a). Time limit at vVO2max and VO2max slow component in swimming. A pilot study in university students. In: J. C. Chatard, (edt.), *Proceedings of the IXth World Symposium on Biomechanics and Medicine in Swimming,* 331-336. Saint-Etienne, France.

Fernandes, R. J., Cardoso, C. S., Soares, S. M., Ascensão, A., Colaço, P. J. & Vilas-Boas, J. P. (2003b). Time limit and VO2 slow component at intensities corresponding to VO2max in swimmers. *Int. J. Sports Med., 24(8),* 576-581.

Fernandes, R., Almeida, M., Morais, P., Machado, L., Soares, S., Ascensão, A., Colaço, P., Morouço, P. & Vilas-Boas, J. P. (2005a). Individual Anaerobic Threshold assessment in a swimming incremental test for VO2max evaluation. In: N. Dikic, S. Zivanic, S. Ostojic, Z. Tornjanski (eds.), *Abstract Book of the 10th Annual Congress of the European College of Sport Science.,* 266. Belgrade, Serbia.

Fernandes, R. J., Billat, V. L., Cruz, A. C., Colaço, P. J., Cardoso, C. S., Vilas-Boas, J. P. (2005b). Has gender any effect on the relationship between time limit at VO2max velocity and swimming economy? *J. Human Mov. Studies., 49,* 127-148.

Fernandes, R. J., Billat, V. L., Cruz, A. C., Colaço, P. J., Cardoso, C. S. & Vilas-Boas, J. P. (2006a). Does net energy cost of swimming affect time to exhaustion at the individual's maximal oxygen consumption velocity? *J. Sports Med. Phys. Fitness., 46(3),* 373-80.

Fernandes, R., Cardoso, C., Silva, J., Vilar, S., Colaço, P., Barbosa, T., Keskinen, K. L. & Vilas-Boas, J. P. (2006b). Assessment of time limit at lowest speed corresponding to maximal oxygen consumption in the four competitive swimming strokes. *Port. J. Sport Sci., 6(2),* 128-130.

Fernandes, R. J., Aleixo, I., Soares, S. & Vilas-Boas, J. P. (2008a). Anaerobic Critical Velocity: A New Tool for Young Swimmers Training Advice (chapter 10). In: N. P. Beaulieu (edt.), *Physical Activity and Children: New Research.*, 211-223. Nova Science Publishers, Inc. New York.

Fernandes, R. J., Keskinen, K. L., Colaço, P., Querido, A. J., Machado, L. J., Morais, P. A., Marinho, D. A. & Vilas-Boas, J. P. (2008b). Time limit at VO2max velocity in elite crawl swimmers. *Int. J. Sports Med., 29*, 145-150.

Gaesser, G. A. & Poole, D. (1996). The slow component of oxygen uptake kinetics in humans. *Exerc. Sport., Sci. Rev.*, 24.

Gastin, P. B. (2001). Energy system interaction and relative contribution during maximal exercise. *Sports Med., 31* (10), 725-41.

Heck, H., Mader, A., Hess, G., Mucke, S., Muller, R. & Hollmann, W. (1985). Justification of the 4-mmol/l Lactate Threshold. Int. *J. Sports Med., 6*, 117-130.

Holmér, I. (1983). Energetics and mechanical work in swimming. In A. P., Hollander; P. A., Huijing; G., de Groot, (Eds.), *Biomechanics and Medicine in Swimming* (154-164). Campaign, Illinois: Human Kinetics Publishers.

Ingham, S. A., Whyte, G. P., Jones, K., Nevill, A. (2002). Determinants of 2.000 m rowing ergometer performance in elite rowers. *Eur. J. Appl. Physiol., 88*, 243-6.

Jones, A. & Doust, J. (1998). The validity of the lactate minimum test for determination of the maximal lactate steady state. *Med. Sci Sports Exerc., 31*, 1299-1306.

Jurimae, J., Maestu, J. & Jiirimae, T. (2001). Blood laciale response to exercise and rowing pcrlbrmancc; relationships in competitive rowers. *J. Hum. Mov. Studies., 41*, 287-300.

Koppo, K. & Bouckaert, J. (2002). The decrease in the VO2 slow component induced by prior exercise does not affect the time to exhaustion. *Int. J. Sports Med., 23*, 262-267.

Lucía, A., Hoyos, J. & Chicharro, J. L. (2001). Physiology of professional road cycling. *Sports Medicine., 31(5)*, 325-337.

Mader, A., Liesen, H., Heck, H; Philippi, H., Rost, R., Schürch, P. & Hollmann, W. (1976). Zur Beurteilung der sportartspezifischen Ausdauerleistungsfähigkeit im Labor. Sportarzt. *Sportmed., 24(4)*, 109.

Mader, A., Madsen, O. & Hollmann, W. (1980). Zur beurteilung der laktaziden energiebereitstellung fur trainings-und wettkampfleistungen im schwimmen. *Leistungssport., 10*, 263-279.

Maestu, J., Jurimae, J. & Jurimae, T. (2005). Monitoring of performance and training in rowing. *Sports Medicine., 35(7)*, 597-617.

Morais, P., Almeida, M., Aleixo, I., Corredoura, S., Colaço, P., Machado, L., Fernandes, R. & Vilas-Boas, J. P. (2006). Oxygen uptake at the lactate threshold in swimming. *Port. J. Sport Sci., 6(2)*, 153-154.

Olbrecht, J. (2000). The science of winning. Planning, periodizing and optimizing swim training. Swimshop. Luton, England.

Olbrecht, J., Madsen, O., Mader, A., Liesel, H. & Hullman, W. (1985). Relationship between swimming velocity and latic acid concentration during continuous and intermittent training exercise. *Int. J. Sports Med., 6(2)*, 74-77.

Papadopoulos, C., Doyle, J., LaBudde, B., Rupp, J., Brandon, L., Benardot, D. & Martin, D. (2003). Relationships between blood lactate parameters and endurance performance. Med. Sci. Sports Exerc., *35(5)*, 498.

Pedro, F. (2006). Aerobic evaluation of middle distance runners (in Portuguese). *Masters Thesis*. Faculty of Sport, University of Porto. Portugal.

Pyke, F. (2000). Introduction. In C. J. Gore (Edt.), Physiological tests for elite athletes (pp. xii-xiv). Australia: Australian Sports Commission.

Pyne, D., Maw, G. & Goldsmith, W. (2000). Protocols for the physiological assessment of swimmers. In C. J. Gore (Edt.), *Physiological tests for elite athletes*, 372-382. Australian Sports Commission. Australia.

Roecker, K., Schotte, O., Niess, A., Hortasmann, T. & Dickhuth, H. (1998). Predicting competition performance in long-distance running by means of a treadmill test. *Med. Sci. Sports Exerc., 30(10)*, 1552-1557.

Santos, P. & Ascencão, A. (1999). Maximal lactate-steady-state in young male runners. International conference book. "Youth Sports in the 21st Century", Michigan.

Soares, S., Fernandes, R. & Vilas-Boas, J. P. (2003). Analysis of critical velocity regression line informations for different ages: from infant to junior swimmers. In: J. C. Chatard (edt.), *Proceedings of the IXth World Symposium on Biomechanics and Medicine in Swimming*, 397-401. Saint-Etienne, France.

Soares, S., Machado, L., Lima, A., Santos, I., Fernandes, R., Correia, M., Maia, J. & Vilas-Boas, J. P. (2006). Velocimetric characterization of a 30 sec maximal test in swimming: consequences for bioenergetical evaluation. *Port. J. Sport Sci.*, *6*, supl. 2,

Soares, S., Aleixo, I., Santos, I., Machado, L., Maia, J. & Vilas-Boas, J. P. (2008). Fatigue thresholds in 30s water and land exercises performed by swimmers. In: J., Cabri, F., Alves, D., Araújo, J., Barreiros, J., Dinis, A., Veloso, (eds.), *Book of Abstracts of the 13th Annual Congress of the European College of Sport Science, 500*. Estoril, Portugal.

Spencer, M. & Gastin, P. (2001). Energy system contribution during 200 to 1500m running in highly trained athletes. *Med. Sci. Sports Exerc., 33(1)*, 157-162.

Svedahl, K. & MacIntosh, B. (2003). Anaerobic threshold: the concept and methods of measurement. *Can. J. Appl. Physiol., 28(2)*, 299-323.

Trappe, S. W. (1996). Metabolic demands for swimming. In J. P., Troup, A. P., Hollander, D., Strasse, S. W., Trappe, J. M., Cappaert, T. A., Trappe (Eds.), *Biomechanics and Medicine in Swimming VII* (127-134). London: E & FN Spon.

Troup, J. (1995). Physiological aspects of swimming. *Abstracts of the XI FINA World Sports Medicine Congress, 65*. FINA, Atenas.

Urhausen, A., Coen, A. B., Weiler, B. & Kindermann, W. (1993). Individual anaerobic threshold and maximum lactate steady state. *Int. J. Sports Med., 14(3)*, 134-139.

Vilas-Boas, J. P., Lamares, J. P., Fernandes, R. & Duarte, J. A. (1997). Relationship between anaerobic threshold and swimming critical speed determined with competition times. In: *Abstract book of the FIMS's 9th European Congress of Sports Medicine*. Porto, Portugal.

Wakayoshi, K., Ikuta, K., Yoshida, T., Udo, M., Moritani, T., Mutoh, Y. & Miyashita, M. (1992). Determination and validity of critical velocity as an index of swimming performance in the competitive swimmer. *Eur. J. Appl. Physiol.*, *64*, 153-157.

Womack, C. J., Davis, S. E., Wood, C. M., Sauer, K., Alvarez, J., Weltman, A. & Gaesser, G. A. (1996). Effects of training on physiological correlates of rowing ergometry performance. *J. Strength Cond. Res.*, *10*, 234-8

We thank José Bragada, from the Polytechnic Institute of Bragança (Portugal), for their review of this paper and for their pertinent suggestions.

In: Encyclopedia of Sports and Athletics
Editors: Jack L. Murray and Emily O. Watson
ISBN: 978-1-61209-959-0

Chapter XI

Performance and Fatigue in an Incremental Running Test on a Track

Ari Nummela**, Erilynn Russo and Tapani Keränen
KIHU - Research Institute for Olympic Sports, Jyväskylä, Finland

Abstract

The present chapter was designed to investigate the performance and fatigue in an incremental 6 x 1000 m running test. Well-trained endurance athletes performed eight non-fatigued sprints from 5 m · s^{-1} to maximal velocity and the 6 x 1000 m running test on a 200-m indoor track. In order to investigate the fatigue induced changes in force production during running, non-fatigued ground reaction forces and ground contact times were compared to the values measured at the end of the last 1000-m run. The performance in the last 1000 m (V_{1000m}) correlated significantly with VO_{2peak} (r = 0.68; P = 0.001), velocity at 4 mM blood lactate level (r = 0.76; P = 0.000), running economy (r = -0.47; P = 0.042), maximal sprint running velocity (r = 0.52; P = 0.023) and anaerobic energy production (r = 0.63; P = 0.004). V_{1000m} was also related to the fatigue at the end of the 6 x 1000 m (r = -0.63; P = 0.004). When fatigued and non-fatigued running were compared at the same velocity, it was observed that ground contact times increased (P = 0.001) and vertical ground reaction forces (P = 0.000) decreased in fatigue. The results showed that the performance in the incremental 6 x 1000 m test on a track is not only related to the traditional endurance performance characteristics, but neuromuscular and anaerobic performance characteristics and fatigue resistance are also important determinants of the incremental running test.

Introduction

Over the past decades there have been numerous attempts to determine the factors that influence distance running performance in athletes. One of the most popular beliefs in

* Corresponding author: Research Institute for Olympic Sports, Rautpohjankatu 6, FI-40700 Jyväskylä, Finland, Phone: +358 40 543 9217, Fax: +358 20 781 1501, E-mail: ari.nummela@kihu.fi

exercise physiology has been that distance running performance is only limited by the ability to transport and consume oxygen during exhaustive exercise. It has been suggested that hypoxia developed in the active muscles during exercise causes fatigue and therefore limits maximal endurance performance. This idea is supported by many previous studies, which have shown a good correlation between maximal oxygen uptake (VO_{2max}) and distance running performance [5, 1, 20]. Although VO_{2max} is a good predictor of distance running performance, some other factors such as fatigue resistance [29], the ability to sustain high $\%VO_{2max}$ or anaerobic threshold [5, 7], running economy [4] and neuromuscular factors [20, 22] have shown to be good predictors of distance running performance. Paavolainen et al. [22] presented a hypothetical model of the variables related to distance running performance. In this model, the traditional model of endurance performance [6] was supplemented with the inclusion of factors relating to the neuromuscular capacity to produce power.

Fatigue is a complex phenomenon that can be defined as a reduction in the maximum force that a muscle can exert [15]. Although the relationship between fatigue resistance and running performance is obvious [1, 2], the relationship between the reduction in the maximum force or velocity and running performance is not so clear. Paavolainen et al. [23] concluded that in a 10 km time trial marked fatigue took place in both high and low calibre runners but the fatigue-induced changes in a maximal 20 m run did not differentiate endurance athletes with different performances in the 10 km time trial. Similarly Nummela et al. [18] observed that muscle fatigue measured by the maximal 20 m sprint and maximal isometric leg press tests were not related to the performance in a 5 km time trial. These results suggest that in 5 and 10 km time trials where the runners can freely choose their pacing strategy the higher calibre runners perform the time trial at faster speed than lower calibre athletes but the degree of fatigue or the amount of reduced force production is not different in low and high calibre athlete at the end of the time trial.

A popular model holds that performance during endurance exercise is limited by the homeostasis failure occurred distal to the neuromuscular junction and it is termed "peripheral fatigue" [10]. Another fatigue model termed "central fatigue" holds that the same homeostatic failure occurs in the brain lowering the central activation of the muscles [13]. These models predict that in the maximal exercises humans continue the exercise mindlessly without any anticipatory system until a catastrophic metabolic failure occurs either in muscle or brain. A complementary model called "central governor model" [27, 17] postulates that central nervous system integrates input from various sources during endurance exercise and prevents the recruitment of skeletal muscles beyond levels of intensity and duration where homeostasis could fail or potential damage could occur to the heart or any other vital organs. It has been proposed that an "internal clock" is used by the brain to generate the knowledge of the distance of the activity still to be covered, so that running velocity and metabolic rate can be altered appropriately during the time trial [26]. Therefore analysing the pacing strategy may allow insight into the muscle fatigue and related physiological and regulatory processes.

It is common that an incremental test protocol and the measurement of VO_{2max}, anaerobic threshold and running economy are used to test endurance athletes. If the results are to have high practical value, the test protocol and the environmental circumstances should imitate the event for which the athlete is training. Therefore, in running events the popularity of the so called field tests in which the incremental test protocol is performed on a track instead of treadmill is increasing.

The aim of the present chapter was to determine the factors related to the maximal distance running performance and fatigue in the incremental running test (6 x 1000 m) on a track. We hypothesized that aerobic endurance characteristics as well as neuromuscular factors are related to the maximal endurance performance in the incremental running test. We also hypothesized that the extent of fatigue at the end of the incremental endurance test is not related to the performance in the test but to the performance in a maximal sprint test like in a 5-km time trial. The fatigue was defined in the present chapter as the difference in maximal running velocity in the non-fatigued (maximal sprint test) and fatigued condition (at the end of the incremental running test).

Methods

Nineteen male endurance athletes (seven distance runners, six orienteers and six triathletes) volunteered as subjects for the present study. All the athletes belonged to the national junior teams and their mean ± SD age, height and body mass were: 20.2 ± 1.0 years, 1.81 ± 0.07 m and 70.2 ± 7.8 kg, respectively. They were fully informed of the procedures and possible risks of the experiments and written informed consent was obtained from each athlete. The informed consent was in accordance with the guidelines of the Ethical Committee of the University of Jyväskylä. The tests were part of the athletes' normal exercise testing and they were in compliance with current Finnish laws regarding the testing of human subjects.

In order to measure ground reaction forces and ground contact times at different running speeds in a non-fatigued state and determine maximal sprinting speed the athletes performed 8 x 60 m sprints with increasing speed. In the test the athletes were able to accelerate 40 m to ensure a normal and steady running gait throughout the 9 m measurement section. The speed of the first run was 5.0 $m \cdot s^{-1}$ and thereafter the speed was increased by 0.40 $m \cdot s^{-1}$ after each run until the sixth run (7.0 $m \cdot s^{-1}$). The running velocity was regulated by small lights placed on the next lane at 4.0 m intervals (Naakka Ltd, Lappeenranta, Finland). The athletes were instructed to adjust their velocity to coincide with the lights, which were switched on and off along the track. The last two runs were asked to run at the maximal velocity of each athlete. Each running bout was separated by two minutes recovery period during which the runners returned to the start of the sprint course. A special 9-m long force platform system was placed at the end of the 60-m run. The system consisted of five two dimensional (2D) and three 3D force platforms (0.9 x 1.0 m each, TR Test Ltd, Jyväskylä, Finland, natural frequency in the vertical direction 170 Hz) and one Kistler 3D force platform (0.9 x 0.9 m, Honeycomb, Kistler, Winterthur, Switzerland, 400 Hz) connected in series and covered with a tartan mat. Each force platform registered both vertical and horizontal components of the ground reaction forces. Vertical and horizontal ground reaction forces were recorded by a microcomputer using an AT Codas A/D converter card (Dataq Instruments Inc, Akron, OH, USA) with a sampling frequency of 1000 Hz. In order to measure running velocity two photocell gates were placed on the 9-m measurement section (Ivar Ltd, Tallinn, Estonia).

After a 15 min recovery from the 8 x 60 m runs, an incremental 6 x 1000 m test was performed on a 200 m indoor track. The initial velocity was 2.78 $m \cdot s^{-1}$ for the orienteers and triathletes and 3.33 $m \cdot s^{-1}$ for the distance runners. Thereafter, the velocity was 3.89, 4.44, 5.00 and 5.56 $m \cdot s^{-1}$. The last 1000-m run was performed at their maximal effort. The running velocity in the submaximal runs was regulated by small lights embedded on the inside of the 200-m indoor track at the intervals of 4.0 m (Naakka Ltd, Lappeenranta, Finland). The athletes were instructed to adjust their velocity to coincide with the lights, which were turned on and off inside the track. The athletes performed a total of five or six runs depending on their maximal aerobic work capacity. Subjects were instructed to run the last 1000 m as fast as possible and were provided with verbal encouragement during the run. At the end of each 200-m lap the athletes ran over the 9-m long force platform system as in the 8 x 60 m runs. At the end of the 1000 m, subjects were asked to run at their maximal effort through the 9-m long measurement section. Vertical and horizontal ground reaction forces were recorded in a similar way as in the 8 x 60 m runs.

Cardio-respiratory parameters (Oxycon Mobile, Viasys Healthcare GmbH, Hoechberg, Germany) were measured continuously during the whole incremental test. In the last maximal 1000 m heart rate, oxygen consumption and carbon dioxide production were averaged (15 s) at the end of each lap. Peak oxygen uptake (VO_{2peak}) was defined as the highest oxygen consumption during the time trial over a 60 second period. The oxygen demand of the last 1000 m was calculated using the oxygen uptake values of the 4 - 5 submaximal 1000 m runs. A linear regression line was used to interpolate oxygen consumption of the submaximal runs to the average velocity of the last 1000 m run. Then the aerobic proportion of the energy production of the last 1000 m was calculated by dividing the measured VO_2 by the calculated demand of the VO_2. Running economy was determined as steady-state VO_2 ($ml \cdot kg^{-1} \cdot km^{-1}$) at the velocity of 3.89 $m \cdot s^{-1}$. Fingertip blood samples (20 μl) for blood lactate analysis (Biosen S_line Lab+, EKF Diagnostic GmbH, Magdeburg, Germany) were taken at the end of each 1000-m run. The velocity at 4 mM blood lactate level (V_{4mM}) was determined from the blood lactate vs. running velocity curve [25].

In order to analyze force time curves 3 - 5 contact phases of each subject were averaged for further analysis. The horizontal force-time curve was used to separate the ground reaction forces into the braking and propulsion phases [14]. The integrals of force-time curves were calculated and divided by the respective time period to obtain the average vertical force for the whole contact phase and for horizontal braking and propulsion phases separately. In order to decrease the effect of the body mass, the average force values were divided by body mass. Ground contact times were determined from the time the applied vertical force exceeded 0 N on the force platform. Fatigue was calculated as the velocity difference between the maximal sprinting velocity and the velocity at the end of the 1000 m ($\%V_{fatigue}$). In order to compare the ground reaction forces and contact times in a non-fatigued and fatigued state, one run from the 8 x 60 m with equal velocity to the end of the 1000 m run was selected for further analysis.

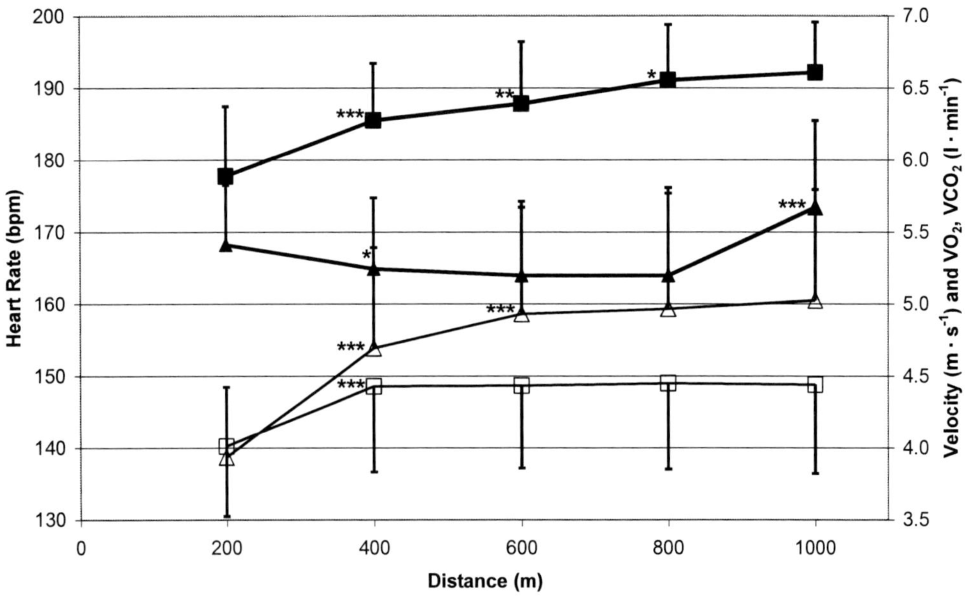

Figure 1. Heart rate (filled squares), running velocity (filled triangles), oxygen uptake (open squares) and carbon dioxide production (open triangles) during the maximal 1000 m run. The asterisks denote the statistical difference compared to the previous value. * $p < 0.05$, ** $p < 0.01$; *** $p < 0.001$

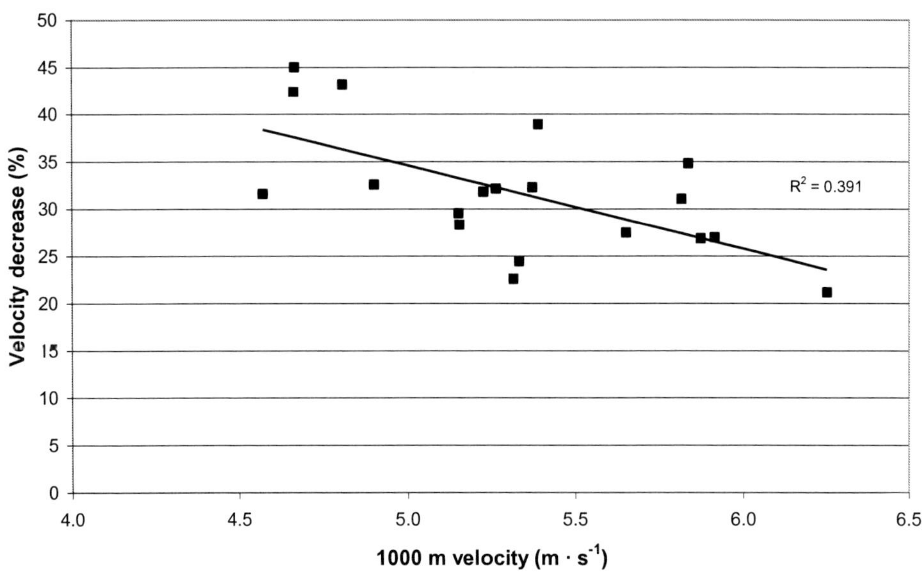

Figure 2. Relationship between the average velocity in the maximal 1000 m run and the difference between maximal velocity in the sprint test and at the end of the maximal 1000 m run.

Standard statistical methods were used to calculate the means, standard deviations and correlation coefficients. A repeated measures analysis of variance (ANOVA) with contrasts (simple) was used to find out the significance of changes of measured parameters during the last 1000-m time trial and to compare the non-fatigued, fatigued and maximal ground reaction forces, ground contact times and velocities. All the statistical analyses were done using SPSSWIN 13.0 (SPSS, Inc., Chicago, ILL, USA).

Table 1. Performance data of 19 endurance athletes

	V_{1000m}	VO_{2max}	La_{peak}	RE	V_{4mM}
	$m \cdot s^{-1}$	$ml \cdot kg^{-1} \cdot min^{-1}$	$mmol \cdot l^{-1}$	$ml \cdot kg^{-1} \cdot km^{-1}$	$m \cdot s^{-1}$
Average	5.33	63.2	11.4	207	4.44
SD	0.48	4.9	2.7	15	0.45

Abbreviations: V_{1000m} = average velocity in the maximal 1000 m; VO_{2peak} = peak oxygen uptake during the maximal 1000 m; La_{peak} = peak blood lactate concentration after the maximal 1000 m; RE = oxygen uptake at 3.89 $m \cdot s^{-1}$; V_{4mM} = velocity at four $mmol \cdot l^{-1}$ blood lactate level; SD = standard deviation.

Table 2. Correlation coefficients between the maximal 1000 m velocity (V_{1000m}) and different performance characteristics and fatigue induced changes in running velocity and stride characteristics at the end of the maximal 1000 m

	r	P
VO_{2max}	0.676	0.001
Anaerobic%	0.629	0.004
La_{peak}	0.448	0.053
RE	-0.469	0.042
V_{4mM}	0.759	0.000
V_{max}	0.516	0.023
$\%V_{fatigue}$	-0.625	0.004
$CT_{fatigue}$	-0.585	0.008
$CT\ Br_{fatigue}$	-0.556	0.013
$CT\ Pr_{fatigue}$	-0.481	0.036
$Fy_{fatigue}$	0.396	0.093
$FxBr_{fatigue}$	0.501	0.028
$FxPr_{fatigue}$	0.201	0.408

Abbreviations: VO_{2max} = peak oxygen uptake during the maximal 1000 m; Anaerobic% = anaerobic energy contribution during the maximal 1000 m; La_{peak} = peak blood lactate concentration after the maximal 1000 m; RE = oxygen uptake at 3.89 $m \cdot s^{-1}$; V_{4mM} = velocity at four $mmol \cdot l^{-1}$ blood lactate level; V_{max} = maximal sprint running velocity; $\%V_{fatigue}$ = difference between the maximal sprint running velocity and the velocity at the end of the 1000 m; $CT_{fatigue}$ = difference in ground contact time between the maximal sprint running test and the end of the 1000 m; $CT\ Br_{fatigue}$ = difference in braking phase of the ground contact time between the maximal sprint running test and the end of the 1000 m; $CT\ Pr_{fatigue}$ = difference in the propulsion phase of the ground contact time between the maximal sprint running test and the end of the 1000 m; $Fy_{fatigue}$ = difference in vertical ground reaction force between the maximal sprint running test and the end of the 1000 m; $FxBr_{fatigue}$ = difference in horizontal ground reaction force during the braking phase between the maximal sprint running test and the end of the 1000 m; $FxPr_{fatigue}$ = difference in horizontal ground reaction force of the propulsion phase between the maximal sprint running test and the end of the 1000 m.

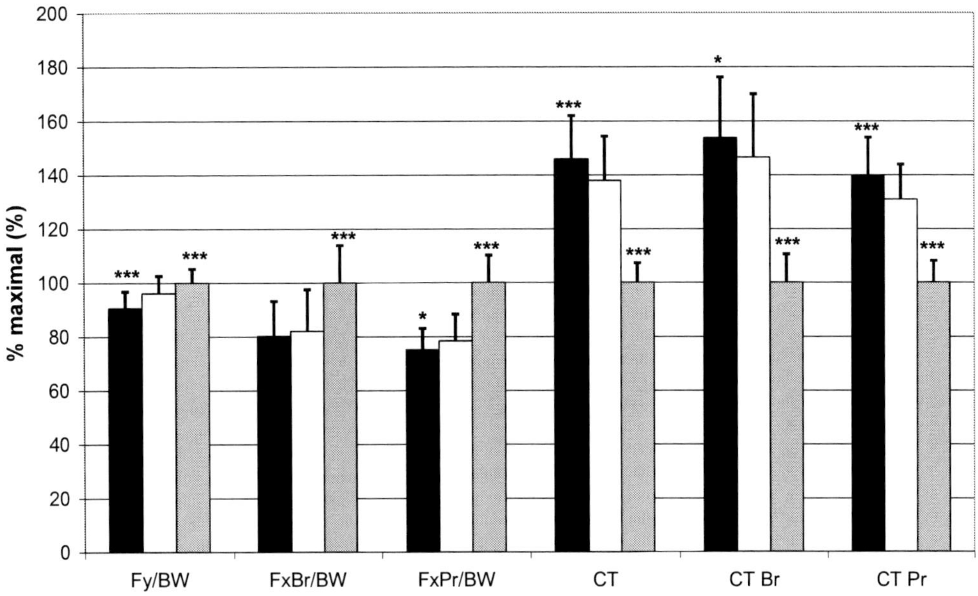

Figure 3. Average vertical forces (Fy/BW), horizontal braking forces (FxBr/BW), horizontal propulsion forces (FxPr/BW), ground contact times (CT), duration of braking phases (CT Br) and the duration of propulsion phases (CT Pr) at the end of the maximal 1000 m (black bars), in the non-fatigued run at the same velocity as at the end of the 1000 m (white bars) and in the maximal sprint running (grey bars). All the values have been related to the values of the maximal sprint run (= 100 %). The values of the fatigued run and maximal sprint run have been compared to the values of the non-fatigued run. * $p < 0.05$; ** $p < 0.01$; *** $p < 0.001$

Results

The averaged performance data is shown in Table 1. The last 1000-m time was 189.2 ± 17.0 s and the proportion of aerobic energy production during the last 1000 m was 87.1 ± 5.8 %. Pacing strategy varied a lot, since the athletes were free to choose their pacing strategy and their experience in track running was not equal. Two athletes increased their velocity throughout the last 1000 m and rest of the athletes had even or negative pacing strategy, which was characterized by an increase in velocity during the last 200-m lap (Figure 1). The average increase in velocity from 800 m to 1000 m was 9.4 ± 7.1 % (P = 0.000) and it was negatively correlated to the proportion of anaerobic energy production (r = -0.57, P = 0.010). Muscle fatigue measured as the velocity difference between the velocity in the maximal sprint test and at the end of the 1000 m ($\%V_{fatigue}$) was 31.7 ± 6.7 %. A significant correlation was observed between V_{1000m} and $\%V_{fatigue}$ as shown in Figure 2. Furthermore, V_{1000m} correlated significantly with VO_{2peak}, V_{4mM}, running economy, maximal sprint running velocity and the proportion of the anaerobic energy production (Table 2). When V_{1000m} was related to the differences in ground contact times and ground reaction forces in the maximal non-fatigued (maximal sprint run) and fatigued (end of the last 1000 m) runs, a significant correlation was observed between the V_{1000m} and the difference in ground contact time ($CT_{fatigue}$) and the horizontal braking force ($FxBr_{fatigue}$) (Table 2). The fatigue index ($\%V_{fatigue}$) was significantly correlated with the VO_{2peak} (r = -0.62, P = 0.005) and V_{4mM} (r = -0.57, P = 0.011).

The results in Figure 3 show that ground contact times increased and vertical ground reaction force and horizontal propulsion force decreased in fatigued compared to non-fatigued run. Heart rate, VO_2 and VCO_2 increased during the 1000-m time trial (Figure 1). VCO_2 increased more than VO_2 during the 1000-m time trial resulting a significant increase in respiratory exchange ratio (RER) from 0.98 ± 0.06 (200 m) to 1.14 ± 0.10 (1000 m) ($P = 0.000$).

Conclusion

In the previous studies, it had been shown that running velocity at maximal oxygen uptake (VO_{2max}) seemed to be the best predictor of performance in middle distance running [12, 24]. Therefore, the average velocity of the last 1000 m run was used as an indicator of running performance in the incremental 6 x 1000 m running test on a track. Di Prampero [6, 7] summarized that VO_{2max}, fractional utilization of VO_{2max} and running economy are the major variables determining the velocity that can be maintained in distance running races. Furthermore, Paavolainen et al. [22, 23] and Nummela et al. [20] have shown that neuromuscular factors may also be important determinants of distance running performance. Therefore, in order to validate the last 1000 m running velocity as an indicator of distance running performance the relationships between V_{1000m} and endurance performance characteristics were determined.

The present results suggest that the last 1000 m in the incremental 6 x 1000 m test on a track can be used to measure distance running performance, since V_{1000m} was significantly correlated with VO_{2max}, V_{4mM} and running economy. The significant correlations between V_{1000m} and maximal sprint running velocity and the proportion of anaerobic energy production suggested that anaerobic and neuromuscular force-velocity characteristics also affect performance in the incremental field test on a track. This supports the model of Paavolainen et al. [22] of distance running performance. In a similar way as VO_{2max} is a measure of the upper limit for aerobic energy delivery, the maximal sprint running velocity may be a measure of the upper limit of the capacity of neuromuscular system to produce power in distance runners as suggested by Nummela et al. [20]. Although maximal sprint running velocity was related to the performance in the last 1000 m, there was no correlation between maximal sprint running velocity and the velocity at the end of the last 1000 m. The reason for this might be that the runners who had the highest maximal running velocities had probably the highest percentages of fast twitch muscle fibres, which are more fatigable than slow twitch muscle fibres. Since faster runners were more fatigued at the end of the test they could not increase their velocity as much as slower runners during the end spurt.

Although the proportion of anaerobic energy production was only 13 % during the last 1000 m in the incremental 6 x 1000 m test, the ability to produce energy by anaerobic pathways affected the performance in the test. The increase in peak blood lactate concentration, VCO_2 and RER during the last 1000 m run also indicated the important role of anaerobic energy production during the last 1000 m run. A significant correlation between V_{1000m} and the proportion of anaerobic energy production suggests that the higher the ability to produce energy by anaerobic pathways, the faster the velocity in the last 1000 m run. Furthermore, a positive but not significant correlation ($r = 0.45$; $P = 0.053$), was observed between V_{1000m} and peak blood lactate concentration after the 6 x 1000 m test. There are also some previous studies which have shown that anaerobic energy yield has an important role in track running performance at distances from 800 m to 5000 m [20, 7, 8].

The average velocity curve of the last 1000 m was similar to the velocity curves measured in longer duration events like a mile and 5000 m [20, 28], which is characterized by fast starts, a period of slower running during the middle of the race, and ended with a significant increase in velocity. At the end of the 1000-m run the athletes could increase their velocity by 9 %, which is much lower than the velocity increase of 34 % in the 5000 m time trial [18]. Although the shape of the velocity curve in the 1000-m run was close to that in the 5000-m run, the huge difference in the increased velocity at the end of the time trial shows that 1000 m is approaching the shorter distances, in which the optimal pacing strategy consists of a faster start followed by slowing down the velocity to the end of the run [28, 9]. The possible reason for the lower velocity increase at the end of the 6 x 1000 m is that muscle fatigue is more severe at the end of the 6 x 1000 m than at the end of the 5000 m.

Muscle fatigue was not measured in the maximal voluntary contraction but a 32 % decrease in running velocity was observed at the end of the 1000-m time trial compared to the maximal sprint test. This is close to the velocity loss of 31 % in 400 m [21] and somewhat higher than the velocity loss of 16 % in 5 km [18] and 23 % in 10 km [23]. Millet and Lepers [15] have observed that after exercise involving running for longer than two hours the loss of strength increases as a non-linear function of the exercise duration. The knee extensor muscle strength loss has been almost 35 % in extremely long running exercises [15]. Therefore, it seems that the greatest force or velocity loss and muscle fatigue can be seen in running exercises lasting 1 - 3 min (400 - 1000 m) and in exercises lasting more than eight hours. The extent of fatigue in the incremental 6 x 1000 m running test is closer to the fatigue in short-term exercises than in 5 or 10-km runs.

The possible reason for the greater velocity loss at the end of 6 x 1000 m compared to 5000 m was that higher percentage of fast twitch muscle fibres and anaerobic metabolism are used in the last 1000 m than in 5000 m [3, 16] and therefore capacity for the end spurt is better after 5000 m than after 1000 m run. This was supported by the findings that in the last 1000 m of the incremental test the decrease in velocity were related to VO_{2max} and V_{4mM} and in 5000 m to the maximal sprinting velocity suggesting that the anaerobic and neuromuscular capacity were more completely used before the end spurt in the 6 x 1000 m than before the end spurt in 5000 m time trial run. The greater contribution of fast twitch muscle fibres in the 1000 m compared to the 5000 m may also be the reason why the V_{1000m} correlated significantly with the muscle fatigue at the end of the 6 x 1000 m ($\%V_{max\text{-}1000m}$) but this was not the case in the 5000-m time trial [18].

The present results confirmed the previous findings that fatigue decreases running velocity, ground reaction forces and increases ground contact times. It is interesting to notice that the ground reaction forces decrease and ground contact times increase similarly in 400 m [21], 1000 m (present results), 10 km [23] and marathon [19], although the causes of muscle fatigue are probably different, for example, in the marathon and 400-m run. The fatigue induced changes were observed both in vertical and horizontal ground reaction forces as well as in braking and propulsion times. Fatigue-induced changes in ground reaction forces and ground contact times were obvious, since in fatigue running velocity decreases and vertical and horizontal components of ground reaction forces and ground contact times are related to running velocity [14, 11]. Therefore, in the present chapter, ground reaction forces and ground contact times were compared in fatigued and non-fatigued running at the same velocity. The results in Figure 3 show that in fatigued running at the end of the 6 x 1000 m test, the changes in ground reaction forces and ground contact times did not only occur as a result of decreased running velocity. These results show that in fatigued running the decreased ability to produce force during ground contact phase is compensated by increasing the time for force production.

Based on the present results it is clear that the incremental running test on a track is a valid method to measure different determinants of distance running performance. It is also clear that distance running performance is influenced not just by factors which are related to oxygen utilization but also by elements which have to do with muscle recruitment by the nervous system and the force production. Thus, the optimal training of distance runners should have a balance between endurance, speed endurance and strength training. Therefore, in the future more studies are needed to investigate the influence of high intensity intervals and strength training on the distance running performance.

The present results show that the performance in the last 1000-m run of the incremental 6 x 1000 m test on a track was related to the traditional determinants of endurance performance as well as maximal sprint running velocity and anaerobic energy production. The results show also that the velocity loss in the 6 x 1000 m was related to the performance in the last 1000 m suggesting that lower calibre runners were more fatigued at the end of the 1000 m than high calibre runners. Finally, the results suggest that the impaired ability to produce force during ground contact phase at the end of 1000-m run was partly compensated by increasing the time for force production.

References

[1] Billat, V., Beillot, J., Jan, J., Rochcongar, P. & Carre, F. (1996). Gender effect on the relationship of time limit at 100% VO_{2max} with other bioenergetic characteristics. *Med Sci Sports Exerc., 28*, 1049-1055.

[2] Billat, V., Faina, M., Sardella, F., Marini, C., Fanton, F., Lupo, S., Faccini, P., De Angelis, M., Koralsztein, J. P. & Dalmonte, A. (1996). A comparison of time to exhaustion at VO_{2max} in elite cyclists, kayak paddlers, swimmers and runners. *Ergonomics., 39*, 267-277.

[3] Busso, T. & Chatagnon, M. (2006). Modelling of aerobic and anaerobic energy production in middle-distance running. *Eur J Appl Physiol., 97*, 745-754.

[4] Conley, D. L. & Krahenbuhl, G. S. (1980). Running economy and distance running performance of highly trained athletes. *Med Sci Sports Exerc., 12*, 357-360.

[5] Costill, D. L., Thomason, H. & Roberts, E. (1973). Fractional utilization of the aerobic capacity during distance running. *Med Sci Sports Exerc., 5*, 248-252.

[6] Di Prampero, P. E. (1986). The energy cost of human locomotion on land and water. Int *J Sports Med., 7*, 55-72.

[7] Di Prampero, P. E. (2003). Factors limiting maximal performance in humans. *Eur J Appl Physiol., 90*, 420-429.

[8] Di Prampero, P. E., Capelli, C., Pagliaro, P., Antonutto, G., Girardis, M., Zamparo, P. & Soule, R. G. (1993). Energetics of best performances in middle-distance running. *Eur J Appl Physiol., 74*, 2318-2324.

[9] Ferro, A., Rivera, A., Pagola, I., Ferreruela, M., Martin, A. & Rocandio, V. (2001). Biomechanical analysis of the 7th *World Championships in Athletics Seville.*, 1999. *IAAF New Studies in Athletics, 16*, 25-60.

[10] Fitts, R. H. (1994). Cellular mechanisms of muscle fatigue. *Physiol Rev., 74*, 49-94.

[11] Hill, D. W. (1999). Energy system contributions in middle-distance running events. *J Sports Sci., 17*, 477-483.

[12] Lacour, J. R., Padilla-Magunacelaya, S., Chatard, J. C. & Arsac, L. (1991). Barthelemy, J.C. Assessment of running velocity at maximal oxygen uptake. *Eur J Appl Physiol., 62*, 77-82.

[13] Lepers, R., Millet, G. Y. & Maffiuletti, N. A. (2001). Effects of cycling cadence on contractile and neural properties of knee extensors. *Med Sci Sports Exerc., 33*, 1882-1888.

[14] Mero, A. & Komi, P. V. (1986). Force, EMG-, and elasticity-velocity relationships at submaximal and supramaximal running speeds in sprinters. *Eur J Appl Physiol., 55*, 553-561.

[15] Millet, G. Y. & Lepers, R. (2004). Alterations of neuromuscular function after prolonged running, cycling and skiing exercises. *Sports Med., 34*, 105-116.

[16] Nicol, C., Komi, P. V. & Marconnet, P. (1991). Fatigue effects of marathon running on neuromuscular performance. I. Changes I muscle force and stiffness characteristics. *Scand J Med Sci Sports., 1*, 10-17.

[17] Noakes, T. D., St Clair Gibson, A. & Lambert, E. V. (2005). From catastrophe to complexity: a novel model of integrative central neural regulation of effort and fatigue during exercise in humans. Summary and conclusions. *Br J Sports Med., 39*, 120-124.

[18] Nummela, A. T., Heath, K. A., Paavolainen, L. M., Lambert, M. I., St Clair Gibson, A., Rusko, H. K. & Noakes, T. D. (2008). Fatigue during a 5-km running time trial. *Int J Sports Med., 29*, 738-745.

[19] Nummela, A., Keränen, T. & Mikkelsson, L. O. (2007). Factors related to top running speed and economy. *Int J Sports Med., 28*, 655-661.

[20] Nummela, A. T., Paavolainen, L. P., Sharwood, K. A., Lambert, M. I., Noakes, T. D. & Rusko, H. K. (2006). Neuromuscular factors determining 5 km running performance and running economy in well-trained athletes. *Eur J Appl Physiol., 97*, 1-8.

[21] Nummela, A., Rusko, H. & Mero, A. (1994). EMG activities and ground reaction forces during fatigued and nonfatigued sprinting. *Med Sci Sports Exerc., 26*, 605-609.

[22] Paavolainen, L., Häkkinen, K., Hämäläinen, I., Nummela, A. & Rusko, H. (1999). Explosive strength-training improves 5-km running time by improving running economy and muscle power. *J Appl Physiol., 86*, 1527-1533.

[23] Paavolainen, L., Nummela, A., Rusko, H. & Häkkinen, K. (1999). Neuromuscular characteristics and fatigue during 10 km running. *Int J Sports Med., 20*, 1-6.

[24] Padilla, S., Bourdin, M., Barthelemy, J. C. & Lacour, J. R. (1992). Physiological correlates of middle-distance running performance. *Eur J Appl Physiol., 65*, 561-566.

[25] Sjödin, B. & Jacobs, I. (1981). Onset of blood lactate accumulation and marathon running performance. *Int J Sports Med., 2*, 23-26.

[26] St Clair Gibson, A., Lambert, E. V., Rauch, L. H. G., Tucker, R., Baden, D. A., Foster, C. & Noakes, T. D. (2006). The role of information processing between the brain and peripheral physiological systems in pacing and perception of effort. *Sports Med., 36*, 705-722.

[27] St Clair Gibson, A. & Noakes, T. D. (2004). Evidence of complex system integration and dynamic neural regulation of skeletal muscle recruitment during exercise in humans. *Br J Sports Med., 38*, 797-806.

[28] Tucker, R., Lambert, M. I. & Noakes, T. D. (2006). An analysis of pacing strategies during men's world record performances in track athletes. *Int J Sports Physiol Perf., 1*, 297-309.

[29] Weston, A. R., Karamizrak, O., Smith, A., Noakes, T. D. & Myburgh, K. H. (1999). African runners exhibit greater fatigue resistance, lower lactate accumulation, and higher oxidative enzyme activity. *J Appl Physiol., 86*, 915-923.

In: Encyclopedia of Sports and Athletics
Editors: Jack L. Murray and Emily O. Watson
ISBN: 978-1-61209-959-0

Chapter XII

Aerobic Exercise Capacity and Its Relationship with Pulmonary Function, Muscle Strength, Physical Activity and Motor Competence in Preterm Born Children: The PREMAFIT-Pilot Study

Tim Takken[1*], Ingrid C. van Haastert[2], Wilco L. Scholman[1], Annelie J. Block[1], Marian J.C. Eijsermans[1], Linda S. de Vries[2] and Paul J. M. Helders[1]

[1]Child Development & Exercise Center, Wilhelmina Children's Hospital, University Medical Center, Utrecht, the Netherlands
[2]Department of Neonatology, Wilhelmina Children's Hospital, University Medical Center Utrecht, the Netherlands

Abstract

Purpose

To describe the aerobic exercise capacity and its relationship with muscle strength and motor competence in fifteen preterm born school-aged children (9 boys; gestational age (GA) 29.7 ± 1.71 weeks; birth weight (BW) 1313 ± 356 gram; age of assessment 7.99 ± 0.35 years).

Methods

Weight, height and skinfolds were measured in a standardized manner. Muscle strength was assessed with a hand-held dynamometer, pulmonary function using a

* Corresponding author: Child Development & Exercise Center, Wilhelmina Children's Hospital, University Medical Center Utrecht, Room KB2.056.0, PO Box 85090, NL 3508 AB Utrecht, The Netherlands., Phone: +31 88 7554030, Fax: +31 88 7555333, E-mail: t.takken@umcutrecht.nl

spirometer, aerobic exercise capacity using a graded treadmill exercise test, and motor competence with the Movement Assessment Battery for Children. In addition, a 3-day physical activity record was filled out.

Results

Aerobic exercise capacity, lower extremity muscle strength and pulmonary function were significantly reduced compared to reference values. Aerobic exercise capacity was associated with pulmonary function and BW.

Conclusion

In our pilot study of preterm born children we found a reduced aerobic exercise capacity and lower extremity muscle strength in our group. Encouragement of active participation in physical activities from early childhood onwards might be important indicated in preterm born children.

Keywords: exercise capacity, prematurity, muscle strength, physical activity

Introduction

With the high survival rates of preterm (PT) born children, there is not only a growing interest in their neuromotor development, but also in their physical functioning and physical fitness. Children with extremely low birth weight (ELBW; <1000 gram) are often smaller in stature compared with their peers. They show poor school performance, motor skill impairments and lower motor proficiency [1].

Several studies have assessed the long term medical, motor and cognitive consequences of premature birth. Studies either reported a lower peak oxygen uptake ($\dot{V}O_{2peak}$) [2-4], or a similar $\dot{V}O_{2peak}$ in PT born children compared with children born at term [5, 6]. It has been suggested that lower performance ability might only be evident in children with ELBW (<1000g), but not in very low birth weight children (VLBW, 1000-1500g)[7]. However, Kriemler et al found a reduced mechanical efficiency in both children with VLBW and ELBW with chronic lung disease [6]. This higher metabolic cost is important for participation, as it may cause early fatigue during prolonged exercise [6].

Possible explanations for the reduced exercise capacity of PT born children are: pulmonary limitation due to reduced soluble gas transfer [8] or exercise-induced bronchoconstriction [6], less metabolically active muscles [9], likely due to a sedentary lifestyle [2, 3], or a lower motor performance [6, 10], mechanical inefficiency and an increased oxygen cost of locomotion [5, 11].

However, relative little is known about the relationship of aerobic exercise capacity with other variables such as muscle strength, physical activity and motor performance in school-aged PT born children. Recently the relationship between a physical inactive lifestyle and a poor motor performance was observed in children [12]. Moreover, a lot of studies have observed a relationship between physical activity and aerobic exercise capacity in various childhood chronic conditions [13-15]. Therefore aim of the current study was firstly to compare muscle strength, pulmonary function, aerobic exercise capacity, physical activity and motor performance in 7 to 8 year old PT born children with reference values, and secondly to study the correlations between these outcomes.

Methods

Participants

Fifteen PT born children (9 boys and 6 girls; gestational age (GA) 29.7 ± 1.71 weeks, birth weight (BW) 1313 ± 356 gram; age of assessment 7.99 ± 0.35 years,) participated in this pilot study. All children were born in 1998. Nine children were preterm born (GA 30-32 weeks) and six were very preterm born (GA < 30 weeks). Six children had a low birth weight (< 2000 gram), six a very low (< 1500 gram) and three an extremely low birth weight (< 1000 gram). Twelve children were appropriate for gestational age and three were large for gestational age.

Initially, 30 children and their parents were approached to participate in this study. These were children who performed a Movement ABC test two years earlier at the age of 5 years during their regular medical follow-up at the Department of Neonatology of our tertiary university hospital. No children with Cerebral Palsy were included in the study. Fifty percent of the children and their parents gave consent to participate. The major reasons not to participate was the amount of travel distance to the hospital and time constraints. There were no significant differences in with respect to BW, GA and Movement ABC score at the age of 5 years between the participants and non-participants.

All procedures were approved by the Medical Ethics Committee of our institution. All patients and parents provided informed consent.

Physical Activity Record

A 3-day activity record was used to estimate energy expenditure (EE) as has been described by Bouchard et al. [16]. On two weekly days and one day in the weekend, the children had to fill out the activity record every 15 minutes. This method estimates the EE using a factorial approach in which the entire day (24 hours) is divided into 96 periods of 15 minutes each. The subjects were instructed to quantify their activity, on a scale of 1–9 (1= sleeping, 9=maximal exercise intensity), in a diary using a list of activities and their categorical values (1 to 9). By summing the activity scores throughout the day, an estimate of the EE was obtained. This value was then expressed per kilogram body mass. The activity record has been shown to be reliable [16].

Anthropometry

Standing body height and weight were measured in a standardized manner using calibrated scales (Seca, Hamburg, Germany) and a wall-mounted measuring stick without shoes and heavy clothing, to the nearest cm, and 100 g, respectively. Frontal occipital head circumference (FOC) was also measured. From the values weight and height, the body mass index (BMI; kg/m^2) was calculated. The values of height, FOC, weight and BMI were compared with reference values for healthy subjects matched for age and sex, and Z-scores were calculated [17].

Body composition was assessed using the sum of 7 skin folds (Σ skin folds) according to the method of Pollack et al [18]. The measurements were taken in triplicate at 7 sites at the right side of the body in accordance with the American College of Sports Medicine guidelines [19], using Harpenden skin fold callipers (Baty International, Burgess Hill, Sussex, U.K.), by an experienced assessor (TT). The sites were biceps, triceps, supra iliacal, sub-scapular, mid-abdominal, medial thigh, and calf. The sum of the mean value of each of the 7 sites was used as an index for subcutaneous adiposity [18].

Muscle Strength

Muscle strength of proximal and distal muscles in the upper and lower extremities were measured with a calibrated hand-held dynamometer (Citec dynamometer type CT 3001, C.I.T. Technics, Groningen, the Netherlands) [20]. Measurements were performed three times consecutively using the 'break method' and the highest value was registered as described previously [20]. In the upper extremity, shoulder abductors, wrist extensors, and grip strength were measured whereas in the lower extremity the hip flexors and knee and dorsal foot extensors were measured. All tests were performed by the same assessor (TT) using the same hand held dynamometer to prevent inter instrument and interobserver bias [21]. Test-retest reliability in hand-held dynamometry in children has been established previously [22, 23].

Pulmonary Function

The pulmonary function studies were performed using a portable spirometer (Microloop, Micro Medical Ltd., Rochester, Kent, UK). It has been shown that the pulmonary values obtained by the Microloop are comparable with the values obtained in a pulmonary function laboratory [24]. Lung function measurements included forced expiratory volume in 1 second (FEV1), and forced vital capacity (FVC). Each subject performed at least 3 forced expiratory maneuvers, using a noseclip, in a standing position. The results were compared with predicted values for healthy subjects matched for age, body height and gender [25]. Pulmonary function can be reliably assessed in young children [26].

Aerobic Exercise Capacity

The child's aerobic exercise capacity was determined by treadmill (Enmill, Enraf, Delft, The Netherlands) exercise testing and a respiratory gas analysis system [27].

Previous studies have shown that exercise capacity (i.e. peak oxygen uptake; $\dot{V}O_{2peak}$) is a reliable and valid measurement in both healthy [28, 29] and diseased children [30, 31]. The $\dot{V}O_{2peak}$ attained during a graded maximal exercise to volitional exhaustion is considered by the World Health Organization as the single best indicator of aerobic fitness [32]. This variable is also a valid indicator of health status [33] and a powerful predictor of mortality in both healthy and diseased individuals [34].

We used a modified version of the Bruce protocol, in which the step duration was reduced to 1.5 min. The initial speed was 2.7 km/hr, and the slope was 10%. Thereafter the speed increased every 1.5 min with 0.7 km/hr and the slope was increased with 1% every 1.5 minute until volitional exhaustion of the patient. The protocol continued until the child voluntary gave up due to exhaustion and despite verbal encouragement of the test leader. During the test, heart rate (HR) and gas exchange variables were measured using a heart-rate monitor (Polar) and a calibrated mobile gas analysis system (Cortex Metamax B^3, Cortex Medical GmbH, Leipzig, Germany). The Cortex Metamax is a valid and reliable system for measuring ventilatory parameters during exercise [35]. The mobile gas analysis system consisted of a facemask, a transmitting unit (containing O_2 and CO_2 gas analyzers), and a receiving unit. The transmitting unit and facemask with tubing (total weight 0.57 kg) were attached to the child with a harness. The receiving unit was connected to a computer, located near the transmitting unit. Metabolic stress test software (Metasoft, Version 2.6, Cortex Medical GmbH, Leipzig, Germany) was used to measure and calculate breath-by-breath minute ventilation ($\dot{V}E$), oxygen uptake ($\dot{V}O_2$), carbon dioxide production ($\dot{V}CO_2$), respiratory exchange ratio (RER = $\dot{V}CO_2/\dot{V}O_2$) and HR.

Absolute peak oxygen uptake ($\dot{V}O_{2peak}$) was taken as the average value over the last 30 seconds during the maximal exercise test. Relative VO_{2peak} ($VO_{2peak/kg}$) was calculated as absolute $\dot{V}O_{2peak}$ divided by body mass. Breathing reserve was calculated as maximum voluntary ventilation (MVV; = FEV1 × 40) - $\dot{V}E$.[36] Predicted $\dot{V}O_{2peak}$ values were obtained from established values from age- and gender- matched Dutch reference values [37].

Motor Performance

The movement assessment battery for children (Movement-ABC) is a performance test to assess the motor competence of a child and to identify substantial motor difficulties [38, 39]. The Movement-ABC is a standardized, discriminative, evaluative and norm-referenced tool for children aged between 4 and 12 years. The test measures three different aspects of motor performance i.e. manual dexterity (MD), ball skills (BS), static and dynamical balance (SDB). Aspects of function with regard to MD are speed and sureness of movement by each hand (MD 1), the coordination of the two hands for the performance of a single operation (MD 2) and hand-eye coordination as it is required in the control of a pen or pencil (MD 3). Aspects of function with regard to BS are the ability to (propel and) catch a moving object (BS 1) and the ability to accurately propel an object into space (BS 2). Finally, aspects with regard to SDB are static control (SDB 1), dynamic balance: the ability to produce (and control) fast and explosive movements (SDB 2) and the ability to move slowly and make spatially precise movements (SDB 3).

The Movement-ABC test consists of eight items for each four age groups: 4- 6, 7-8, 9-10 and 11-12^{+} years. In this study the age-band 7-8 was used. Percentile scores of the child's motor abilities, derived from raw subscores or a total impairment score (TIS: ranging from 0-40; the lower the score, the better the performance), were compared with a normative age-matched sample of children [38]. A TIS score equal to or below the 5th percentile indicates that a child has a severe disturbance in motor performance. A TIS score between the 5th and the 15th percentile indicates that the child is at risk for this disturbance. A TIS score above the 15th percentile is considered adequate [38].

Statistics

Statistical analyses were performed using the Statistical Package for the Social Sciences for Windows (version 12.0, SPSS Inc, Chicago, Ill). One-sample T-tests were used to test differences between patients and reference values. Correlations were calculated using Pearson's correlation coefficient for parametric values and Spearman's correlation for non-parametric values. Non-parametric statistics were used when variables were not normally distributed according to the Shapiro-Wilk test. Alpha level was set at $p < 0.05$ for all analyses.

Results

All children completed all tests. Body height and weight, BMI and FOC are displayed in Table 1. Average sum of the 7 skin folds was 56.7 ± 24.6 mm, and was significantly correlated with BMI ($r=0.82$, $p<0.0001$).

All children were attending regular schools. None of the children underwent any eye corrections or wore glasses. Two children used bronchodilatory medication (short-acting β2 antagonists) on a regular basis, however the children and their parents were instructed not to use any medication on the day of assessment, until the tests were over.

Every child participated in physical education classes with an average of 1.68 ± 0.38 hours per week. Twelve children participated in regular sports, with a mean of 1.13 ± 0.35 hours per week. Thirteen children used an active mode of transportation to and from school (walking or cycling). From the 15 participants in our study, 11 returned the 3-day physical activity record (7 boys and 4 girls). The average daily EE was 47.07 ± 3.4 Kcal/kg. There was a significant correlation between the hours of sports per week and the daily EE derived from the physical activity record ($r=0.56$, $p = 0.048$). More participation in sport activities was related to a higher EE.

Table 1. Patient characteristics

	Mean ± SD (range)	Z-score	P-value
Body height (m)	1.33 ± 0.6 (1.23 - 1.47)	0.17 ± 1.1	NS
Body weight (kg)	26.3 ± 4.5 (19.2 - 33.4)	-0.14 ± 1.26	NS
BMI (kg/m^2)	14.83 ± 1.36 (12.8 - 17.3)	-0.41 ± 1.26	NS
FOC (cm)	52.4 ± 1.9 (48 - 55)	-0.30 ± 1.15	NS

Legend: BMI = body mass index; FOC= Frontal Occipital head Circumference.

Z-scores for muscle strength were -0.22 ± 0.85 for the shoulder abductors (NS), -0.37 ± 0.77 for the wrist extensors (NS), -0.81 ± 0.86 for the grip strength (p=0.004), -1.57 ± 0.8 for the hip flexors (p=0.0001), -1.17 ± 0.58 for the knee extensors (p=0.0001), and 0.06 ± 1.13 for the foot dorsal flexors (NS).

A reduced pulmonary function was observed, mean FEV_1 was 1.38 ± 0.3 mL, which was 81.6 ± 15.9 % of predicted ($P < 0.0001$). The FVC was 1.59 ± 0.33 L, which was 79 ±13 % of predicted ($P < 0.0001$) in PT born children. FEV1/FVC ratio was 87.5 ± 10.9, which was 102.3 ± 13.2% of predicted.

All children performed the treadmill exercise test to volitional exhaustion. Peak heart rate (HR_{peak}) was 176 ± 22.3 (range 138-203) and peak Respiratory Exchange Ratio (RER_{peak}) 1.06 ± 0.08. Ten children had a HR_{peak} >180 (HR_{peak} > 90% of predicted) and eleven a RER_{peak} > 1.0. The HR_{peak} of the boys was significantly higher compared to the girls (186 ±18.7 vs 161 ± 19.8 beats per min; $p < 0.05$).

Mean Z-scores for $\dot{V}O_{2peak}$ and $\dot{V}O_{2peak}$/kg were significantly lower compared to healthy children (Table 2). Five children had a Z-score for $\dot{V}O_{2peak}$ below -2 SD. There was no significant difference in Z-score for $\dot{V}O_{2peak}$, $\dot{V}O_{2peak}$ /kg and endurance time between boys and girls. Peak $\dot{V}E/\dot{V}O_2$ was 91.4 ±14.4% of predicted ($p = 0.13$) and peak $\dot{V}E/\dot{V}CO_2$ was 100.96 ± 13.7 % of predicted (NS). Ventilatory anaerobic threshold occurred at 69 % ± 13.6 (range 53 – 94%) of their $\dot{V}O_{2peak}$, and at 56% ± 12 (range 33 - 75%) of their predicted $\dot{V}O_{2peak}$. The mean breathing reserve (BR) was 58 ± 24.1 %; two children, with severe bronchopulmonary dysplasia (BPD) in their history, showed a pulmonary limitation at peak exercise (BR < 0). Children with a HR_{peak} >180 or a RER_{peak} >1.0 still had a significantly reduced $\dot{V}O_{2peak}$, and $\dot{V}O_{2peak}$/kg.

The mean percentile score on the Movement-ABC was 56 ± 33 (range 9 –96), indicating a normal motor performance. However, two children had scores < P5 and three children between P5-15 on ball skills. One child had a balance skill score <P5 and one child had a score of P5-15 for manual dexterity. Scores on motor performance were neither significantly associated with GA, nor with BW.

Table 2. Exercise capacity in preterm born children compared to reference values

	Mean ± SD (range)	Z score mean ± SD	P-value
$\dot{V}O_{2peak}$ (L/min)	1.07 ± 0.22 (0.765 - 1.43)	-1.1 ± 0.73	< 0.0001
$\dot{V}O_{2peak}$/kg (ml/kg/min)	41.35 ± 8.67 (28.4 - 53.7)	-1.08 ± 1.3	< 0.09
Endurance time (min)	8.93 ± 2.23 (5.43 - 14.25)	-2.57 ± 1.88	< 0.0001
HR_{peak} (beats/min)	176.07 ± 22.3 (138 – 203)	-2.77 ± 2.42	< 0.0001
$\dot{V}E_{peak}$ (L/min)	40.36 ± 11.97 (24.8 - 58.0)	-1.78 ± 1.50	< 0.0001

Legend: $\dot{V}O_{2peak}$: peak oxygen uptake, HR_{peak}: peak heart rate, $\dot{V}E_{peak}$: peak ventilatory exchange.

Correlations

The correlations between various variables can be appreciated from Table 3. In addition, BW was significantly correlated with current weight (r=0.70, p=0.005) and Movement ABC percentile score was significantly correlated with BMI (r=0.567, p<0.05).

Table 3. Correlations between cardiopulmonary fitness, muscle strength and motor competence

	BW	MABC	Pulmonary Function	$\dot{V}O_{2peak}$	$\dot{V}O_{2peak}$/kg	Physical activity	Muscle strength
BW	1	NS	NS	r=.55	NS	NS	NS
MABC	NS	1	NS	NS	NS		Ball skills-grip strength r=.562
Pulmonary Function	NS	NS	1	FEV1 r=.62, FEV1/FVC r=.62	NS	NS	FVC-gripstrength r=.54, FEV1/FVC-kee extensor r=.64
$\dot{V}O_{2peak}$	r=.55	NS	FEV1 r=.62 FEV1/FVC r=.62	1	r=.53	NS	Knee extensors r=.58
$\dot{V}O_{2peak}$/kg		NS	NS	r=.53	1	NS	NS
Physical activity	r=.71	Ball skills (r=.647)	NS	NS	NS	1	NS
Muscle strength	NS	Ball skills-grip strength r=.56	FVC-grip strength r=.54, FEV1/FVC-kee extensor r=.64	Knee extensors r=.58	NS	NS	1

Legend: NS: not significant, BW: birth weight, MABC: movement ABC, $\dot{V}O_{2peak}$: peak oxygen uptake, FEV1: Forced Expiratory Volume in 1 sec, FVC: Forced Vital Capacity, FEV1/FVC: ratio of the FEV1 to the FVC of the lungs.

Discussion

The main finding in this pilot study was the significantly reduced aerobic exercise capacity in 15 PT born children of 7-8 years of age. One third of our children had an aerobic exercise capacity lower than minus two standard deviations when compared to reference values. A reduced $\dot{V}o_{2peak}$ was also reported in other studies [2, 9, 40], but other studies reported no significant difference in $\dot{V}o_{2peak}$ between prematurely born children and children born at term [5, 6, 41, 42]. These differences might be explained by the heterogeneity of the characteristics of the included subjects such as BW, pulmonary function and age at assessment.

$\dot{V}O_{2peak}$ was also significantly related to HR_{peak}, suggesting that some children terminated the test for other reasons than cardiovascular limitations [43]. The negative correlation between breathing reserve and $\dot{V}o_{2peak}$/kg endorses this suggestion. Children with the lowest breathing reserve were able to perform with a higher intensity and had the highest $\dot{V}o_{2peak}$/kg. There is an indication that the reason for the five children to terminate the exercise test before they had reached their maximal level, was due to muscular fatigue. Even in the children with a $HR_{peak} > 180$ or a $RER > 1.0$, a significantly reduced $\dot{V}o_{2peak}$ and $\dot{V}o_{2peak}$/kg was observed. This indicates that the reduced exercise capacity was not simply the result of premature (sub-maximal) termination of the exercise test. The reason why girls gave up at a lower HR_{peak} than boys is unclear. Data from our own laboratory shows that there is no significant difference in HR_{peak} between boys and girls during peak exercise [44].

From current literature it is well known that a reduced aerobic capacity has an important impact on general health and well being in childhood as well as in adolescence [45, 46]. We observed significantly reduced muscle strength in knee and hip muscles as well as in grip strength, which is in accord with Rogers et al who found a reduced muscle strength in ELBW patients in late adolescence [3]. However, others did not find a reduced muscle strength in ELBW-born adolescents [1]. Differences in measurement method and patient selection might explain these controversial findings. The significant correlation between grip strength and ball skills on the Movement-ABC suggests that a reduced muscle strength of the hand might influence performance on ball skill tasks.

Keller et al [10] found a deficient neuromotor control in ELBW children. Reduced muscle strength in the lower extremities might be related to these problems in motor control and subsequently leading to muscular fatigue during exercise activities in these children [47]. The moderate correlation between knee extensor strength and $\dot{V}o_{2peak}$ might partly explain this phenomenon. However, there was no significant correlation between muscle strength and HR_{peak}.

The reduced pulmonary function is in accordance with previous studies of PT born children with or without BPD [2, 6, 8, 40]. $\dot{V}o_{2peak}$ and pulmonary function were significantly related, suggesting a relationship between oxygen uptake and pulmonary function. Vrijlandt et al [48] showed that prematurely born adolescents still had subtle reductions in pulmonary function and exercise capacity at the age of 19 years.

Pulmonary function improves with age, but adolescents who were born prematurely might still have a reduced pulmonary function due to airway obstruction and a lower diffusion capacity [48]. Assisted ventilation, a higher oxygen concentration, the absence of lung fluid, maternal factors (e.g. smoking, stress, substance abuse) or placental malfunctioning influence intra-uterine lung development and can cause an airway obstruction in the small airways and a reduction in soluble gas transfer in children leading to BPD [8]. This was the case in two children of our sample.

From studies of motor development it is known that many prematurely born children show a different developmental trajectory, but a catch-up at the age of 18 months [49]. As there are no conclusive data on the developmental course of aerobic capacity in these children, it is unknown whether they also show a catch-up effect in this area and at what age. It is also unknown which factors are pivotal in influencing the developmental course on exercise capacity and whether exercise and/or nutritional interventions are effective. A long-term follow-up study showed subtle reductions in exercise capacity and pulmonary function in a group of prematurely born adolescents at the age of 19 [48]. Moreover, another study reported a reduced participation in physical activities during late adolescence in ELBW teens [3]. Therefore, we encourage prematurely born children to participate in physical activities and sports from early childhood onwards, to improve exercise capacity and physical fitness. The final period of gestation is important for the development of lungs, bones and muscles. Several studies showed that that a passive range of motion exercise program in premature infants resulted in increased weight gain, bone width, and bone mineral density [50, 51]. These studies indicated that exercise interventions should start soon after birth.

There are several limitations of this study. Firstly, there were only 15 PT born children with a heterogeneous neonatal status included and compared to norm-referenced outcomes. A selection bias can not be ruled out. However, the majority of the findings are in accord with other published studies. Secondly, the use of reference values can be disputed, although they provide a robust benchmark against which patients can be compared. The use of a relative small control group can result in a selection bias of active children who enjoy exercising and physical activities which will give an 'above average' norm.

Conclusion

In conclusion, in this pilot-study we found a reduced exercise capacity and lower extremity muscle strength in our group of prematurely born children of 7-8 years of age. Aerobic exercise capacity was associated with pulmonary function and BW. No association was found between aerobic exercise capacity and motor performance.

Longitudinal studies are needed to find out whether the reduction in aerobic exercise capacity is transient, if so at what age these children show a catch-up effect and which factors are pivotal in improving aerobic exercise capacity in these group. Although there is no evidence until now that exercise interventions may improve aerobic exercise capacity in prematurely born children, encouragement of active participation in physical activities and sports might be important in these children.

References

[1] Small, E; Bar-Or O; van Mil E; Saigal S. Muscle function of 11- to 17-year- old children of extremely low birthweight. *Pediatric Exercise Science.*, 1998, 10, 327-36.

[2] Kilbride, HW; Gelatt, MC; Sabath, RJ. Pulmonary function and exercise capacity for ELBW survivors in preadolescence: effect of neonatal chronic lung disease. *J Pediatr.*, 2003, 143(4), 488-93.

[3] Rogers, M; Fay, TB; Whitfield, MF; Tomlinson, J; Grunau, RE. Aerobic capacity, strength, flexibility, and activity level in unimpaired extremely low birth weight (<or=800 g) survivors at 17 years of age compared with term-born control subjects. *Pediatrics.*, 2005, 116(1), e58-65.

[4] Smith, LJ; van Asperen, PP; McKay, KO; Selvadurai, H; Fitzgerald, DA. Reduced exercise capacity in children born very preterm. *Pediatrics.*, 2008, 122(2), e287-93.

[5] Baraldi, E; Zanconato, S; Zorzi, C; Santuz, P; Benini, F; Zacchello, F. Exercise performance in very low birth weight children at the age of 7-12 years. *Eur J Pediatr.*, 1991, 150(10), 713-6.

[6] Kriemler, S; Keller, H; Saigal, S; Bar-Or, O. Aerobic and lung performance in premature children with and without chronic lung disease of prematurity. *Clin J Sport Med.* 2005, 15(5):349-55.

[7] Falk, B; Eliakim, A; Dotan, R; Liebermann, DG; Regev, R; Bar-Or, O. Birth weight and physical ability in 5- to 8-yr-old healthy children born prematurely. *Med Sci Sports Exerc.*, 1997, 29(9), 1124-30.

[8] Mitchell, SH; Teague, WG. Reduced gas transfer at rest and during exercise in school-age survivors of bronchopulmonary dysplasia. *Am J Respir Crit Care Med.*, 1998, 157(5 Pt 1), 1406-12.

[9] Pianosi, PT; Fisk, M. Cardiopulmonary exercise performance in prematurely born children. *Pediatr Res.*, 2000, 47(5), 653-8.

[10] Keller, H; Ayub, BV; Saigal, S; Bar-Or, O. Neuromotor ability in 5-to 7-year-old children with very low or extremely low birthweight. *Dev Med Child Neurol.*, 1998, 40(10), 661-6.

[11] Hebestreit, H; Bar-Or, O. Exercise and the child born prematurely. *Sports Med.*, 2001, 31(8), 591-9.

[12] Wrotniak, BH; Epstein, LH; Dorn, JM; Jones, KE; Kondilis, VA. The relationship between motor proficiency and physical activity in children. *Pediatrics.*, 2006, 118(6), e1758-65.

[13] Takken, T; Henneken, T; van de Putte E; Helders, P; Engelbert, R. Exercise testing in children and adolescents with chronic fatigue syndrome. *Int J Sports Med.* 2007, 28(7):580-4.

[14] Janz, KF; Dawson, JD; Mahoney, LT. Tracking physical fitness and physical activity from childhood to adolescence: the muscatine study. *Med Sci Sports Exerc.*, 2000, 32(7), 1250-7.

[15] Takken, T; Van der Net, J; Kuis, W; Helders, PJ. Physical activity and health related physical fitness in children with juvenile idiopathic arthritis. *Annals of the Rheumatic Diseases.*, 2003, 62(9), 885-9.

[16] Bouchard, C; Tremblay, A; LeBlanc, C; Lortie, G; Savard, R. A method to assess energy expenditure in children and adults. *American Journal of Clinical Nutrition.* 1983, 37, 461-7.

[17] Gerver, W; De Bruin, R. Peadiatric Morphometrics, a reference manual. Utrecht, the *Netherlands: Bunge*, 1996.

[18] Pollack, ML; Schmidt, DH; Jackson, AS. Measurement of cardio-respiratory fitness and body composition in the clinical setting. *Compr Ther.*, 1980, 6(9):12-27.

[19] Latin, RW. Surface anatomy. In: Roitman JL; editor. ACSM's resource manual for guidelines for exercise testing and prescription. Third edition ed. Baltimore: *Williams and Wilkins*, 1998. 89-100.

[20] Beenakker, EA; van der Hoeven, JH; Fock, JM; Maurits, NM. Reference values of maximum isometric muscle force obtained in 270 children aged 4-16 years by hand-held dynamometry. *Neuromuscul Disord.*, 2001, 11(5), 441-6.

[21] Click Fenter, P; Bellew, JW; Pitts, T; Kay, R. A comparison of 3 hand-held dynamometers used to measure hip abduction strength. *J Strength Cond Res.*, 2003, 17(3):531-5.

[22] Brussock, C; Haley, S; Munsat, T; Bernhardt, D. Measurement of isometric force in children with and without Duchenne's muscular dystrophy. *Phys Ther.* 1992, 72:105-14.

[23] Stuberg, WA; Metcalf, WK. Reliability of quantitative muscle testing in healthy children and in children with Duchenne muscular dystrophy using a hand-held dynamometer. *Phys Ther.*, 1988, 68, 977-82.

[24] Liistro, G; Vanwelde, C; Vincken, W; Vandevoorde, J; Verleden, G; Buffels, J. Technical and functional assessment of 10 office spirometers: A multicenter comparative study. *Chest.*, 2006, 130(3), 657-65.

[25] Rosenthal, M; Bain, SH; Cramer, D; Helms, P; Denison, D; Bush, A; et al. Lung function in white children aged 4 to 19 years: I--Spirometry. *Thorax.*, 1993, 48(8), 794-802.

[26] Arets, HG; van der Ent, CK. Flow/volume measurements from childhood to adulthood. *Monaldi Arch Chest Dis.*, 2000, 55(4), 348-52.

[27] Bruce, RA; Blackmon, JR; Jones, JW; Strait, G. Exercise testing in adult normal subjects and cardiac patients. *Pediatrics.*, 1963, 32(II), 742-56.

[28] Boileau, RA; Bonen, A; Heyward, VH; Massey, BH. Maximal aerobic capacity on the treadmill and bicycle ergometer of boys 11-14 years of age. *Journal of Sports Medicine and Physical Fitness.*, 1977, 17(2), 153-62.

[29] Rowland, TW. Does peak VO_2 reflect VO_2max in children?: evidence from supramaximal testing. *Med Sci Sports Exerc.*, 1993, 25(6), 689-93.

[30] Takken, T; van der Net, J; Helders, PJM. Aerobic exercise testing in juvenile rheumatoid arthritis (JRA) patients. *Clinical Exercise Physiology.*, 2002, 4(1), 38-43.

[31] Takken, T; van der Net, J; Helders, PJ. The reliability of an aerobic and an anaerobic exercise tolerance test in patients with juvenile onset dermatomyositis. *J Rheumatol.*, 2005, 32(4), 734-9.

[32] Shephard, RJ; Allen, C; Benade, AJ; Davies, CT; Di Prampero, PE; Hedman, R; et al. The maximum oxygen intake. An international reference standard of cardiorespiratory fitness. *Bull World Health Organ.*, 1968, 38(5), 757-64.

[33] Blair, SN; Cheng, Y; Holder, JS. Is physical activity or physical fitness more important in defining health benefits? *Med Sci Sports Exerc.* 2001, 33(6 Suppl):S379-99.

[34] Myers, J; Prakash, M; Froelicher, V; Do, D; Partington, S; Atwood, JE. Exercise capacity and mortality among men referred for exercise testing. *N Engl J Med.* 2002, 346(11), 793-801.

[35] Meyer, T; Georg, T; Becker, C; Kindermann, W. Reliability of gas exchange measurements from two different spiroergometry systems. *Int J Sports Med.*, 2001, 22(8), 593-7.

[36] Wasserman, K; Hansen, JE; Sue, DY; Casaburi, R; Whipp, BJ. *Principles of Exercise testing and Interpretation.* 3th Edition ed. Baltimore, MD, USA: Lippincott, Williams & Wilkins, 1999.

[37] Binkhorst, RA; van 't Hof, MA; Saris, WHM. Maximale inspanning door kinderen; referentiewaarden voor 6-18 jarige meisjes en jongens [Maximal exercise in children; reference values girls and boys, 6-18 year of age]. *Den-Haag: Nederlandse Hartstichting*, 1992.

[38] Henderson, SE; Sugden, DA. Movement Assesment Battery for Children: Kent: *The Psychological Corporation.*, 1992.

[39] Smits-Engelsman, BCM; Movement, ABC. *Nederlandse handleiding* [Movement ABC. Dutch Manual]. Lisse, the Netherlands: Swets & Zeitlinger, 1998.

[40] Barker, M; Merz, U; Hertl, M; Heimann, G. School-age lung function and exercise capacity in former very low birth weight infants. *Pediatric Exercise Science.* 2003, 15:44-55.

[41] Gross, SJ; Iannuzzi, DM; Kveselis, DA; Anbar, RD. Effect of preterm birth on pulmonary function at school age: a prospective controlled study. *J Pediatr.*, 1998, 133(2), 188-92.

[42] Svien, LR. Health-related fitness of seven- to 10-year-old children with histories of preterm birth. *Pediatr Phys Ther.*, 2003, 15(2):74-83.

[43] Wagner, PD. New ideas on limitations to VO2max. *Exerc Sport Sci Rev.*, 2000, *28(1)*, 10-4.

[44] Van Leeuwen, PB; Van Der Net, J; Helders, PJM; Takken, T. Exercise parameters in healthy Dutch children [in Dutch, English summary]. *Geneeskunde en Sport.*, 2004, 37(5), 126-32.

[45] Andersen, LB; Harro, M; Sardinha, LB; Froberg, K; Ekelund, U; Brage, S; et al. Physical activity and clustered cardiovascular risk in children: a cross-sectional study (The European Youth Heart Study). *Lancet.*, 2006, 368, 299-304.

[46] Carnethon, MR; Gidding, SS; Nehgme, R; Sidney, S; Jacobs, DR; Jr; Liu, K. Cardiorespiratory fitness in young adulthood and the development of cardiovascular disease risk factors. *Jama.*, 2003, 290(23), 3092-100.

[47] Keller, H; Bar-Or, O; Kriemler, S; Ayub, BV; Saigal, S. Anaerobic performance in 5- to 7-yr-old children of low birthweight. *Med Sci Sports Exerc.*, 2000, 32(2), 278-83.

[48] Vrijlandt, EJ; Gerritsen, J; Boezen, HM; Grevink, RG; Duiverman, EJ. Lung function and exercise capacity in young adults born prematurely. *Am J Respir Crit Care Med.* 2006, 173(8):890-6.

[49] van Haastert, IC; de Vries, LS; Helders, PJ; Jongmans, MJ. Early gross motor development of preterm infants according to the Alberta Infant Motor Scale. *J Pediatr. 2006*, 149(5):617-22.

[50] Moyer-Mileur, LJ; Brunstetter, V; McNaught, TP; Gill, G; Chan, GM. Daily physical activity program increases bone mineralization and growth in preterm very low birth weight infants. *Pediatrics.*, 2000, 106(5):1088-92.

[51] Nemet, D; Dolfin, T; Litmanowitz, I; Shainkin-Kestenbaum, R; Lis, M; Eliakim, A. Evidence for exercise-induced bone formation in premature infants. *Int J Sports Med.*, 2002, 23(2), 82-5.

In: Encyclopedia of Sports and Athletics
Editors: Jack L. Murray and Emily O. Watson
ISBN: 978-1-61209-959-0

Chapter XIII

Self Selection of Athletes into Sports via Skeletal Ratios

Arthur D. Stewart[1*], Philip J. Benson[2], Tim Olds[3], Michael Marfell-Jones[4], Alasdair MacSween[5] and Alan M. Nevill[6]

[1]Centre for Obesity Research and Epidemiology, Robert Gordon University, St Andrew Street, Aberdeen, AB25 1HG, UK

[2]School of Psychology, College of Life Sciences and Medicine, University of Aberdeen, AB24 2UB, UK

[3]School of Health Sciences, University of South Australia, City East Campus, GPO box 2471, Adelaide, SA, Australia 5001.

[4]School of Health Sciences, Universal College of Learning, Private Bag 11022, Palmerston North, New Zealand

[5]School of Health and Social Care, Teesside University, Middlesbrough, TS1 3BA, UK.

[6]School of Sport, Performing Arts and Leisure, University of Wolverhampton, Gorway Road, Walsall, WS1 3BD, UK

Abstract

This study examined differences in physique and skeletal dimensions between 1146 elite Caucasian athletes classified into endurance, strength, speed, upper body or combined sports categories and controls, to test the hypothesis that athletes of certain types of sport would exhibit a distinct morphology commensurate with their task. Participants were measured by experienced anthropometrists using an internationally-recognised protocol to describe physique. This involved calculating the anthropometric somatotype in terms of fatness, musculoskeletal robustness and linearity. Further skeletal measures were acquired sufficient to describe an array of morphological indices: crural index (tibial height / femur length), skelic index (leg length / sitting height), androgyny index (biacromial breadth / bicristal breadth) and brachial index (forearm length / upper arm length). Significant inter-group differences in indices prevailed after adjustment for age. Endurance athletes had a high crural index and low brachial index, relative to

[*] Corresponding author: E-mail a.d.stewart@rgu.ac.uk, Phone +44 (0)1224 262895 FAX +44 (0)1224 262828

controls. A low skelic index appears characteristic of female strength athletes while a low brachial index is typical of female endurance and strength athletes. Bayesian cluster analysis has shown the crural index in particular is a discriminant in phenotypic categorisation, in addition to the primary somatotype components of endomorphy, mesomorphy and ectomorphy. These findings are congruent with biomechanical imperatives to maximise force and/or minimise energy expenditure offering sports-specific advantage. Because the skeletal relationships do not respond to the conditioning stimulus in the same way adipose and muscle tissue do, the observed inter-group differences suggest a self-selection of athletes into sports in which they are likely to excel.

Keywords: Caucasian, athlete, skeletal proportions

Introduction

Drivers for physique specialisation in humans and our precursors have hitherto included factors which are thermoregulatory (where body surface area and proportions appear to alter with climatic adaptation), or biomechanical (where certain proportions may favour agility in difficult terrain), load carrying, speed of locomotion or protection against injury (Bramble and Lieberman, 2004; Porter, 1999; Trinkaus, 1986). Commensurate with subsequent advances in technology and medicine, in the Western world, is the erosion of the link between morphology and survival. In such an urbanised environment, a persuasive argument can be marshalled to suggest that, in the 21st century, the evolutionary forces that shaped human morphology have largely disappeared. While these forces of natural selection may be redundant, elite athletes display morphological adaptations via self-selection by choosing sports to which they are anatomically suited and conditioning their bodies appropriately with increasingly sophisticated and specific training methods.

Although world-class athletes' morphology has attracted scientific enquiry since the 1928 Amsterdam Olympics, it was 32 years later at the Rome Olympics before the first systematic morphological study of track and field athletes was widely publicised (Tanner, 1964). This drew attention to physique differences between different ethnic groups, and between athletes from different sports. Discriminant analysis showed differences between groups in terms of proportions and somatotype, rated photoscopically for endomorphy (roundness or fatness), mesomorphy (musculo-skeletal robustness) and ectomorphy (linearity). Somatotype profiles have formed a rich literature, and large diverse data sets have been comprehensively catalogued, providing a range of evidence for physique variation and specialisation (Carter and Heath, 1990). Notwithstanding this, more recently, ethnicity has proved less robust as a criterion for differentiation of physique, due to hybridisation of populations.

Elite athletes' skeletal dimensions have also proved helpful in predicting body mass in hominid skeletal remains, because their extreme fitness more closely approximates the physical conditioning of earlier humans (Ruff, 2000a). Ruff's approach pooled data from different ethnic groups and postulated a physique which optimised power and speed as being most adaptive, resembling those of athletes from sporting events such as decathlon in men and pentathlon in women.

Physique specialisation is one of several factors determining performance in competitive sport, where the most successful athletes could be expected to acquire morphology commensurate with their performance task (Carter, 1985). The rewards of competitive sport over the last century or so - in terms of personal acclaim, financial inducement and national prestige - have provided sufficient incentive to drive what has been described as a 'morphological arms race' (Norton and Olds, 2001). In some sports, the rate of increase in size of participants is 2-6 times greater than those of the populations from which they are drawn (Olds, 2001). More is worthy of consideration, however, than size itself. Body tissues can be theoretically grouped as 'active' or 'ballast' whether they contribute to or retard force or power production respectively, while relative strength has been shown to scale to mass raised to the power 0.69, if composition is assumed to be constant (Carter, 1985). While soft tissue can be readily modified by adaptation to appropriate training stimuli, the same is not true of skeletal proportions; these are largely genetically determined and remain largely constant in adults. Although body shape variation is understood to show continuous variation, skeletal proportions appear to exhibit a 'race specificity' (Feldesman and Fountain, 1996; Holliday and Ruff, 2001; Ruff, 2000b) when groups from different geographical areas are compared. For instance, this has been graphically depicted in terms of longer limbs in Afro-Caribbean compared to Caucasian athletes in the same track and field events (Tanner, 1964). The rise to global dominance by East African endurance runners has been partly explained by preferential physique in terms of optimised force production and movement. Differing leg morphology and inertial properties, between Senegalese and Italian sprinters, has also been reported (Rahmani, Locatelli and Lacour, 2004). The longer, lighter legs of the Senegalese incurred a lower level of inertial work. By comparison, the Italians needed to generate more force in order to run at the same speed. This approach was taken further by the calculation of ground support forces by the world's fastest runners across eight distances (Weyand and Davis, 2005). They noted that early studies had overestimated the mechanical power requirement for lifting and accelerating the body and limbs during running. However, the larger forces during faster running combined with the constant force-area relationship of skeletal muscle demand more muscle to generate and transmit such forces to the ground. Weyand and Davis argued that for those of the same stature and composition, more tissue may be biologically necessary for attaining faster speeds.

While morphology may explain performance differences between groups, to date, study samples have either focused on specific ethnic group comparisons or involved experimentation of biomechanical parameters with small samples. Given the wealth of data available on elite athletes, it is surprising that relatively little is known of sports involving more complex movements. A further difficulty is introduced by the extreme specialisation of certain sports which focus on certain aspects of physique. This requires a categorisation system which can be generated to group similar influences together, so that observations can be made with larger samples. Therefore, this study aimed to compare skeletal proportions of elite athletes from a range of different sports, while focusing on a large and relatively-homogeneous sample. Specifically, it was hypothesised that a) proportional differences would be observed between different sporting categories and that b) these differences would be in addition to those of sexual dimorphism. If found, such differences might give some indication of criteria for selectivity, representing a competitive advantage for certain sports.

Methods

Participants (829 male and 317 female adult competitive athletes) were assessed for mass, skinfolds, girths, lengths and breadths by standardised procedures in a 39-measurement protocol (Marfell-Jones, Olds, Stewart and Carter, 2006) by experienced criterion anthropometrists and anthropometric somatotype calculated according to the method of Carter and Health (1990). Local ethical permission was obtained from participating universities and informed consent was obtained from all subjects. Athletes from the United Kingdom, Australia and New Zealand were included if they were of national or international standard. Due to the predominant ethnicities of the three host countries, the sample was almost exclusively Caucasian.

Sporting categories were developed in order to produce meaningful group sizes for comparative purposes. Specific criteria for conditioning which would be likely to influence physique were developed from primary movement imperatives and assigned according to a decision chart summarised in Figure 1.

Endurance (n=235) – where locomotor efficiency emphasising the major postural muscles is dominant – included running, cycling (time trial and road), orienteering, cross country skiing, and rowing. *Speed* (n=338) – where sprinting and/or very rapid body segment movement is involved – included sprint running (1500m and less), hurdling, javelin, diving, rugby (backs), touch rugby, badminton, track cycling, Australian rules football and martial arts. *Combined* (n=231) – where basic locomotion was accompanied by additional speed or strength requirements – included gymnastics (female) dance, softball, handball, fencing, hockey, soccer, volleyball, tennis. *Strength* (n=132) – where absolute strength and / or power requirement is more important than relative strength, relative power or locomotion – included bodybuilding, rugby forwards, powerlifting, gymnastics (male), wrestling, shot put and hammer throwing. *Upper Body* (n=102) – where the sport requirement favours the development of upper body muscles and/or where the body weight is supported so the postural muscles are de-emphasised – included kayaking, canoeing, dragon boat racing, rock climbing, swimming. *Control* (n=108) – subjects who were healthy, and possibly physically active, but not competitive in sport. Athletes whose sport required no clear specific physique specialisation such as cricket, golf, yachting and shooting were excluded. Categorical assignation was agreed between members of the research team using these criteria prior to analysis.

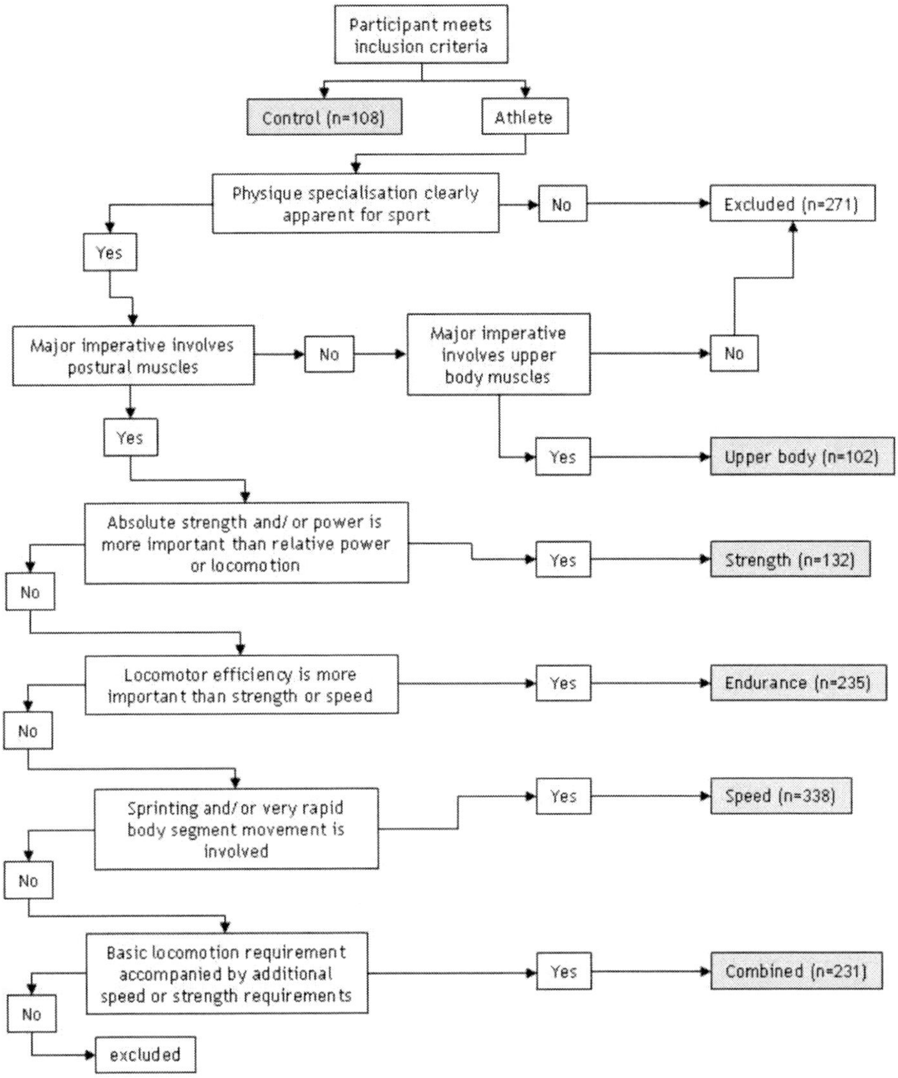

Figure 1. Categorisation of athletic groups.

Segment length measurements which summarised the major relationships of the skeletal development were made on the right side of the body using a segmometer or wide spreading calliper (Rosscraft Innovations Inc., Canada) to 0.1 cm. Stature and sitting height were measured to 0.1 cm with the head in the Frankfort plane and following inspiration. Data were converted into ratios defined as follows: The *crural index* is a measure of tibia length in relation to femur length, defined as the height of the tibiale laterale (a) with the subject standing, divided by the trochanterion – tibiale laterale length (b). The *brachial index* is a measure of the length of the forearm in relation to the upper arm and is defined as the radiale–stylion length (c) divided by the acromiale – radiale length (d) . The *androgyny index* is essentially shoulder breadth in relation to pelvic breadth, defined as the biacromial breadth (e) divided by the bicristal breadth (f). The *skelic index* describes leg length in relation to torso length and is defined as the derived total leg length (stature minus sitting height) divided by sitting height. These ratios are depicted in Figure 2.

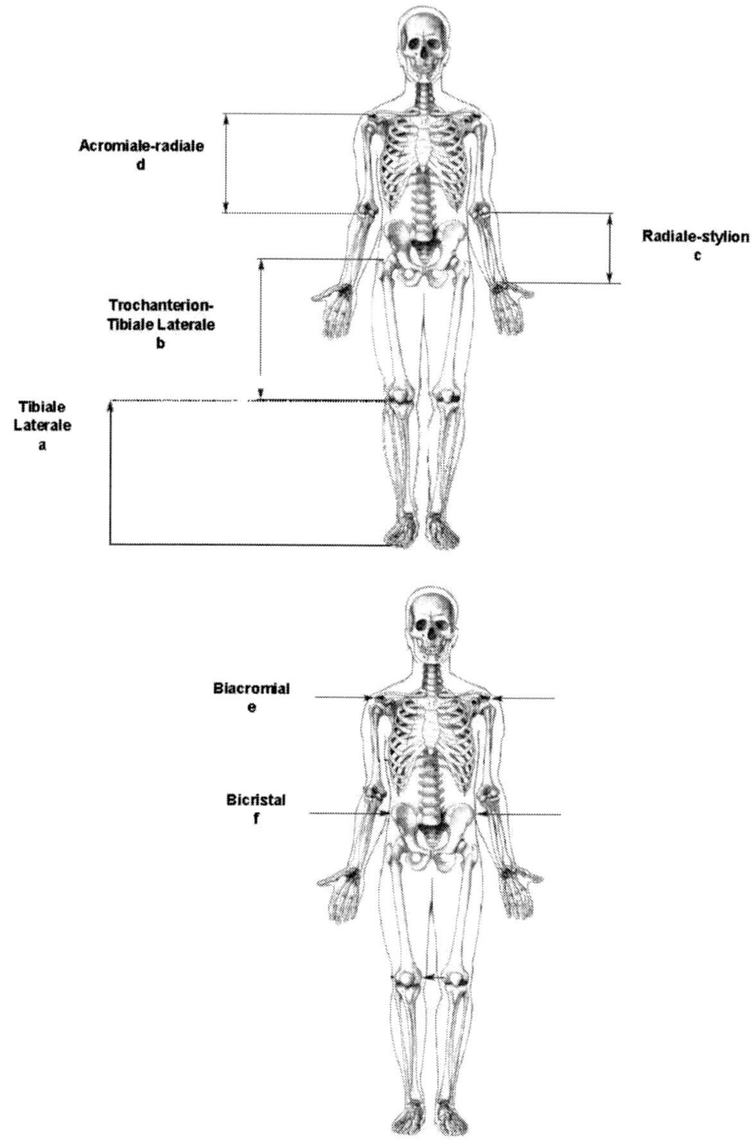

Figure 2. Skeletal measurements and derived ratios. The *crural index* is height of the tibiale laterale (a), divided by the trochanterion – tibiale laterale length (b). The *brachial index* is radiale – stylion length (c) divided by the acromiale – radiale length (d). The *androgyny index* is the biacromial breadth (e) divided by the bicristal breadth (f). The *skelic index* is the derived total leg length (stature minus sitting height) divided by sitting height (not shown). All landmarks and definitions were measured using the International Society for the Advancement of Kinanthropometry's protocol (Marfell-Jones, Olds, Stewart and Carter, 2006). Diagram reproduced with permission.

All landmarks and definitions were measured using the protocol of the International Society for the Advancement of Kinanthropometry (Marfell-Jones, Olds, Stewart and Carter, 2006). This involves anatomically-defined landmarks and systematic procedures, together with exam-based quality assurance of precision and accuracy of data. Technicians assembling the current data had intra-tester technical error of measurement below 1% and averaging 0.4%

for skeletal data. The widespread use of this protocol has enabled data pooling which in turn allowed comparison of large groups of specialist competitive athletes.

Skeletal indices were entered into a general linear model using SPSS Version 14 (Chicago, IL) with gender and sport category as fixed factors and identifying any interaction. Age was entered as a covariate because controls were significantly older than sporting groups and the effect of a secular trend in height could mean potential differences arising from the effect of stature. As a further check on patterns of physique, all anthropometric somatotype and skeletal data were entered into unsupervised cluster analysis. Bayesian decision theory provided a maximum posterior probability classification of individuals that was maximally probable with respect to the data and model (Cheeseman and Stutz, 1996; Wallace and Dowe, 1999). Sport category and sex were not entered as factors. The resulting class membership thus determined whether the skeletal ratios contributed to phenotypic variation beyond that associated with the three somatotype categories of endomorphy, mesomorphy and ectomorphy.

Results

There were significant differences in skeletal ratios between sporting categories and by sex as shown in Figures 3 to 6. For the crural index, 9.1% variation was explained by sport category, age and gender. Age was negatively associated with crural index, indicating that, in younger athletes, crural index was greater ($P<0.001$). For the androgyny index, 17.3% of the variation was explained by sport category and gender ($P<0.001$), but age was not significant ($P=0.83$). In all sports categories, males had greater values. For the skelic index, 4% of variation was explained by sport category ($P<0.01$) and gender ($P<0.001$) but not age ($P = 0.45$). For the brachial index, 5.3% of variation was explained by age ($P<0.05$), sport and gender ($P<0.001$). Interaction between sex and sport (all $P < 0.05$ except brachial index, $P = 0.08$) suggested that the observed sporting differences did not follow the same pattern for males and female athletic groups.

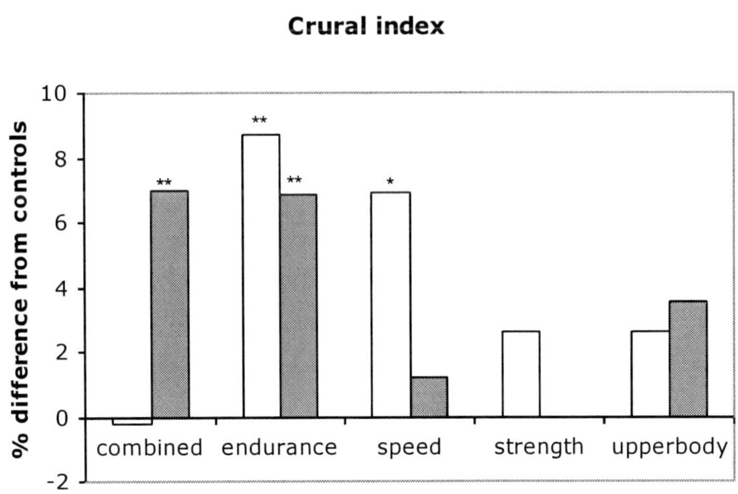

Figure 3. Age-adjusted crural index of athletic groups showing males (shaded) and females (white) * $P<0.05$ ** $P<0.01$, all comparisons being two tailed.

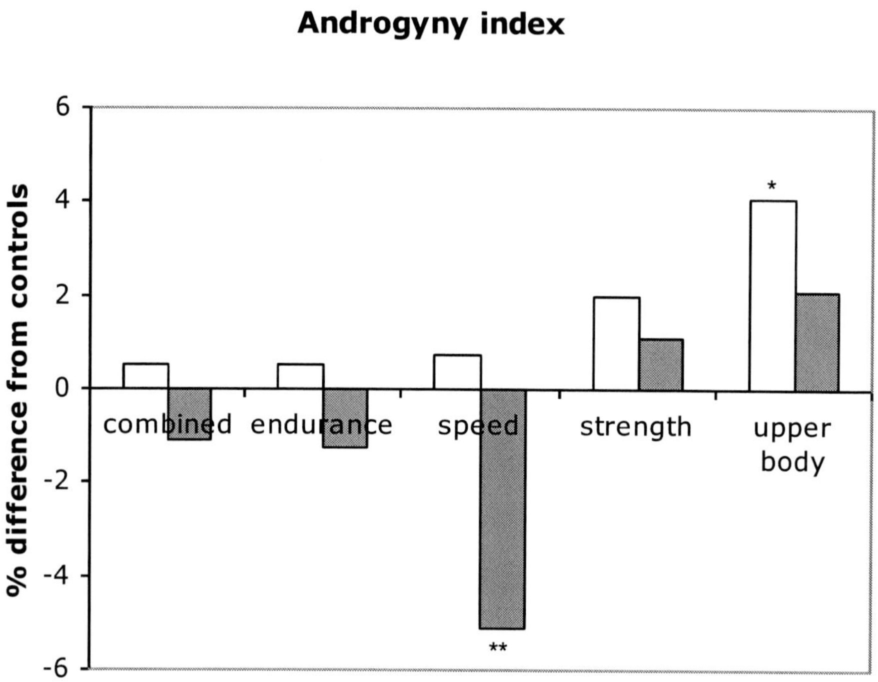

Figure 4. Age-adjusted androgyny index of athletic groups showing males (shaded) and females (white) * P<0.05 ** P<0.01, all comparisons being two tailed.

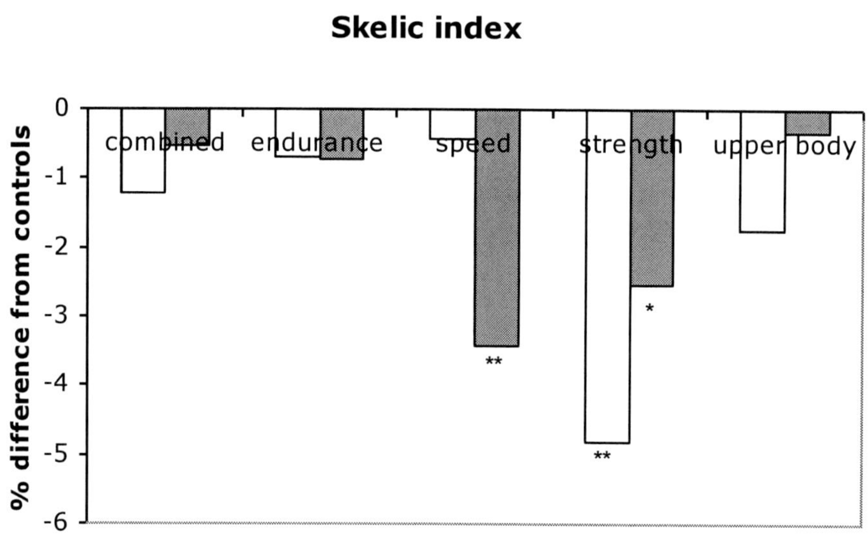

Figure 5. Age-adjusted skelic index of athletic groups showing males (shaded) and females (white) * P<0.05 ** P<0.01, all comparisons being two tailed.

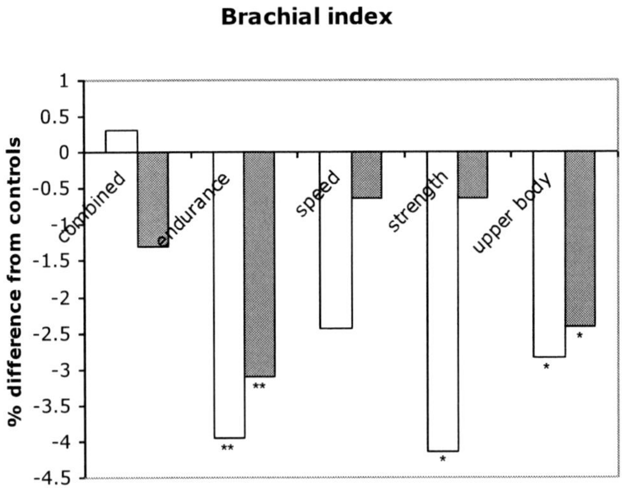

Figure 6. Age-adjusted brachial index of athletic groups showing males (shaded) and females (white) * P<0.05 ** P<0.01, all comparisons being two tailed.

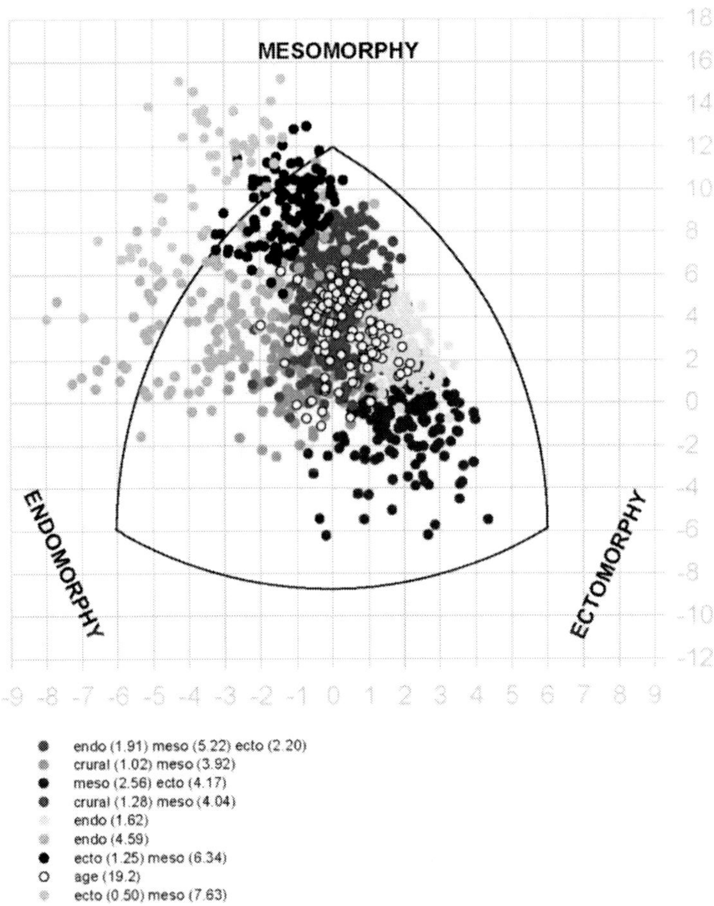

Figure 7. Physique class membership of Bayesian analysis plotted on conventional somatochart (Carter and Heath, 1990). Mean values of statistically-influential class attributes are shown for each category. Endomorphy, mesomorphy and ectomorphy are rated using anthropometric somatotype.

Of the skeletal ratios described, only the crural index was selected in the Bayesian cluster analysis as a discriminant of the larger sample, in addition to the established somatotype categories of endomorphy, mesomorphy and ectomorphy. Significant class attributes are depicted in Figure 7 and Table 1. (Note that the crural index here is not age-adjusted).

Table 1. Here we show that while the computed somatotype components describe physique, the crural index (Davenport, 1933) represents an additional discriminant in describing physique variation across our adult sample. A dominant crural index in classes 2 and 4 illustrates the importance of relative limb length in athletes trained for endurance and strength. A smaller crural index may be advantageous for general agility, whereas a higher value may determine mechanically advantageous take-off technique in long-jump and high-jump events (Alexander, 1990) and in basketball, in tandem with development of commensurate muscle power to maximise femoral leverage Ackland et al., 1997). Sex and sport composition within each class was reconstructed by referring to individuals' details in the original database. Overall body mass (M = 73.7, SD = 14.6 kg) and stature (M = 176.6 cm, SD = 10.4cm).

Table 1. Athletes distinguished by attribute

Group	Attributes	Description
1 ●	endo (1.91) meso (5.22) ecto (2.20)	N = 176, 99% male, 36% speed, 22% endurance Low endomorphy with high mesomorphy; heavier (77.1kg) and marginally taller (178.2cm)
2 ●	crural (1.02) meso (3.92)	N = 144, 65% female, 26% control, 24% combined, 20% endurance Equal tibial height and femur length with low mesomorphy; lighter (66.8kg) and shorter (172.9cm)
3 ●	meso (2.56) ecto (4.17)	N = 141, 51% female, 38% speed, 26% endurance, 23% combined Very low mesomorphy with high ectomorphy; smaller mass (63.3kg) with average stature
4 ●	crural (1.28) meso (4.04)	N = 122, 53% male, 42% endurance, 24% speed, 21% combined Tibia height significantly greater than femur length, with large upper body; slightly below average mass (70.5kg) and stature (175.8cm)
5 ●	endo (1.62)	N = 125, 100% male, 33% endurance, 25% speed, 23% combined Low endomorphy; tall male athletes (184.0cm) only marginally heavier than sample average (75.0kg)
6 ●	endo (4.59)	N = 115, 57% female, 30% control, 17% endurance, 16% combined Endomorphy almost twice the sample mean; average weight but shorter in stature (170.6cm)
7 ●	ecto (1.25) meso (6.34)	N = 114, 99% male, 36% speed, 34% strength Low ectomorphy with high mesomorphy; heavy males (82.9kg) of average stature
8 ○	age (19.2)	N = 98, 83% male, 84% speed Younger male runners (database mean 25.4 years); lightweight (66.8kg) and shorter in stature (172.8cm)
9 ●	ecto (0.50) meso (7.63)	N = 56, 84% male, 64% strength Predominantly heavy male strength athletes; significantly greater body mass (96.3kg) but average height

Discussion

All four ratios remained significantly different after adjusting for age, suggesting that sporting prowess benefits from certain skeletal characteristics that are proportional. Taken together, these show signs of a preferred "morphotype" for the sporting categories described. The phenomenon of differential skeletal ratios has not been reported hitherto in a large athletic sample. It is reasonable to assume that athletes will select to compete in sports for which they are anatomically suited. In doing so, they may excel by fulfilling a biomechanical imperative of energy efficiency or power production, via considerations of segmental mass and lever arms, which have different determinants in different sports. For instance, while running at a given speed, an advantage may be offered by a higher crural index which concentrates the mass more proximally on the moving limb thus decreasing its resistance arm. The low crural index of Neanderthals compared with modern humans has been attributed to the imperatives of locomotion and load carrying over difficult terrain, safeguarding knee ligaments against injury (Porter, 1999). In a similar fashion, male and female strength athletes appear to combine similar attributes of relatively short and distally-abbreviated legs with wide shoulder girdles which may favour force production and load bearing at the expense of speed.

Consideration of the possible contribution of endurance running to human evolution has identified leg morphology among many factors affecting locomotion where greater leg length increases sustainable speed and contact time, reducing energy expenditure over a distance as a result of lower cadence and greater stride length (Bramble and Lieberman, 2004). This is supported by comparison of different animal species, where effective limb length explained 98% of the energy cost of locomotion (Pontzer, 2007). However our data suggest the effect may not be due to leg length *per se*, but also the relative position of the knee joint and the concomitant alteration in both the segmental (thigh and shank) and overall lower limb Moment of Inertia (MI). In the present study, endurance athletes had similar leg proportions to controls (quantified by the skelic index). However, their crural index was greater ($P<0.001$). This has the effect of moving the knee joint proximally in endurance athletes relative to controls. As the greater balance of the mass of the lower limb lies in the thigh segment, this change may explain the greater speed and efficiency of running achieved through greater segmental angular acceleration. Greater angular acceleration is facilitated by reduced lower limb MI without compromising proximal muscle power (torque), as given by the angular motion version of Newton's second law $T = I.\alpha$, where T is torque in Nm, MI is moment of inertia in $kg.m^{-2}$, and α is angular acceleration in $rad.s^{-2}$. [MI is dependent on the square of the distance between the centre of mass of the rotating limb segment and the axis of rotation]. As the main bulk of the primary muscles of running (hamstrings and quadriceps) and hence lower limb mass, lies proximal to the knee, the effect of any increase in crural index is mechanically profound in the lower limb. The effect of altering mass distribution in the lower limb and hence segmental I, has been previously observed by runners strapping 3.6 kg of additional weight to the waist, upper thigh, shank or ankle (Myers and Steudel, 1985). Moving this additional weight from the ankle to the hip reduced MI and also reduced running energy expenditure by 15%. However, a more recent experimental study of kinematics and moments of inertia of 27 healthy adults found no effect of the crural index on moments during walking, suggesting that postural adjustments might moderate locomotor forces (Gruss, 2007). Running, especially for the maximal performance sought by the athletes of the present study may appear to introduce different criteria which become significant once the forces and velocity become great enough.

The predicted muscle mass exponent (the power to which the muscle circumference scales to mass) from thigh measurements has been shown to be 0.96 in endurance and 1.49 in speed athletes (Nevill, Stewart, Olds and Holder, 2004), suggesting endurance athletes rely less on muscular and more on gravitational force to accelerate their limbs than speed athletes. The present study provides skeletal data suggesting a further energy saving by a more proximal location of their knee joint. Using group mean limb circumferences and lengths with a fixed-density cylindrical model, endurance athletes effectively have the centre of mass of their extended limb moved proximally by about 1.7 cm, enabling a lighter distal segment to be accelerated more rapidly with less energy expenditure. The significance of age in the model suggests that more recent generations of athletes appear to have longer distal lower limb segments, possibly as a consequence of alterations in environmental influences such as nutrition. Paradoxically, the effect of age on the brachial index is positive, suggesting younger athletes have distally abbreviated upper limb segments. Endurance athletes also showed distal abbreviation relative to controls, effectively moving the centre of mass of the extended arm 0.4 cm distally. The reason for this is unclear. A counterbalance effect of opposing pendulum movement of arms and legs of similar relative proportions may confer a small energy saving, although style variation, via differential arm flexion and torso rotation, could negate this.

It has been suggested that the androgyny index could discriminate successful athletes in bodybuilding for aesthetic reasons and a capacity to increase muscle mass on the torso (Fry, Ryan, Schwab, Powell and Kraemer, 1991). Beyond this, a broad shoulder girdle may enable greater leverage or reach in some upper-body sports such as rock climbing or canoeing. Conversely, competition rules of the International Powerlifting Federation may discriminate against larger athletes whose grip may be required to be narrower than the optimal functional position (Gilbert and Lees, 2003). In addition, a smaller brachial index might be an advantage in strength sports requiring full elbow extension by reducing the work required, as demonstrated in the female, but not male, strength athletes.

Previously, we described mass exponents for athlete data sets for girths (Nevill, Stewart, Olds and Holder, 2004) and skinfolds (Nevill, Stewart, Olds and Holder, 2006). Such surrogates of adipose and muscle tissue respond directly to the stressors of specialist training and high energy expenditure. By contrast, adult skeletal size and proportions are relatively unaffected by such training, but have considerable effects on the biomechanics of movement and work. Since an individual is not at liberty to alter these dimensions, (unlike those relating to soft tissue masses and proportions in an adult), selective processes are driven by them in elite sport. The data specifically illustrate that a high or low crural index is responsible for distinct phenotypes. High values are typically represented in male and female endurance, female speed and male combined sports physiques, while low values are typical of controls and female combined sports athletes. While the skeletal ratios show highly significant differences between groups (figures 3 - 6), the degree of correspondence between crural index in phenotype (figure 7 and table 1) and sporting categorisation is modest. There are two explanations for this. One is that skeletal proportion limitation can, to an extent, be negated by other factors in the sports performance such as physiological fitness, psychological attributes and skill. The other is that our principle-based categorisation of sports into groups inevitably has limitations. If our criteria for sports categorisation were to be changed, the findings would likely alter. Nevertheless, the differences found here could be logically explained by our categorisation. We further concede modelling the limbs on the basis of cylindrical or conical models of an isotropic body tissue to estimate the effect on centre of mass may be too simplistic for suggesting biomechanical models, since adaptive remodelling of bone and adaptations of connective tissue alter tissue density non-uniformly. However, mathematical modelling of athletic performance combining actual athlete dimensions was beyond the scope of the present work.

This notwithstanding, our findings which effectively locate relative joint positions differently on a generic skeletal template for different sporting categories may well have possible explanations in biomechanical theory. This suggests a reduction in energetic cost of transport (i.e. per unit distance) with increasing leg length in other animals, but available data are equivocal (Steudel, 1996). Estimating muscle masses required to maintain equilibrium in selected extant taxa (Hutchinson, 2004) found none with extensor muscles exceeding 7% body mass acting across any joint, suggesting a limit for how muscle is apportioned within a limb. While the present study did not address this, we would surmise that the relative development of primary force-producing muscles in human athletes is more variable, as a possible means of exacerbating or compensating for the effect of skeletal proportions.

The fact that our sporting categories, relative to controls show different effects on skeletal proportions by gender, as well as gender interactions for sport (when controls are treated as a sports category) is of specific interest. It might seem reasonable to hypothesise that an identical exercise stimulus for males and females would result in broadly similar drivers for selectivity, and broadly similar differences by sport from controls, however our observations require a different explanation. Some findings are undoubtedly the result of different exercise adaptation arising from different activities (e.g. rhythmic gymnastics only in females), or differences in the relative representation within a sporting category (e.g. rugby being more prevalent in males than females) or alternatively differences in the extent of the selective process necessary for international representation. However, the data set is sufficiently large to be able to suggest, despite the shortcomings of differing gender prevalence in some sports, there appears to be a strong influence of selectivity based on the skeletal proportions described here.

Conclusion

Accepting the limitations of categorisation, our data suggest two conclusions. Firstly, there appears strong evidence of self-selection of athletes into sports to which they are anatomically suited because the skeletal proportions vary significantly between groups. Secondly, the crural index in particular is influential in phenotypic variation within an athletic sample. While the genotypic variation of the sample was limited to predominantly Caucasian athletes, a future study may consider athletes of any ethnic group in order to acquire an even larger sample. Future biomechanical research may align these findings with lab-derived movement data and virtual sports performances. Given the value placed on sporting success, understanding the nature of any competitive advantage offered by morphology will become an important focus for future research effort. Considering the fact that it requires perhaps 10 years to produce athletes of Olympic calibre, a further priority will be to recognise potentially successful adult morphology from the skeleton of the growing athlete.

References

Ackland, TR; Schreiner, AB; Kerr, DA. Absolute size and proportionality characteristics of World Championship female basketball players. *Journal of Sports Sciences.,* 1997, 15, 485-490.

Alexander, RM. Optimum take-off techniques for high and long jumps. *Philosophical Transactions of the Royal Society of London Biological Sciences.,* 1990, 329, 3-10.

Bramble, DM; Lieberman, DE. Endurance running and the evolution of Homo. *Nature.*, 2004, 432, 345-352.

Carter, JEL. Morphological factors limiting human performance. In: Clarke DH, Eckert HM, editors. *Limits of Human Performance.* American Academy of Physical Education Papers No 18, Champaign: Human Kinetics; 1985, 106-117.

Carter, JEL; Heath, BH. *Somatotyping: Development and applications.* Cambridge UK: Cambridge University Press; 1990.

Cheeseman, P; Stutz, J. In: UM; Fayyad. G; Piatetsky-Shapiro. P; Smyth. R; Uthurusamy. editors. *Advances in Knowledge Discovery and Data Mining* Cambridge. MA: AAAI Press/MIT Press., 1996, 61-83.

Davenport, CB. The crural index. *American Journal of Physical Anthropology,* 1933. 17, 333-353.

Feldesman, MR; Fountain, RL. "Race" specificity and the femur/stature ratio. *American Journal of Physical Anthropology.,* 1996, 100, 207-224.

Fry, AC; Ryan, AJ; Schwab, RJ; Powell, DR; Kraemer, WJ. Anthropometric characteristics of body-building success. *Journal of Sports Sciences.,* 1991, 9, 23-32.

Gilbert, G; Lees, A. Maximum grip width regulations in powerlifting discriminate against larger athletes. In: Reilly T, Marfell-Jones M, editors. *Kinanthropometry VIII* London: Routeledge, 2003, 175-180.

Gruss, LT. Limb length and locomotor biomechanics in the genus homo: An experimental study. *American Journal of Physical Anthropology.,* 2007, 134, 106-116.

Holliday, TW; Ruff, CB. Relative variation in human proximal and distal limb segment lengths. *American Journal of Physical Anthropology.,* 2001, 116, 26-33.

Hutchinson, JR. Biomechanical modelling and sensitivity analysis of bipedal running ability. Extant Taxa. *Journal of Morphology.,* 2004, 262, 421-440.

Marfell-Jones, M; Olds, T; Stewart, A; Carter, JEL. *International Standards for Anthropometric Assessment.* Potchefstroom, South Africa. International Society for the Advancement of Kinanthropometry; 2006.

Myers, MJ; Steudel, K. Effect of limb mass on the energetic cost of running. *Journal of Experimental Biology.,* 1985, 116, 363-373.

Nevill, AM; Stewart, AD; Olds, T; Holder, R. Are adult physiques geometrically similar?: the dangers of allometric scaling using body mass power laws. *American Journal of Physical Anthropology.,* 2004, 124, 177-182.

Nevill, AM; Stewart, AD; Olds, T; Holder, R. Modelling the relationship between adiposity and body size reveals the limitation of BMI. *American Journal of Physical Anthropology.,* 2006. 129, 151-156.

Norton, K; Olds, T. Morphological evolution of athletes over the 20th century: causes and consequences. *Sports Medicine.,* 2001, 31, 763-783.

Olds, T. The evolution of physique in rugby union players in the twentieth century. *Journal of Sports Sciences.,* 2001, 19, 253-262.

Pontzer, H. Effective limb length and the scaling of locomotor cost in terrestrial animals. *Journal of Experimental Biology.,* 2007, 210, 1752-1761.

Porter, AMW. Modern human, early modern human and Neanderthal limb proportions. *International Journal of Osteoarchaeology.,* 1999, 9, 54-67.

Rahmani, A; Locatelli, E; Lacour, J. Differences in morphology and force/velocity relationship between Senegalese and Italian sprinters. *European Journal of Applied Physiology.,* 2004, 91, 399-405.

Ruff, CB. Body mass prediction from skeletal frame size in elite athletes. *American Journal of Physical Anthropology.,* 2000a, 113, 507-517.

Ruff, CB. Body size, body shape, and long bone strength in modern humans. *Journal of Human Evolution.,* 2000b, 38, 269-290.

Saltin, B; Larsen, H; Terrados, N; Bangsbo, J; Bak, T; Kim, CK; Svedenhag, J; Rolf, CJ. Aerobic exercise capacity at sea level and at altitude in Kenyan boys, junior and senior runners compared with Scandinavian runners. *Scandinavian Journal of Medicine and Science in Sports.,* 1995, 5, 209-221.

Steudel, K. Limb morphology, bipedal gait, and the energetics of hominid locomotion. *American Journal of Physical Anthropology.,* 1996, 99, 345-355.

Tanner, JM. *The physique of the Olympic athlete.* London: George Allen & Unwin; 1964.

Trinkaus, E. The Neandertals and modern human origins. *Annual Review of Anthropology.,* 1986, 15, 193-218.

Wallace, CS; Dowe, DL. Minimum message length and Kolmogorov complexity. *The Computer Journal.,* 1999, 42, 270-283.

Weyand, PG; Davis, JA. Running performance has a structural basis. *Journal of Experimental Biology.,* 2005, 208, 2625-2631.

In: Encyclopedia of Sports and Athletics
Editors: Jack L. Murray and Emily O. Watson

ISBN: 978-1-61209-959-0

Chapter XIV

Aerobic Exercise in Patients with Chronic Kidney Disease

Irfan Moinuddin and David J. Leehey
Hines Veterans Affiars Hospital, Hines, IL, US and
Loyola University School of Medicine, Maywood, IL, US

Abstract

Patients with chronic kidney disease (CKD) have increased cardiovascular morbidity and mortality. They are frequently deconditioned as a result of inactivity, malnutrition, and abnormal muscle function In advanced CKD, hyperparathyroidism, acidosis, and severe catabolism/malnutrition contribute to debility. Patients with CKD often have cardiovascular risk factors such as inadequate blood pressure control, impaired fasting glucose (or overt diabetes), impaired insulin secretion and/or insulin resistance, abnormal lipid profiles, decreased testosterone and/or estrogen levels, and poor quality of life. Other non-traditional risk factors, such as sympathoactivation, inflammation, oxidative stress, and endothelial dysfunction, are also thought to increase cardiovascular morbidity and mortality. In addition to physical disease, CKD is associated with abnormal mental health, including depression, anxiety, and a feeling of helplessness and lack of well-being.

Aerobic exercise has been proposed to have beneficial effects in CKD. This chapter seeks to define the mechanisms whereby aerobic exercise may benefit such patients. The type, duration, and recommended intensity of exercise will be discussed. While aerobic exercise is relatively safe for most CKD patients, the potential pitfalls of aerobic exercise and concerns about its safety will be addressed. The effects of exercise in the adult non-dialysis CKD population and end-stage renal disease (ESRD) population on dialysis will be clarified. Home exercise, and interdialytic versus intradialytic aerobic exercise will be discussed. Children with CKD are also susceptible to muscle weakness, low aerobic capacity, and abnormal fat composition; the impact of aerobic exercise in the pediatric CKD population will also be discussed. The effect of aerobic exercise on muscle weakness, weight loss, graft loss, and mortality in CKD patients post-transplantation will be illuminated. Finally, emphasis will be placed on areas novel to aerobic exercise and CKD requiring further research.

Introduction

The morbidity and mortality associated with chronic kidney disease (CKD) are primarily due to atherosclerosis and cardiovascular disease, which may be in part due to inflammation and oxidative stress. Aerobic exercise has been shown to be beneficial in the normal population and is thought to be similarly beneficial in CKD. What are the mechanisms whereby aerobic exercise may exert its beneficial effects? Aerobic exercise increases muscle mass, reverses the catabolism of uremia, improves aerobic capacity (increased oxygen consumption, increased left ventricular systolic function), decreases inflammation, decreases oxidative stress, and corrects endothelial dysfunction, as will be discussed. Although resistance (strength) training is also thought to have benefits in CKD [1], [2] and is often used in conjunction with aerobic training (or even prior to aerobic exercise in patients with severe muscle weakness), we will focus on aerobic training in this chapter.

Reversal of muscle atrophy and muscle dysfunction is an important benefit of both aerobic exercise and resistance training. This benefit is mediated by an exercise-induced increase in insulin-like growth factors (IGFs). Muscle atrophy is initiated by caspase-3, which dismantles actomyosin. Subsequently, actin and myosin are degraded by the ubiquitin-proteasome, which is catalyzed by E1, E2, E3, and E4 enzymes. E3 ligase (atrogin-1) is upregulated in muscle atrophy. IGF, via phosphoinositide-3 kinase/mTOR, inhibits the caspase/ubiquitin/atrogin cascade and is thus anabolic. In addition, tumor necrosis factor-alpha (TNF-alpha) inhibits IGF and stimulates caspase and ubiquitin. Exercise downregulates TNF-alpha as well as interleukin-6 and angiotensin II, and ameliorates metabolic acidosis, growth hormone resistance, amino acid depletion, and protein malnutrition [3]. Myostatin mRNA decreases and mRNA for insulin-like growth factors increases with interdialytic aerobic exercise [4]. Sakkas et al. found that aerobic exercise corrected fiber atrophy, increased cross-sectional fiber area, and improved capillarization [5]. Kouidi et al report that interdialytic aerobic exercise resulted in improved muscle architecture (increased type II fibers and decreased type I fibers), increased muscle fiber area, increased cross-sectional area of the vastus lateralis, and increased mitochondrial density [6].

What type of aerobic exercise might provide the best intervention in CKD? It has been postulated that physical activity that does not cause muscular microinjury (which can lead to inflammation) is particularly beneficial. One study of athletes showed that swimming reduced C-reactive protein (CRP), a commonly utilized marker of inflammation, far more than cycling, soccer, running, or controls [7]. However, another study of healthy subjects found that jogging and aerobic dancing were less likely than other forms of aerobic exercise to be associated with elevated inflammatory markers after adjustment for confounding factors such as age, race, sex, BMI, smoking, and health status [8]. Almost any method of increased activity is likely to be beneficial; choice of activity should be based on tolerance level and practicality. For most people, consistent and persistent simple walking is probably suitable. Even household chores such as gardening can be useful [9]. Patients should start at a moderate difficulty level and progressively increase the time to thirty minutes for three days a week or more [10].

Aerobic exercise is generally safe in all stages of CKD. However, a few caveats should be noted. Intradialytic aerobic exercise (see below) has been shown to be safe in the first two hours of dialysis; after two hours, cardiac decompensation may preclude exercise [11]. There have also been several reports of adverse renal events caused by exercise. A 26 year old woman developed perirenal hematoma after hula-hooping [12]. After running a 200-meter sprint event, a 33-year old man developed bilateral diffuse enlargement of the kidneys, which improved after a month [13]. Exercise is still uncommon in CKD patients and physical inactivity is usual in this population. Kontos et al. recently tried to elucidate the barriers and facilitators to physical activity. Barriers include fatigue, depression, transportation, time, and equipment. Facilitators include sources of motivation, desire to improve, actual improvement, formal prescription and incorporation into the treatment plan [14].

Aerobic Exercise and Non-Dialysis CKD

Aerobic exercise in non-dialysis patients with CKD improves symptom scores, sickness impact profiles, and health-related quality of life[15]. Boyce et al. found that four months of exercise training in sixteen non-dialysis CKD subjects resulted in the following findings: a) decreased blood pressure (systolic and diastolic), b) increased peak oxygen consumption, c) unchanged hemoglobin, lipids, and left ventricular mass and function, and d) no effect on declining glomerular filtration rate (GFR) [16]. Clyne et al. report that aerobic exercise in non-dialysis CKD patients was associated with increased maximum exercise capacity and decreased heart rate but was not associated with improved hemoglobin, GFR, blood pressure, or echocardiographic findings [17]. Eidemak et al. studied patients with moderate to severe CKD (GFR range 10-43 mL/min) and found that aerobic exercise increased maximum work capacity but had no effect on declining GFR [18]. Heiwe et al. studied the elderly population (average age 76 years, average GFR 18 mL/min) and demonstrated that aerobic exercise increased muscle strength and functional capacity [19]. Pechter et al. found that aquatic exercise in mild to moderate CKD decreased blood pressure, decreased proteinuria, decreased products of lipid peroxidation, and increased glutathione; mean GFR increased from 62.9 to 67.1 mL/min [20]. Physical activity correlated with elevated GFR in an analysis of The Third National Health and Nutrition Examination Survey (NHANES III)[21].

Aerobic Exercise and Hemodialysis Patients

Intradialytic

Intradialytic aerobic exercise has been shown to be safe in the first two hours of dialysis; after two hours, cardiac decompensation may preclude exercise[11]. Intradialytic cycling, with normalization of hematocrit, has been shown to improve peak oxygen consumption and quality of life[22]. Storer et al. have shown that intradialytic cycling increases peak oxygen consumption, power, endurance time, quadriceps strength, and improves fatigability[23]. Macdonald et al. report increased power and increased physical function with intradialytic cycling but were unable to show a change in lean mass or insulin-like growth factor[24]. Dialysis efficacy and physical functioning improve with intradialytic cycle ergometer exercise[25].

Anderson et al. report that intradialytic exercise bicycle training resulted in decreased blood pressures; however, this effect waned with detraining [26]. Sakkas et al. recruited eighteen patients to undergo a program of intradialytic aerobic exercise; of eighteen patients, nine completed the study and were biopsied. They found that aerobic exercise corrected fiber atrophy, increased cross-sectional fiber area, and improved capillarization [5].

Exercise plus intradialytic parenteral nutrition (IDPN) improves albumin fractional synthetic rate in chronic hemodialysis patients[27]. Intradialytic aerobic plus strength training in Australia has recently been shown to improve functionality in sit to stand, step in place, and arm curl. In addition, phosphate levels declined and urea clearance increased [28].

Interdialytic

Aerobic exercise on non-dialysis days has been shown to be associated with improved quality of life, decreased depression, and decreased anxiety [29]. Regular life-readiness activities, such as household chores and gardening, are also associated with improved physical functioning and improve quality of life [9]. Goldberg et al. report that the benefits of exercise can occur without a change in body weight [30]. In a subsequent study, they again showed that interdialytic aerobic exercise increases maximum aerobic capacity, decreases blood pressure, decreases depression, increases hemoglobin, decreases triglycerides, increases HDL, and increases insulin sensitivity [31]. Shalom et al., in a study of interdialytic aerobic exercise, report that compliance was very poor and though work capacity was increased, there were no improvements in psychological well-being, blood pressure, hematocrit, or left-ventricular ejection fraction [32].

Molsted et al., in a study of interdialytic aerobic exercise, report increased aerobic capacity and improved scores on SF36 (Medical Outcomes Short Form 36) but report lack of effect on blood pressure or lipids [33]. Of 22 patients in the exercise group, eleven dropped out, eight because they did not have time or because they regretted enrolling in the study and 3 because of medical complications. Kouidi et al report that aerobic exercise on non-dialysis days resulted in increased type II fibers, increased muscle fiber area, increased VO_2, and increased exercise time [6]. Mustata et al. report that 3 months of interdialytic exercise improved arterial stiffness but did not have an impact on insulin resistance. Overall participation was 80% [34].

Koufaki et al. report that interdialytic cycling in ESRD patients resulted in increased VO_2. Of thirty four patients, eighteen completed the six month training. Reasons for dropping out included injury, loss of interest, noncompliance, transportation problems, surgery, frailty, and death [35]. These investigators also demonstrated that aerobic exercise is associated with better nutritional status, as evidenced by increased subjective global assessment (SGA)[36]. Kouidi et al. have shown that interdialytic aerobic exercise increases muscle fiber cross-sectional area of the vastus lateralis [6]. A comparison of two equivalent 3-month studies, one on interdialytic aerobic exercise and one on interdialytic resistance training, reveals equal improvements in peak leg strength [37,38]. Myostatin mRNA decreases and mRNA for insulin-like growth factors increases with interdialytic aerobic exercise [4].

Cardiac rehabilitation after coronary bypass in dialysis patients is associated with 35% decreased risk of all-cause mortality and 36% decrease risk of cardiac death. However, only ten percent of dialysis patients undergoing coronary bypass get cardiac rehabilitation [39].

Intradialytic versus Interdialytic Exercise in Patients with ESRD on HD

Although interdialytic exercise has been reported to be superior to intradialytic exercise, patients generally have greater difficulty in complying with the interdialytic prescription and intradialytic exercise prescription usually has fewer dropouts. One study compared three kinds of rehabilitation: A) aerobic exercise and strength training on non-dialysis days, B) aerobic exercise on dialysis days, C) unsupervised moderate exercise program at home, and D) controls. They found that group A was most effective as evidenced by increased peak oxygen consumption, anaerobic threshold, and exercise time. However, group A had a higher dropout rate [40]. Kouidi et al. studied intradialytic versus interdialytic aerobic exercise. They reported that interdialytic aerobic exercise is associated with increased exercise time, increased peak VO_2, a perception of improved health, and increased numbers of employed patients; however, interdialytic exercise had a greater dropout rate [41]. Painter et al. compared independent exercise versus in-center cycling; they reported that both were effective at improving quality of life although the effect was most pronounced with those whose initial functioning capacity was low [42, 43].

Exercise and Renal Transplantation

Cardiorespiratory fitness is reduced in uremic adults; it improves slightly with transplantation but it remains reduced compared to age and gender matched controls. It has been suggested that reduced cardiorespiratory fitnsess is correlated with inactivity, metabolic syndrome, and atherosclerotic burden [44].

Transplant patients tend to be physically inactive. Reasons for physical inactivity include lack of motivation, mind occupied with other things to do, weather, fatigue, poor health, and shortness of breath. Facilitators include expectation that health will get better and mobility, strength, and energy will increase. Encouragement from physicians and exercising with others are other facilitators [45].

Home based exercise (walking or cycling) did not improve blood pressure in transplant recipients, caused an improvement in HDL, and increased METS slightly but fitness remained low. Cardiovascular risk remained high [46].

Rehabilitation in adult renal transplant patients increases flexibility, range of motion, and peak expiratory flow [47]. With exercise, quadriceps strength increases, peak work rate and aerobic capacity/oxygen consumption increases and muscle fiber architecture improves, with decreased myosin type I and increased myosin type IIa[48]. In addition, six months after renal transplantation, improvement is seen in left ventricular function (ejection fraction and wall motion) [49].

Glucose metabolism tends to deteriorate in renal transplant patients. Aerobic exercise effectively improves glucose metabolism in such patients. In a study by Sharif et al., 44% of impaired glucose tolerance (IGT)) became normal and 58% or new onset diabetes after transplantation (NODAT) improved to IGT or to normal[50].

Finally, urinary creatinine excretion (as an indicator of muscle mass) has been shown to be a predictor of mortality and graft loss in renal transplant recipients, and exercise has been proposed as a way of preserving muscle mass so as to decrease mortality and prevent graft loss[51].

Aerobic Exercise and Pediatric CKD

Exercise capacity in pediatric patients with end-stage renal disease is impaired markedly. Alayh et al. demonstrated that in pediatric patients on peritoneal dialysis quadriceps strength is decreased and there is increased fat in muscles that contributes to decreased physical functioning and muscle strength [52]. Weaver et al. have shown that stages three and above pediatric CKD, hemodialysis and transplant patients all have decreased oxygen consumption/aerobic capacity; in addition, VO_2 had an inverse correlation with creatinine, triglycerides, CRP and diastolic dysfunction[53]. There is no difference between pediatric patients on hemodialysis and peritoneal dialysis in treadmill time, aerobic capacity, and oxygen consumption at anaerobic threshold[54].

Transplantation does improve muscle oxygen metabolism and aerobic capacity to a limited extent in uremic children[55]; however even after transplantation, VO_2 and muscle strength remains significantly below the norm, exercise capacity remains low, and these children remain physically inactive, much of which correlates with increased fat in muscle[56].

There are no studies that have prospectively used exercise as an intervention in pediatric CKD, pediatric hemodialysis, pediatric peritoneal dialysis, or pediatric transplant patients to date; such studies are greatly needed.

Adverse Role of Inflammation

Low-grade chronic inflammation, characterized by high serum levels of CRP and interleukin-6 (IL-6), has been associated with protein-energy malnutrition and decreased survival [57,58,59]. A correlation between nutritional indices and acute-phase reactant protein levels has been documented [60, 61]. Chronic hemodialysis patients with high serum IL-6 levels lost body weight by more than 4% over three years; serum albumin and creatinine were also low [62]. IL-6 promotes cancer cachexia [63]. It has been reported that there is an association between acute-phase reactant proteins and cardiovascular disease. In the Physicians Health Study, a single CRP measurement was shown to have high predictive power for future myocardial infarction in apparently healthy men [64].

Inflammation in non-Dialysis CKD

Stenvinkel et al., in a study of non-dialysis CKD patients with a mean GFR of 7 mL/min, demonstrated that 44% suffered from malnutrition and 32% had an active acute phase response, as evidence by increased levels of CRP [57]. Barzilay et al., in a cross-sectional analysis, showed that in non-dialysis CKD, microalbuminuria is associated with age, elevated systolic blood pressure, and markers of systemic inflammation, including CRP[65].

Inflammation in Hemodialysis Patients

CKD and uremia are strongly associated with elevated inflammatory markers; in uremia, this association has been termed the Malnutrition-Inflammation Complex Syndrome (MICS) [66,67,68,69,70]. In one study of 845 hemodialysis patients, 35% had elevated CRP. The study reported a strong inverse relationship between both serum albumin and creatinine and the odds of death; no such relationship was found for CRP [71]. However, many other studies in hemodialysis patients have shown that CRP was as strong a predictor of morbidity/mortality as hypoalbuminemia [58,59,62,72,73]. In hemodialysis patients, CRP is associated with an increased risk of hospitalization [73]. Also, it has been reported that among hypoalbuminemic patients, the degree of hypoalbuminemia correlated with elevation of CRP, alpha2-macroglobulin, ferritin, and serum amyloid A [59,74,75,76]. It is of note that analbuminemic rats have a normal life span and normal renal function so it is probably the cause of hypoalbuminemia and not hypoalbuminemia itself that leads to higher mortality [77].

The kidney is the major site of elimination of many cytokines, which may be at least in part the cause of inflammation in renal failure. In addition, the dialysis process itself can be pro-inflammatory [78]. Finally, T-helper type 1 (TH1) cells promote interferon-gamma, interleukin-12 (IL-12), and TNF-alpha, which are inflammatory cytokines. T-helper type 2 (TH2) cells promote other interleukins such as IL-4, IL-5, IL-6, and IL-10, which are anti-inflammatory. CKD is characterized by a shift in the TH1/TH2 balance towards TH1[79].

Aerobic Exercise and Inflammation in CKD

There is a paucity of studies that have looked at the effects of aerobic exercise on inflammation in renal failure. This may be because it is often viewed that abnormal muscle function makes exercise impractical in patients with CKD. However, in dialysis patients, aerobic exercise training can achieve favorable improvements in muscle atrophy and fiber hypertrophy [80]. The aerobic exercise capacity of people on hemodialysis is half the expected value for healthy individuals; dialysis patients often report limitation in tasks such as walking several blocks or climbing stairs. One study, albeit in the general population, notes that one must expend 1500 kcal/wk in order to attenuate atherosclerosis/inflammation [81]. Uremic myopathy may limit aerobic capacity in hemodialysis patients [82]. Therefore, a good rehabilatation program will ideally combine both aerobic training and strength training. For some people with orthopedic compromise, non-weight bearing activities may be utilized, and for people with severe deconditioning, resistive training should be initiated prior to aerobic exercise [83, 84, 85].

A cross-sectional study by Hung et al. reported elevated cytokines, including CRP, in the dialysis population but failed to ascertain a correlation between physical activity and cytokines, performance, or functionality [86]. However, the lack of associations in population studies do not contradict benefits which may be achieved by exercise programs in such patients.

Effect of Exercise on Albuminuria and Progression of CKD

Diabetic patients with CKD and overt albuminuria typically develop progressive kidney failure. Therefore, there is much interest in the effects of exercise on albuminuria and progression of kidney disease. Since exercise is associated with a decrease in inflammation, the relationship between inflammation and progression of kidney disease is first considered. In a cross-sectional analysis of coronary heart disease data from different years of follow-up, it was concluded that there is a significant relation between inflammation and microalbuminuria (urinary excretion of small amounts of albumin). Because of the cross-sectional nature of the study, causality could not be established, but the authors speculated that inflammation probably precedes microalbuminuria [65]. One study in type 2 diabetes established that markers of endothelial dysfunction and inflammation were strongly associated with increases in urinary albumin excretion and thus could be involved in the pathogenesis of CKD. Endothelial dysfunction causes an increase in inflammatory activity, potentially creating a vicious cycle of inflammatory activity and endothelial dysfunction [87]. Cytokines and inflammatory markers may mediate glomerular and renal damage and thus be involved in the pathogenesis of albuminuria and renal failure [88].

In view of the evidence linking inflammation, albuminuria, and progression of CKD, one would suspect that exercise would also decrease albuminuria and slow down the rate of progression of renal failure. Studies in rats have shown a beneficial effect of aquatic exercise on the rate of progression of CKD [89], but these findings could not be reproduced with land-based exercise in either rats or humans (median GFR 25 ml/min/1.73 m^2) [90, 91]. However, the human studies failed to note an improvement in blood pressure or plasma lipids, and the improvement in aerobic performance was small. It is of note however that a study of mild to moderate renal failure subjects noted enhanced GFR and diminished proteinuria with aquatic exercise [20], which is consistent with the previously quoted findings in experimental animals. Thus, there could be differences between the effects of land-based and aquatic exercise on kidney function.

Inflammation, Obesity, Leptin, and CKD

Inflammation is also related to obesity. Macrophages invade fat in response to an unknown signal and form giant cells; hence, adipose tissue is the site of active inflammation, characterized by elevated cytokines and leptin. Chronic inflammation and acute infection are associated with anorexia and cachexia, probably through the actions of cytokines and leptin on the hypothalamus. Fasting/starvation leads to declining leptin levels, which in turn leads to increased appetite, decreased energy expenditure, diminished thyroid hormone production, inhibition of the reproductive axis, and apoptosis in the thymus. However, despite elevated cytokines and leptin, appetite is not decreased in obesity/metabolic syndrome. This may be because of hypothalamic resistance and concurrent activation of the peripheral immune system (immune cells have leptin receptors). Thus, a vicious cycle of inflammation in adipose tissue leading to leptin production coupled with hypothalamic resistance and activation of the inflammatory process, may lead to further leptin production.[92].

Similarly, adipose tissue secretes IL-6, which is associated with insulin resistance, inflammation, and the hepatic acute phase response. IL-6 causes decreased food intake and increased energy expenditure; deletion of IL-6 in mice leads to obesity. Thus, obesity leads to IL-6 production and concurrently induces CNS IL-6 resistance, which exacerbates obesity and further increases IL-6 levels [92].

It is suggested that macrophage invasion of fat and inflammation-related gene expression precedes the development of insulin resistance. It may be hypothesized that inflammation also precedes CKD, which in turn worsens inflammation and leads to a vicious cycle. Research regarding the effects of aerobic exercise and strength training on leptin in obese diabetic patients with CKD is of particular interest. Aerobic exercise in the general population has been shown to decrease BMI and leptin [93].

Exercise, Oxidative Stress and Endothelial Dysfunction

Most cardiovascular risk factors such as smoking, hypercholesterolemia, hypertension, diabetes mellitus, and renal failure are associated with endothelial dysfunction and oxidative stress. Inflammation produces free radicals and therefore gives rise to oxidative stress. In addition, spontaneous leukocyte activation in CKD may generate free radicals and promote oxidative stress [94]. CKD is an important cause of oxidative stress, as evidenced by the observation that oxidative stress parameters normalize after kidney transplantation with complete recovery of renal function [95]. Finally, the antioxidant activity of HDL in CKD is reduced [96].

One of the major mechanisms leading to endothelial dysfunction is increased oxidative stress. Oxidative stress causes nitric oxide (NO) breakdown; consequently, endothelial cells lose their ability to protect the vessel wall and become atherosclerosis promoters. One study showed that flow-mediated dilation (FMD) was lower in non-dialysis CKD following 5 minutes of ischemia when compared with controls and was even lower in hemodialysis patients. Vitamin C enhanced FMD in HD patients but not in non-dialysis CKD [97]. ADMA (asymmetric dimethyl-L-arginine) accumulates and inhibits NO synthase leading to endothelial dysfunction and increased cardiovascular risk [98, 99]. Arterial stiffness, as measured by pulse wave velocity, improves with the use of a bicycle ergometer during hemodialysis [100].

Does exercise training affect oxidative stress? Although strenuous exercise acutely increases oxidative stress, most studies have shown increased resistance to oxidative stress with chronic exercise [101,102]. Plasma reduced glutathione content has been shown to increase with training distance in long distance runners during a training season and after 20 weeks of physical training in previously sedentary men [103]. It has been reported that endurance exercise in combination with vitamin E reduces oxidative stress (reduced lipid hydroperoxide), improves aerobic fitness, and reduces blood pressure and weight in older adults recruited from a retirement community [104]. Many studies have documented reduced malondialdehyde (MDA) with chronic endurance exercise [105,106,107,108,109].

Much less is known about the effects of exercise on oxidative stress in CKD patients. Aquatic exercise diminishes proteinuria, enhances GFR, decreases products of lipid peroxidation and increases reduced glutathione in subjects with mild to moderate renal failure[20].

Novel Area: Sympathoactivation

It has been postulated that ESRD patients are characterized by sympathoactivation at rest and exaggerated sympathoexcitatory response to exercise, as evidenced by increased norepinephrine levels during exercise [110,111]. Total peripheral vascular resistance was found to be elevated in pediatric renal transplant patients [112]. In rats with reduced renal mass, there is heightened sensitivity to alpha-1-adrenergic mediated contractility, depressed sensitivity to endothelium mediated relaxation; furthermore, exercise decreases oxidative stress, improves endothelial dysfunction (relaxation in response to acetylcholine), and decreases sensitivity to phenylephrine [113].

Sympathoactivation is not thought to be central; rather it is thought to be due to the exercise pressor reflex, mediated by sensory nerve endings in muscle. These sensory nerve endings constitute the metaboreceptors, which respond to chemical stimuli, and the mechanoreceptors, which respond to stretch.

In congestive heart failure, sympathoactivation is characterized by chemosensitivity mediated by decreased NO and increased angiotensin II. Exercise blunts metaboreceptors by increasing NO and decreasing angiotensin II. Mechanoreceptors are thought to be exaggerated[114]. A similar finding is expected in ESRD. However, Park et al. found that static handgrip exercise did not increase muscle sympathetic nerve activity despite a hypertensive response to exercise [115].

Conclusions

Despite much evidence for benefits of exercise in all stages of chronic kidney disease, hemodialysis, peritoneal dialysis, pediatric CKD, and renal transplant recipients, regular exercise in these populations remains very uncommon. This is probably due, in part, to the fact that most of the scientific literature on exercise and CKD is grounded in studies involving few numbers of patients (usually less than a hundred). Moreover, exercise has not been shown to have an impact on survival and mortality. Large, multi-institutional randomized double blind studies are needed before renal rehabilitation or even regular exercise will become a routine part of the medical care of patients with CKD.

References

[1] Castaneda, C; Gordon, PL; Uhlin, KL; Levey, AS; Kehayias, JJ; Dwyer, JT; Fielding, RA; Roubenoff, R; Singh, MF. Resistance training to counteract the catabolism of a low-protein diet in patients with chronic renal insufficiency. A randomized, controlled trial. *Ann Intern Med.,* 2001, 135, 965-976.

[2] Castaneda, C; Gordon, PL; Parker, RC; Uhlin, KL; Roubenoff, R; Levey, AS. Resistance training to reduce the malnutrition-inflammation complex syndrome of chronic kidney disease. *Am J Kidney Dis.,* 2004, 43(4), 607-616.

[3] Adams, GR; Vaziri, ND. Skeletal muscle dysfunction in CRF: effects of exercise. *Am J Physiol Renal Physiol.,* 2006, 290(4), F753-61.

[4] Kopple, JD; Cohen, AH; Wang, H; et al. Effect of exercise on mRNA levels for growth factors in skeletal muscle of hemodialysis patients. *J Ren Nutr.,* 2006, 16(4), 312-324.

[5] Sakkas, GK; Sargeant, AJ; Mercer, TH; Ball, D; Koufaki, P; Karatzaferi, C; Naish, PF. Changes in muscle morphology in dialysis patients after 6 months of aerobic exercise training. *Nephrol Dial Transplant.*, 2003, 18(9), 1854-61.

[6] Kouidi, E; Albani, M; Natsis, K; Megalopoulos, A; Gigis, P; Guiba-Tziampiri, O; Tourkantonis, A; Deligiannis, A. The effects of exercise training on muscle atrophy in haemodialysis patients. *Nephrol Dial Transplant.,* 1998, 13, 685-699,.

[7] Dufaux, B; Order, U; Greyer, H; Hollmann, W. C-reactive protein serum concentrations in well-trained athletes. *Int J Sports Med.,* 1984, 5, 102-106,

[8] King, DE; Carek, P; Mainous, AG. 3rd; Pearson WS: Inflammatory markers and exercise: differences related to exercise type. *Med Sci Sports Exerc.,* 2003, 35(4), 575-581.

[9] Tawney, K; Tawney, P; Hladik, G; Hogan, SL; Falk, RJ; Weaver, C; Moore, DT; Lee, MY. The life readiness program: a physical rehabilitaton program for patients on hemodialysis. *Am J Kidney Dis.*, 2000, 36, 581-591.

[10] Kutner, NG. How can exercise be incorporated into the routine care of patients on dialysis? *Int Urol Nephrol.*, 2007, 39, 1281-1285.

[11] Moore, GE; Painter, PL; Brinker, KR; Stray-Gundersen, J; Mitchell, JH. Cardiovascular response to submaximal stationary cycling during hemodialysis. *Am J Kidney Dis.*, 1998, 31(4), 631-637.

[12] Park, SK; Kum, H; Lhee, HY; Lee, KB. Development of a perirenal hematoma after hula-hooping. *Yonsei Med J.,* 2007, 48(5), 868-870.

[13] Matsumura, N; Yamamoto, K. Bilateral diffuse enlargement of the kidneys after exercise. *Intern Med.*, 2006, 45(8), 567.

[14] Kontos, PC; Miller, K; Brooks, D; et al. Factos influencing exercise participation by older adults requiring chronic hemodialysis: a qualitative study. *Int Urol Nephrol.,* 2007, 39, 1303-1311.

[15] Fitts, SS; Guthrie, MR; Blagg, CR. Exercise counseling and rehabilitation counseling improve quality of life. *Nephron.,* 1999, 82(2), 115-21.

[16] Boyce, ML; Robergs, RA; Avasthi, PS; Roldan, C; Foster, A; Montner, P; Stark, D; Nelson, C. Exercise training by individuals with predialysis renal failure: cardiorespiratory endurance, hypertension, and renal function. *Am J Kidney Dis.,* 1997, 30(2), 180-192.

[17] Clyne, N; Ekholm, J; Jogestrand, T; Lins, LE; Pehrsson, SK. Effects of exercise training in predialytic uremic patients. *Nephron.,* 1991, 59(1), 84-9.

[18] Eidemak, I; Haaber, AB; Feldt-Rasmussen, B; Kanstrup, IL; Strandgaard, S. Exercise training and the progression of chronic renal failure. *Nephron.,* 1997, *75*, 36-40,.

[19] Heiwe, S; Tollback, A; Clyne, N. Twelve weeks of exercise training increases muscle function and walking capacity in elderly predialysis patients and healthy subjects. *Nephron.*, 2001, 1, 48-56.

[20] Pechter, U; Ots, M; Mesikepp, S; Zilmer, K; Kullissaar, T; Vihalemm, T; Zilmer, M; Maaroos, J. Beneficial effects of water-based exercise in patients with chronic kidney disease. *Int J Rehabil Res,* 2003, 26, 153-156.

[21] Finkelstein, J; Joshi, A; Hise, MK. Association of physical activity and renal function in subjects with and without metabolic syndrome: a review of the Third National Health

and Nutrition Examination Survey (NHANES III). *Am J Kidney Dis.*, 2006, 48(3), 372-382.

[22] Painter, P; Moore, G; Carlson, L; Paul, S; Myll, J; Phillips, W; Haskell, W. Effects of exercise training plus normalization of hematocrit on exercise capacity and health-related quality of life. *Am J Kidney Dis.*, 2002, 39(2), 257-265.

[23] Storer, TW; Casaburi, R; Sawelson, S; Koppel, JD. Endurance exercise training during haemodialysis improves strength, power, fatigability and physical performance in maintenance haemodialysis patients. *Nephrol Dial Transplant.*, 2005, 20, 1429-1437.

[24] Macdonald, JH; Marcora, SM; Jibani, M; Phanish, MK; Holly, J; Lemmey, AB. Intradialytic exercise as anabolic therapy in haemodialysis patients – a pilot study. *Clin Physiol Funct Imaging.*, 2005, 25, 113-118.

[25] Parsons, TL; Toffelmire, EB; King-VanVlack, CE. Exercise training during hemodialysis improves dialysis efficacy and physical performance. *Arch Phys Med Rehabil.*, 2006, 87(5), 680-687.

[26] Anderson, JE; Boivin, MR; Jr; Hatchett, L. Effect of exercise training on intradialytic ambulatory and treatment-related blood pressure in hemodialysis patients. *Ren Fail.*, 2004, 26(5), 539-44.

[27] Pupim, LB; Flakoll, PJ; Ikizler, TA. Exercise improves albumin fractional synthetic rate in chronic hemodialysis patients. *Eur J Clin Nutr.*, 2007, 61, 686-689. 2007.

[28] Bennett, PN; Breugelmans, L; Agius, M; et al. A haemodialysis exercise programme using novel exercise equipment: A Pilot Study. *J Ren Care.*, 2007, 33(4), 153-8.

[29] Kouidi, E; Lacovides, A; Iordanidis, P; Vassiliou, S; Deligiannis, A; Lerodiakonou, C; Tourkantonis, A. Exercise renal rehabilitation program (ERRP): Psychological effects. *Nephron.*, 1997, 77, 152-158.

[30] Goldberg, A; Hagberg, J; Delmez, J; Carney, RM; McKevitt, PM; Ehsani, AA; Harter, HR. The metabolic and psychological effects of exercise training in hemodialysis patients. *Am J Clin Nutr.*, 1980, 33(7), 1620-8.

[31] Goldberg, AP; Geltman, EM; Gavin, JR; 3rd; Carney, RM; Hagberg, JM; Delmez, JA; Naumovich, A; Oldfield, MH; Harter, HR. Exercise training reduces coronary risk and effectively rehabilitates hemodialysis patients. *Nephron.*, 1986, 42, 311-316.

[32] Shalom, R; Blumenthal, JA; Willaims, RS; McMurray, RG; Dennis, VW. Feasibility and benefits of exercise training in patients on maintenance dialysis. *Kidney Int.* 1984, 25, 958-963.

[33] Molsted, S; Eidemak, I; Sorensen, HT; Kristensen, JH. Five months of physical exercise in hemodialysis patients: effects on aerobic capacity, physical function, and self-rated health. *Nephron Clin Pract.*, 2004, 96(3), c76-81.

[34] Mustata, S; Chan, C; Lai, V; Miller, JA. Impact of an exercise program on arterial stiffness and insulin resistance in hemodialysis patients. *J Am Soc Nephrol.*, 2004, 15, 2713-2718.

[35] Koufaki, P; Nash, PF; Mercer, TH. Assessing the efficacy of exercise training in patients with chronic disease. *Med Sci Sports Exerc.*, 2002, 34(8), 1234-1241,.

[36] Koufaki, P; Mercer, TH; Naish, PF. Effects of exercise training on aerobic and functional capacity of patients with end-stage renal disease. *Clin Physiol Func Im.*, 2002, 22, 125-134.

[37] Headley, S; Germain, M; Mailloux, P; Mulhern, J; Ashworth, B; Burris, J; Brewer, B; Nindl, B; Coughlin, M; Welles, R; Jones, M. Resistance training improves strength and

functional measures in patients with end-stage renal disease. *Am J Kidney Dis.,* 2002, 40(2), 355-364.

[38] Mercer, TH; Koufaki, P; Naish, PF. Exercise training improves functional capacity, nutritional status,and self-reported activity of daily living in peritoneal dialysis patients. *Med Sci Sports Exerc.,* 33, S254. 2001.

[39] Kutner, NG; Zhang, R; Huang, Y; Herzog, CA. Cardiac rehabilitation and survival of dialysis patients after coronary bypass. *J Am Soc Nephrol.,* 2006, 17, 1175-1180.

[40] Konstantinidou, E; Koukouvou, G; Kouidi, E; Deligiannis, A; Tourkantonis, A. Exercise training in patients with end-stage renal disease on hemodialysis: comparison of three rehabilitation programs. *J Rehabil Med.,* 2002, 34, 40-45,

[41] Kouidi, E; Grekas, D; Deligiannis, A; Tourkantonis, A. Outcomes of long-term exercise training in dialysis patients: comparison of two training programs. *Clin Nephrol.*, 2004, 61 suppl: s31-s38.

[42] Painter, P; Carlson, L; Carey, S; Paul, S; Myll, J. Low-functioning hemodialysis patients improve with exercise training. *Am J Kidney Dis*., 2000, 36(3): 600-8.

[43] Painter, P; Carlson, L; Carey, S; Paul, S; Myll, J. Physical functioning and health-related quality of life changes with exercise training in hemodialysis patients. *Am J Kidney Dis*., 2000, 35(3), 482-92.

[44] Armstrong, K; Rakhit, D; Jeffriess, L; et al. Cardiorespiratory fitness is related to physical inactivity, metabolic risk factors, and atherosclerotic burden in glucose-intolerant renal transplant recipients. *Clin J Am Soc Nephrol.,* 2006, 1, 1275-1283.

[45] Sanchez, Z; Cashion, A; Cowan, P. Perceived barriers and facilitators to physical activity in kidney transplant recipients. *Prog Transplant.,* 2007, 17(4), 324-331.

[46] Painter, P; Hector, L; Ray, K; et al. Effects of exercise training on coronary heart disease risk factors in renal transplant recipients. *Am J Kidney Dis.,* 2003, 42(2), 362-369.

[47] Korabiewska, L; Lewandowska, M; Juskowa, J; Bialoszewski, D. Need for rehabilitation in renal replacement therapy involving allogeneic kidney transplantation. *Transplant Proc.,* 2007, 39, 2776-2777.

[48] Van den Ham, E; Kooman, J; Schols, A; et al. The functional, metabolic, and anabolic responses to exercise training in renal transplant and hemodialysis patients. *Transplantation.,* 2007, 83(8), 1059-1068.

[49] Stokkel, M; Duchateau, CS; Jukema, W; deFijter, HW. Noninvasive assessment of left ventricular function prior to and 6 months after renal transplantation. *Transplant Proc.*, 2007, 39, 3159-3162.

[50] Sharif, A; Moore, R; Baboolal, K. Influence of lifestyle modification in renal transplant recipients with postprandial hyperglycemia. *Transplantation.,* 2008, 85(3), 353-358.

[51] Oterdoom, LH; van Ree, RM; de Vries, APJ; et al. Urinary creatinine excretion reflecting muscle mass is a predictor of mortality and graft loss in renal transplant recipients. *Transplantation.,* 2008, 86(3), 391-398,.

[52] Alayh, G; Ozkaya, O; Bek, K; et al. Physical function, muscle strength and muscle mass in children on peritoneal dialysis. *Pediatr Nephrol.,* 2008, 23, 639-644.

[53] Weaver, Jr; D; Kimball, T; Knilans, T; et al. Decreased maximal aerobic capacity in pediatric chronic kidney disease. *J Am Soc Nephrol.,* 2008, 19, 624-630.

[54] Pattaragarn, A; Warady, B; Sabath, R. Exercise capacity in pediatric patients with end stage renal disease. *Perit Dial Int.,* 2004, 24, 274-280.

[55] Matsumoto, N; Ichimura, S; Hamaoka, T; et al. Impaired muscle oxygen metabolism in uremic children: Improved after renal transplamtation. *Am J Kidney Dis.,* 2006, 48(3), 473-480.

[56] Painter, P; Krasnoff, J; Mathias, R. Exercise capacity and physical fitness in pediatric dialysis and kidney transplant patients. *Pediatr Nephrol.,* 2007, 22, 1030-1039.

[57] Stenvinkel, P; Heimburger, O; Paultre, F; Diczfalusy, U; Wang, T; Berglund, L; Jogestrand, T. Strong association between malnutrition, inflammation, and atherosclerosis in chronic renal failure. *Kidney Int.,* 1999, 55, 1899-1911,

[58] Yeun, JY; Levine, RA; Mantadilok, V; Kaysen, GA. C-Reactive protein predicts all-cause and cardiovascular mortality in hemodialysis patients. *Am J Kidney Dis.,* 2000, 35(3), 469-476,

[59] Zimmermann, J; Herrlinger, S; Pruy, A; Metzger, T; Wanner, C: Inflammation enhances cardiovascular risk and mortality in hemodialysis patients. *Kidney Int.,* 1999, 55, 648-658,

[60] Kaysen, GA; Yeun, J; Depner, T. Albumin synthesis, catabolism and distribution in dialysis patients. *Miner Electrolyte Metab.,* 1997, 23, 218-224,

[61] Gabay, C; Kushner, I: Acute-phase proteins and other systemic responses to inflammation. *N Engl J Med.,* 1999, 340(6), 448-454.

[62] Kaizu, Y; Kimura, M; Yoneyama, T; Miyaji, K; Hibi, I; Kumagai, H. Interleukin-6 may mediate malnutrition in chronic hemodialysis patients. *Am J Kidney Dis.,* 1998, 31, 93-100,

[63] Strassmann, G; Fong, M; Kenney, JS; Jacob, CO. Evidence for the involvement of interleukin 6 in experimental cancer cachexia. *J Clin Invest,* 1992, 89, 1681-1684,

[64] Ridker, PM; Cushman, M; Stampfer, MJ; Tracy, RP; Hennekens, CH. Inflammation, aspirin, and the risk of cardiovascular disease in apparently healthy men. *New Eng J Med,* 1997, 336(14), 973-979,

[65] Barzilay, JI; Peterson, D; Cushman, M; Heckbert, SR; Cao, JJ; Blaum, C; Tracy, RP; Klein, R; Herrington, DM. The relationship of cardiovascular risk factors to microalbuminuria in older adults with or without diabetes mellitus or hypertension: the cardiovascular health study. *Am J Kidney Dis,* 2004, 44(1), 25-34,

[66] Kalantar-Zadeh, K; Ikizler, TA; Block, G; Avram, MM; Kopple, JD. Malnutrition-inflammation complex syndrome in dialysis patients: causes and consequences. *Am J Kidney Dis,* 2003, 42(5), 864-881,

[67] Galle, J; Seibold, S; Wanner, C. Inflammation in uremic patients: what is the link? *Kidney Blood Press Res.,* 2003, 26, 65-75,

[68] Caglar, K; Hakim, R; Ikizler, T. Approaches to the reversal of malnutrition, inflammation, and atherosclerosis in end-stage renal disease. *Nutr Rev.,* 2002, 60(12), 378-387,

[69] Pupim, LB; Ikizler, TA. Uremic malnutrition: new insights into an old problem. *Semin Dial,* 2003, 16(3), 224-232,

[70] Kalantar-Zadeh, K; McAllister, CJ; Lehn, RS; Lee, GH; Nissenson, AR; Kopple, JD. Effect of malnutrition-inflammation complex syndrome on EPO hyporesponsiveness in maintenance hemodialysis patients. *Am J Kidney Dis.*, 2003, 42, 761-773.

[71] Owen, WF; Lowrie, EG. C-reactive protein as an outcome predictor for maintenance hemodialysis patients. *Kidney Int.,* 1998, 54, 627-636,

[72] Bergstrom, J. Nutrition and mortality in hemodialysis. *J Am Soc Nephrol,* 1995, 6(5), 1329-1341,

[73] Ikizler, TA Wingard, RL; Harvell, J; Shyr, Y; Hakim, RM. Association of morbidity with markers of nutrition and inflammation in chronic hemodialysis patients: a prospective study. *Kidney Int,* 1999, 55, 1945-1951,

[74] Kaysen, GA; Chertow, GM; Adhikarla, R; Young, B; Ronco, C; Levin, NW. Inflammation and dietary protein exert competing effects on serum albumin and creatinine in hemodialysis patients. *Kidney Int.*, 2001, 60(1), 333-40.

[75] Kaysen, GA; Rathore, V; Shearer, GC; Depner, TA. Mechanisms of hypoalbuminemia in hemodialysis patients. *Kidney Int,* 1995, 48, 510-516.

[76] Kaysen, GA; Stevenson, FT; Depner, TA. Determinants of albumin concentration in hemodialysis patients. *Am J Kidney Dis.,* 1997, 29, 658-668,

[77] Kaysen, GA. Hypoalbuminemia in dialysis patients. *Semin Dial.,* 1996, 9, 249-256,

[78] Horl, WH. Hemodialysis membranes: interleukins, biocompatibility, and middle molecules. *J Am Soc Nephrol.,* 2002, 13(Suppl 1), S62-71.

[79] Carrero, JJ; Yilmaz, MI; Lindholm, B; Stenvinkel, P. Cytokine dysregulation in chronic kidney disease: How can we treat it? *Blood Purif.*, 2008, 26, 291-299.

[80] Mercer, TH; Koufaki, P; Naish, PF. Nutritional status, functional capacity and exercise rehabilitation in end-stage renal disease. *Clin Nephrol,* 2004, 61(Suppl. 1), S54-S59,

[81] Hambrecht, R; Niebauer, J; Marburger, C; Grunze, M; Kalberer, B; Hauer, K; Schlierf, G; Kubler, W; Schuler, G. Various intensities of leisure time physical activity in patients with coronary artery disease: effects on cardiorespiratory fitness and progression of atherosclerotic lesions. *J Am Coll Cardiol.*, 1993, 22, 468-477,

[82] Moore, GE; Parsons, DB; Stray-Gunderson, J; Painter, PL; Brinker, KR; Mitchell, JH. Uremic myopathy limits aerobic capacity in hemodialysis patients. *Am J Kidney Dis.,* 1993, 22, 277-287,

[83] Painter, P. The importance of exercise training in rehabilitation of patients with end-stage renal disease. *Am J Kidney Dis.,* 1994, 24 suppl 1, S2-S9.

[84] Painter, PL. End Stage Renal Disease. In: Skinner, JS, ed. *Exercise Testing and Exercise Prescription for Special Cases*. 2nd edition. Media, PA: Williams & Wilkins; 1993, 351-362.

[85] Evans, N; Forsyth, E. End-stage renal disease in people with type 2 diabetes: systemic manifestations and exercise implications. *Phys Ther.,* 2004, 84(5), 454-463.

[86] Hung, AM; Chertow, GM; Young Belinda, S; Carey, S; Johansen, KL. Inflammatory markers are unrelated to physical activity, performance, and functioning in hemodialysis. *J Ren Nutr.,* 2002, 12(3), 170-176.

[87] Stehouwer, CD; Gall, MA; Twisk, JW; Knudsen, E; Emeis, JJ; Parving, HH. Increased urinary albumin excretion, endothelial dysfunction, and chronic low-grade inflammation in type 2 diabetes: progressive, interrelated, and independently associated with risk of death. *Diabetes.,* 2002, 51, 1157-1165.

[88] Klahr, S. Mechanisms of progression of chronic renal damage. *J Nephrol.,* 1999, 12(suppl 2), S53-S62.

[89] Heifets, M; Davis, T; Klahr, S. Exercise training ameliorates progressive renal disease in rats with subtotal nephrectomy. *Kidney Int.,* 1987, 32, 815-819.

[90] Bergamaschi, CT; Boim, MA; Moura, LA; Picarro, JC; Schor, N. Effects of long-term training on the progression of chronic renal failure in rats. *Med Sci Sports Exerc.,* 1997, 29(2), 169-174,

[91] Eidemak, I; Haaber, AB; Feldt-Rasmussen, B; Kanstrup, IL; Strandgaard, S. Exercise training and the progression of chronic renal failure. *Nephron.,* 1997, 75, 36-40,

[92] Wisse, BE. The inflammatory syndrome: the role of adipose tissue cytokines in metabolic disorders linked to obesity. *J Am Soc Nephrol,* 2004, 15, 2792-2800.

[93] Pischon, T; Hankinson, SE; Hotamisligil, GS; Rifai, N; Rimm, EB. Leisure-time physical activity and reduced plasma levels of obesity-related inflammatory markers. *Obes Res.,* 2003, 11(9), 1055-1064.

[94] Yoon, JW; Patel, W; Vaziri, ND. Spontaneous leukocyte activation and oxygen-free radical generation in end-stage renal disease. *Kidney Int.,* 2007, 71(2), 167-73.

[95] Antolini, F; Valente, F; Ricciardi, D; Fagugli, RM. Normalization of oxidative stress parameters after kidney transplant is secondary to full recovery of renal function *Clin Nephrol.,* 2004, 62(2), 131-137.

[96] Moradi, H; Patel, MV; Elahimehr, R; Vaziri, ND. Impaired antioxidant activity of HDL in chronic kidney disease. *Transl Res.,* 2009, 153(2), 77-85.

[97] Ghiadoni, L; Cupisti, A; Huang, Y; Mattei, P; Cardinal, H; Favilla, S; Rindi, P; Barsotti, G; Taddei, S; Salvetti, A. Endothelial dysfunction and oxidative stress in chronic renal failure. *J Nephrol,* 2004, 17, 512-519.

[98] Kielstein, JT; Boger, RH; Bode-Boger, SM; Frolich, JC; Haller, H; Ritz, E; Fliser, D. Marked increase of asymmetric dimethylarginine in patients with incipient primary chronic renal disease. *J Am Soc Nephrol,* 2002, 13, 170-176.

[99] Zoccali, C; Benedetto, FA; Maas, R; Mallamaci, F; Tripepi, G; Malatino, LS; Boger, R. CREED Investigators: Asymmetric dimethylarginine, C-reactive protein, and carotid intima-media thickness in end-stage renal disease. *J Am Soc Nephrol.,* 2002, 13, 490-496,

[100] Toussaint, ND; Polkinghorne, KR; Kerr, PG. Impact of intradialytic exercise on arterial compliance and B-type natriuretic peptide levels in hemodialysis patients. *Hemodial Int.,* 2008, 12, 254-263.

[101] Polidori, MC; Mecocci, P; Cherubini, A; Senin, U. Physical activity and oxidative stress during aging. *Int J Sports Med.,* 2000, 21, 154-157.

[102] Kostka, T; Drai, J; Berthouze, SE; Lacour, JR; Bonnefoy, M. Physical activity, fitness and integrated antioxidant system in healthy active elderly women. *Int J Sports Med.,* 1998, 19, 462-467.

[103] Evelo, CT; Palmen, NG; Artur, Y; Janssen, GM. Changes in blood glutathione concentrations, and in erythrocyte glutathione reductase and glutathione S-transferase activity after running training and after participation in contests. *Eur J Appl Physiol Occup Physiol,* 1992, 64, 354-8,

[104] Jessup, JV; Home, C; Yarandi, H; Quindry, J. The effects of endurance exercise and vitamin E on oxidative stress in the elderly. *Biol Res Nurs.,* 2003, 5(1), 47-55,

[105] Fatouros, JG; Jamurtas, AZ; Villiotou, V; Pouliopoulou, S; Fotinakis, P; Taxildaris, K; Deliconstantinos, G. Oxidative stress responses in older men during endurance training and detraining. *Med Sci Sports Exerc.,* 2004, 36(12), 2065-2072,

[106] Metin, G; Gumustas, MK; Uslu, E; Belce, A; Kayseriliogfu, A. Effect of regular training on plasma thiols, malondialdehyde and carnitine concentrations in young soccer players. *Chin J Physiol.,* 2003, 46(1), 35-39,

[107] Kobe, H; Nakai, A; Koshino, T; Araki, T. Effect of regular maternal exercise on lipid peroxidation levels and antioxidant enzymatic activities before and after delivery. *J Nippon Med Sch,* 2002, 69(6), 542-548.

[108] Lawler, JM; Hu, Z; Green, JS; Crouse, SF; Grandjean, PW; Bounds, RG. Combination of estrogen replacement and exercise protects against HDL oxidation in post-menopausal women. *Int J Sports Med,* 2002, 23(7), 477-483,

[109] Sharman, JE; Geraghty, DP; Shing, CM; Fraser, DI; Coombes, JS. Endurance exercise, plasma oxidation and cardiovascular risk. *Acta Cardiol,* 2004, 59(6), 636-642,

[110] Blake, JW; Solangi, KB; Herman, MV; et al. Left ventricular response to exercise and autonomic control mechanisms in end-stage renal disease. *Arch Intern Med.,* 1989, 149, 433-436.

[111] Kettner, A; Goldberg, A; Hagberg, J; et al. Cardiovascular and metabolic responses to submaximal exercise in hemodialysis patients. *Kidney Int.,* 1984, 26, 66-71.

[112] Matteucci, MC; Giordano, U; Calzolari, A; et al. Total peripheral vascular resistance in pediatric transplant patients. *Kidney Int.,* 2002, 62, 1870-1874.

[113] Shelkovnikov, S; Summers, SM; Elahimehr, R; et al. Effect of exercise training on aortic tone in chronic renal insufficiency. *Am J Hypertens.*, 2008, 21(5), 564-9.

[114] Stickland, MK; Miller, JD. The best medicine: exercise training normalizes chemosensitivity and sympathoactivation in heart failure. *J Appl Physiol.* 2008, 105, 779-781.

[115] Park, J; Campese, VM; Middlekauff, HR. Exercise pressor reflex in humans with end-stage renal disease. *Am J Physiol Regul Integr Comp Physiol.,* 2008, 295, R1188-R1194.

In: Encyclopedia of Sports and Athletics
Editors: Jack L. Murray and Emily O. Watson
ISBN: 978-1-61209-959-0

Chapter XV

Effects of Plyometric Training Followed by Short-Term Specific Detraining and Reduced Training Periods on Explosive Strength, Agility and Speed Variables in Early Pubertal Male Basketball Players

E. Santos and M.A. Janeira
Faculty of Sport Sciences, University of Porto, Porto, Portugal

Abstract

The aims of the present study were: a) to identify the effects of plyometric training on explosive strength [squat jump (SJ), countermovement jump (CMJ), mechanical power (MP)], agility (AG), and 20-m sprint speed (20 m) variables in young basketball players; and b) to understand the effects of short-term specific detraining and reduced plyometric training on the previously achieved gains.

The sample consisted of nineteen male basketball players (13-14 years old; weight, 61.26.74 kg; height, 175.46.77 cm). The adopted structure was based upon two fundamental phases. First, subjects were submitted to an 8-week plyometric training program (standing jumps, multiple jumps, box drills, depth jumps, jumps with extra-loads), three times a week. At the end of this period, the subjects showed statistically significant increases in all the assessed variables ($p < 0.05$).

Subsequent to the plyometric training application, subjects were randomly assigned to one of two groups: a reduced training group (RT, n=9) and a specific detraining group (SDT, n=10). During the following four weeks, the former performed a single plyometric training session and the latter ceased plyometric activity. Both groups kept on regular basketball practice. In this period, RT group significantly increased ($p < 0.05$) SJ, CMJ, and S20 values, while SDT group showed statistically significant enhances ($p < 0.05$) on 20 m and AG test. The RT and SDT groups maintained the values of the remaining variables. At the end of this period, no statistically significant differences were observed between RT and DTR groups in all the evaluated variables. In conclusion, a) the outcomes highlight the efficacy of the plyometric training design; b) the reduced training program and the specific detraining indistinctly contribute to the explosive strength levels maintenance; and c) basketball training has an obvious power in the maintenance and sustainability of motor performance at least taking into account the applied training program.

Keywords: Plyometrics; Explosive Strength; Specific Detraining; Reduced Training; Basketball

Introduction

Given its peculiar characteristics, the basketball game places the athletes before a wide range of technical and tactical demands usually pointed out as decisive in higher sport performance levels. However, the particularities of these demands do not seem to be unique on the conceptual universe of sport performance. Thus, the multi-faced expression of the athletes' physical condition clearly contributes to the performance levels enhancement and to its maintenance throughout the season, constituting a precious basement upon which will raise the technical and tactical building of the team.

In this context, muscular strength is a fundamental capacity to an enhanced basketball player's performance and the strength training periodization has proved to be an indispensable topic as far as the competition teams' annual planning is concerned. The main objective is to optimize the athletes' strength gains since this factor seems to contribute unequivocally to the attainability of higher levels of sport performance. This idea has been corroborated both by training methodologists and coaches, and by physiologists and experts on biomechanics (NSCA, 1988; Klausen, 1990; Sale, 1991; Bompa, 1994; Pauletto, 1994; Fleck & Kraemer, 1997).

Performance in basketball has been associated to both technical skills properly applied in the different tactical game situations and to strength, speed, and agility aspects (Stone & Steingard, 1993). Despite the particular characteristics of the different competition levels requiring adequate attention, the main attribute of this game seems to be the ability to perform the game fundamentals (technical and tactical) in a faster and more explosive way, maintaining low fatigue levels.

The basketball particular constraints put the players before an exclusive set of demands usually adjusted to a peculiar morfotype. Guards, forewords and centers are requested to do tasks quite different during the game. However, modern basketball is a game of personal initiatives, unknown strategies where every player must be capable of fine performances in multiple tasks and situations. Demands become higher. Such a behavior implies technical, tactical and strategic particularities as well as high cardio-respiratory levels and different strength types and levels, according to the different game situations.

Given the technical demands, the diversity and multiplicity of functions which players have to perform as well as the kind of work required in the different court areas, basketball implies three basic forms of strength: maximal strength, muscular endurance and explosive strength/power. Players are seldom asked to applied maximal strength during a basketball game. Nevertheless, it seems to play an important and decisive role on some players' actions or movements, while blocking, recovering from balanced positions, as well as on the maintenance of every position particularly during defense blocks.

On the other hand, muscular endurance expressing the adequate manner athletes are able to apply a sub-maximal strength level repeatedly also highlights the important role of this strength component when considered in the basketball game temporal context. This strength component reveals itself mostly on the defensive work and on the technical-tactical actions that are repeatedly performed during the game (e.g., legs movements to reach and maintain centers position). Depending on the competitive level, a basketball lasts in average 90 minutes. Thus, it is easy to understand the relevance of muscular endurance in what concerns all the technical particularities of this sport.

Basketball is essentially a game with explosive characteristics. Strength application is often used in a dynamic, explosive and repetitive way. These characteristics demand power and express in a unique way the velocity of this sport. That is the case of shooting, rebounding and dunking. Accelerations, decelerations and fast changes of direction are as well constantly repeated movements all through the game, which demand more explosive strength levels.

Plyometrics can be assumed as a muscular strength training method based upon a set of exercises, which enable the muscle to attain high level of explosive power. Plyometric training has thus gradually become known and accepted by the coaches who wanted to develop explosive strength levels in their athletes in short periods (e.g., 8 to 12 weeks).

Most basketball technical skills imply a variety of tasks that require leg explosive power. Therefore, coaches have turned to plyometrics for strength development. They include it in their normal training programs. Besides, if plyometrics are implied in a great deal of athletic tasks in team sports, and basketball requires many countermovement actions it would be interesting to know how young athletes respond to such a training routine.

Furthermore, it is not known how plyometric training induces changes in different aspects of explosive strength, and which is the response of young athletes both to a reduced plyometric training program and to a detraining period of short duration.

Therefore, the main purposes of our study were:

(i) to identify the effects of plyometric training on different levels of explosive strength: running speed, shuttle-run, squat jump, countermovement jump and mechanical power;
(ii) to assess the effects of specific detraining and reduced plyometric training program on the gains previously obtained.

Material and Methods

Subjects

The subjects for the study were 19 young basketball players (age 13/14 years old; height 175.4±6.77 cm, and weight was 61.2±6.74 kg). Their maturation status was assessed according to Tanner's (1962) criteria for secondary sexual characteristics and corresponded to status 3 and 4.

Design of the Study

The structure adopted for the consecution of this study was based upon two different phases. On the first one, and after the initial evaluation, the subjects were submitted to a plyometric training program (jumps in place, bounds, depth jumps and plyometric exercises with extra-loads). The duration of the training was 8 weeks with 3 workouts per week. At the end of this period, an intermediate evaluation was made. On the second phase, immediately after the 8 weeks of training, the subjects were randomly assigned to one of two groups. One group (SDT, n=10) accomplished a 4 weeks specific detraining period maintaining, however, the regular basketball workouts; the other subjects (RT, n=9), during the same period, performed a reduced plyometric training program, simultaneously with the regular basketball training. The adopted training structure was similar to the first one, with the same levels of intensity but a reduction in frequency (once a week) and volume. At the end of this period, a final evaluation took place.

Testing Procedures

On the three different moments of evaluation (T0, T1, and T4), subjects were tested on the following explosive strength indicators: running speed - 20m dash (Carvalho, 1993); agility (AG; Marques et al., 1990); squat jump - SJ, countermovement jump – CMJ, and mechanical power – MP (Bosco, 1994).

Statistical Analysis

Ordinary statistical methods were used for the calculation of means and standard deviations. A repeated-measures t-test was used to assess the presence or the absence of gains on the first 2 moments of evaluation. An independent-measures t-test was used when the two groups were constituted and on the third moment of evaluation. Differences were considered significant at 5%.

Results

Effects of Plyometric Training

The results obtained from the pre- to the post-training show statistically significant differences in all the studied variables (Table 1). The most important gains were observed in the running speed, agility and squat jump indicators.

From these results emerges the following interpretation:

- the plyometric training program structure (duration, selected exercises, volume, intensity, frequency, as well as recovery intervals between sets and between exercises), naturally observing the training principles and the methodological orientations well-advised in a study of that nature, revealed efficient as far as the improvement of the subjects' leg explosive strength is concerned. Our results are in agreement with other basketball investigations (Brown *et al.*, 1986; Häkkinen, 1993; Wagner & Kocak, 1997; Matavulj *et al.*, 2001) and like these authors, we can state that:

- the efficacy of the training exercises employed in our investigation is evident.

The improvements obtained in our study can also be attributed though in a subjective and empirical way, to the large approval demonstrated by the athletes to the suggested training program. To that adhesion probably contributed the unusual character of the exercises, as well as their diversity and in some way the feeling of improvement in what concerns the motor availability for the basketball game.

On the other hand, as we concentrate exclusively on the gains obtained by the individuals on the different indicators of explosive strength, it seems important to refer the possible contribution of that kind of training to the improvement of performance in basketball. As we know, the basketball game is an activity essentially explosive that appeals to the fast and agile aspects of the athletes and which simultaneously appeals to the need of jumping, jumping higher and in a continued way, in every situation of game.

The indicators of explosive strength selected in our study thus clearly demonstrate the efficacy of the training program and its increments when juxtaposed to the game technique will obviously express the higher levels of output.

Table 1. Results of the comparison of means for the explosive strength indicators, from pre- to the post-training

Tests (n=19)	T0	T1	t	p
Running speed (20m) (seconds)	3.44±0.2	3.32±0.2	5.472	**0.000**
AG (seconds)	18.79±1.0	17.87±0.9	6.825	**0.000**
SJ (cm)	28.40 ± 4.2	31.60 ± 3.6	-4.835	**0.000**
CMJ (cm)	32.90 ± 5.4	34.60 ± 4.7	-2.104	**0.025**
MP ($w \cdot kg^{-1}$)	23.52 ± 3.5	25.79 ± 4.4	-2.876	**0.005**

Table 2. Results of means comparison on explosive strength indicators during specific detraining period (SDT group)

Tests (n=10)	T1	T4	t	p
Running speed (20m) (seconds)	3.27±0.1	3.22±0.1	2.623	**0.014**
AG (seconds)	17.88±0.7	18.02±0.8	-0.914	0.192
SJ (cm)	31.20 ± 2.1	33.10 ± 3.7	-1.733	**0.006**
CMJ (cm)	34.60 ± 3.4	36.80 ± 5.1	-2.648	**0.013**
MP ($w \cdot kg^{-1}$)	26.18 ± 4.2	26.16 ± 2.8	-1.545	0.784

Effects of Specific Detraining and Reduced Plyometric Training

The final comparison within each sub-group sends us to the following tables of results:

1. in SDT group we found statistically significant differences only as far as the values of running speed, the squat jump and the countermovement jump are concerned (Table 2).

2. in RT group the statistically significant differences were found exclusively on the values of the running speed and agility indicators (Table 3).

The differences previously related, although statistically significant, have given rise to a certain perplexity, namely in SDT group, whose behavior in what concerns the studied variables is different from the one referred to in literature (Häkkinen *et al.*, 1981; Häkkinen & Komi, 1985a; 1985b; Hoffman *et al.*, 1991a, 1991b; Ingle *et al.*, 2006).

On the other hand, it seems clear that as far as the group submitted to a reduced plyometric training is concerned, the efficacy of that training program was corroborated since we pretended to maintain the explosive strength levels previously obtained. Actually, its utilization surpassed one's expectations since the indicators of running speed and agility present, at the end, statistically significant gains.

The literature analysis on detraining and reduced plyometric training with respect to the strength indicators namely the explosive strength ones is scarce concerning studies carried out with athletes. In both cases, studies have concentrated on sedentary populations with somewhat experience in strength training, and they have appealed to the assessment of explosive strength indicators (Häkkinen *et al.*, 1981; Häkkinen & Komi, 1985a; 1985b; Colliander & Tesch, 1991) and the assessment of isometric strength indicators (Graves *et al.*, 1988).

In a general way, the results of those studies concerning detraining and reduced plyometric training seem to express the concept of reduction and maintenance on the different strength indicators assessed. Although the possible comparisons between the values available in literature and those of the present study cannot be established owing to the different samples, it seems important to refer the following:

- the tendency to the improvement and maintenance of the different explosive strength levels, on the studied sub-groups, independently of the reduced plyometric training and the absence of specific physical training.

Anyhow, the subjective and integrated interpretation of these values allows us to clarify certain aspects considered relevant on the framing of our study. If on the one hand these indicators are connected as far as the multifaceted strength expression is concerned, and if they legitimate the efficacy of the reduced plyometric training application, on the other hand, they do not seem consistent with the references in literature, which suggest an usual reduction during the absence of specific physical training.

Table 3. Results of means comparison on explosive strength indicators during reduced plyometric training (RT group)

Tests (n=9)	T1	T4	t	p
Running speed (20m) (seconds)	3.39±0.2	3.31±0.2	2.354	**0.023**
AG (seconds)	17.87±1.2	17.63±1.1	2.082	**0.036**
SJ (cm)	31.90 ± 4.9	32.20 ± 5.5	-0.408	0.347
CMJ (cm)	34.70 ± 6.0	34.80 ± 5.9	-0.291	0.389
MP ($w \cdot kg^{-1}$)	25.43 ± 4.9	23.51 ± 4.8	2.054	0.371

It is probable that beyond the results found in SDT group, there will also be matters related to the probable increased contribution of the specific training in basketball and simultaneously in the reduced number of assessed individuals.

Specific Detraining vs. Reduced Plyometric Training

The whole results attained on both sub-groups, at the end of four weeks of specific detraining and reduced plyometric training, made us believe that those sub-groups would reveal themselves essentially different, at least by the light of some of the assessed indicators. As we know, as far as SDT group is concerned, the improvements occurred on the indicators of running speed, squat jump and countermovement jump, while in RT group those improvements took place exclusively on the running speed and agility.

This being the case, we have decided to test the former hypothesis and the results clearly evidenced that no statistically significant differences occurred on the various indicators of explosive strength (Table 4).

As we can verify, the similarity between the two sub-groups is evident. However, a more careful analysis presents some details initially concealed. Although that similarity is a fact, it is certain that concerning the specific detraining group, the final values on the different tests of explosive strength, with the exception of agility, were always superior to those found on the same occasion on the reduced plyometric training group.

The two aspects previously referred (similarity between groups; superior results as far as the SDT group strength indicators are concerned), constitute, in our opinion, the most important aspect of this second part of our study. Thus, those evidences clearly suggest that specificity of training in basketball is by itself a guarantee on the maintenance of the explosive strength gains, based upon the unique framing of demands that express the fast and powerful dimension of that game.

In face of that combination of facts, it seems licit to suggest the omission of a reduced plyometric training on the athletes' basketball preparation, at least as far as those ages are considered and only in a four-week training period.

Table 4. Results of means comparison for explosive strength indicators between SDT and RT groups, at the end of 4 weeks

Tests (n=19)	SDT (n=10)	RT (n=9)	t	p
Running speed (20m) (seconds)	3.22±0.1	3.31±0.2	-1.516	0.148
AG (seconds)	18.02±0.8	17.63±1.1	0.907	0.377
SJ (cm)	33.10 ± 3.7	32.20 ± 5.5	0.430	0.673
CMJ (cm)	36.80 ± 5.1	34.80 ± 5.9	0.814	0.427
MP ($w \cdot kg^{-1}$)	26.16 ± 2.8	23.51 ± 4.8	1.485	0.156

Conclusion

From this study, emerge the following conclusions:

(i) the results highlight the efficacy of the plyometric training design;

(ii) the reduced training program and the specific detraining indistinctly contribute to the explosive strength levels maintenance;
(iii) basketball training has an obvious power in the maintenance and sustainability of motor performance at least taking into account the applied training program.

References

Bompa, T. O. (1994). *Theory and methodology of training*. Dubuque, Iowa: Kendall-Hunt Publishing Company.

Bosco, C. (1994). *La Valoración de la Fuerza con el Test de Bosco*. Barcelona: Editorial Paidotribo.

Brown, M. E., Mayhew, J. L. & Boleach, L. W. (1986). Effect of plyometric training on vertical jump performance in high school basketball players. *Journal of Sports Medicine and Physical Fitness*, *26*, 1, 1-4.

Carvalho, C. (1993). Desenvolvimento e treinabilidade da força em jovens em fase pubertária. *Estudo em alunos do 8º ano de ambos os sexos em escolas de Vila Real*. PhD thesis, UTAD, Vila Real, Portugal.

Colliander, E. B. & Tesch, P. A. (1992). Effects of detraining following short term resistance training on eccentric and concentric muscle strength. *Acta Physiologica Scandinavica, 144*, 23-29.

Fleck, S. J. & Kraemer, W. J. (1997). *Designing Resistance Training Program*. (2nd edition). Champaign, ILL: Human Kinetics Books.

Graves, J. E., Pollock, M. L., Legget, S. H., Braith, R. W., Carpenter, D. M. & Bishop, L. E. (1988). Effect of reduced training frequency on muscular strength. *International Journal of Sports Medicine, 9*, 316-319.

Häkkinen, K. (1993). Changes in physical fitness profile in female basketball players during the competitive season including explosive type strength training. *Journal of Sports Medicine and Physical Fitness*, *33*, 19-26.

Häkkinen, K. & Komi, P. V. (1985a). Changes in electrical and mechanical behavior of leg extensor muscles during heavy resistance strength training. *Scandinavian Journal Sports Science, 7*, 55-64.

Häkkinen, K. & Komi, P. V. (1985b). Effect of explosive type strength training on electromyographic and force production characteristics of leg extensor muscles during concentric and various stretch-shortening cycle exercises. *Scandinavian Journal Sports Science, 7*, 65-76.

Häkkinen, K., Komi, P. V. & Tesch, P. A. (1981). Effect of combined concentric and excentric strength training and detraining on force-time, muscle fiber and metabolic characteristics of leg extensor muscles. *Scandinavian Journal Sports Science, 3*, 50-58.

Hoffman, J. R., Fry, A. C., Howard, R., Maresh, C. M. & Kraemer, W. J. (1991a). Strength, Speed and Endurance Changes During the Course of a Division I Basketball Season. *Journal of Applied Sport Science Research*, *5*, 144-149.

Hoffman, J. R., Maresh, C. M., Armstrong, L. E. & Kraemer, W. J. (1991b). Effects of off-season and in-season resistance training programs on a collegiate male basketball team. *Journal of Human Muscle Performance*, *1*, 48-55.

Ingle, L., Sleap, M. & Tolfrey, Keith (2006). The effect of a complex training and detraining programme on selected strength and power variables in early pubertal boys. *Journal of Sports Sciences*, *24(9)*, 987-997.

Klausen, K. (1990). Exercise. Strength and weight-training. In T. Reilly, N. Secher, P. Snell, & C. Williams (Eds.), *Physiology of Sports* (41-67). London: E. & F. N. Spon.

Marques, A., Costa, A., Maia, J., Oliveira, J. & Gomes, P. (1990). Aptidão física. In F. Sobral, & A. Marques (Coords.) *FACDEX - Desenvolvimento somato-motor e factores de excelência desportiva na população escolar portuguesa* (volume 1, 33-51). Lisboa: Ministério da Educação.

Matavulj, D., Kukolj, M., Ugarkovic, D., Tihanyi, J. & Saric, S. (2001). Effects of plyometric training on jumping performance in junior basketball players. *Journal of Sports Medicine and Physical Fitness*, *41*, 159-164.

NSCA (1988). Strength training and conditioning for basketball. *A coaches guide*. Lincoln: NSCA Journal.

Pauletto, B. (1994). Strength training for basketball. *Champaign,* ILL: Human Kinetics Publishers.

Sale, D. G. (1991). Testing strength and power. In J.D. MacDougall, H.A. Wenger, & H.J. Green (Eds.), *Physiological Testing of the High-Performance Athlete* (pp. 21-106). Champaign, ILL: Human Kinetics Books.

Stone, W. J. & Steingard, P. M. (1993). Basketball Injuries. Year-round conditioning for basketball. In P. Steingard (Ed.), *Clinics in Sport Medicine* (12, 173-191). Phyladelphia: W.B. Saunders Company.

Tanner, J. M. (1962). *Growth at adolescence*. Oxford: Blackwell Scientific Publications.

Wagner, D. R. & Kocak, M. S. (1997). A multivariate approach to assessing anaerobic power following a plyometric training program. *Journal of Strength and Conditioning Research*, *11*, 251-255.

In: Encyclopedia of Sports and Athletics
Editors: Jack L. Murray and Emily O. Watson
ISBN: 978-1-61209-959-0

Chapter XVI

Home Country Disadvantage for United States Championship Boxers

Jason E. Warnick*, Andrew Johnson and W. Daniel Martin
Department of Behavioral Sciences, Arkansas Tech University, US

Abstract

The home-field advantage is a topic of much debate in the research literature. This experiment attempted to assess whether there was an advantage for boxers performing in a home country in championship bouts due to judging bias. Official records of all championship bouts in 2006 were analyzed to see if the number of judges that shared the champion's home country was associated with a bout's outcome. It was found that the increased number of judges from a champion's home country produced a disadvantage for the champion when the bout occurred in the United States. These findings are discussed in the context of psychological reactivity.

Keywords: Boxing; Pugilism; Athletic Competition

Introduction

Many variables have been identified to play a role in the outcome of an athletic performance, besides training regimen and ability. For example, in many sports increased age is associated with a decline in athletic performance (*boxing*: Warnick & Warnick, 2007; *baseball*: Schulz, Musa, Staszewski, & Siegler, 1994; *running*: Starkes, Weir, Singh, Hodges, & Kerr, 1999; Fair, 2007). Similarly, losing weight immediately prior to an athletic event is associated with negative athletic performances (*amateur wrestling*: Horswill, Hickner, Scott, & Costill, 1990; *amateur boxing*: Hall & Lane, 2001). Positive athletic performance has been associated with variables like wearing red uniforms (Hill & Barton, 2005) and having a

* Corresponding author: Department of Behavioral Sciences, Arkansas Tech University, 407 West Q St., Russellville, AR 72801 USA, E-mail: jwarnick@atu.edu.

record of previous success in the sport (Landis, 2001; Warnick & Warnick, 2007; Warnick & Warnick, 2009).

Much of the research into the variables affecting an athletic event's outcome has focused on the advantages associated with contests occurring at a home field or in a home country. In group sports, home teams, when compared to visiting teams, have a significantly greater chance of winning the contest (*baseball*: Courneya, 1990; Pollard, 1986; *basketball*: Schwartz & Barsky, 1977; Silva & Andrew, 1987; *soccer*: Brown, Van Raalte, Brewer, Winter, Cornelius, & Andersen, 2002; Pollard, 1986; *hockey*: Schwartz & Barsky, 1977). A similar effect has been seen for athletes performing in individual competitions at home (*amateur wrestling*: McAndrew, 1993). Further, the home country effect has been found to occur in international athletic events like the Olympic Games (Balmer, Nevill, & Williams, 2001; 2003) and the World Cup (Brown et al., 2002). While the home advantage effect is a complex phenomenon, it is believed that it is primarily the result of two variables.

Table 1. List of Titles Contested During the Year 2006 by Weight Division

Heavyweight	WBC, WBA, IBF, WBO
Cruiserweight	WBC, WBA, IBF, WBO
Light Heavyweight	WBC, IBF, WBO, IBO
Super Middleweight	WBC, WBA, IBF, WBO, IBO
Middleweight	WBC, WBA, IBF, WBO
Super Welterweight	WBC, WBA, IBF, WBO IBO
Welterweight	WBC, WBA, IBF, WBO
Junior Welterweight	WBO
Lightweight	WBC, WBA, IBO
Junior Lightweight	WBC, WBA, IBF, WBO, IBO
Featherweight	WBC, WBA, IBF, WBO, IBO
Junior Featherweight	WBC, WBA, WBO, IBO
Bantamweight	WBC, WBA, IBF, WBO
Junior Bantamweight	WBC, WBA, IBF
Flyweight	WBC, IBF, WBO
Junior Flyweight	WBC, WBA, IBF, WBO
Minimumweight	WBC, WBA

Abbreviations: WBC = World Boxing Council; WBA = World Boxing Association, IBF = International Boxing Federation; WBO = World Boxing Organization; IBO = International Boxing Organization.

One of the variables associated with the home advantage effect is the psychological state that accompanies performing in front of a supportive audience (Bray, Jones, & Owen, 2002). Under normal conditions, this psychological state has been shown to be associated with increased levels of self-efficacy (Bray et al., 2002; Bray & Widmeyer, 2000) and self-confidence (Bray et al., 2002; Terry, Walrond, & Carron, 1998; Thuot, Kavouras, & Kenefick, 1998) and decreased levels of state anxiety (Bray et al., 2002; Terry et al., 1998). However, this relationship is context dependent as performing at home during high-stakes contests (e.g., championship events) is associated with decreased chance of victory (Baumeister & Steinhilber, 1984; Wright & Jackson, 1991; Wright & Voher, 1995). This is believed to be the result of the negative psychological states, like increased self-monitoring and over-cautiousness (Wallace, Baumeister & Vohs, 2005), that accompany meaningful athletic events.

The second variable that is believed to contribute to the home advantage effect is officiating bias. For example, soccer referees have been found to award extra time to a home team if they are losing (Sutter & Kocher, 2004). Similarly, judges for subjectively scored sports, like ice-skating, have been shown to give more favorable scores to athletes from their home country (Seltzer & Glass, 1991).

The current study sought to investigate a potential home advantage-like effect in championship boxing contests by seeking evidence for potential judging biases. Official records of all championship bouts in 2006 were analyzed to see if the number of judges that shared the champion's home country was associated with a bout's outcome.

Method

The information for all championship boxing bouts (i.e., World Boxing Council, World Boxing Association, World Boxing Organization, International Boxing Federation, International Boxing Organization) occurring in 2006 was obtained from *The Boxing Record Book* (Fight Fax Inc, 2007; see Table 1 for listing of titles contested). The following information was taken for each bout: the bout's result, the champion's previous win and loss record, the opponent's previous win loss record, the champion's home country, the opponent's home country, the home country of each judge, the scoring of each round for every judge, the country where the bout occurred. Bouts that ended in a draw or ended due to disqualification were not included in the analyses. Chi-square, correlation and logistic regression analyses were employed to determine whether there was a home country bias that associated with a judges scoring.

Results

For bouts occurring in the United States, the champion was more likely to win the bout if he was not from the United States, $\chi^2(1) = 6.02, p = 0.014$. For bouts occurring outside of the United States, the champion was more likely to win the bout if he was fighting in his home country, $\chi^2(1) = 5.85, p = 0.016$. Analyses of bouts going to the judges' scorecards revealed a similar pattern of results. For bouts occurring in the United States, the champion was more likely to win the bout if he was not from the United States, $\chi^2(1) = 3.74, p = 0.053$. For bouts occurring outside of the United States, the champion was more likely to win the bout if he was fighting in his home country, $\chi^2(1) = 6.17, p = 0.013$.

For bouts going to the judges' scorecards, there was a significant correlation between the number of judges that share the champion's home country and the champion losing the bout, $r(65) = 0.20$, $p = 0.011$. A stepwise logistic regression analysis was conducted on the following variables: 1) number of champion's previous victories, 2) number of champion's previous defeats, 3) number of opponent's previous victories, 4) number of opponent's previous losses, 5) number of judges sharing the champion's home country and 6) number of judges sharing the opponent's home country. The regression model was significant [χ^2 (1) = 5.056, p = 0.025] and indicated the number of judges sharing the champion's home country was a significant predictor of the bout outcome (see Table 2). The classification table for this model is shown in Table 3.

Including the bouts that ended without going to the judges' scorecards (e.g., knockout, technical knockout) into the analysis produced a similar series of results. There was a significant correlation between the number of judges that share the champion's home country and the champion losing the bout, r (118) = 0.19, p = 0.043. A stepwise logistic regression analysis conducted using the above listed variables produced a significant regression model [χ^2 (1) = 3.915, p = 0.048] and indicated the number of judges sharing the champion's home country was a significant predictor of the bout outcome (see Table 4). The classification table for this model is shown in Table 5.

For bouts occurring in the United States, there was a significant correlation between the number of judges that share the champion's home country and the champion losing the bout, r (25) = 0.504, p = 0.01. However, for bouts occurring outside of the United States, there was no relationship between the number of judges that share the champion's home country and the bout's result, r (40) = 0.067, p = 0.681.

Table 2. Logistic Regression Analysis Output

Variables	B	SE	Wald's χ^2	df	p-value	e^{β} (Odds ratio)
Constant	1.47	0.39	14.45	1	<0.001	4.35
Number of Judges Sharing Champion's Home Country	-0.54	0.24	4.94	1	0.026	0.58

Table 3. Regression Model Classification Table

	Predicted Win		
Observed Win	Loss	Win	**Percentage Correct**
Loss	5	13	27.8
Win	4	43	91.5
			Total: 73.8

Table 4. Logistic Regression Analysis Output

Variables	B	SE	Wald's χ^2	df	p-value	e^{β} (Odds ratio)
Constant	1.13	0.25	20.28	1	<0.001	3.10
Number of Judges Sharing Champion's Home Country	-0.38	0.19	3.95	1	0.047	0.68

Table 5. Regression Model Classification Table

	Predicted Win		
Observed Win	Loss	Win	**Percentage Correct**
Loss	6	29	17.1
Win	5	78	94.0
			Total: 71.2

Discussion

This study attempted to assess whether judges from the same country as boxing champions exhibited evidence of scoring bias. The findings revealed that the increased number of judges from a champion's home country produced a disadvantage for the champion, as this was associated with more rounds being scored for the opponent. This association was only seen for bouts occurring in the United States.

These findings both support and further a previous study investigating the home advantage effect in professional boxing. In that study, Balmer and colleagues (2005) that found European boxing champions enjoyed an increased probability of winning when fighting in their home country. The current study supports this finding by showing there were a greater number of victories for champions fighting in their home country for bouts occurring outside of the United States. However, there does not appear to be any evidence of judging bias in these bouts as the number of judges from the champion's home country is not associated with the bout's outcome. This suggests that this home advantage effect is likely due to factors not associated with the bout's officiating, like the psychological factors associated with performing for a supportive audience.

The current study's findings for bouts occurring in the United States are novel and will need to be further investigated as many potential hypotheses can be found to explain the pattern of results. In the United States, boxing has received much attention as being influenced by corruption (see Newfield, 1995). Boxing judges in the United States may be displaying a form of psychological reactance by not wanting to show any evidence of bias, thus judging the opponent more favorably. The judges are in an environment that mimics the conditions associated with the Hawthorne effect (Mayo, 1949). That is, they are aware that their scoring will be public record. Further, being involved in the sport, they are likely to be aware of the public's perception that corruption influences the outcome of boxing contests. Boxing judges may be reacting, either consciously or unconsciously, in a manner that is attempting to correct for potential bias towards the champion.

The findings that champions are at a home disadvantage in the United States may also be a component of the country's long history of racial and ethnic discrimination. Many studies have shown that people attempt to correct for perceived discrimination against a particular group by favoring that group (i.e., reverse discrimination; Dutton, 1973; Dutton & Lake, 1973). The judges in the current study may be attempting to reverse the ethnocentric appeal to favor the champion from one's home country.

As the current study solely analyzed archival data, future studies will need to test this reactivity hypothesis by administering psychological measures to boxing judges in the United States and abroad. However, until shown otherwise, the current findings could be seen as an appeal for more comprehensive education of boxing officials. In the United States, the Association of Boxing Commissions currently conducts training seminars for referees and judges. One component of this training is to prepare a judge to be mentally prepared for a bout. This should likely be expanded to include a discussion on biased scoring and the Hawthorne effect. Analysis of the training efficacy should be employed to improve future educational protocols.

Conclusions

The current study sought to investigate whether there was a home advantage effect in championship boxing contests. Official records of all championship bouts for one year were analyzed to determine if the number of judges from the champion's home country was correlated with a bout's outcome. The findings revealed that the increased number of judges from a champion's home country produced a disadvantage for the champion. However, this was only found for bouts occurring in the United States. These findings are likely due to psychological reactivity due to the negative media portrayal of boxing being a corrupt sport. Further education should be offered to boxing judges in an attempt to reduce this biased scoring.

References

Balmer, N. J., Nevill, A. M. & Lane, A. M. (2005). Do judges enhance home advantage in European championship boxing? *Journal of Sports Sciences, 23*, 409-416.

Balmer, N. J., Nevill, A. M. & Williams, A. M. (2001). Home advantage in the Winter Olympics (1908-1998). *Journal of Sports Science, 19*, 129-139.

Balmer, N. J., Nevill, A. M. & Williams, A. M. (2003). Modeling home advantage in the Summer Olympic Games. *Journal of Sports Science, 21*, 469-478.

Baumeister, R. F. & Steinhilber, A. (1984). Paradoxical effects of supportive audiences on performance under pressure: The home field disadvantage in sports championships. *Journal of Personality and Social Psychology, 47*, 85-93.

Bray, S. R., Jones, M. V.,& Owen, S. (2002). The influence of competition location on athletes' psychological states. *Journal of Sport Behavior, 25*, 231-242.

Bray, S. R. & Widmeyer, W. N. (2000). Athletes' perceptions of the home advantage: An investigation of perceived causal factors. *Journal of Sport Behavior, 23*, 1-10.

Brown, T. D., Van Raalte, J. L., Brewer, B. W., Winter, C. R., Cornelius, A. E. & Anderson, M. B. (2002). World cup soccer home advantage. *Journal of Sport Behavior, 25*, 134-144.

Courneya, K. S., (1990). Importance of game location and scoring first in college baseball. *Perceptual and Motor Skills, 71*, 624-626.

Dutton, D. G. (1973). Reverse discrimination: The relationship of amount of perceived discrimination toward a minority group on the behavior of majority group members. *Canadian Journal of Behavioural Science, 5*, 34-45.

Dutton, D. G. & Lake, R. A. (1973). Threat of own prejudice and reverse discrimination in interracial situations. *Journal of Personality and Social Psychology, 28*, 94-100.

Fair, R. C. (2007). Estimated age effects in athletic events and chess. *Experimental Aging Research, 33*, 37-57.

Fight Fax Inc. (2007). *The boxing record book* (Vol. 24). Maple Shade, NJ: Fight Fax Inc.

Hall, C. J. & Lane, A. M. (2001). Effects of rapid weight loss on mood and performance among amateur boxers. *British Journal of Sports Medicine, 35*, 390-395.

Hill, R. A. & Barton, R. A. (2005). Psychology: Red enhances human performance in contests. *Nature, 7040*, 293.

Horswill, C. A., Hickner, R. C., Scott, J. R. & Costill, D. L. (1990). Weight loss, dietary carbohydrate modifications, and high intensity, physical performance. *Medicine & Science in Sports & Exercise, 22*, 470-476.

Landis, R. S. (2001). A note on the stability of team performance. *Journal of Applied Psychology, 86*, 446-450.

McAndrew, F. T. (1993). The home advantage in individual sports. *The Journal of Social Psychology, 133*, 401-403.

Mayo, E. (1949). *Hawthorne and the Western Electric Company: The social problems of an industrial civilization*. London: Routledge.

Newfield, J. (1995). *Only in America: The life and crimes of Don King*. New York: Morrow.

Pollard, R. (1986). Home advantage in soccer: A retrospective analysis. *Journal of Sport Sciences, 4*, 237-248.

Schulz, R., Musa, D., Staszewski, J. & Siegler, R. S. (1994). The relationship between age and major league baseball performance: Implications for development. *Psychology and Aging, 9*, 274-286.

Schwartz, B. & Barsky, S. F. (1977). The home advantage. *Social Forces, 55*, 641-661.

Seltzer, R. & Glass, W. (1991). International politics and judging in Olympic skating events: 1968-1988. *Journal of Sport Behavior, 14*, 189-200.

Silva, J. M. & Andrew, J. A. (1987). An analysis of game location and basketball performance in the Atlantic Coast Conference. *International Journal of Sport Psychology, 18*, 188-204.

Starkes, J. L., Weir, P. L., Singh, P., Hodges, N. J. & Kerr, T. (1999). Aging and the retention of sport expertise. *International Journal of Sports Psychology, 30*, 283-301.

Sutter, M. & Kocher, M. G. (2004). Favoritism of agents – The case of referees' home bias. *Journal of Economic Psychology, 25*, 461-469.

Terry, P. C., Walrond, N. & Carron, A. V. (1998). The influence of game location on athletes' psychological states. *Journal of Science and Medicine in Sport, 1*, 29-37.

Thuot, S. M., Kavouras, S. A. & Kenefick, R. W. (1998). Effect of perceived ability, game location, and state anxiety on basketball performance. *Journal of Sport Behavior, 21*, 311-321.

Wallace, H. M., Baumeister, R. F. & Vohs, K. D. (2005). Audience support and choking under pressure: A home disadvantage? *Journal of Sports Sciences, 23*, 429-438.

Warnick, J. E. & Warnick, K. (2009). Specification of variables predictive of victories in the sport of boxing. II. Further characterization of previous success. *Perceptual and Motor Skills, 108*, 137-138.

Warnick, J. E. & Warnick, K. (2007). Specification of variables predictive of victories in the sport of boxing. *Perceptual and Motor Skills, 105*, 153-158.

Wright, E. F. & Jackson, W. (1991). The home-course disadvantage in golf championships: Further evidence for the undermining effect of supportive audiences on performance under pressure. *Journal of Sport Behavior, 14*, 51-60.

Wright, E. F. & Voyer, D. (1995). Supporting audiences and performance under pressure: The home-ice disadvantage in hockey championships. *Journal of Sport Behavior, 18*, 21-28.

In: Encyclopedia of Sports and Athletics
Editors: Jack L. Murray and Emily O. Watson

ISBN: 978-1-61209-959-0

Chapter XVII

Aerobic Capacity Testing and its Public Health Implications

L. Lochte[*]
University of Bristol, Bristol Royal Hospital for Children,
Department of Social Medicine & ALSPAC, Oakfield House,
Oakfield Grove, Bristol, BS8 2BN, United Kingdom

Abstract

According to a recent World Health Organization report, children and adolescents worldwide are physically inactive during 50% of a normal week (http://www.euro.who.int/Document/e82923.pdf) and the low physical activity level tracks into adult life, with one-third of the disease burden in adulthood being related to such youth behaviour as physical inactivity (http://www.who.int/features/factfiles). Current public health policy lacks routine management of asthmatic child patients; therefore, public health promotion for the future referral of paediatric and adolescent asthmatic patients to chest clinics with standardized equipment available for aerobic capacity testing is urgently recommended.

Milgrom & Taussig affirmed that all asthmatic children should be questioned about their "exercise habits and exercise tolerance," and those with a concerning history should have an exercise test. Such recommendations address populations of asthmatic youth in the global community.

Numerous scores of physical activity exist. One was validated recently and originates from a questionnaire concerned with the frequency and extent of vigorous physical recreational and sports activity after school.

Early detection of physical inactivity and low aerobic capacity addressed by relevant public health policy implementations can be expected to reduce individual and public health care costs by preventing morbidity, disability, and mortality from such chronic respiratory diseases as paediatric asthma.

[*] Corresponding author: Lene Lochte, 6 Kaermindevej, 3460 Birkerod, Copenhagen, Denmark. Phone: +45 40 98 83 90. Fax: +45 45 82 99 50. Email: le@lochte.org

Increasing paediatric asthma is one consequence of physical inactivity [1]. Asthmatic children often suffer exercise-induced asthma (EIA) and various disease severities accordingly, and more than three-fourths of asthmatic children reported respiratory symptoms to accompany physical activity [2]. Yet, even with their high burden of symptoms, the asthmatic children showed the same level of physical activity as that of healthy children [3]. The children and adolescents thereof were representatives of a national asthmatic youth population and further demonstrated increased BMI and low aerobic capacity [3]; such evidence calls for recommendations of *cardiorespiratory evaluation* and rehabilitation of asthmatic children who suffer exercise-related symptoms. Exercise prescriptions for rehabilitation must be individualized based on objective criteria such as the aerobic capacity, and the flexibility of the programmes offered should be designed according to disease severity.

EIA must always be controlled in the management of childhood asthma. Appropriate medical treatment and encouragement by family and peers of the child are of critical importance for the child's participation in a prescribed exercise programme. Some types of sports exert high asthmogeneity related to the accompanying increase in minute ventilation and climatic conditions associated with the particular activity [4,5] and such knowledge facilitates appropriate physical activity selection. Therefore, the ideal exercise programme for asthmatic children entails activities associated with low levels of minute ventilation according to the pathogenesis of EIA. Breathing through the nose rather than the mouth or through a mask reduces the loss of heat and moisture and has shown to minimize EIA [6]; rather than avoiding physical activity and sports, care should be taken to guide and assist asthmatic children to participate in appropriate sports along with their peers.

Moreover, the child's psychological coping strategy with the asthmatic disease is at least as important as the medical variables [7]. Such evidence needs to be implemented along with acknowledgments suggesting that asthmatic children, even with optimal medical treatment, do not necessarily experience good "quality of life." Milgrom & Taussig [8] affirmed that all asthmatic children should be questioned about their "exercise habits and exercise tolerance" and those with a concerning history should have an exercise test. Such recommendations address populations of asthmatic youth in the global community.

The submaximal test of *aerobic capacity* (mLO_2/min/kg) is one method for cardiorespiratory evaluation of asthmatic children. The validity of the submaximal exercise test depends upon a predictable relationship between oxygen consumption and heart rate response [9,10]. Lochte et al. [3] recently validated the so-called *predicted aerobic capacity* (PAC) test of maximal oxygen uptake from such submaximal exercise. Aerobic capacities were highly consistent in childhood through adolescence over 4 years [3] and 10 years [11] and thus provide epidemiological capability.

Contrary to laboratory assessment, the submaximal exercise test overcomes many of the limitations of the VO_2max test, and is thus a noninvasive method that can accurately estimate the aerobic capacity of the individual child to further serve the cardiorespiratory and general health assessment of asthmatic youth.

According to the British Thoracic Society's 1997 guidelines [12], further recommendations concerning patient, partnership and psychosocial issues were included, which represent a change up through the 1990s. The benefits of patient education were demonstrated by evidence, and self-management plans are currently issued to enhance the commitment of patients and parents. In 1997, an early asthma policy for schools was published [13]. The

National Asthma Education and Prevention Programme [13] clearly advised that the goal should be to "meet patients' and their families' expectations of and satisfaction with asthma care."

Today, the updated consensus GINA guidelines confirm such earlier expert advocacy, in particular with respect to asthma control [14]. Periodic assessments by the school physician and/or health care professionals are of vital importance to asthmatic children; unfortunately, such assessments often suffer low priority. The role of the multidisciplinary team around asthmatic children has increased commensurate with the increasing prevalence of paediatric asthma. Therefore, public health promotion must aim at uniform involvement of asthmatic children and their parents, schoolteachers and sports coaches in the continuous assessment of the functional ability of the children in everyday school and leisure time life to recognize early signs of physical or psychosocial deconditioning.

In consequence, the public health implications for asthmatic child populations are the targeting of regular, standardized monitoring of both the *respiratory function* and the *aerobic capacity* with the purpose of reaching the widest possible disease spectrum among asthmatic children.

Additionally, the evaluation of patient perception of improvement, especially *quality of life* and the ability to engage in desired activities, must be monitored. Preferably, such measurement is conducted by epidemiological questionnaire surveys or in applied settings such as the school for the promotion of improved quality of life and reduced psychosocial implications of asthma.

Current public health policy lacks such routine management of asthmatic child patients; therefore, my urgent recommendation bears on the public health promotion nationwide for the future referral of paediatric and adolescent asthmatic patients to chest clinics with standardized equipment available for aerobic capacity testing.

Important revision of the "regular daily physical activity guidelines" for the young was launched by the commencement of the year 2000; and, according to the current public health endorsement, young people must participate in physical activity of moderate intensity for 60 minutes per day [15,16].

Numerous scores of physical activity exist. One was validated more recently [17] and originates from a questionnaire concerned with the *frequency* and *extent* of vigorous physical recreational and sports activity after school [18]. The two questions on physical activity were adopted in a previous population-based Scandinavian study [19] and are currently embodied in the WHO cross-national social survey of "Health Behaviour in School-Aged Children" (HBSC) [20].

Hence, early detection of physical inactivity and low aerobic capacity addressed by relevant public health policy implementations can be expected to reduce the individual and public health care costs [21] by preventing morbidity, disability and mortality from such chronic respiratory disease as paediatric asthma.

References

[1] Nystad, W; Stigum, H; Carlsen, KH. Increased level of bronchial responsiveness in inactive children with asthma. *Respir Med.*, 2001, 95, 806-10.

[2] Lochte, L. Exercise capacity of asthmatic children validation in clinical context. *Thesis*, Copenhagen, University of Copenhagen, 2001, 70. ISSN: 1600-7379. Available from: URL: http://akademia.com.gmta.info/?q=node/323

[3] Lochte, L; Angermann M, Larsson B. Cardiorespiratory fitness of asthmatic children and validation of predicted aerobic capacity. *The Clinical Respiratory Journal* 2009. 3: 42-50. Available from: URL: http://dx.doi.org/10.1111/j.1752-699X.2008, 00107.x

[4] Carlsen, KH. Exercise induced asthma in children and adolescents and the relationship to sports. *Pediatr Allergy Immunol.*, 1998, 9, 173-80.

[5] Cypcar, D, Lemanske, RF. Jr. Asthma and Exercise. *Clin Chest Med.*, 1994, 15, 351-68.

[6] Shturman-Ellstein, R; Zeballos, RJ; Buckley, JM; Souhrada, JF. The beneficial effect of nasal breathing on exercise-induced bronchoconstriction. *Am Rev Respir Dis.*, 1978. 118, 65-73.

[7] Strunk, RC; Mrazek, DA; Fukuhara, JT; Masterson, J; Ludwick, SK; LaBrecque, JF. Cardiovascular Fitness in Children With Asthma Correlates With Psychologic Functioning of the Child. *Pediatrics*, 1989, 84, 460-4.

[8] Milgrom, H; Taussig, LM. Keeping children with exercise-induced asthma active. *Pediatrics*, 1999, 104, 1-5.

[9] Minor, MA; Johnson, JC. Reliability and Validity of a Submaximal Treadmill Test to Estimate Aerobic Capacity in Women with Rheumatic Disease. *J Rheumatol.*, 1996, 23, 1517-23.

[10] Harrison, MH; Bruce, DL; Brown, GA; Cochrane, LA. A comparison of some indirect methods for predicting maximal oxygen uptake. *Aviat Space Environ Med.*, 1980, 51, 1128-33.

[11] Rowland, TW. Maturation of Aerobic Fitness. In: Rowland TW, editor. *Developmental Exercise Physiology*. Human Kinetics, Champaign, IL, 1996, 73-96.

[12] British Thoracic Society. The British guidelines on asthma management. 1995: review and position statement. *Thorax*, 1997, 52, S1-10.

[13] National Asthma Education and Prevention Program. Highlights of the Expert Panel Report 2: *Guidelines for the Diagnosis and Management of Asthma*. Bethesda, MD: US Department of Health and Human Services, Public Health Service, National Institutes of Health. National Heart, Lung, and Blood Institute; 1997. Publication No. 97-4051A.

[14] Global Strategy for Asthma Management and Prevention, *Global Initiative for Asthma (GINA)* 2008. Available from: URL: http://www.ginasthma.org.

[15] Biddle, S; Cavill, N; Sallis, J. Policy framework for young people and health-enhancing physical activity. In: Biddle S, Sallis J, Cavill N, editors. *Young and Active? Young people and health-enhancing physical activity—evidence and implications*. London: Health Education Authority, 1998, 3-16.

[16] Riddoch, C. Relationship between physical activity and health among young people. In: Biddle S, Sallis J, Cavill N, editors. *Young and Active? Young people and health-enhancing physical activity—evidence and implications*. London: Health Education Authority., 1998, 17-48.

[17] Booth, ML; Okely, AD; Chey, T; Bauman, A. The reliability and validity of the physical activity questions in the WHO Health Behaviour in Schoolchildren (HBSC) Survey: a population study. *Br J Sports Med.*, 2001, 35, 263-7.

[18] Hickman, M; Roberts, C; de Matos, MG. Exercise and leisure-time activities. In: Currie C, Hurrelmann K, Settertobulte W, Smith R, Todd J, editors. Health and Health

Behaviour among Young People. *Health Behaviour in School-aged Children: a WHO Cross-National Study (HBSC) International Report.* Copenhagen: World Health Organization, 2000, 73-82.

[19] Nystad, W. The physical activity level in children with asthma based on a survey among 7-16-year-old school children. *Scand J Med Sci Sports*, 1997, 7, 331-5.

[20] Currie, C; Gabhainn, SN; Godeau, E; Pickett, W; Ritcher, M; Roberts, C; et al. Health Behaviours- Physical Activity. In: Currie C, Gabhainn SN, Godeau E, Roberts C, Smith R, Currie D, et al., editors. *Inequalities in Young People's Health. Health Behaviour in School-Aged Children.* International Report from the 2005/2006 Survey. Copenhagen, World Health Organization Europe, 2008: 105–8. Available from: URL: http://euro.who.int/Document/E91416_Ch2_3.pdf/.

[21] Sears, MR. Epidemiological Trends. In: Kalinger MA, Barnes PJ, Persson CGA, editors. *Asthma Its Pathology and Treatment.* New York: Marcel Dekker, 1991, 1-49.

In: Encyclopedia of Sports and Athletics
Editors: Jack L. Murray and Emily O. Watson
ISBN: 978-1-61209-959-0

Chapter XVIII

From 'Motivational Climate' to 'Motivational Atmosphere': A Review of Research Examining the Social and Environmental Influences on Athlete Motivation in Sport

Richard Keegan[1], Chris Harwood[2], Christopher Spray[2] and David Lavallee[3]
[1]University of Lincoln, UK
[2]Loughborough University, UK
[3]Aberystwyth University, UK

Abstract

This chapter is intended to provide a comprehensive review of the various theories of social and environmental factors that influence athletes' motivation in sport. In order to achieve this, a short historical review is conducted of the various ways in which motivation has been studied over the past 100 years, culminating in the 'social-cognitive' approach that undergirds several of the current theories of motivation in sport. As an outcome of this brief review, the conceptualisation and measurement of motivation are discussed, with a focus on the manner in which motivation may be influenced by key social agents in sport, such as coaches, parents and peers. This discussion leads to a review of Deci & Ryan's (2000) self-determination theory (SDT), which specifies that environments and contexts which support basic psychological needs (competence, relatedness and autonomy) will produce higher quality motivation than environments which frustrate of exacerbate these needs. The research establishing the ways in which key social agents can support these basic needs is then reviewed, and the review depicts a situation wherein SDT has precipitated a way of studying the socio-environmental influences on motivation that has become quite piecemeal and fragmented. Following this, the motivational climate approach (Ames, 1992) specified in achievement-goals theory (AGT – Nicholls, 1989) is also reviewed. This section reveals a body of research which is highly consistent in its methodology and findings. The following two sections reflect recent debates regarding the nature of achievement goals and the way they are conceptualised (e.g., approach-avoidance goals and social goals), and the implications of this for motivational climate research are discussed. This leads to a section reviewing the current issues and concerns in the study of social and environmental influences on athlete motivation. Finally, future research directions and ideas are proposed to facilitate, precipitate and guide further research into the social and environmental influences on athlete motivation in sport. Recent studies that have attempted to address these issues are reviewed and their contribution is assessed.

Introduction

In the consideration of how social and environmental influences may affect the motivation of athletes, it may be helpful to define and delineate some of these important concepts. As soon as that is established, a number of theories of the way human motivation operates, or is regulated, also become relevant. These include achievement goal theory (Nicholls, 1989), trichotomous (Elliot & Church, 1997) and 2x2 achievement goals (Elliot & McGregor, 2001), self-determination theory (Deci & Ryan, 1985, 2000), and social goals (Urdan & Maehr, 1995; Wentzel, 1993).

This chapter seeks to overview and synthesise the current knowledge base into a foundation from which informed research can be constructed. Firstly, the concept of motivation, and its historical development, is outlined and explained, with key definitions provided. Secondly, the broadest and arguably most inclusive theory is overviewed and explained: Deci and Ryan's (1985, 2000) self-determination theory (SDT). This represents the closest attempt at a grand-unifying theory of human motivation. SDT will be presented both in terms of its contribution to the way motivation is conceptualised/measured and the way motivation is determined/regulated. Thirdly, achievement goal theory (AGT) is described and its history and development are traced. AGT has made a significant contribution to the study of human motivation in achievement contexts, and also offers a specific model of social and environmental influences on motivation in the form of 'motivational climate' (Ames, 1992). Fourthly, approach-avoidance theory (Elliot & McGregor, 2001) is described and explained; its historical development, as well as attempts to reconcile it with AGT, are described and analysed. Fifth in this sequence, the contribution of social goals (Urdan & Maehr, 1995; Wentzel, 1993), and their derivation from AGT is examined and explored, and throughout these sections an assessment is made of the ways in which these theoretical mechanisms and constructs might contribute to an analysis of the ways in which social (interpersonal and inter-group) and environmental (properties of the environment such as the nature of the sport, resources available, career stage, etc.) influences can be motivationally relevant/impactful. Finally, a series of recent qualitative studies are introduced and reviewed, and their implications for this area of research are examined. During this coverage, the important issues in the study of social and environmental influences on motivation are made clear and their relevance is assessed.

A Brief History of the Study of Motivation

Defining Motivation

Motivation is one of the most discussed constructs in psychology, both in scientific study and lay interpretations. Deci and Ryan (1985) succinctly summarise that motivation concerns the 'why' question in behaviour, while the title of Deci's (1995) paper coined a glib but highly appropriate definition: "Why we do what we do." In this interpretation, motivation refers to the reasons behind a behaviour, or absence of behaviour. In contrast, according to Maehr (1984), the study of human motivation "begins and ends with the study of behaviour" (p. 132). This is because, to date, scientists have been unable to design and produce a 'motivation-o-meter,' meaning that an individual's motivation must be *inferred* by measuring behavioural indices such as: i) attention, ii), effort, iii) choice of behaviours (and levels of challenge), iv) likelihood/consistency of behaviours, v) persistence following difficulty/failure, vi) bodily/facial expressions and vii) enjoyment, which *taken together* closely reflect the ideas that motivational researchers have used to operationalise motivation (Atkinson & Birch, 1970; 1978; Bolles, 1975; Eccles *et al.,* 1983; Ekman & Friesen, 1975). Historically, however, merely studying human behaviour proved to be problematic, and the emergence of theories to infer what *processes* occur in order to produce motivated behaviours became necessary.

Behaviourism and Physiological Needs

In the early days, internal processes were believed to be simple physiological needs which could be inferred by manipulating inputs, such as food and rewards or punishments, and observing 'outputs' (i.e., classic behaviourism). However, this approach could not account for apparently spontaneous behaviours that were exhibited with no apparent relation to physiological needs – examples include play and exploration. Likewise, the behaviourist approach could not explain highly complex behaviours, such as the learning and production of language. Despite being ultimately flawed, behaviourism was the beginning of a vast and growing literature on human motivation and represented the first attempts to systematically study human behaviour (Skinner, 1953; Watson, 1913). However, in conceptualising human motivation as purely 'mechanistic' – based on physiological needs and responses – the behaviourist approach failed to incorporate the complicated cognitive processes occurring between 'input' and 'output.'

To try and address this criticism, a number of 'instincts' were hypothesised to explain such behaviours, including suckling, play, locomotion, socialising or exploring, fight and 'mother offspring' (McDougall, 1926). The list of 'instincts' necessary to explain all human behaviours grew exponentially, perhaps reaching 6000 (Bernard, 1924; Dunlap, 1919). Additionally, a tautology was identified wherein 'instinct' arguments tended to explain a particular behaviour by naming an instinct after it. For example, the statement: "People are aggressive because they have an instinct to fight" does not actually explain why the behaviour occurred or why the instinct exists. As such, it became clear that human motivation could not be adequately explained by instinct theories or physiologically derived drive theories – it simply proved too complicated for such explanations.

The Cognitive Era

In the 1930's, Tolman promoted the idea that unobservable variables (or cognitions) played a mediating role between stimulus and response (Tolman, 1932). As such, humans were believed to have complete control over their behaviours; meaning that behaviours are deliberate choices based on the processing of information from internal (e.g. memories) and external (e.g. situations) sources; so called 'free-will.' This approach was conceived as managing/controlling a constant flow of motivation – for example: "Sound motivational theory... should assume that motivation is constant, never ending, fluctuating and complex and that it is an almost universal characteristic of practically every organismic state of affairs" (Maslow, 1954; p.69). From this perspective, the ground was laid to conceptualise cognitive processes as the central determinant of motivated action, examining how the individual deployed and managed their motivational resources. Weiner's (1990) review described how the main cognitive theories of motivation are based on interrelated cognitions, such as causal attributions (e.g. Weiner, 1985), self-efficacy (e.g. Schunk, 1991; Pajares & Miller, 1994), goals (Locke & Latham, 1990), expectations (Seligman, 1975) and subjective task values (e.g. Wigfield & Eccles, 1992). However, in order to produce testable hypotheses and explainable results, researchers using a purely cognitive approach tended to emphasise one particular aspect of motivation over another, losing generalisability and explanatory power (Wigfield, Eccles, & Rodriguez, 1998). For example, the majority of cognitively-derived motivation research manipulates variables such as success and failure feedback (Weiner, 1990), ignoring other variables (Reeve, 2009). The cognitive approach has also been criticised for failing to readily explain *why* a person may want to achieve and succeed, and for not systematically addressing the value attached to such outcomes (i.e., where do people's beliefs, values, desires etc. come from in the first place? Roberts & Treasure, 1992). A cognitive approach can also be argued to assign too much determining power to the individual, and not enough to 'inputs' (Elliot, 2005) or external variables (social norms, etc.). Put simply, a purely cognitive approach became too concerned with describing internal processes and forgot the original question of *why* (Deci & Ryan, 1985; 2000), which concerns outcomes and their associated values. In order to understand more about why behaviours are undertaken, it became important to understand how we come to define success and failure, and how we learn the value of these outcomes – through social processes.

The Social Cognitive Approach

The term 'social cognitive' covers a wide conceptual area, and as such many theories have been included under its remit. Fundamentally, the approach assumes that: "…variation in behaviour may not be the result of high or low motivation, as has been assumed in previous theories, but rather the manifestation of different perceptions of what is the appropriate goal within that social context." (Roberts, 1993; p.416); notice how Roberts here focuses on the *perceptions* of the social context, rather than the social context itself. Reeve (2009; p.43), however, gives an even simpler definition: "ways of thinking guided by exposure to other people." Hence, motivation – seen as effort, persistence, behavioural choice, preferred level of challenge and enjoyment/immersion – is not merely a function of satisfying some innate appetite, nor is it determined by a simple process of perceiving and processing information in the brain, but rather, motivation can be viewed as a function of: a) situational task requirements (e.g. the specific achievement domain); b) their perception and processing by the individual; c) socially learned ideas about the values of possible task outcomes; and also d) the immediate social indices of value in the possible task outcomes. Whilst all of these levels can be examined separately, a fuller understanding will come from examining all the levels together and their interactions and combinatory influences (Elliot & Thrash, 2002; Nicholls 1984; 1989). This combination of influences also seems to reflect both the 'evolutionary baggage'; accumulated as scientific thinking progressed from mechanistic, through cognitive to social-cognitive theory; and also an increasingly central role in the study of motivation for the idea of *how* valuable/desirable outcomes are defined (e.g., demonstrating ability/competence/success - Duda & Whitehead,1998; Elliot & Dweck, 2005).

As such, the social cognitive perspective gave rise to a wide variety of 'mini theories' (as opposed to grand unifying theories) – each addressing particular domains of activity, such as work (Locke & Latham, 1984), school (Weiner, 1979), coping with stress (Lazarus, 1966) and dealing with depression (Seligman, 1975). In each instance the ways in which success/failure were defined, and then pursued/avoided (respectively), became central considerations. Even in recent work regarding academic (and sporting) achievement contexts, Elliot and his colleagues (Elliot & Dweck, 2005) have highlighted the importance of placing competence at the centre of the achievement goal concept (note: not the entire study of motivation in sport). A key theme seems to emerge across all these research programmes and theories, pertaining to the ways in which un/desirable outcomes are defined and then pursued/avoided. Before moving on to discuss the ways in which motivated actions are defined and/or valenced (e.g., as desirable or otherwise), it is first useful to examine the ways in which motivation itself is conceptualised, measured and studied – such that we may understand what is being influenced by the social and environmental determinants being discussed in this chapter.

Conceptualising and Measuring Motivation

In its broadest sense, motivation has been defined as: "the hypothetical construct used to describe the internal and/or external forces that produce the initiation, direction, intensity and persistence of behaviour" (Vallerand & Thill, 1993; p.18). This definition emphasises two key points. Firstly, that motivation is hypothetical – it cannot necessarily be thought of as real or independently observable. The following discussion of how motivation is conceptualised and measured reinforces this point. Secondly, a key component of motivation is the "external forces", and yet these forces are arguably very difficult to define and measure; a point which has arguably led researchers to focus on evaluating participants' *perceptions* of external influences, rather than the social and interpersonal aspects of the environment that might be considered to constitute an "external force." This chapter aims to (a) identify and understand these external forces (b) in as full and comprehensive a manner as possible.

Deci and Ryan's (1985; 2000) self-determination theory (SDT), which is actually a meta-theory containing four sub-theories, makes two important contributions to the study of motivation. Firstly, it provides researchers with a conceptualisation of 'good', 'bad' and 'non-existent' motivation – in the forms of intrinsic regulation, extrinsic regulation, and amotivation, respectively. SDT also posits several levels in-between (Ryan & Connell, 1989; Ryan & Deci, 2002); these will be explained shortly (this section), and these aspects of SDT are explicitly derived from Organismic Integration Theory (OIT - Deci & Ryan, 1985; 1991). Secondly, SDT offers a mechanism/model of the ways in which motivation can be influenced. This mechanism takes the form of three psychological needs (Basic Needs Theory – Deci & Ryan, 1985, 1991), which can be met in a number of different ways by the environment and the individual's interaction with the environment. Like food and water, these needs are no sooner satiated than they become salient again shortly afterwards and, like food and water, environments which do not allow the individual to cater for these needs lead to maladaptive consequences. Deci and Ryan are relatively candid in outlining that, in meeting or undermining these needs, the interaction between person and environment can be relatively complex (a "person-environment dialectic" - see below, p.8). Whilst they are packaged up into a single theory at times, the conceptualisation/measurement aspects will be discussed here, followed by the proposed mechanisms of motivational regulation.

As already discussed, motivation is relatively difficult to "see", and whilst a range of behaviours and facial/bodily expressions can be assessed, it would be almost impossible to reliably capture these in a way that was consistent between participants and observers. Instead, research has focused on designing and validating questionnaires to measure subjective perceptions of motivation, and these have generally supported a conceptualisation based around the amount of external inducement required/perceived in order to complete a given task, or participate in a certain activity (Vallerand & Fortier, 1998). On the one hand, *intrinsic motivation* can be defined as the impetus to perform and activity for its own sake – for the pleasure and satisfaction inherent in participating in a task (Deci, 1975; Deci & Ryan, 1985) – i.e., no external inducement is required (or perceived). On the other hand, *extrinsic motivation* (or more specifically, *external regulation*) refers to engaging in an activity as a means-to-an-end and not for its own sake (Vallerand & Fortier, 1998), or instrumental behaviours, which are motivated by expected outcomes or contingencies (inducements) not inherent in the activity itself (Ryan & Deci, 2008). In addition, SDT conceptualises a state of *amotivation* – not having any intention or energy directed towards action – and also several different levels/types of extrinsic motivation, including: *introjected* (avoiding external disapproval, seeking external approval); *identified* (relating to internally held but learned values/contingencies); and *integrated* (relating to behaviours that have become so internalised that they can be deemed to satisfy psychological needs – see also Ryan & Deci, 2008; p.8). Behaviours that are more intrinsically motivated will continue even after the 'ends' associated with them are achieved (e.g., continuation of exercise after achieving desired target(s) – Vallerand, 1997). They will also produce experiential rewards such as enjoyment and pleasure, as opposed to palpable external rewards (money, approval, etc. – Berlyne, 1971; Deci & Ryan, 1985). As such, intrinsically motivated behaviours also carry improved longer term outcomes, as they are strongly associated with pleasure, enjoyment and positive subjective experiences, and very rarely associated with perceptions of pressure, tension, anxiety, or undermined personal autonomy – yet the opposite is apparent for more extrinsic forms of motivation (Frederick-Recascino & Ryan, 1995; Vansteenkiste, Soenens & Lens, 2008).

The above conceptualisation of motivational regulation types raises several questions in relation to measurement. Firstly, do these different forms of motivational regulation represent a single uni-dimensional continuum (e.g., intrinsic = 10/10, amotivation = 0/10), or can they all be experienced, to different degrees, simultaneously (the multidimensional approach – Deci, 1975; Harter, 1981). Research consensus seems to support the multi-dimensional conceptualisation by demonstrating factorial independence, and different profiles of antecedents and consequences for each form of regulation (Deci & Ryan, 1991; Deci, Vallerand, Pelletier & Ryan, 1991; Vallerand, 1993; 1997). To further complicate this issue, there are also questionnaires containing three different forms of intrinsic motivation (to know, towards accomplishment, and to experience stimulation – Pelletier *et al.,* 1995; Vallerand *et al.,* 1992; 1993). This range and complexity in forms of motivational regulation means that researchers wishing to measure motivation using these questionnaires must choose very carefully between available questionnaires, in relation to what they are trying to detect. For example, an experiment comparing the effects of reward structures in a boring task is unlikely to require the differentiation between three forms of intrinsic motivation.

A second question relates to the level of generality at which the constructs of IM/EM are measured. Are intrinsic (IM), extrinsic (EM) and amotivation (AM) properties of the individual in general (i.e., personality), are they relevant to specific tasks/activities, at certain points in time, or are they measured in relation to contexts (e.g., generally in this team/class)? In designing the Hierarchical Model of Intrinsic and Extrinsic Motivation (HMIEM), Vallerand (1997; 2007) specified that these construct exist at all three levels: *global* (e.g., ever-present from the viewpoint of the actor, and usually taken to mean personality/traits), *context* (distinct spheres of activity, such a school, sport, relationships), and *situational* (the motivation experienced whilst engaged in an activity). In principle, global and contextual measures should be expected to exhibit temporal stability (i.e., test-retest reliability), whereas situational measures should not. Partly as a consequence of this, the vast majority of questionnaires for measuring intrinsic and extrinsic motivation are designed to assess the contextual, or quasi-contextual, level (e.g., Intrinsic Motivation Inventory - McAuley, Duncan & Tammen, 1989; Sport Motivation Scale – Pelletier *et al.*, 1995; The Motivational Orientation in Sport Scale – Weiss, Bredemeier & Shewchuk, 1985). This tendency is because test-retest reliability is a highly valued property for questionnaires (Rousson, Gasser & Seifert, 2002), which seems to rule out situational measures (in fact, a scale that claims to have test-retest reliability is arguably not a situational measure at all). Additionally, global measures are rare because personality/orientation type scales have already been developed in different spheres and represent close analogues of what a global intrinsic-extrinsic scale might measure (Vallerand & Fortier, 1998).

It is in this regard that the measurement of motivation still exhibits some divergent ideas and inconsistencies. For example, the IMI (McAuley *et al.,* 1989) does not return measures of IM and EM, but rather subjective ratings of interest/enjoyment, perceived competence, pressure/tension, effort/importance, perceived choice, value/usefulness and relatedness – with the latter three subscales being deployed much less frequently. As a general tendency, interest/enjoyment is taken to represent IM, whilst pressure/tension is taken to represent EM, but this is not strictly in accordance with the conceptualisations of IM and EM given above. Other measures, such as the Task Reaction Questionnaire (TRQ – Mayo, 1977) have also been criticised for including items that refer to determinants (e.g., perceived competence) and consequences (e.g., concentration) of IM, as well as not offering any indication of the scale's factorial structure (Guay, Vallerand & Blanchard, 2000; Vallerand & Fortier, 1998). The IMI contains exactly the same problems, and both Deci and Ryan (1987) and Markland and Hardy (1997) warn against confounding antecedents, motivational states and consequences into a single measure, not least because they almost guarantee positive results (i.e., significant findings) without necessarily allowing researchers to differentiate between causes and effects. Guay *et al.* (2000) developed the Situational Motivation Scale (SIMS) to try and overcome some of these issues, but even then only four (intrinsic, identified, external and amotivation) out or 6 possible subscales emerged (integrated and introjected were missing). In addition, the questionnaire method still requires participants to stop what they are doing to fill it in, presumably interrupting the motivated state and forcing participants to reflect on, and so potentially change, their motivation. Measuring motivation at the situational level of generality is necessarily complicated, and perhaps even impossible if the rigours of validity and reliability are to be fully applied. Upon reviewing the various scales available, it becomes clear that there is very little consensus on the best way of measuring IM/EM, especially when considering the levels-of-generality, life domains (work, school, sport), and cultural/linguistic differences. By way of emphasising this point, Meyer, Faber and Xu (2007) reviewed the various questionnaires that have been used in the study of motivation between 1930-2005, identifying 230 questionnaires relating to the measurement of motivation, 155 of which were specifically for measuring motivation in some form. In summarising this section, a case can be made that arguments surrounding measurement issues (validity, reliability etc.) and domain relevance (e.g., the workplace, academic settings, sport settings) have contributed to a degree of disarray in the conceptualisation and measurement of IM/EM. The sheer number and variability of scales available contributes to a degree of incompatibility between findings – a point first noted by Murray (1938):

> Some use physiological techniques, others present batteries of questionnaires. Some record dreams and listen for hours to free associations, others note attitudes in social situations. These different methods yield data which, if not incommensurate, are, at least, difficult to organise into one construction (Murray 1938; p.6).

The heavy use of questionnaires and correlations (including structural equation modelling, multiple regressions, mediation analyses etc.) has also been criticised by Harwood *et al.* (2008) as problematic and often uninformative. Nonetheless, by understanding how motivation is conceptualised, observed and experienced, it becomes possible to make better informed appraisals of how key social protagonists (i.e., coaches, parents and peers) may influence the motivation of athletes. Notably, all of the following theories addressing the mechanisms for determining motivation have been quite consistently linked to measures of IM/EM, and so in addressing how the behaviours of social agents may affect athlete motivation, it is necessary to understand both what is meant by motivation (as described above), and also the mechanisms through which motivationally relevant behaviours may influence this motivation (the following sections).

Self Determination Theory – Mechanisms and Models

Overview of Self-Determination Theory

As noted previously, SDT is actually made up of four theories – Organismic Integration Theory (OIT), Causality Orientation Theory (COT), Cognitive Evaluation Theory (CET) and Basic Needs Theory (BNT). OIT refers to the above-explained conceptualisation of motivation in terms of the degree to which the motivated behaviour is perceived to originate from internal sources, or from external inducements. COT refers to a general stable tendency of individuals to act in either autonomous or controlled ways; i.e., the extent to which people's behaviours emanate from themselves, or whether they depend on rewards, deadlines, and externally construed values in order to generate action. Alternatively, if neither tendency is present, the amotivation is likely to dominate (Deci & Ryan, 1985). As Weiss and Amorose (2008) summarise: "COT represents one of the least studied portions of the SDT framework in the context of sport and physical activity" (p.136), perhaps not least because the attention of researchers studying this seems to be drawn to attribution theory (Weiner, 1986) which is very similar and arguably more expansive, including a broader explanatory framework, and addressing both trait (orientation) and state conceptualisations.

CET refers to the social-cognitive developments in motivational research, emphasising the subjective meaning (*functional significance* – Deci & Ryan, 1985) attributed to tasks, environments and interactions; specifying that this perceptual-cognitive process will ultimately determine the impact of such external events. CET emerged from an expansive body of research into feedback and rewards which had often produced contradictory findings, for example rewards/positive feedback undermining motivation (at the time this was viewed as contradictory, in the light of behaviourist ideas, although more recently such a finding is commonplace). This led researchers to re-examine individual differences in terms of orientations, preferences, and needs; leading to a re-emphasis on the cognitive processes in motivation.

Finally, BNT posits three basic psychological needs; competence, relatedness and autonomy. *Competence* represents "a need to feel effective in dealing with and mastering one's environment" (Markland & Vansteenkiste, 2008; p.91; Harter, 1978; White, 1959). *Relatedness* refers to "a concern about connections with others and the quality of our interpersonal relationships" (Allen & Hodge, 2006; p.268; Ryan, 1993), whilst *autonomy* refers to the degree to which athletes "engage in the activity for their own valued reasons and feel that they have freely chosen to be involved" (Allen & Hodge, 2006; p. 267); or as DeCharms (1968) denotes: the desire to be self-initiating in the regulation of one's actions.

Deci, Vallerand, Pelletier and Ryan (1991) summarised their position, that: "motivation, performance, and development will be maximised within social contexts that provide people the opportunity to satisfy their basic psychological needs for competence, relatedness, and autonomy" (p. 327-328 – also specified in Ryan & Deci, 2008; p.13). To the extent that social contexts do not allow satisfaction of the three basic psychological needs, they will diminish motivation, impair the natural developmental process, and lead to alienation and poorer performance. In addition (although perhaps not mutually exclusive), Deci and Ryan (1985; Ryan & Deci, 2002) propose that humans have innate tendencies towards psychological growth, integration of the self and behavioural self-regulation, including a tendency for behaviours to progress towards to the integrated/intrinsic end of the spectrum if environmental conditions are conducive.

A particular aspect of this theory that has remained relatively unexplored is the person-environment dialectic or "organismic-dialectic" (Deci & Ryan, 2000; p.228). This dialectic denotes a continual interaction between an active, integrative human nature and social contexts that either nurture or impede the organism's natural needs/tendencies. The dialectical view was reached following tensions between the humanistic and cognitive theories, which place an emphasis on intra-individual difference, and the behavioural/situational theories which place an emphasis on 'inputs', such as stimuli, rewards, punishments, contingencies etc. (Ryan & Deci, 2002). According to SDT, the problem cannot be fully addressed by either approach, but rather by considering the ongoing interactions between the two. This postulate of SDT remains theoretically plausible, but has rarely been explicitly addressed in research as it is difficult to envisage a methodology that might adequately evaluate such a complex system (although it has been examined in other areas, e.g., Mischel, 1968).

As already alluded to, OIT and BNT arguably represent the most significant and most researched aspects of SDT. COT has been paid quite little attention (for reasons described above), whilst CET has been quite widely researched, but is often less associated with the SDT label, addressing as it does, aspects of feedback and rewards. Overall, research into CET seems to be supporting the above stipulation that the degree to which environments, tasks, interactions and relationships support/deny athletes' basic needs will determine the effects on motivation (Weiss & Amorose, 2008). As a result of this analysis and to comply with general usage in the literature, SDT will hereafter be used to refer to BNT (unless otherwise stated), while IM/EM will be used to refer to OIT and the way in which motivation is conceptualised/measured.

Research into SDT – The Effects of Supporting Psychological Needs

Reviews such as Reeve (2009), Vallerand (2007) and Weiss and Amorose (2008) present a relatively coherent picture, suggesting that when athletes perceive that their psychological needs are being supported, the results are almost universally positive in terms of producing more self-reported intrinsic motivation, and producing positive affective and behavioural responses. Vallerand (2007) reviewed this research in relation to how it had been conducted at three different levels of analysis: situational, contextual and global, whereas Reeve (2009) chose to review the literature in relation to the ways in which autonomy, competence and relatedness needs could be supported, respectively. In contrast, Weiss and Amorose (2008) attempted to briefly summarise the literature in relation to coach, peer and parent influences, but this was perhaps the most ambitious classification system, as the research available only facilitated the presentation of general themes and ideas, as opposed to a comprehensive review of the influences and effects of each social agent.

Even within the broadly consistent SDT literature occasional caveats exist, such as the interesting research conducted by Kast and Connor (1988), Pittman, Davey, Alafat, Wetherill and Kramer (1980) and Ryan, Mims and Koestner (1983). In these studies, positive-controlling feedback (e.g., "Well done, you did exactly what I told you and it worked!") – which supported competence but undermined autonomy needs – produced less adaptive outcomes than genuine praise or informational feedback, and could not be separated from a 'no feedback' condition. This playoff, cancelling out the effects of competence support, highlights a degree of interactivity between the basic needs and the ways in which the environment meets them. Henderlong and Lepper (2002; p.784) surmise: "Though it is often easy to make predictions about the effects of informational versus controlling statements relative to one another, it is typically much more difficult to make absolute predictions about whether the net effects are likely to be positive, negative, or neutral relative to a control condition." In many ways, these difficulties permeate research into SDT (see below), although more attention is invariably paid to positive findings where the tenets of SDT are more clearly supported – and this is arguably much easier to detect at the contextual level of analysis than the situational.

At the contextual level, Allen and Howe (1998) assessed the relationship between perceived coaching behaviours and self-rated competence perceptions in female hockey players. In line with SDT, praise was positively associated with perceived competence, but in direct contradiction of SDT, encouragement and information following skill-errors were negatively associated with perceived competence. This appears to be a problematic finding, and Weiss and Amorose's attempt to account for it might be considered rather speculative: "It is conceivable that the players in Allen and Howe's study perceived an emphasis on performance [competitive] oriented climates [which was not measured] and that coaches' encouragement plus instruction after errors was interpreted within that social context" (p.125 – parentheses added). The suggestion, derived from Wilko's (2004) unpublished study, is that a competitive motivational climate may lead an individual receiving instruction following an error to interpret this action as criticism, or highlighting the error in a public way – perhaps even acting as a punishment rather than a reinforcer – whereas in a perceived mastery context [emphasising improvement and individual development], instruction would be interpreted as helpful and positive, especially following an error. Viewed critically, these minor inconsistencies can be argued to reflect SDT's all-encompassing nature as a 'grand' theory, which at times becomes cumbersome to apply and interpret. This situation can occasionally cast the scientist as a puzzle solver (reconciling results with theories, as Weiss and Amorose attempted above) rather than as a theory-tester. As a rule-of-thumb, SDT (and many other theories) seems to lose predictive accuracy (and conceptual clarity) at the situational level, where multiple behaviours and interactions can occur concurrently and have combinatorial effects (an observation echoed by Henderlong & Lepper, 2002; with specific regard to praise having mixed effects). At the more general contextual and global levels, where participants' general perceptions of an activity (or themselves) are measured, findings tend to be more readily reconciled with SDT.

The Global Level-of-Generality

The global level of generality in Vallerand's HMIEM has attracted remarkably little research interest. As Vallerand (2007; p.72) comments: "Very little research has focused on motivation and determinants and consequences at the global level . . . [and] . . . no research appears to have examined how global social factors may affect global motivation." One can speculate that this is for (at least) two main reasons. Firstly, research at the contextual level of generality tends to subsume variables that might otherwise be labelled as global. Differentiating between these two levels can be difficult and, indeed, Vallerand's (2007) chapter appears to question the distinction in the subsection labelled "Two or three levels of generality?" (p.74).

This difficulty may reflect both the genuine uncertainty in determining whether a variable is contextual or global, as well as reflecting the disproportionate prevalence of studies examining the contextual level of generality. Secondly, the global level of analysis tends to contain both intrapersonal/personality variables (relatively omnipotent – hence 'global') aas well as 'global' social variables. Whilst social global variables are difficult to define, intrapersonal global variables tend to have been studied in different domains of motivation research, which are often not immediately reconcilable with SDT. For example, whilst Need-for-Achievement (NAch) and Fear-of-Failure (FoF – Atkinson, 1957; McClelland, Atkinson, Clark, & Lowell, 1953) can be measured as global/personality variables, they are not easily converted into 'need for relatedness' or 'need for autonomy', and indeed these concepts are rarely measured directly (Guiffrida, Gouveia, Wall & Seward, 2008). Instead, the participant's perception that these needs have been met/undermined (i.e., need satisfaction) is more frequently measured, and then correlated with motivational outcomes (e.g., Deci, Ryan, Gagne *et al.*, 2001; Kasser & Ryan; 1999; Reinboth & Duda, 2006; Reinboth, Duda & Ntoumanis, 2004), but this does neglect that different individuals may experience the needs for competence, relatedness and autonomy to different degrees, in terms of urgency/salience, and thus react differently to different social environments.

The Contextual Level-of-Generality

Vallerand's (2007) chapter identified several factors that that were proposed to occupy the contextual level: the coach (Pensgaard & Roberts, 2002; Mageau & Vallerand, 2003), perceived motivational climate (Ames, 1992; Duda & Hall, 2001), and sport/scholarship structures (Amorose & Horn, 2000; 2001). It is unclear why the coach is classified as a contextual variable in this formulation, as the coach can presumably influence motivation situationally (with immediate behaviours and interactions), or globally (in the coach's role as relatively omnipresent social agent during all sporting involvements). Likewise, it is unclear why sport/scholarship structures might be classified as exclusively contextual influences, when these are unlikely to change year-on-year and so might be argued to constitute social-global influences. As outlined shortly, most measures of perceived motivational climate do use question stems addressing a generic level, e.g., "on this team...", which is arguably quite suitable for the contextual level of generality (e.g., PMCSQ-2 – Newton, Duda & Yin, 2000); so perhaps perceived motivational climate may well be classified as a social contextual variable.

At the contextual level, self-report measures of contextual IM have been positively associated with affective consequences such as increased satisfaction and enjoyment (Briére *et al.,* 1995; Pelletier *et al*., 1995) and reduced burnout (Cresswell & Eklund, 2005; Hodge, Lonsdale & Ng, 2008; Lemyre, Treasure & Roberts, 2006); cognitive consequences such as increased concentration (Briére *et al.,* 1995; Pelletier *et al*., 1995) and imagery style (Wilson, Rodgers, Hall & Gammage, 2003); and behavioural consequences such as self-reported intention to participate in sport (Chatziserantis *et al*., 2003; Sarrazin *et al*., 2002) as well as teacher-rated effort/engagement in PE (Weiss & Ferrer-Caja, 2000). It is not clear, on the basis of the existing research, which variables from the contextual level of generality could be argued to support the needs for competence, autonomy and relatedness, respectively – not least because the perceived degree to which these needs have been met tends to constitute a starting point for research – indeed perceived need satisfaction becomes a key variable in itself (as noted above), with the antecedents of need satisfaction receiving significantly less empirical attention.

One theoretical proposition that has been tentatively supported is the 'top-down' effect, with features of the contextual level influencing situational indices. For example, Gagné *et al.* (2003) found that gymnasts who rated themselves as intrinsically motivated at the contextual level were generally more intrinsically motivated when sampled for situational motivation before training ($0.22 \leq r \leq 0.50$), although it is worth noting that such a finding is quite unsurprising. Throughout the rest of the study, once participant attrition was accounted for, only one significant correlation was apparent between contextual and situational variables (parent autonomy support associated with situational identified regulation, but not the other forms). A study by Blanchard, Mask, Vallerand, Sablonière and Provencher (2007) also found weak but statistically significant correlations ($0.20 \leq r \leq 0.44$) between contextual motivation (for basketball) and situational motivation (following matches). Once again, however, whilst providing support for Vallerand's (1997) HMIEM, very little is unveiled about what specific variables and perceptions led to contextual IM/IM, or what specific situational factors moderate/mediate the impact of these contextual factors on situational motivation.

Recent studies at the contextual level have, however, suggested that the degree to which the basic needs for competence, autonomy and relatedness are met, when measured as contextual-level variables, mediates the relationship between antecedents , such as perceived coach autonomy support (again, contextual measure), and outcome variables such as motivational orientation (Amorose & Anderson-Butcher, 2007) or subjective well-being/vitality (Adie, Duda & Ntoumanis, 2008 – *also* measured as generalised, contextual constructs). As above, such findings provide support for theory, SDT in this case, but they give very little detail about what leads athletes to feel that coaches support/prevent autonomy, competence or relatedness and so whilst theoretically relevant, these studies do not provide the sort of specificity needed to train future coaches or parents, nor do they offer anything more than an overview of a rich, fluid and deeply complex system of motivational processes.

The Situational Level-of-Generality

Like the global level, the situational level has received little relatively empirical attention, particularly in sport. Vallerand's (2007) review simply highlights four concepts which he proposes can be considered situational: rewards and awards, competition, feedback (positive/negative) and choice. Research on rewards contributed in no small part to the conception of SDT, or at least CET. As such, Deci, Koestner and Ryan (1999, 2001) were able to conduct meta-analytic reviews revealing that any rewards which are contingent upon participation, effort or achievement undermine IM, but unexpected and non-contingent rewards appeared to have no effect. Initial research into competition suggested it was detrimental to IM (Deci, Betley, Kahle, Abrams & Porac, 1981), but it subsequently became clear that those who won, or felt they performed well in competitions had significantly higher IM than losers and participants who felt they performed poorly (Vallerand, Gauvin & Halliwell, 1986; Weinberg & Ragan, 1979). In addition, the findings of Tauer and Harackiewicz (2004) suggested that competing as part of a team was relatively beneficial to IM. Positive feedback generally increases IM, whereas negative feedback is generally detrimental to IM (Vallerand & Reid, 1988). However, interactions with other variables (e.g., controlling praise – as mentioned earlier – Deci *et al.*, 1981), led Henderlong and Lepper (2002) to conclude that praise could be beneficial, detrimental or inconsequential for IM *depending on other factors*. Choice is generally beneficial to IM (Dwyer, 1995; Goudas, Biddle, Fox & Underwood, 1995) but only on the condition that it is perceived to be a genuine choice, and not a forced choice (Patall, Cooper & Robinson, 2008; Reeve, Nix & Hamm, 2003). A genuine choice leaves all options open, for example "what would you like to do today?" whereas a forced choice usually only offers 2-3 options, some/none of which may be desirable to the participant; e.g., "would you like to listen to classical or country music this afternoon?"

Overall, despite Vallerand's (2007) careful analysis, it remains extremely difficult to differentiate between situational, contextual and global level variables – and indeed many research studies do not specify which level their measures relate to. It might be helpful to differentiate between intrapersonal and social-environmental varieties of each, as well as seeking additional clarity about how each level interacts. For example, how many times must a specific behaviour be observed at the situational level before it influences (or even becomes) a contextual variable? If a coach is always smiling, tolerant of skill failures and welcoming, at what point does this become represented as a contextual variable (e.g., positive coach affective style)? Thus, whilst the situational level arguably contributes the building blocks of the contextual level and occurrences at the situational level appear most likely to predict immediate motivated behaviours, at this time very little is known about the specific influences at each level, and how they interact in order to produce perceptions and/or influence IM/EM.

Supporting Basic Psychological Needs

Reeve (2009) arranged his discussion of SDT not around levels of generality, but instead around the ways in which each psychological need can be supported or undermined. Care is required in interpreting this summary for the following reasons: 1) the review is a little (necessarily) abstract in places; 2) the review overlooks the potential interactivity between antecedents in determining outcomes; and 3) it does not differentiate between behaviours occurring at the global, contextual or situational levels of generality.

Reeve's (2009) review nonetheless offers an initial insight into the ways that social agents (and environments) can support, or undermine, psychological needs. The considerations identified in Table 1 could be enacted by coaches, parents, teachers, peers or, indeed, experimenters. This review is informative, but it also highlights the relative paucity of knowledge built up in this area. Whilst numerous studies are conducted under the auspices of SDT, a fuller awareness of issues regarding level-of-generality, the interaction between variables (from different levels) and the mechanisms by which need satisfaction mediates motivational outcomes are all undermined by the predominance of questionnaire methodologies, correlating quite general perceptions and leading to, at best, rules of thumb.

A preference can be identified in the extant literature for measuring the degree to which participants perceive that their psychological needs are met, and the way this precipitates motivational consequences.

Table 1. A summary of ways in which basic psychological needs have been shown to be supported in studies. Adapted from Reeve (2009; p.145-164)

Basic psychological need	General antecedent	Specific variations	Studies supporting link
Autonomy	Offering choices	'Forced' versus 'genuine'	•Patall et al. (2008) •Reeve et al. (2003) •Williams (1998); •Zuckerman, Porac, Lathin, Smith & Deci (1978) •Flowerday & Schraw (2003) •Flowerday, Schraw & Stevens (2004) •Moller, Deci & Ryan (2006)
Autonomy	Autonomy supportive style Versus Controlling style	Nurtures recipient's inner motivational resources - rather than seeking compliance	•Deci, Schwartz et al. (1981) •Flink et al. (1990) •Reeve et al. (1999)
		Informational language – as opposed to controlling language	•Assor, Roth & Deci (2004) •Ryan (1982) •Soenens, Vansteenkiste, Duriez, Luyten & Goossens (2005)
		Providing explanations and rationales – rather than relying on unquestioning compliance	•Deci, Eghrari, Patrick, & Leone (1994) •Koestner, Ryan, Bernieri & Holt (1984) •Newby (1991) •Reeve, Jang, Hardre & Omura (2002) •Sansone, Weir, Harpster & Morgan (1992) •Sansone, Wiebe, & Morgan (1999)
		Acknowledge/accept negative affect associated with task– as opposed to ignoring or punishing it	Not evidenced but suggested by: •Deci, Speigel, Ryan, Koestner & Kauffman (1982) •Reeve et al. (1999) •Reeve & Jang (2006)
Competence	Optimal challenge	Level of task must be '**optimal**' as opposed to too difficult or too easy	•Csikszentmihalyi, Rathunde & Whalen (1993) •Csikszentmihalyi & Csikszentmihalyi (1988) •Keller & Bless (2008)
Competence	Feedback	**Positive feedback** supports competence but negative feedback undermines it	•Anderson et al (1976) •Blank et al (1984) •Deci (1971) •Dollinger & Thelen (1978) •Vallerand & Reid (1984)
Competence	Task structure	**Clear goals and structure** – and support in progressing	•Hokoda & Fincham (1996) •Hollembeak & Amorose (2005) •Ntoumanis (2005) •Taylor & Ntoumanis (2007)
Competence	Tolerance of failures	Social environment is **permissive of failures** and does not punish them	•Clifford (1988, 1990)
Relatedness	Perceptions of a social bond	Beyond mere involvement Must know and accept "the real me" Knowledge of specifics appears to be lacking	•Deci & Ryan (1995) •Wheeler, Reis & Nezlek (1983) •Carstensen (1993)

This methodological tendency bypasses the identification of social and environmental features that may lead to these needs being met – but it does support the idea that when psychological needs are (perceived to be) met, the consequences are generally positive in terms of adaptive behaviours, cognitions and positive affect (Adie, Duda & Ntoumanis, 2008; Coatsworth & Conroy, 2009; Gillet, Berjot & Gobance, 2009; Reinboth & Duda, 2006; Reinboth, Duda & Ntoumanis, 2004). Supporting this link at the contextual level of generality is useful, and supports Vallerand's (1997) HMIEM as well as supporting a key tenet of SDT, but it does leave a lot to be discovered – not least because it would still be rather difficult to convey to coaches, parents and peers exactly how they should support these needs such that their specific athletes perceive their needs to be met, and experience positive motivational outcomes as a result. Research aimed at bridging this gap between theoretical ideas and detailed behavioural recommendations may well be fruitful and pertinent in this moment of motivational research.

Achievement Goal Theory

Overview of Achievement Goal Theory

Achievement goal theory (AGT - Nicholls, 1989) evolved alongside SDT, but in the sport and educational domains AGT has arguably become the dominant theory in explicitly examining the idea of how success/failure in achievement contexts is defined. Achievement contexts are defined by the presence of some evaluative elements and so can include school, sports, and sometimes exercise/health (Roberts, 2001). The debate is ongoing as to whether the subjective definition of success/failure used in AGT should extend to any aspects of the achievement context, or whether it should focus exclusively on competence, and much of the existing research also considers other non-competence concerns, such as self presentation or social status (Elliot & Dweck, 2005). Maehr and Nicholls (1980; p.262) proposed that: "Achievement motivation should be defined in terms of its purpose or meaning for people rather than in terms of overt behaviours or the characteristics of situations in which the behaviour occurs." This focus on subjective meaning became the lynchpin of achievement goal theory. Nicholls (1984, 1989) asserted that an individual's internal sense of competence was pivotal in achievement contexts and that importantly, the meaning of competence could be defined in at least two different ways:

> Achievement behaviour is defined as behaviour directed at developing or demonstrating high rather than low competence. It is shown that competence can be conceived in two ways. First, ability can be judged high or low with reference to the individual's *own past performance or knowledge*. In this context, gains in mastery indicate competence. Second, ability can be judged as capacity *relative to that of others*. In this context, a gain in mastery alone does not indicate high competence. To demonstrate high capacity, one must achieve more with equal effort or use less effort than do others for an equal performance. (Nicholls, 1984; p. 328 – italics added)

Hence, individuals are *task involved* when improvements in, or the mastering of, a skill or task provide them with a sense of competence (and subsequent satisfaction). Alternatively, an individual is *ego involved* when their sense of competence depends upon demonstrating superior performance to others (e.g., genuinely superior or an equal performance to their competitor with less effort exhibited). These two definitions of competence can be applied at the involvement level-of-analysis, the situational/contextual level (climate), and the pre-dispositional level (orientation), as well as being two separate definitions in their own right.

Developmental Processes

Nicholls' contribution to achievement goal theory emerged from developmental ideas surrounding how young children develop through process whereby children gradually become able to differentiate the concept of ability from effort, task difficulty and luck (Nicholls & Miller, 1984). Initially, between 5 and 7 years of age, Nicholls proposed that children did not differentiate between the concepts of ability/capacity and effort. Tasks which children are uncertain of completing were viewed as difficult, requiring more effort and so completion would provide children with a sense of achievement and competence. In effect, the limitation of ability in restricting what effort could produce is not realised and so, in the mind of a 5-year old, effort and ability were one-and-the same. Thus, achieving-by-trying would be the same as achieving-through-ability. This undifferentiated definition of competence was arguably the earliest (or even the purest) form of task involvement. Ironically it represents a mindset that Nicholls and all achievement goal theorists seek to re-introduce and reinforce in older, cognitively more sophisticated, athletes.

In Nicholls' conception, as children mature they move through a series of cognitive-developmental stages whereby, at 11 or 12 years-of-age, children are able to conceptualise ability as a relatively stable capacity, separate from effort (Fry, 2001). Children with a differentiated understanding of competence understand that difficult tasks are often those that only few can complete, and that this is a relatively good heuristic/rule-of-thumb for appraising task difficulty and one's own level of achievement. As such, children begin to understand that ability (on the specific task), perhaps more than effort, determines whether achievement tasks are successfully completed. Fundamentally, during this phase-of-development children realise that the outcome of a task is a *product* of ability/capacity and effort (and sometimes luck). Low ability/capacity can undermine compelling effort, and likewise lack-of-effort can produce underperformance in the more able athletes. Hence, the role of effort can become a double-edged-sword (Covington & Omelich, 1979), with some tasks demanding effort in order to maximise capacity/ability and increase the likelihood of success, some tasks where low effort expenditure and success-through-ability can combine to 'look good', and others where the likelihood of success is minimal, regardless of effort, so effort is best not expended.

Nicholls proposed that when children achieve the more sophisticated definition of competence they are capable of being ego-involved, by focusing on interpersonal comparisons of ability, and perhaps even overemphasising the role of ability in task outcomes. It should be noted, however, that these findings were originally achieved in an academic setting, and it should not necessarily be assumed that the same results would be found in sport (Fry & Duda, 1997; Smith, Smoll & Cummings, 2009). The complexity of the task and instructions has been cited as reasons why younger children may have failed to 'differentiate' (Heyman *et al.,* 2003) as some of the studies involved rather complex experimental procedures (e.g., Nicholls, 1978; Nicholls & Miller, 1983). Additionally, the salience of concepts such as ability and effort are proposed to be much more salient in sport than academic settings (Smith *et al.,* 2009). Score keeping, performance statistics, league standings and the awarding of trophies all amplify the salience of ability, whilst grimacing, exclamations, sweating/breathing and fatigue are all highly salient signs of effort exertion in sport, which are not as salient in academic settings. In addition, Smith *et al.*'s (2009) re-analysis of Fry and Duda's (1997) findings suggested that 9 and 11 year-old children did not differ significantly in their ability to differentiate effort from ability in sport, and that the majority of children at both ages were able to differentiate. Finally, studies such as Cumming, Smith, Smoll, Standage & Grossbard (2008) and Smoll, Smith and Cumming (2007) have validated perceived motivational climate questionnaires with younger athletes. These studies could also be taken as support for the notion that children below 12 can differentiate between effort and ability. Hence, the decision to exclude athletes under the age of 12 from studies (e.g., Vazou *et al.,* 2005) may not be as well substantiated as previously argued.

Overall, Nicholls' body of work is persuasive in establishing how maintaining optimal motivation in sport revolves around producing task-involvement (particularly once children have become capable of ego involvement) by encouraging a focus on effort, improvement and intrapersonal comparisons. On occasion, task involvement is referred to as 'less/un-differentiated', and ego involvement as more differentiated; this nomenclature could easily be interpreted as meaning task involvement is less sophisticated. However, in adults this may be a misnomer, as the strong salience of an ego/performance definition may imply that there is more cognitive effort and sophistication required in separating out results from ability, and realising the role of effort in both immediate performance and subsequently improved performances. As a further consideration, the differentiation process is, according to Nicholls, completed around the time that athletes transition to secondary school, which coincides with the time many athletes transition from sampling sports to specialising into a single sport (Côté, *et al.,* 2003 and Wylleman *et al.,* 2004). This transition is also likely to play a significant role in the ways children define, interpret and value success/failure.

A Related (but Separate) Theory: Dweck's Implicit Theories

During the development of AGT (through a series of seminars in the 1970's at the University of Illinois), whilst Nicholls was studying developmental processes surrounding ability/competence, Carol Dweck's work focused on why children of equal ability reacted differently to success and failure on tasks (in terms of withdrawal versus increasing effort). Based on their research, Dweck and her colleagues (Diener & Dweck, 1978; 1980; Dweck, 1975) proposed specific individual differences that lead to the pursuit of different goals. These individual differences in belief or 'implicit theories-of-ability' (ITA) have become known as *implicit theories.* According to Dweck (1999), attributes of the self, other people, places, and the world-in-general can be conceived: a) as fixed, uncontrollable factors; or, alternatively b) as malleable and controllable factors that are open to development. The first approach has been termed an *entity theory*, the second an *incremental theory*, and individuals can be described as entity or incremental theorists depending on their views of attributes within a given achievement domain (sport, school, work), or even activities within that domain.

Dweck proposed that entity theorists are more likely to endorse performance/ego goals, whereas incremental theorists are more likely to pursue task/mastery goals. This is because performance goals serve to demonstrate or prove one's stable ability (or avoid displaying the inadequacy of one's fixed and unchangeable ability), whereas one form of the task goal is to develop/improve one's malleable ability. Hence, individuals can interpret achievement settings differently depending on their underlying implicit theories. It is also likely that, by reinforcing or challenging such beliefs, coaches, parents and peers will influence a player's conception of ability (improvable versus fixed) within a certain achievement domain and therefore influence their interpretations of what constitutes competence within that situation (Gottfried, Fleming & Gottfried, 1994; Kamins & Dweck, 1999; Mueller & Dweck, 1999). This is a potentially important (and relatively under-represented) aspect of the socially determined 'motivational climate.'

There is an issue of measurement with regard to the study of ITAs, identified by Weiner (1995). Dweck, Chiu and Hong (1995) used three Likert-scaled items to measure implicit beliefs, but Weiner observes that "the wording of the items overlaps significantly" (p.319) in order to ensure strong reliability, but that this also compromises the validity and utility of the measure. Another approach is to use forced-choice indicators, along the lines of: "Do you believe that practice on this task will improve your level of performance?" [Yes/No]. The problem with this is that, when given more choices (e.g., Dweck et al., 1995), participants often endorsed *both* conceptions of ability. Hence, measuring ITAs seems to be rather difficult, so instead researchers have tended to try and manipulate these beliefs regarding a specific task by changing the instructions given to participants (e.g., Jourden, Bandura & Banfield, 1991; Niiya, Crocker & Bartmess, 2004). One difficulty with this is that the only available option for observing whether such a manipulation 'works' is to look at the experimental results (usually free-time task choice, effort, or persistence) – as the above measures of ITA (i.e., as a manipulation check) seem to be compromised from the outset.

Levels of Application

According to AGT (Nicholls, 1984; 1989) the states of task and ego involvement are induced by a combination of relatively stable intrapersonal traits ("orientation") with the specific pragmatic and social situations in which the achievement task is defined ("climate"). Duda (1993) suggested that this orientation – proneness to one-or-the-other goal involvement – is a product of socialisation experiences within achievement domains. Hence, it is possible to argue that the "climates" experienced by the developing sports participant influence that participant's subsequent "orientation" – although the interplay between these constructs is still relatively unknown except to say that they correlate strongly, and frequently (see below). The central point, however, is that achievement goal theory conceptualises two contrasting definitions of competence (task versus ego) at three different levels of analysis: i) involvement – the immediate here and now, ii) orientation – intrapersonal predispositions to either/both kinds of goal involvement and iii) climate – the situational factors that interact with orientation in determining immediate goal involvement (Nicholls, 1989 – although note that in the vast majority of cases, participants' perceptions of the climate are measured, and these often bear little relation to objectively observable events - Cumming, Smith, Smoll &

Grossbard, 2007; Papaioannou, Marsh & Theodorakis, 2004; Morgan, Sproule, Weigand & Carpenter, 2005).

Numerous psychometric instruments exist in order to measure the endorsement of each definition of competence at all three levels, in different domains (sport, PE, exercise - Duda & Whitehead, 1998). It is important to note, however, that the researchers responsible for the emergence of approach-avoidance goals (discussed shortly) do not conceptualise these three levels of analysis but rather a vast set of interacting intrapersonal antecedents and situational antecedents that combine to produce a goal-involvement state. Hence, goals are not analogised between levels but restricted to the level of involvement (although this 'involvement' can last weeks and months as opposed to moments, as Nicholls' definition would denote – i.e., Elliot, 1999). In the two-by-two theory of achievement goals, 'involvement' (termed *goal adoption*) spans both the situational and contextual levels), meaning that intrapersonal and environmental/social 'goals' are instead conceptualised as antecedent variables.

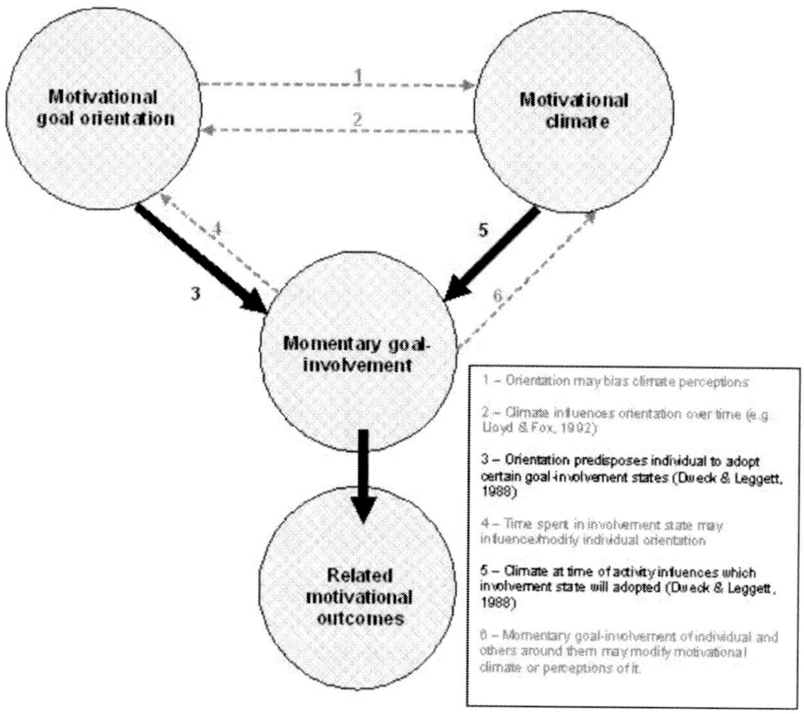

Figure 1. A representation of Nicholls' (1984; 1989) traditional AGT framework. Theoretical links between goal orientations (e.g., personality / trait), motivational climates (contextual + situational determinants) and momentary goal involvement, leading to potential influences on motivational outcomes. Thick arrows indicate relationships indicated by Nicholls. Dashed arrows indicate other potential relationships.

This difference between Nicholls' and Elliot's formulations raises the question of whether it is acceptable to apply achievement goal constructs to each level. For example, in Elliot's (1999; 2005) hierarchical model of approach and avoidance motivation (detailed shortly) intrapersonal traits and preferences are likely to be relatively stable and may readily be modelled as a 'goal orientation.' Indeed, Elliot and Thrash (2002) would appear to have adopted this approach in modelling neuro-anatomical variations and personality variables as approach and avoidance 'temperaments' that influence the adoption of mastery, performance-approach and performance-avoidance goals (although their 2001 paper argues against this approach in relation to modelling performance and mastery orientations). In either case, a number of antecedent variables are collapsed to form a summary construct. However, there is some intuitive sense in having consistency of concepts between levels, particularly for coaches and practitioners attempting to convey or apply these influential psychological principles. Whether this is a satisfactory argument for maintaining this representational framework is yet to be determined.

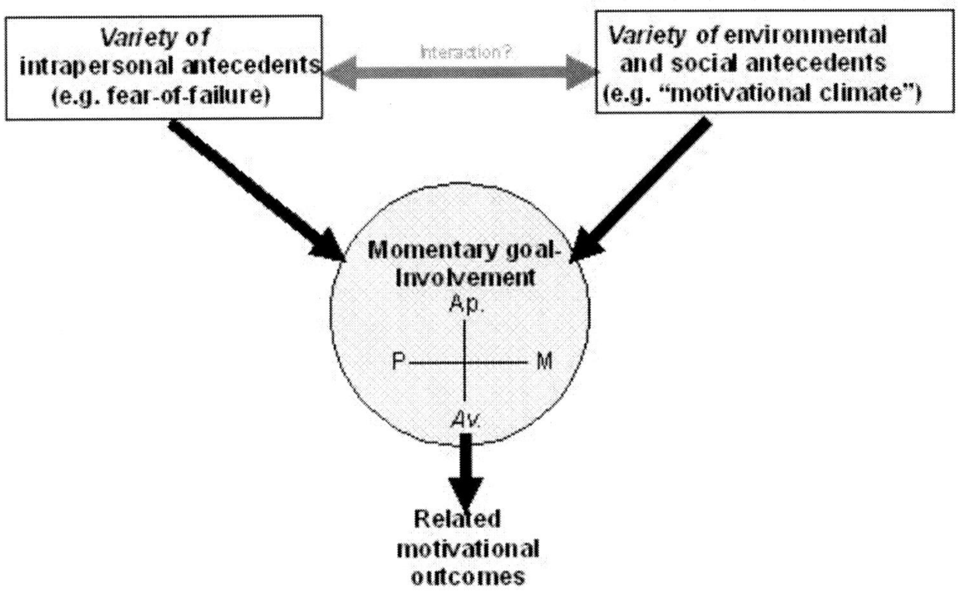

Figure 2. Elliot's (1999) alternative conceptualisation of achievement goal structures; the hierarchical model. Notably there is no 'goal orientation' concept, only antecedents. P = Performance/ego definition of competence, M = Mastery/task definition of competence, Ap. = Approach-valenced (seeking to demonstrate competence), Av. = Avoidance-valnced (seeking to avoid demonstrating incompetence). For further explanation of this goal framework see the following section.

Theoretical Predictions and Findings

Nicholl's (1984; 1989) dichotomous achievement goal theory dictates that individuals in a state of mastery involvement will display a positive and adaptive pattern of motivational responses; cognitive, affective and behavioural. These participants are predicted to positively engage in the achievement situation, demonstrating effort, persistence and choosing challenging tasks (Nicholls, 1984). Further, individuals with a high mastery orientation/disposition would also have positive beliefs about sport, for example, viewing effort and hard work are the main causes of success in sport (Duda & Nicholls, 1992; Duda & White, 1992; Roberts & Ommundsen, 1996). These individuals would also believe that the purpose of sport is to foster mastery, co-operation and social responsibility, which reduces the implications of failure to the self and therefore should facilitate increased enjoyment and satisfaction (Duda, Chi, Newton, Walling & Catley, 1995; Ntoumanis & Biddle, 1999). Further, individuals who are more predisposed towards mastery involvement view the opposition as co-operative in creating the chance for personal development and challenge, so will endorse relatively high moral values and frown upon cheating (Duda, 1992; 2001; Roberts, 2001; Roberts, Treasure & Kavussanu, 1996). In contrast, performance/ego oriented individuals should show the either opposite pattern or, in some cases, no consistent pattern.

Whilst correlational links between task/mastery versus ego/performance definitions of competence at the *climate* level and important associated variables are discussed shortly, research examining achievement goal *orientations* and goal *involvement* states demonstrates almost exactly the patterns predicted above, but given that these does not form the focus of this chapter (which focuses on environmental and social influences), orientations and involvement-states are kept separate from the current analysis. The interested reader is referred to reviews by Duda and Whitehead (1998) and Harwood, Spray and Keegan (2008).

Approach-Avoidance Achievement Goals

The distinction between approaching the desirable and avoiding the aversive has been a part of theorising in motivation since the inception of psychology as a scientific discipline (Elliot, 1999). Indeed, Nicholls' (1984) original writing also examined the notion that individuals in achievement settings can be concerned with avoiding the demonstration of incompetence. Traditionally AGT has placed the concept of perceived competence in a position of vital importance, as described earlier, and Nicholls (1984) suggested that individuals with *low perceived competence* can belong to one of three different categories when placed in achievement situations: a) individuals committed to demonstrating competence *despite* perceptions of inadequacy [approach]; b) individuals committed to *avoiding demonstrating incompetence* [avoidance]; and c) individuals who are *not committed* to avoiding demonstrating low ability [amotivation?]. Note that in these definitions 'demonstrating' competence may mean either normatively (i.e., ego) *or* in a self-referenced (i.e., task) manner. It is only recently, however, that this assertion by Nicholls has been revisited. The goal of avoiding demonstrating incompetence is proposed to be adopted when the likelihood of demonstrating competence is undermined (Nicholls, 1984; p.332). However, it is possible that participants may begin a task with this goal in mind, without having to 'lose' the prospect of demonstrating competence first.

In addition, it is also notable that the constructs of perceived high-or-low ability were considered as functionally isomorphic with approach-versus-avoidance motivational tendencies by some theorists (Kukla, 1972; Meyer, 1987). Thus the moderating influence of perceived competence in Nicholls' (1989) achievement goal theory may have already been incorporating aspects of approach and avoidance tendencies in a convoluted manner, and Elliot (1994, 1997) asserted that this may have delayed progress in achievement goal theory by providing 'false positive' results regarding perceived competence – which has often been proposed as a mediator between goals and outcomes, rather than as a goal itself, in the form of the approach-avoidance distinction.

Whilst Nicholls (1984) had alluded to the avoidance of demonstrating incompetence, Dweck's (1986) conceptualisation (described earlier) also proposed that individuals possessing low perceived ability, *and* who view human attributes/skills as a fixed entities, are more likely to want to avoid negative judgments of competence and seek to gain positive judgments of their fixed and unchangeable ability. Dweck and Leggett (1988) described how children with 'entity' theories (in the domain of intelligence) were most likely to exhibit challenge-avoidant goals – choosing easy tasks where they could do well and thus avoid the inevitable mistakes on more difficult tasks. However, the concept of seeking to avoid demonstrating incompetence was largely ignored in the research that followed, which focused overwhelmingly on approach motivation (often termed 'achievement motivation'), examining the implications of seeking to *demonstrate competence* in task/mastery versus ego/performance terms (Duda, 2001; Duda & Hall, 2001). More recently, Elliot and colleagues (Elliot, 1997, 1999; Elliot & Church, 1997) have (re)introduced the concept of avoidance goals i.e., striving to avoid displaying inadequacy, chiefly in the *educational* achievement domain.

Elliot (1997, 1999) argued that inconsistent findings in the achievement goal literature concerning the motivational implications of ego/performance goals were, *in part,* a result of the failure to distinguish 'approach' and 'avoidance' forms of this goal definition ("in part" because he also cited the failure of AGT to focus more exclusively on competence, thus allowing social and self-presentational concerns to confuse matters, as well as a failure to distinguish between goals – in the form of involvement/adoption - and the numerous antecedents of goals – as opposed to 'orientations'). Moreover, Elliot argued the relevance of a mastery-avoidance goal in which the individual is concerned with, *and strives to avoid,* demonstrating incompetence in a self-referenced (e.g., deterioration relative to previous scores) or technical (poor technique) manner (Elliot 1999).

Elliot and Covington (2001) and Elliot and Thrash (2002) also illustrate the fundamental importance of the approach-avoidance distinction in the history of psychological study, and more specifically in the study of motivation and motivated behaviour. There is a compelling case that approach-based or 'hedonic' systems and avoidance-based or 'survival' systems operate simultaneously on numerous intrapersonal levels ranging from neurophysiological (Gray, 1990), emotional predisposition (Tellegen, 1985; Watson & Clark, 1993; Clark & Watson, 1999), general personality (e.g. neuroticism versus extroversion, McCrae & Costa, 1987; Costa & McCrae, 1992) and cognitive predispositions (Cacioppo *et al.,* 1997). Further, these bivariate systems at different cognitive and affective levels can be modelled together into a consistent two-factor model that predicts related motivational and affective outcomes across *different domains* (Elliot & Thrash, 2002; Gable, Reis & Elliot, 2003). Additionally this evaluative process appears to be supported by neurological structures in the brain, independent from those that support perception and higher cognition (see Cacioppo *et al.,* 1996; Elliot & Covington, 2001). The evaluative processing that leads to approach or avoidance predispositions is purported to take place "in a matter of milliseconds" (Bargh & Chartrand, 1999, p.475). Consequently, the consideration of approach-avoidance motivation may well be important for the development of an achievement goal theory, but it is certainly important in any study of human motivation and motivated behaviour.

Elliot's Concurrent Contribution – The Focus on Competence

Elliot and colleagues also argue that the achievement goal construct should focus solely on *competence*, the demonstration of it and the avoidance of demonstrating a lack of it (Elliot & Thrash, 2001). As such, valence and definition are the sole components of an (momentary/involvement type) achievement goal, whereas measures of goals that utilise Nicholls' and Dweck's conceptualisations go beyond the definition and valence of competence and extend to tap indices of self-evaluation and social status. For example, in measures such as the Task-Ego Orientations in Sport Questionnaire (TEOSQ – Duda & Nicholls, 1992) and Perceptions of Success Questionnaire (POSQ – Roberts & Balague, 1989; 1991; Treasure & Roberts, 1994), individuals are asked to indicate what makes them feel successful in general (inviting responses regarding more than just competence), or they are predisposed to a focus on how others judge their competence. This is also exemplified in the POSQ, which asks: "when playing sport, I feel successful when [I show other people I am the best / I am clearly superior]", whilst the TEOSQ asks: "I feel most successful in sport when [I can do better than my friends / I'm the best]." Such wordings do not necessarily relate *exclusively* to competence as opposed to social concerns, as the two can be significantly inter-related (Skinner & Piek, 2001), i.e., demonstrating physical competence can be associated with increased popularity and status, and vice versa – and these item wordings do not discriminate between these issues. Hence, according to Elliot such self-worth and self-presentational concerns should not be included in the conceptualisation and measurement of a goal, because it becomes unclear whether these concerns impact upon motivational processes and outcomes and how they may combine with a (competence based) achievement goal. Such a refinement arguably makes it easier to reconcile AGT with SDT, as it would focus AGT into the consideration of competence needs, rather than (sometimes awkwardly) relating to all three of SDT's psychological needs (competence, autonomy and relatedness).

Core Theoretical Predictions

Approach-avoidance considerations were initially incorporated into a hierarchical model of achievement goals in which multiple antecedents of goal striving and goal adoption (the lower tier of the hierarchy) combined to produce *three* types of momentary goal/involvement-state: *mastery* (approach) in which the concern is to demonstrate self-referenced competence, *performance-approach* in which the concern is to demonstrate competence relative to others, and *performance-avoidance* in which the concern is to avoid demonstrating incompetence relative to others - these formed the higher tier of the hierarchical model (Elliot, 1997; Elliot & Church, 1997). Subsequently, the mastery goal was also split into approach and avoidance forms, providing a full 2x2 crossing of approach and avoidance forms over performance and mastery goals (see Figure 3 - Elliot, 1999; Elliot & McGregor, 2001). This created four possible achievement goals (performance-approach, performance-avoidance, mastery-approach and mastery-avoidance) that were construed as "concrete cognitive representations that serve a directional function in motivation by guiding the individual toward or away from specific possible outcomes" (Elliot & Thrash, 2001, p.143). For example, a sport participant may be concerned that they will do poorly in relation to the other participants (performance-avoidance goal), or poorly in relation to a previous performance, or perhaps fail to achieve a desirable technique or skill (mastery-avoidance goal). The participant may well be concerned with wanting to win an event or race (performance-approach goal) or simply to 'play well' from a technical perspective and improve on his or her own previous performances (mastery-approach goal).

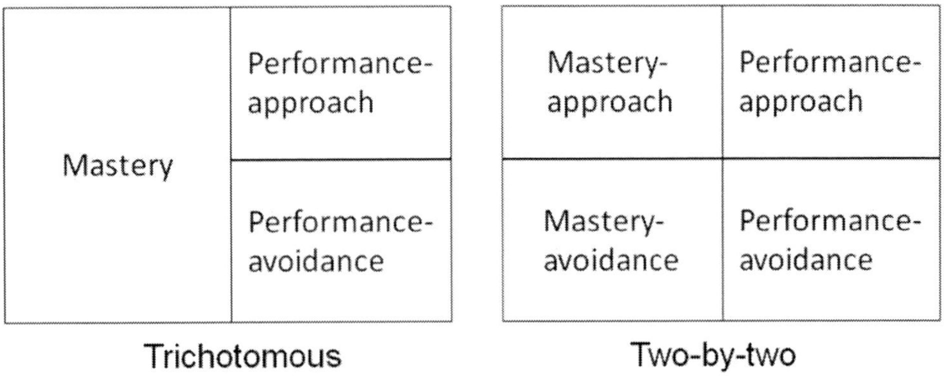

Figure 3. A representation of the trichotomous and 2x2 goal frameworks.

In Elliot and McGregor's (2001) 2x2 framework, a goal is neither an intrapersonal predisposition to adopt goals nor a socially emphasised desirable outcome, but instead a cognitive representation that serves to direct behaviour. Each of the four goals can be pursued for a host of different *reasons* (antecedents). These reasons provide the *energising force* for behaviour, whereas the goals themselves *channel* this energy toward or away from specific desirable and aversive possibilities respectively. Theoretically, the reasons for pursuing a goal and the goal itself interact, forming 'goal complexes' that determine motivational outcomes and processes (although the number of potential goal complex combinations is immense). Key antecedents/'reasons', can be intrapersonal - such as implicit theories of ability (cf. Dweck & Leggett, 1988), competence expectancies (Nicholls, 1989), need for achievement (Atkinson, 1957; McClelland, Atkinson, Clarke & Lowell, 1953), need for approval (Rogers, 1961; Hall & Lindzey, 1985), fear of failure (Atkinson, 1957), and perceived competence (i.e., *not* a moderator – Elliot & Church, 1997; Lopez, 1999) - as well as situational factors such as perceived motivational climate (cf. Ames, 1984b). Therefore, individuals may experience sport settings very differently depending on the goal(s) adopted and the intrapersonal and situational *reasons* for goal adoption (see Elliot, 1999).

An additional consideration is that, in Elliot's conceptualisation, it is possible for each of the four types of concern (i.e., goals) to be *simultaneously* salient to differing degrees. In this construction of the theory, achievement goals are considered neither orthogonal (i.e., Nicholls' goal orientations) nor bipolar (i.e., Dweck's state goals). Individuals can pursue different goals at the same time. In support of this, positive associations may be found empirically among all four goal involvement states (see Conroy, Elliot & Hofer, 2003).

Both the trichotomous and 2x2 frameworks facilitate the testing of predictions in terms of both antecedents of the four goals and their achievement-related consequences despite the fact that the numerous individual and environmental factors potentially underpinning achievement goal pursuit will impact on processes and outcomes in diverse ways. This is one of the benefits of moving from cognitive theories to social-cognitive theories as described earlier. Theoretically, mastery-approach goals are underpinned by success-oriented factors such as need-for-achievement and incremental beliefs and are thus predicted to bring about generally positive outcomes, particularly in terms of positive affect and self-determination experienced in sport. Performance-avoidance goals, in contrast, are rooted in failure-oriented antecedents such as fear-of-failure and low self-esteem. These are thought to lead to a host of negative processes and outcomes such as high state anxiety, lower self-determination, and impaired performance. Performance-approach goals are complex given that they can potentially be underpinned by factors that orient an athlete to success or failure. For example, a sports participant pursuing performance-approach goals underpinned by a strong fear-of-failure may work hard and persist on a short-term basis, but is likely to experience greater anxiety and lower self-determination than another participant pursuing performance-approach goals underpinned by a strong need-for-achievement and high competence expectancy. Finally, mastery-avoidance goals are likely to be a product of fear-of-failure, incremental beliefs, low perceptions of competence, perfectionism and situational cues that highlight self and task improvement but also the possibility of failure rather than success (Elliot, 1999).

The consequences of pursuing the above-listed goals will depend on their antecedent/reasons profile. Mastery-avoidance goals underpinned by fear-of-failure may lead to more negative consequences than if underpinned by incremental beliefs or perfectionism. In general, it was postulated that the motivational impact of adopting mastery-avoidance goals will be less positive than that of mastery-approach goals but more positive than that of performance-avoidance goals (Elliot, 1999; Elliot & McGregor, 2001). Empirical findings to date have largely supported the proposed relationships between goal-states, antecedents and consequences (Elliot, 2005) although the conceptual overhaul of achievement goals that has accompanied the introduction of approach and avoidance goals has slowed down empirical proceedings while new theoretical aspects are debated and modified research methods/paradigms are introduced to accommodate the examination of proposed antecedent-goal-consequence relationships.

On occasion, researchers have touched upon ways in which approach-avoidance goals can be conceptualised at the socio-environmental level. Barkoukis *et al.* (2007) used the Learning and Performance Orientations in Physical Education Classes Questionnaire (LAPOPECQ - a dichotomous measure of perceived motivational climate; Papaioannou, 1994) to predict trichotomous goal-adoptions and found that the subscale 'worry about mistakes' (a performance-climate subscale) was a positive predictor of both mastery- and performance-avoidance goals. Church, Elliot and Gable (2001) also studies motivational climate in college classes, gain using the trichotomous model of approach-avoidance goals, and found that interesting material/style (mastery), emphasis on evaluation and assignment scores (mastery), and perceived harsh evaluation (performance-avoidance) were aspects of the environment that could be associated with the trichotomous framework. Overall, however, in the years since these ideas were first proposed, relatively little research has been conducted to establish the ways that approach and avoidance goals can be promoted/stimulated in the social context.

Social Goals

Whilst Nicholls' (1984, 1989) most recognised formulations of AGT focused on task and ego goals, his work prior to (Maehr & Nicholls, 1980), and following (Jarvinen & Nicholls,

1996) his most seminal work discussed ways of conceptualising competence other than the task and ego conceptions. For example, even in achievement contexts such as sport, an individual could strive to have a good relationship with others or to be accepted by others. Maehr and Nicholls (1980) included a social approval goal orientation in addition to task and ego goal orientations in their original theoretical framework. They suggested that a social approval goal orientation emphasises the desire for acceptance by significant others (in this case, through conformity to norms while displaying maximal effort). However, this social approval goal was largely ignored in the research that followed. Urdan and Maehr (1995) called for the resurrection of social goal orientations and highlighted their importance in achievement behaviour; suggesting a wide range of social goal orientations reflecting the wide variety of potential social bonds. These goal orientations included social welfare (i.e., to benefit the larger society by becoming a productive member), social responsibility (i.e., to be conscientious), and social affiliation (i.e., to feel a sense of belonging). Stuntz and Weiss (2003) claimed that there is a multitude of conceptually and meaningfully distinct types of social relationship, and so there must be a corresponding variety of potential social goals. On the basis of this, they also suggest that the 'social approval orientation' originally included in AGT only partially addressed the desire to maintain positive social relationships, even before it was largely ignored during ensuing period of research that focused on task and ego goals.

Social goals are most frequently specified in relation to peer relationships, which can be broadly divided into two categories: friendship/affiliation and peer acceptance/group membership (Allen, 2003; 2006; Bukowski & Hoza, 1989). Friendship/affiliation describes a close, mutual dyadic relationship between two individuals, while peer acceptance/group membership refers to a group-level construct of acceptance or liking by the peer group. Specifically in the sporting domain, positive team interactions, friendship and social support from peers have been linked to sport enjoyment, motivation, expectations of success, and future participation intentions (e.g.,Scanlan, Carpenter, Lobel, & Simons, 1993; Weiss & Smith, 2002). Proponents of social goals research argue that task and ego goal orientations alone are insufficient to explain achievement behaviours in sport, because task and ego goals by definition cannot include the range of social definitions of success in achievement situations (Urdan & Maehr, 1995; Weiss & Ferrer-Caja, 2002) – especially if Elliot's suggestions are applied regarding the strict restriction of task and ego goals to issues of competence, as distinct from self-presentational and social concerns.

Allen (2006) has reported that friendships and group memberships are key motivating factors in sport, whilst Ullrich-French and Smith (2006) noted that the quality of friendship and peer acceptance also influenced motivational variables such as enjoyment and perceived competence. Allen (2003) validated a questionnaire that modelled social competence (an indication of effectiveness in interactions with other people - Howes & James, 2002) in a notably similar way to the dichotomous achievement goals, with social affiliation goals (familiarity, attachment, mutual benefit) contrasting with social status goals (e.g. How many friends do I have? How many people think I'm good?). This may prove an interesting framework in which to examine 'social competence' given the recent suggestion to re-focus achievement goals onto the concept of competence.

The consideration of social goals is certainly important when considering how key social protagonists are able to influence athlete motivation, and the exclusion of social considerations in this context as not-relating-to-competence (i.e., Roberts, 2001) could prove a costly oversight. There is indirect support for such a conceptualisation in the research presented by Wentzel (2005) examining peer influences on motivation (chiefly in the academic context). Wentzel describes how peer group membership (e.g. as a 'popular', a 'jock' or a 'goth') - which may be analogised to holding social status - carried no relationships with academic achievements or personal characteristics (in the same way that performance 'orientations' often produce equivocal results in relation to important outcome variables - Wentzel & Caldwell, 1997). Indeed, those with the highest 'status' orientations/memberships (e.g. the 'populars') were often described as having undesirable personal characteristics such as being exclusionary, discriminatory and lacking pro-social skills (Parkhurst & Hopmeyer, 1998). In contrast, simply having an affiliated dyadic friendship at school, in line with social affiliation goals, was linked with numerous positive outcomes including self-confidence, sociability, independence, altruism and decreased aggression (Wentzel, Barry & Caldwell, 2004), as well as improved grades and test scores (Berndt & Keefe, 1995; Wentzel, *et al.*, 2004) and increased engagement in school activities (Berndt & Keefe, 1995; Ladd, 1990). This finding may mirror the many positive outcomes linked with mastery orientations/involvement states.

In a recent sport-based study Stuntz and Weiss (2003) found that social goals could be more influential than achievement goals in predicting unsportsmanlike play. Thus firstly, social competence should certainly not be excluded from achievement goal research, especially when considering motivational climates which are heavily socially determined. Secondly, it is perhaps worth entertaining the idea that 'social competence' might operate in a similar fashion to task/sport competence, with a mastery (affiliation) definition and a performance (status) definition. At the very least, the analysis of qualitative data should not exclude social influences on motivation (as is sometimes recommended e.g. Elliot, 1997; 1999) but rather categorise them separately. Nicholls (1984) omitted social approval goals from his conceptualisation on the grounds that 'social goals' was a motivational topic in its own right and blending them with task or ego goals could confound our understanding of motivation (Nicholls, Cheung, Lauer, & Patashnick, 1989). However, it may be the case, particularly when studying socially induced motivational states, that the study of social goals is essential in order to produce a more complete understanding of sport motivation, and this is increasingly the case in sport (Harwood *et al.*, 2008).

Achievement Goal Climates

The study of what was termed *situational factors* has formed an important strand of AGT, with the most notable contribution arising from Carole Ames' initial work (also integral at the Illinois seminar series during the 70s). This section will begin with an overview of Ames' own research before moving onto a broad discussion of the literature on *motivational climate* – the construct that emerged from Ames' work. Subsequently, a number of future directions for motivational climate research are proposed.

Ames' Approach

Whilst the initial work on motivational climate is credited to Ames and her colleagues (Ames, Ames & Felker, 1977; Ames, 1984a), her early work did not draw on AGT per se but examined the influences of the environment (rewards structures, incentives) on motivational processes (e.g., attributions following success and failure). Ames *et al.* (1977) examined the behaviours of 40 sixth-grade boys following success and failure in competitive and non-competitive situations. Boys were placed in matched-ability pairs and assigned to either fail or succeed. Under competitive conditions, only the 'winner' received a reward but under non-competitive conditions both could chose a prize for participating. Competitive conditions led to significant increases in self-punitive behaviours following failure (rating self as lower ability and undeserving of reward) but 'ego-enhancing' behaviours were shown following success (rating self as higher ability and deserving of rewards). No differences in attribution were found in the non-competitive condition. In a later study, Ames (1984a) created a 'competitive' goal structure by testing children in pairs against each other, and 'individualistic' goal structure by testing children on their own and encouraging them to improve their scores. The outcome (high versus low success) was manipulated by changing the number of solvable puzzles a child was given. Following testing, children were asked questions about what they were thinking during the tasks. In the competitive condition, children tended to link their own *ability* to the outcomes, whereas, in the individualistic condition, children attributed outcomes (success/failure) to *effort*. Further, the individualistic condition led children to 'self-instruct' (e.g. "I need to take my time over this", "I'm going to think carefully about this") more than the competitive condition. In Ames' own words these children "behaved much like Diener and Dweck's (1980) mastery-oriented children and reflected what Nicholls has called task involvement." (p.485). These differences in behaviour as a function of *situational conditions* (cf. goal/reward structures) suggested that differing reward structures influence the salience of various informational sources in self-evaluations of ability, the affective impact of success and failure and subsequent perceptions of ability

From here, Ames (1984b) defined qualitatively different 'motivational systems' in children, which bore a more than passing resemblance to the conceptualisations of task and ego involvement. Although not directly grounded in achievement goal theory, the competitive and individualistic conditions (as well as co-operative goal structures that formed her work) are closely analogised to what were later termed 'performance involving' (i.e., ego) and 'mastery involving' (e.g., task) climates, respectively.

Ames and Archer (1988) and Ames (1992a) continued investigating these performance-versus-mastery involving classroom environments proposing that situational cues, chiefly controlled by the teacher, will influence the salience of different achievement goals. In non-classroom settings, significant others and important social agents were proposed to determine goal salience by the nature of their "instructional demands" (1992a; p.262). Further, Ames (1992b) asserted that the subjective meaning, or individual's perception of the motivational environment was the critical factor in predicting subsequent achievement goals and patterns of behaviour. This body of literature aided researchers in defining two types of motivational climate: a *mastery climate* where the criteria for evaluation are self-referenced and people are viewed as competent when they have made progress, accomplished a task or learned something new; or a *performance climate* where the criteria for evaluation are heavily other-referenced and the emphasis is upon outperforming others and, notably, *making as few mistakes as possible* (Blumenfeld, 1992).

Based on Epstein (1989), Ames (1992a) then described specific classroom structures that were likely to invoke 'mastery' or 'performance' climates; these six achievement structures were 'task' (design of tasks), 'authority' (location of decision-making), 'recognition' (distribution of rewards), 'grouping' (manner and frequency of grouping), 'evaluation' (standards for performance) and 'time' (pace of learning). The initial letters of the six structures create the acronym TARGET – and using each structure, a performance or mastery climate could be emphasised by the teacher or other salient social agents. A task-climate would include collaborative tasks, democratic leadership, recognition for effort/improvement, mixed ability groupings, private and individual evaluation, and sufficient time for everyone to learn. An ego-climate would include competitive tasks, autocratic leadership, recognition of normative ability, segregation by ability, normative and public evaluation, and time for only the more advanced students to complete a task. In most coaching environments, however, the above behaviours are likely to occur interchangeably depending on the circumstances (Keegan *et al.*, 2009; 2010).

Manipulations of Situational Goal Structures in Sport

Through manipulating the criteria derived from the TARGET framework, early research attempted to create environmental conditions that would foster mastery or performance involvement in participants. Examples of these studies included Duda and Chi (1989; basketball), Marsh and Peart (1988; aerobics classes), Lloyd and Fox (1992; fitness classes) and Theeboom De Knop and Weiss (1995; children's martial arts classes). All four of these studies supported theoretically specified links between 'climate' and participants' behaviours or cognitions. In Lloyd and Fox's (1992) six-week study, low-performance oriented participants in the performance-involving climate became more performance-oriented over the course of the study and high-performance oriented participants in the mastery climate became less performance-oriented. This is one of very few studies demonstrating an influence of climate upon goal orientation. Such a theoretical link between climate and orientation has been suggested on a number of occasions (Treasure & Roberts, 1995; Duda, 1992; 1993; Nicholls, 1989) but experimental investigations of sufficient length have been scarce. More recently, studies by Smith, Smoll and Cumming (2007; 2009) have demonstrated reductions in anxiety and changes in goal-orientation in relation to perceptions of the motivational climate.

Whilst notable for their field-based, experimental designs, several difficulties exist that undermine the interpretation of these experimental studies in relation to Nicholls' assertions concerning the interactional nature of achievement striving (e.g. Figure 5.4.1). Firstly, in some cases no account was taken of the independent effect of participants' goal orientations on motivational outcomes, and so limited insight can be gained into the relative influence of dispositional and situational characteristics on mastery and performance involvement. Secondly, no measure was taken of participants' *perceptions* of the climate, perhaps misguidedly assuming that the climate manipulation was uniformly interpreted and applied by participants within each condition. Further, no measures of mastery and performance involvement were taken to determine degrees of situational change in achievement goals. Nevertheless, such studies laid down a marker for the testing of achievement goal theory in true-to-life settings and it is unfortunate that this line of research has stuttered slightly in the intervening period (instead focusing on participants' perception of the motivational climate). This design gave way to what has since become the most dominant means of assessing 'situational factors' in achievement goal theory – the measurement of *perceived* motivational climate.

Perceived Motivational Climate in Sport and Physical Education

Following Ames' (1992b) assertion that the perception of the motivational environment was critical, a number of questionnaires emerged to assess the perceived situational and contextual goal emphases in sport and physical education settings. These included: the Learning and Performance Orientations in Physical Education Classes Questionnaire (LAPOPECQ – Papaioannou, 1994; 1995; 1997), the Physical Education Class Climate Scale (PECCS – Goudas & Biddle, 1994), L'Echelle de Perception du Climat Motivational (EPCM - Biddle, Cury, Goudas, Sarrazin, Famose, & Durand, 1995), the Perceived Motivational Climate in Sport Questionnaire (PMSCQ - Seifriz, Duda & Chi, 1992), PMCSQ-2 (Newton & Duda, 1993) and the Motivational Climate Scale for Youth Sports (MCSYS - Smith, Cumming & Smoll, 2008). These questionnaires, their strengths, weaknesses and associated findings are reviewed in Harwood *et al.* (2008) and Duda and Whitehead (1998). However, in succinctly summarising the sub-factors of these scales: i) effort; ii) learning/skill-improvement; iii) perceived important role; iv) cooperative learning; and v) 'mistakes-are-part-of-learning' are all key themes of a mastery climate; whereas: i) interpersonal comparison (and rivalry); ii) punishment/fear of mistakes; iii) unequal treatment of players; and iv) 'achieving-without-effort' are consistent themes of performance climates. Notionally, any individual leading or participating in sporting activities can influence the motivational climate by differentially emphasising the above themes and it is immediately clear that coaches/teachers, parents and peers are important social protagonists of such climates.

Whilst the development of these questionnaires has contributed significantly to our understanding of the role played by perceptions of contextual influences on motivation, the measurement of motivational climate remains controversial. In addition to what is presented here, Duda and Whitehead (1998) provide a comprehensive summary and critique of the different measures of perceived motivational climate, their origins and properties, and the conceptual appropriateness of certain scales. Ideas for advancements in measurement and other methodological issues will follow shortly. First, however, it is important to summarise what has been learned from the research that has employed these scales (cf. Ntoumanis & Biddle, 1999).

Correlates of Perceived Motivational Climate

In a similar vein to research investigating dispositional goal orientations (Duda & Nicholls, 1992), interest has been equally high in the motivational, affective and behavioural *correlates* of perceived mastery/performance climates in sport and PE. An overview of this research is presented below. Correlates are listed using Roman numerals.

I. *Beliefs about causes of sporting success*: According to theory, a task/mastery emphasis will be linked to belief that *effort* is necessary for success while an ego/performance emphasis will link to beliefs that success stems from greater (i) *ability* (finite and unchangeable), and possibly (ii) deception or 'gamesmanship.'
The evidence available supports both of these links between perceived climate and sport participants' beliefs about causes of success (Seifriz, Duda & Chi, 1992; Treasure & Roberts, 1998; 2001; Newton & Duda, 1995; Carpenter & Morgan, 1999) although *causality* cannot be established from such correlational data. However, the implications are still important, as participants in a (perceived) performance climate are likely to believe that their potential to succeed is limited by ability (this is believed to both undermine their motivation to continue following failures, and promote the use of deception or foul-play in order to succeed) as increasing effort is not believed to increase the chances of succeeding (see earlier sections). Conversely, participants in (perceived) mastery climates are likely to ascribe failure to a lack of effort and try harder. There is no link between mastery climate and deception beliefs, so these sport performers are unlikely to resort to deception when faced with failure. Thus, arguments for *creating* climates high in task/mastery cues are supported by the existing evidence.

II. *Beliefs about the purpose of sport*: Sport is regularly cited as an eminent vehicle for the learning of life skills and adaptive coping strategies. However, the evidence available suggests that this perception is only likely when a mastery climate is perceived by participants (Ommundsen & Roberts, 1999; Ommundsen, Roberts & Kavusannu, 1998) as only mastery climates link to the belief that sport serves the purpose of improving and challenging ourselves. Performance climates, on the other hand, appear to link to the belief that sport is for the enhancement of social status. Thus, *if* children are encouraged to participate in sport in order to become 'better people', *then* the current evidence specifies that a mastery climate should be prominent so that participation does not become an exercise in linking an (apparently unchangeable) ability-level to social status.

III. *Positive affect – enjoyment, intrinsic interest and satisfaction*: Theoretically, a focus on task/mastery should promote challenge and autonomy, and cause sport participation to be seen as the end in itself (intrinsic motivation and enjoyment), whilst a focus on ego/performance should promote the idea that the activity is a means-to-an-end: the demonstration of superior ability. This should create pressure and tension and reduce positive affect. The evidence, to date, shows a clear link between perceptions of mastery climates and positive affect in sport participants – meaning that (perceived) mastery climates tend to be more enjoyable, involving and interesting (Balague, Duda & Crespo, 1999; Dorobantu & Biddle, 1997; Kavussanu & Roberts, 1996; Liukkonen, Telama & Biddle, 1998; Newton, Duda & Yin, 2000; Parish & Treasure, 2003; Treasure & Roberts, 2001; Whitehead, Andrée & Lee, 2004). The proposed negative relationship between perceived performance climate and positive affect is only supported in some of the studies (Balaguer *et al.,* 1999; Liukkonen *et al.,* 1998; Parish & Treasure, 2003; Treasure & Roberts, 2001; Whitehead *et al.,* 2004), meaning that performance climates are unlikely to promote positive experiences for sport participants, and may even reduce enjoyment. This discrepancy in findings concerning perceived performance climates may be caused by the failure of current measures to differentiate between the approach and avoidance aspects of climate; i.e., a climate emphasising winning and success may be more adaptive than one emphasising avoiding loss or deselection.

IV. *Negative affect – pressure, tension, anxiety, distress and worry*: The majority of studies examining this correlate suggest that a perceived mastery climate *either* does not relate to negative affective experiences for participants (Escarti & Gutierrez, 2001; Ntoumanis & Biddle, 1998a; b), *or* that a mastery emphasis *reduces* negative affect (Newton *et al.,* 2000; Papaioannou & Kouli, 1999; Pensgaard & Roberts, 2000; Walling, Duda & Chi, 1993). In contrast all the above-listed studies also reported a positive association between perceptions of a performance climate and anxiety, worry, distress, and dissatisfaction with the team. Hence, when participants perceive performance climates, they are usually prone to experience negative feelings, while those perceiving a mastery climate are usually not. On current evidence, therefore, one could argue that the creation of a mastery climate by important social agents should lead to less negative affect than a strong performance (comparative, win-at-all costs) climate.

V. *Perceived competence*: A number of studies (Balaguer, Duda, Atienza & Mayo, 2002; Balaguer, Duda & Crespo, 1999; Digelidis, Papaioannou, Laparidis, & Christodoulidis, 2003; Escarti & Gutierrez, 2001; Goudas & Biddle, 1994; Kavussanu & Roberts, 1996; Liukkonen, Telama & Biddle, 1998; Ommundsen & Roberts, 1999; Sarrazin, Vallerand, Guillet, Pelletier & Cury, 2002; Standage, Duda & Ntoumanis, 2003a; b) have all supported the theoretically positive link between a perceived mastery climate and perceived competence, whereas no association emerged in ten of these studies between a perceived performance climate and perceived competence. Cury, Da Fonseco, Rufo & Sarrazin (2002) – using the PECCS - reported a negative association between perceived performance climate and perceived competence, as did Sarrazin *et al.* (2002). The central conclusion that can be drawn from this research is that perceptions of a mastery climate appear to link strongly with participants' perceived competence which is not the case for perceptions of a performance climate. In fact, in some cases a perceived performance climate is linked with lower perceptions of competence.

VI. *Adoption of learning versus competitive strategies*: Roberts and Treasure (1992) suggest that a task/mastery emphasis promotes internal standards of comparison and striving for improvement leading participants to seeking challenging tasks, persist and participate more in training Conversely, an ego/performance emphasis promotes interpersonal comparisons, which are relatively unstable outcomes and therefore result in the use of *varied learning strategies* (e.g. no association). Gano-Overway and Ewing (2004), Yoo (1999), Xiang and Lee (2002), and Magyar and Feltz (2003); Ntoumanis, Biddle and Haddock (1999), Ommundsen and Roberts (2001), Ommundsen, Roberts and Kavussanu (1998) and Treasure and Roberts (2001) have reported that sport participants who perceive a mastery climate use more adaptive strategies and learning strategies while playing and training. No link between perceived performance climate and strategy use existed in the majority of these studies. Negative associations with performance climates include Magyar and Feltz (2003), who found that a perceived performance climate *reduced* the tendency of participants to confidently accept tuition from their coach, and Ryska, Yin and Boyd

(1999), who found a link between perceived performance climates and self-reported self-handicapping (avoiding difficult tasks). Ntoumanis, Biddle and Haddock (1999) reported that participants reporting a performance climate also indicated a tendency towards avoidance and emotional-focused (venting, anger) methods of coping as opposed to solution focused coping and seeking social support, which occurred in a perceived mastery climate.

VII. *Goal orientations*: A number of studies have supported a link between perceptions of climate and participants' own respective goal orientations (e.g., Digelidis *et al.,* 2003; Standage *et al.,* 2003; Williams, 1998; Xiang & Lee, 2002). In establishing the direction of this link (i.e., goal orientation-biases-perception vs. climate-influences-goal orientation) we can draw from *intervention* studies that have been conducted. Lloyd and Fox (1992) and Todorovich and Curtner-Smith (2002) are two examples of studies where changing the climate has been shown to influence participants' goal orientations over time. However, it is certainly plausible that within a given situation or sporting context, a participant's goal orientation/disposition may cognitively bias their selection and perceptions of motivational cues in the climate. In other words, individuals may be more sensitive to cues or behaviours that correspond to their own goal orientations. For example, a high performance/low mastery oriented athlete may seek out any behaviours of a coach that relate to winning, social evaluation and public recognition even if such behaviours do not accurately represent the behaviours, or intended messages of the coach (or parent, or peers). Indeed, this athlete may report a 'high performance/low mastery' climate when the coach may be intending to offer numerous mastery cues that the athlete simply ignores or fails to process. Further research is still required to carefully investigate such issues (Duda, 2001), although a cluster of recent studies demonstrated very low within-class agreement regarding perceptions of the motivational climate (Cumming, Smith, Smoll & Grossbard, 2007; Papaioannou, Marsh & Theodorakis, 2004; Morgan, Sproule, Weigand & Carpenter, 2005), meaning the 'objective' climate may bear little or no relation to what is subjectively perceived. In the immediate here and-now, orientation is likely to bias climate perception, but in the longer term it seems that climates can influence orientations which may prove significant in the applied arena (Duda, 1993).

VIII. *Moral development*: Theory suggests that a mastery approach links to concern over effort and improvement so opponents are seen as allies in testing and improving skill, meaning foul play and cheating is considered amoral and unsportsmanlike. In contrast, theory suggests a performance climate emphasises winning at all costs and so foul-play/cheating are considered acceptable means to this end - promoting the use of foul play, deception and rule-breaking (Duda *et al.,* 1991; Ommundsen, Roberts, Lemyre & Treasure, 2003). The current evidence is coherent with achievement goal theory and consistent with parallel research into goal orientations, reviewed by Harwood *et al.*, 2008); revealing a strong body of evidence that supports the link between perceived mastery climate and higher moral standards in sport (respect for the rules, officials and opposition; avoiding cheating or intentionally injurious behaviours). Ommundsen, Roberts, Lemyre and Treasure (2003), Fry and Newton (2003), Gano-Overway, Guivernau, Magyar, Waldron and Ewing (2005), Boixadós, Cruz, Torregrosa and Valiente (2004) and Miller, Roberts and Ommundsen (2004) all reported a link between perceived mastery climate and positive moral beliefs and standards. Similarly, Ommundsen, Roberts, Lemyre and Treasure (2003), Fry and Newton (2003), Kavussanu, Roberts and Ntoumanis (2002), Boixadós, Cruz, Torregrosa and Valiente (2004) and Miller, Roberts, Ommundsen (2004) reported a link between a perceived performance climate and lower moral standards.

IX. *Motor learning/development*: An under-explored yet valuable line of research has tentatively illustrated how the creation of mastery climates (e.g., using the TARGET framework) results in enhanced motor learning, relative to performance climates and 'traditional' methods (Theeboom, De Knop & Weiss, 1995; Valentini & Rudisill, 2004a; b). Although not explicitly suggested in the theory, Papaioannou and Kouli (1999) discuss this finding in terms how reduced confidence and increased anxiety attributable to performance climates *should* reduce motor learning and performance through cognitive distraction and inappropriate muscle tension. Alternatively, a task climate enhances the potential for motor learning through optimal learning strategies, positive experiences, higher persistence (Whitehead *et al.,* 2004) as well as higher perceived competence.

X. *Flow experiences*: Jackson and Roberts (1992) found that participants with a high task orientation tended to experience flow states more often (i.e., effortless excellent, being 'in the zone'). Similarly, Kowal and Fortier (2000) found that participants who perceived a mastery climate also reported increased experiences of flow, whereas a perceived performance climate showed no relationship to the reporting of flow.

Summary of Motivational Climate Research

In summarising the above findings, there appears to be a strong case that the perception of an environment emphasising/promoting mastery conceptions is likely to produce numerous adaptive and desirable consequences for the participation and development of sports performers. In contrast, when participants perceive performance climates there seem to be less frequently positive or adaptive motivational patterns displayed. In fact perceived performance climates are often correlated with undesirable beliefs and patterns of behaviour. It is imperative that future research establishes the direction of causality in these relationships, in order to determine whether the creation of climates high in mastery cues (for example) leads to the perception of a mastery climate and the numerous associated positive motivational consequences listed above, or whether participants' own orientations and preferences influence what they perceive, rendering the objectively observable behaviours of coaches, parents and peers almost irrelevant, in quite a lonely and solipsistic state-of-affairs which might be labelled cognitive-cognitive, as opposed to social-cognitive. The most likely answer to this question would appear, intuitively, to be a complex interaction of personal traits with objectively observable behaviours in determining participants' perceptions, and subsequent motivational outcomes.

Key Conceptual Issues

Key Social Agents in Influencing Motivation

There is a growing requirement to understand which social agents significantly influence the athlete's motivation at different stages of the athletic career. From the previous summary of questionnaires that measure perceived motivational climate, it is possible to identify coaches/teachers, parents (mother/father) and peers as common determinants of motivational climate. Other influences identified to date also include National Governing Body reward structures and 'sporting heroes' (Carr & Weigand, 2001). It is also important to establish whether national governing bodies, selection/development policies and wider social cultures can affect a sporting motivational climate (Harwood & Swain, 2001) and if they do, how much? And is this knowledge helpful?

Given the potential and identified limitations of some of the above climate scales in isolation, the following sections looks more closely at how: i) instructors (coach/teacher), ii) parents and iii) peers can influence motivation by synthesising findings both from sport and PE and also more mainstream social psychology. These social agents are singled out because their immediacy and salience to sport participants is likely to be greater, and therefore they are likely to have the strongest influences on motivation and other related outcomes.

The Instructor – Coaches and Teachers

Much of the research examining motivational climate has done so at a relatively general level (e.g. 'outcome-without-effort orientation' in the LAPOPECQ – it is not clear which social agents determine this). However, overall it is possible to assert that the instructor can: i) differentially emphasise learning and personal mastery (e.g. LAPOPECQ, PECCS) versus normative performance (e.g. PMCSQ-2, EPCM); ii) induce fear of mistakes (e.g. EPCM, PMCSQ-2) or alternatively convey that mistakes are part of learning (e.g. PMCSQ-2); and additionally coaches/instructors can iii) treat the normatively more able players preferentially (e.g. PMCSQ-2) as opposed to involving every player and making them feel valued (e.g. PMCSQ-2). Instructors can also: iv) contribute to an intra-team rivalry and competition for places (e.g. PMCSQ-2) or alternatively promote co-operative learning (e.g. PMCSQ-2). There is also evidence that coaches/instructors can influence perceived motivational climate by: v) conveying the belief that success is a result of ability and not effort (e.g. LAPOPECQ) or promoting effort and hard work as the route to excellence (e.g. PMCSQ, PMCSQ-2). The Motivational Climate Scale for Youth Sport replicated this pattern but does not contain discrete subscales, in order to facilitate comprehension by young athletes (Smith *et al.*, 2007)

Firstly, not all of the observed instructor influences on motivational climate relate directly to the idea of competence. For example, un/equal recognition and success from ability/effort beliefs are, arguably, indirectly linked to an individual's achievement-goal state, in the same way that antecedent variables are linked to goal states in Elliot and Church's (1997) hierarchical model. Thus, it is important to establish whether instructors' influences on participants' definition and valence of competence should be the sole focus of questionnaires assessing perceived motivational climate, or whether an antecedents approach should be taken in line with Elliot and colleagues' recommendations.

Secondly, while the contrasting themes listed may represent a strong synthesis of concepts from the existing research, it is important to establish *how* these themes/ideas are presented and interpreted; through behaviours displayed, beliefs and values conveyed, or by affective responses to situations; in order for future intervention work to be effective. To this end, items within each of the listed scales contain stems such as "on this team the coach gets mad when...", which would be considered an affective response; "on this team coach believes...", which would be considered a (conveyed) belief/value; and "on this team the coach takes failing students out of drills/the coach helps players improve their skills", which qualify as demonstrable behaviours that influence motivational climate. Thus, the separate consideration of affective responses, beliefs and values conveyed and behaviours demonstrated is important within each climate subscale, not least because an absence of one or the other mechanism (e.g. behaviour without affect or belief) is unlikely to be as effective.

Parents

The favoured scale concerning parents' contributions to motivational climate is the PIMCQ-2 (White, 1996; 1998; White, Duda & Hart, 1992), which measures 'learning/enjoyment climate', 'worry conducive climate' and 'success without effort climate' and *can* be applied to both the father and the mother (e.g. Carr & Weigand, 2001; White, 1998). Immediately it is apparent that there is not such a richness of subscales as with instructors, where is it possible to dichotomise different subscales into performance-versus-mastery emphases. Additionally, conceptual and empirical weaknesses exist with this scale (Duda & Hall, 2001), suggesting that any findings from it should be interpreted cautiously. Further, on reflection, the items of the scale are often difficult to classify into mechanisms (behaviours, beliefs or affective style), for example; "my mother makes me worry about failing" – is this a behaviour, belief of affective style? Given the tremendous influence of parents in children's development and socialisation, it may also be necessary to consider influences beyond the performance situation (training/competing).

Pomerantz, Grolnick and Price (2005) are relatively thorough in their review of what parents can do to influence their children's definitions of, and orientations towards, competence and motivation (albeit not specifically addressing sport). Behaviourally, they suggest parents should be involved in their children's pursuits in order to promote learning, foster closeness/relatedness with the child and reinforce self-esteem by communicating belief in the child by investment, and also that the activity is valued. Several studies have now suggested that parental involvement in academic pursuits leads to enhanced academic achievement (Keith *et al.,* 1993; Pomerantz & Eaton, 2001; Senechal & LeFevre, 2002). Pomerantz *et al.* also recommend that parents provide a structure for learning/improvement for the child, by offering guidance, expectations and specific feedback – basically providing assistance in a manner that facilitates children's skill acquisition; this could be termed 'competence support' (Grolnick, 2003). This support is also linked to heightened achievement and task engagement, even in very young children (Hokoda & Fincham, 1995; Winsler, Diaz, McCarty, Atencio & Chabay, 1999). It is also a beneficial behaviour to promote autonomy in child as opposed to controlling them (Grolnick, 2003) which tends to involve attending whilst not controlling, allowing exploration and mistakes, and encouraging children to generate their own strategies for novel/difficult tasks. In contrast, controlling behaviours include commands, directives, instructions and perhaps punishments (including the withdrawal of affection) which reduce autonomy. Autonomy support is also linked to increased task engagement (Kelley, Brownell & Campbell, 2000), increased perceived competence (Grolnick, Ryan & Deci, 1991) and graded achievement (Hess & McDevitt, 1984). Additionally, parents can emphasise and reinforce effort and hard work, or take a more 'entity-based' approach (cf. Diener & Dweck, 1978; 1980), conveying the belief that skill and ability are fixed attributes and unchangeable. This aspect is reconcilable with parental 'learning climates' and 'success without effort' climates found in existing climate scales. The reinforcement of effort over stable ability has been linked to increased perceived competence (Kamins & Dweck, 1999), subsequent mastery orientations (Hokonda & Fincham, 1995) and the child's own incremental/entity beliefs (Kempner & Pomerantz, 2003).

In terms of beliefs and values, there is evidence that parents who believe their children to be competent encourage more optimal outcomes in the child, although there is a caveat here in that the parental appraisal of competence depends heavily on the child's actual ability and additionally, inaccurate parental beliefs are seen as patronising (Miller, Manhal & Mee, 1991; Peet, Powell & O'Donnell, 1997). It is however, important for parents to value the particular achievement activity (school, sport) as this provides additional incentive for the child to seek competence in this domain (Pomerantz *et al.,* 2005). In terms of affective style, it appears that children who have secure bonds with the parents (thus meeting the need for relatedness) are more able to then seek competence and autonomy in achievement domains (Allen, Marsh, McFarland, McElhaney & Land, 2002). Hence, creating and maintaining a secure attachment to a child (cf. Ainsworth *et al.,* 1978) and also keeping this attachment relatively independent of achievement activities (e.g. love is not dependent on success) is optimal for children's development. This deeper understanding of how parents can influence children's motivation may be important when interpreting interview data and conceptualising climate on the basis of questionnaire subscales.

Fredricks and Eccles (2005; p.4) proposed three main mechanism by which parents may influence their child's participation in sport: "(a) by being a role model either as a coach or by participating in athletics themselves; (b) by interpreting their children's experience and giving them messages about their athletic ability and the value of participating in sport; and (c) by providing emotional support and positive athletic experiences for their children's involvement in sport." In particular, parents' ratings of their child's sporting ability significantly correlate with changes in the child's attitude to sport as they grow older (Fredricks & Eccles, 2002), and parents' beliefs in relation to gender roles in sport also associated with self-rated competence and value-beliefs of children (Fredricks & Eccles, 2002). Whilst this research represents an important contribution to our understanding of whether, and in what respects, parent attitudes influence athlete motivation, it would still be difficult to offer parents advice on how best to act around their athletes, or how to endorse certain key values. The understanding of specific behaviours, the contexts they occur in, and their subsequent impact/influence remains a missing link in this body of research. It would seem that to increase understanding in this area, researcher need to 'unpack' such conclusions as "One possible explanation is that parents convey these beliefs to their child *through both subtle and more overt messages* about their children's abilities and the value the parents themselves attach to their children's participation" (Fredricks & Eccles, 2005; p.22 – italics added). What are these subtle/overt messages? How are they conveyed? Where and when does this happen? Are the outcomes consistent or does it depend on other considerations?

Recent qualitative studies have examined the roles of parents in more detail, identifying such behaviours as additional coaching/instruction, feedback and commentary, emotional responses and emotional intensity, autonomy support, controlling behaviours, maintaining focus, social support (Gould, Lauer, Rolo, Jannes & Pennisi, 2008; Holt, Black, Tamminen, Mandigo & Fox, 2008; Holt, Tamminen, Black, Mandigo & Fox, 2009) and the 'conditionality' of support - whether parents emphasise a return for their 'investment' or assure the athlete that their support is unconditional (Gould *et al.*, 2008; see also Assor, Roth & Deci, 2004). These developments represent an initial response to the above questions, but there remains a requirement to study athletes outside the 17-25 university/collegiate (i.e., specialisers) population, and likewise it would arguably be very helpful if such findings could be synthesised and understood jointly, as opposed to being conducted in relation to different phenomena and with different emphases (e.g., social support, defining parental influences, testing/expanding SDT etc.). By carrying out qualitative research with a specific focus on motivation, researchers may contribute significantly to the motivational literature as well as the above-described research examining the ways that parents may influence their child's overall involvement in sport.

Peers – Team-Mates and Classmates

In contrast to coach-athlete and parent-athlete influences, peer relationships are more numerous and therefore more multifaceted. On the one hand, team-mates and competitors can influence how a player defines and seeks competence. On the other, players also participate in sport in order to establish and build friendships and seek social validation. In terms of task/sport competence, existing questionnaires can be cited showing how team/class-mates can differentially endorse success-as-learning versus success-as-outperforming-others involvement(e.g. LAPOPECQ, PECCS), and important roles versus neglect and avoidance (PMCSQ-2 – note that these subscales may relate more to social competence than sport/task competence). In terms of 'social competence', Smith (1999; 2003) has shown that performers often participate in order to spend time with their best friend and the quality of relationships often influences motivation (participation, persistence) independently of task/sport competence. When studying social-environmental influences on motivation, which are inherently influenced by key social agents, such considerations cannot be overlooked.

In a more holistic approach, Vazou *et al.* (2005) used qualitative methods to establish: i) improvement emphasis; ii) equality emphasis; iii) relatedness support; iv) concern over mistakes (or lack of); v) co-operation and teamwork; vi) success-from-effort emphasis; vii) intra-team competition; viii) success-from-ability emphasis; ix) autonomy support; x) evaluations/assessments of competence; and xi) intra-team conflict as the key dimensions of a sporting motivational climate with adolescent children from various sports and levels. These different aspects of peer climate all relate in some way to task/sport competence, 'social competence' or both. For example, the 'success-from-effort/ability' dimensions reported clearly related to sporting competence, whereas relatedness support and co-operation/teamwork dimensions may relate more significantly to building either the number or quality of social relationships.

Finally in this section, the factors influencing how players define (and seek to demonstrate) competence may interact quite significantly. For example, it may be difficult to make new friends on a team where a player is poor and the standard is high as team-mates may not wish to relate to a poor player. Likewise, a highly competitive player may not wish to persist long or foster relationships in a group where the sport is played chiefly for fun in the knowledge that none of the players are going to 'make-it.' Additionally, peers may gravitate towards a player who is normatively competent and successful (e.g. wishing to pick up hints and tips), leading to numerous but shallow friendships, whereas less able players may unite in their adversity and form one or two deeper, mutually beneficial friendships. It may also be necessary to examine the issues surrounding *quality of relationships* with certain social agents (e.g., how likely are we to be influenced by the behaviour or values of coaches/peers that we do not *like*). If a certain social agent is not valued by an athlete, then that agent's perceived mastery and/or performance involving behaviour may carry little or no motivation-related salience whatsoever. Hence, the argument for considering social aspects and the possibility of 'social competence' as a motivation in sporting contexts is strong. Whilst it has been raised in relation to peer-influences on motivation, this does not preclude its examination concerning coaches and parents, as this is particularly likely to be one factor that changes over the career of an athlete.

Level of Influence – Situation, Contexts and Socialisation

There remains an issue of whether climate measures are examining a specific situation (e.g. training, pre-competition) or the context of being 'in this team.' On the one hand, situational influences are theorised to have the strongest influence on goal involvement (cf. Nicholls, 1984; 1989), but on the other hand the context is likely to be easier to measure (e.g. away from competitions/training venues, less interruption) and more stable over time, especially if researchers measure general perceptions of the motivational climate. Equally, it is possible that longer-term contextual considerations may also influence momentary motivation. The temptation to find a happy-medium may have led researchers to develop scales that (arguably) confound the separate analytical levels of situation and context together. However, from the point of view of conducting good research and promoting more informed applied practice, it is necessary to address this issue.

The conceptual difficulties surrounding analytical levels highlight the central question: 'what is a motivational climate?' According to Nicholls' (1984; 1989) theory, the concept should be restricted to situational influences, i.e., here immediate here-and-now. This would involve specific coaching and parenting behaviours and reactions in specific situations. However, as previously noted, many measures of motivational climate depart from this in two key areas: Firstly, they measure perceived motivational climate as opposed to specific and objectively observable situational indices, and secondly questionnaires tap the more abstract contextual level; with items asking "on this team/when I play sport, the coach gets mad when/the coach believes…." When playing regularly under the same coach then this may come to resemble the situational level that Nicholls' theory specifies. However, the additional consideration of parents and peers (and other extra-personal variables) reveals this confusion of analytical levels to be a significant problem. Suddenly, the situations where motivation can be influenced expands from the training pitch and match day (relatively specific situations) to include time at home, pre and post match discussions, time at school and even time travelling to and from events (the more general sport context). The influence of parents in particular is likely to be reduced at the situational level but vastly important in a more general context.

Peers, on the other hand, may have significant influences in the specific performance situations and also more generally (e.g., at school as well). Hence, the social and environmental influences on motivation concern an ostensibly larger conceptual span than just training and competition. In the light of recent reviews (e.g. Harwood *et al.,* 2008) and a conceptual overhaul of achievement goal theory (e.g. Elliot, 1999), there is a growing argument for moving beyond Nicholls' original conceptualisation of situation-specific influences on goal involvement and seeking to examine what key social agents can do in relation to the broader sporting context in order to foster stronger motivation, persistence, and mastery-based definitions of competence. The counterargument to including socialisation in a climate model would be that longer term parental and peer influences contribute to an internalised goal-orientation (i.e. intrapersonal adoption tendency), such as fear-of-failure and need-for-achievement, and not situational goal climate (Wentzel, 1999). It is tremendously difficult to separate these without adequate research accompanied by theoretical debate and clarification.

Another possible solution to the difficult issues regarding which level-of-analysis is most suitable for measures of goal-climate is to take the approach that Elliot (1997, 1999) has introduced with reference to goal-orientation. Instead of conceptualising a goal-orientation as a relatively independent cognitive structure/schema, Elliot proposes multiple intrapersonal antecedents of goal-adoption. This may also be a beneficial approach to take with goal-climates. For example, the behaviours, beliefs and affective styles of coaches, parents and peers may not directly relate to a dichotomous goal-climate *per se*, but rather they may be interpersonal antecedents of goal adoption. It is certainly worth entertaining this prospect in the light of recent developments within AGT.

Approach vs. Avoidance Climates

It is important to reiterate that motivational climate research to date has been based upon Ames, Dweck and Nicholls' two-goal conceptualisations. The propensity of mastery and performance climates to invoke approach or avoidance goals has not been adequately studied. Nevertheless, while certain items on existing scales may correspond to some of Elliott's dimensions (e.g., mastery, performance, approach and avoidance), there is perhaps a need to conceptualise aspects of motivational climate in a manner that explicitly corresponds with the 2x2 approach-avoidance framework (Papaioannou, Milosis, Kosmidou, & Tsigilis, 2007). Research that identifies the precise constituents of 2x2 (mastery/performance x approach/avoidance climates), could be expected to further our understanding of human motivation, particularly the construct of avoidance motivation that remains understudied within achievement goal theory (Spray & Keegan, 2005).

Developmental Considerations

Nicholls' (1989) research led to the proposition that around 11 years-of-age children become capable, for the first time, of being truly 'ego involved.' However, anecdotal reports, or even a quick trip to the park on a Sunday, would provide examples of children much younger than 11 exhibiting patterns of behaviours consistent with ego involvement (Fry, 2001; Fry & Duda, 1997). This is a tension that requires research attention to resolve it. If true ('Nichollsian') ego-involvement can only be experienced from eleven years of age then do the contents of the social environment matter much during this time; are children oblivious to competitive and pressurising cues below the age of 11? Alternatively, it is possible that the same cues and behaviours are noted by pre-11 and post-11 year old athletes, but they may be interpreted differently following 'differentiation'. In either case, identifying the specific motivationally relevant behaviours of key social agents would facilitate the subsequent study of their impact. This is arguably more informative than simply excluding athletes younger than 12, which has been the approach in much of the achievement goals research to date (e.g., Vazou, Ntoumanis & Duda, 2005 – although see Smith *et al.,* 2007 for a study using athletes below 12 years of age).

Perceived Motivational Climate

As described herein, the vast majority of research in this area has deployed questionnaires such as the Perceived Motivational Climate in Sport Questionnaire (-1: Seifriz, Duda & Chi, 1992; and -2: Newton, Duda & Yin, 2000), the LAPOPECQ (Papaioannou, 1994; 1995; 1997), the PECCS (Goudas & Biddle, 1994), and the EPCM (Biddle, Cury, Goudas, Sarrazin, Famose & Durand, 1995). All of these are measures of *perceived* motivational climate, in relation to dichotomous AGT (Nicholls, 1989). This is generally justified two ways. Justification X: (often unspoken) is the convenience of deploying two questionnaires to the same participant – one tapping their perceptions of the climate, and the other assessing a variable that is theoretically likely to be linked with climate perceptions (this justification is addressed below). Justification Y is that measuring perceived motivational climate is theoretically/empirically better than trying to take an objective measure of the motivational climate. One supporting argument (Y_1) is best voiced by Treasure, Duda, Hall, Roberts, Ames and Maehr (2001), in their 'rebuttal' of Harwood, Hardy and Swain (2000): "Ames (Ames, 1992a; 1992b; Ames & Archer 1988), Maehr (Maehr & Braskamp, 1986; Maehr & Midgley, 1991) and colleagues... ...have *repeatedly shown* that it is the subjective interpretation of the environment, or perceived motivational climate, that we must examine to understand the meaning of achievement endeavours" (p.319 – italics added). In order for this statement to be convincing, it is necessary to understand what is meant by "repeatedly shown." Has the case been conclusively demonstrated? Have subjective perceptions been shown to conclusively contribute more to our empirical understanding than the measurement (or manipulation) of situational indices?

Y_1 is, in fact, not supported by the papers quoted: a careful reading of the five papers cited reveals that three of them are reviews and book chapters specifying and reinforcing theoretical tenets (not research findings); these discuss but do not *demonstrate* the above claim. Rather, they are the authors' interpretations and conjectures speculating about the potential meaning of their own ongoing work (which is good, but it does not constitute a demonstration). The remaining two are indeed, original research papers, but they do not *demonstrate* the claim made in Y_1. Instead, it is simply assumed by their methodology (measuring the children's perceptions of climate) but there is no explicit comparison of 'perceived' versus 'actual' climate in terms of their predictive accuracy. What emerges is a point that has been repeatedly assumed (or at best, repeatedly argued) rather than "repeatedly shown." This should not be taken as evidence that "subjective interpretations" are the only avenue for exploration in studying motivational climate.

A second supporting argument (Y_2) is the finding of Papaioannou (1994) that, despite sharing the same class environment, the variability in perceptions of motivational climate between pupils in the same class was even greater than the variability between classes. Hence, the subjective perception of the class environment must be more important than the objective class environment. Whilst initially quite convincing, it is worth noting that this finding was not the central outcome of the study but was instead picked up some time after publication. This reasoning also leads to a logical absurdity, that rather than training coaches to create motivating atmospheres, scientists and practitioners should simply instruct the athletes themselves to interpret any coach/parent/peer behaviours as optimally motivating (task/mastery/approach-oriented/friendly). On this foundation, supporting argument Y_3 is established: an array of studies supporting achievement goals by demonstrating that generalised perceptions of a task climate have invariably correlated with adaptive motivational outcomes, whilst perceptions of an 'ego' climate have either shown no correlation, or been associated with maladaptive motivational patterns. An example of this argument is as follows: [to question the importance of this research] "contradicts research from 14 studies, with a total sample of 4,484, showing a large effect [using meta-analysis techniques] for a mastery climate on positive psychological outcomes such as satisfaction, positive attitudes, and intrinsic motivation (Ntoumanis & Biddle, 1999). To reduce this effect to "small" would require 85 studies with zero effects!" (Biddle, Duda, Papaioannou & Harwood, 2001; p.466). And since this assertion, many more studies have been conducted adding weight to this case. This is a considerable and impressive body of evidence. However, the task of reducing this "large" effect to small/zero does not necessarily require 85 studies showing no result (which may never be published anyway as 'no result' studies are hardly ever submitted for publication). All that is required is a brief perusal of the literature on cognitive biases, such as social desirability bias (Crowne & Marlowe, 1960), confirmation bias (Wason, 1960; 1966), the lucid fallacy (Taleb, 2007), and the confabulation of Gazzaniga's split brain patients (Gazzaniga, 1998) – amongst other effects. All of these observations suggest a tendency for participants to demonstrate an inherent need to appear logically consistent (both to themselves and others). Hence, there is just as much chance that participants filling in these questionnaires unconsciously try to produce a pattern of responses that is internally consistent (and perhaps partially based on a stereotype or a belief they hold, or worse still, the experimenter's explanation/expectations). Whichever variable is being measured, the 'code' would not be especially difficult to crack as there are only usually two options - 'competitive emphasis' and/or 'personal/effort emphasis' – followed by a questionnaire assessing something 'nice' (enjoyment, intrinsic motivation, moral behaviour) and/or something 'nasty' (unhappiness, extrinsic motivation, rule-breaking/immoral behaviour). As such, answering the first few questions would make it almost impossible for the participant to appear inconsistent in answering the rest. If a respondent likes competition, their responses will reflect that, and if they loath competition, their responses will reflect that. Even if one is not cautioned by this problem, we can also consider the problem of the 'selective perception' bias, the tendency for personal preferences and expectations to affect perception (Hastorf & Cantril, 1954). In the light of this effect, it should not be surprising that the strongest and most consistent correlations are between achievement goal orientation, and perceptions of motivational climate (as reviewed in Harwood, Spray & Keegan, 2008 and Ntoumanis & Biddle, 1999). It is important to enquire how different the constructs are when measuring 'goal orientation' and 'perceived goal climate.' If two constructs are measured with remarkably similar questionnaire items, are frequently highly correlated, and appear to correlate with a highly similar constellation of other variables, how different are they? In measuring 'perceived motivational climate' how close are we *in reality* to measuring 'achievement goal orientation' and making inferences about coach/teacher behaviours that, in fact, are being "actively perceived" by the participants in a rather selective manner? To what extent was Papaioannou's (1994) result simply a reflection of increased variability in the *orientations* of the children within each class? These cognitive biases appear to pose serious problems for both Y_2 and Y_3.

Returning to Justification X, which might be labelled the 'convenience' justification for measuring perceived motivational climate, this too requires a degree of critical examination. Whilst pragmatic limitations are common in science, and absolutely should not become impediments to progress (Giacobbi, Poczwardowski, & Hager, 2005), scientists must always critically assess the methods they deploy, and never resort to faithfully following the methodological specifications put forward by others (Feyerabend, 1975). As such, the contribution of research using measures of perceived motivational climate, as reviewed in Harwood *et al.* (2008), must be recognised as a significant contribution - not least as it has produced quite consistent findings highlighting the importance of perceived situational and contextual influences in determining athlete motivation. However, the reason for examining perceived subjective interpretations must be recognised as a pragmatic limitation, and not a theoretical imperative. As noted above, if treated as a theoretical imperative and taken to its logical extreme this approach would entail that there is no need to train coach and parents in order to optimise the athletic experience, but rather simply instruct the athlete to interpret all behaviours from these social agents as kind, helpful, positive and mastery-involving. Instead, it is worth considering whether the pragmatic limitation posed in studying a complex social and environmental context (which currently forces a retreat into measuring simplified and abstract subjective perceptions) may perhaps be addressed by using a 'bottom-up' approach, and examining the unique, combined and interactive influences of specific behaviours and exchanges in determining athletes' motivation. Difficult? Yes. Impossible? No.

As a result of this simultaneously dense, disparate, intimidating and yet sometimes uninformative literature (especially regarding pragmatic applied recommendations), a pressing need has been identified for research that: a) increases the applicability of the above-discussed theories (thus also increasing their testability); and b) allows scientists to make practical recommendations based on the extensive research and relatively consistent findings discussed here. To quote Harwood *et al.* (2008) on the matter, it constitutes "a research area that probably represents the most salient advances that we can make as academics" (p.185).

Recent Developments

In response to many of the above developments, criticisms, debates and questions, Keegan et al. (2009, 2010, in submission) conducted a series of qualitative studies with athletes at different stages of their careers. The first of these (Keegan et al., 2009) qualitatively explored the motivational climate perceived by young athletes at the start of their participation in sport (termed *sampling*), whilst the subsequent two studies investigated the same phenomenon in middle-career (termed *specialising*) and elite athletes (termed *investment* or *mastery*) respectively. All three studies examined the ways in which athletes perceived their coaches, parents and peers could influence their motivation, positively or negatively. A key element of this series of investigations was that none of the above-described theories of motivational regulation (AGT, SDT, 2x2, social goals) were adopted in advance, but rather all were kept in mind: a kind of 'theoretical agnosticism' advocated by Henwood and Pidgeon (2003). This was contrasted against previous qualitative studies that had explicitly (or implicitly) adopted a single theory as their guiding principle. For example, Pensgaard and Roberts (2002) and Vazou *et al.* (2005) explicitly accept AGT *a priori*, as guiding the questions and analysis ("the motivational perspective adopted in this study [achievement goal theory] determined the variables and concepts focused upon, and it also guided the interpretation" – Pensgaard & Roberts, p.55), whilst Vazou *et al.* deductively coded raw data themes (quotes) into task and ego categories, *before* conducting a more conventional inductive content analysis within each category. This theory-led approach can also be argued to occur implicitly at times; for example, in Mallett and Hanrahan's (2004) qualitative study, financial reward was associated exclusively with an ego climate as a function of status and normative reward, when it could be argued that elite athletes need to be paid in order to give up work and train full time to develop their skills. Likewise, Krane *et al.* (1997) clustered 'training-through-injury' and issues surrounding body-shape and disordered eating under an ego-climate on the grounds that they are maladaptive behaviours, when (rightly or wrongly) they could be considered to contribute to improved task performance (e.g., judges scores) depending, perhaps, on the level of competition. To become 'theoretically agnostic,' processes of private reflection, group reflection, peer review and consensus validation were heavily utilised in order to challenge the influence of existing theories and preconceptions during the analysis. By removing the 'guiding' role of theories, the Keegan *et al.* studies returned rich data reflecting the complexity of the social milieu; and whilst the interested onlooker may wish to 'cherry-pick' themes in relation to their favoured theory, the results took the form of a comprehensive list of highly specific (situational rather than contextual) motivationally impactful behaviours, as exhibited by the coaches, parents and peers of developing athletes.

In all three Keegan *et al.* studies, the influences of social agents were related to the specific roles they fulfil in relation to the athlete, which varied as the athletes progressed, developed and matured. The analysis indicated that the influences of coaches related most strongly to the manner in which they perform their roles of instruction and assessment, whereas parents' influences were most salient in terms of the way they support participation and learning. Both parents and coaches exerted influences through their leadership styles, affective responses and pre-performance behaviours. In support of this notion, within the *initiation/sampling* and *specialising* studies (2009 and 2010, respectively), the influences of coaches and parents were most similar where their roles converged, and differed most noticeably where their roles were different. In both these studies, peers influenced motivation through competitive behaviours, collaborative behaviours, evaluative communication and through their social relationships. These similarities between career-phases were interpreted in terms of the common characteristics between each: the key social agents, their relationships and the achievement contexts remain relatively consistent between the two career stages, with an increasing focus on skill development and fewer sports being the main differences (Côté & Hay, 2002a; b; Wylleman *et al.,* 2004). The study of elite athletes (Keegan *et al.*, in submission) suggested a markedly decreased influence from parents, whose role became becoming increasingly distal, and limited to emotional and moral support, whilst coaches and peers were reported to be focal influences. Themes of feedback/evaluation, and pre-performance motivating behaviours were common to all social agents (to a lesser extent with parents), whilst the coach-athlete and peer-athlete relationships appeared to be important in *both* moderating the motivational impact of behaviours *and* directly influencing motivation.

The most salient theme through all three studies in terms of promoting motivation was 'positivity' – which included any behaviours that incite approach-type motivation (e.g., building confidence, highlighting positive consequences), positive affect/emotion, friendship, collaboration, and, of course, praise. In contrast, behaviours which were associated with negativity were generally linked to undermining motivation. At the general level, behaviours invoking avoidance-type motivation (e.g., emphasising punishments and negative consequences, a fault-finding evaluative style), negative affect/emotion (such as anger or sadness), conflict, rivalry, and, of course, criticism, all seemed to be associated with an increased propensity for reduced motivation. Less prominent in the three studies, but certainly notable, were a cluster of ideas surrounding facilitation: making it possible for the athlete to practice, learn, improve, or achieve. This might include an autonomy-supportive leadership style, offering useful, relevant and overtly justified advice (at opportune moments), facilitating/encouraging practice, creating tasks/games that allow athletes of any ability level to engage and improve, providing transport, equipment and moral support, or collaborating with peers (for example, to help them learn a skill). There appeared to be a very fine line between this facilitative, autonomy supportive approach, and the giving of unsolicited instructions or opinions – which was sometimes described as being controlling, judgemental or disparaging, and thus undermining autonomy (even if the provider was convinced they are being helpful or has the best intentions). Coaches who exhibited a controlling leadership style, parents who became over-involved or who made their love/support contingent upon sporting success, and peers who refused to collaborate or who willingly cultivated links between normative ability and social popularity were all potentially linked with detrimental effects on athlete motivation, as they could be viewed as undermining the athlete's own need for autonomy. Finally, affiliation and close relationships were also almost invariably associated with adaptive motivation from athletes. The main exception to this appeared to be that when an athlete likes their coach/parent/peers, they sometimes wished to avoid "letting them down." However, for the main part, feelings of mutual closeness and commitment with one's coach, and experiences of friendship and group belonging amongst the peer group were frequently associated with positive motivational patterns.

There were other more subtle themes over-arching three studies: First, a complex interactivity between motivationally-relevant behaviours and their impact on motivation. The authors were quite emphatic in reporting that it was almost impossible to establish any direct and exclusive correspondence between the behaviour of a coach, parent or peer and the impact on athlete motivation. The influence of all motivationally-relevant behaviours from these key social agents seemed to be moderated by other factors such as: a) the behaviours immediately preceding the event; b) co-occurring behaviours – i.e., *'it's not what you said, it's the way (or moment, or place) you said it'*; c) the consistency of the behaviour in relation to the person concerned and in comparison to others; d) the relationship between the athlete and protagonist; and e) other contextual or environmental variables (e.g., training vs. competition, stage-of-season). This could either be considered as unnecessarily complicated (in comparison to a simple dichotomous, trichotomous or four-goal model), or it could be viewed as a first step towards deconstruction of the motivational climate: which has been called for in studies such as Smith, Smoll and Cumming (2007), who commented on the need to "clarify relations between particular intervention elements and various outcome measures" (p. 54). Elliot (1999) also speculated: "it is also possible that some of the antecedent variables combine together to jointly and interactively predict achievement goal adoption" (p.176).

Conclusion

As a result of conducting the above studies, Keegan et al. (2010) coined the term *motivational atmosphere* in order to reflect the apparent supercomplexity of the social milieu in determining athlete motivation. For example, whilst climates can exist within an atmosphere, the atmosphere itself is much bigger and more complex than the climate, which meteorologically (and perhaps fittingly) is usually taken to mean the averaging out of weather conditions over a period of time. Research reflecting this complex interactivity is, on the basis of the preceding chapter, long overdue and, most importantly, methodological approaches now exist to facilitate such research. The findings of the Keegan et al. studies may also act as a foundation for future research, allowing new studies to progress by examining the situational level-of-generality at a moment-to-moment level, rather than relying on generalised perceptions (which, at best, represent the contextual level-of-generality and which arguably guarantee the finding of generic associations between variables). In order to more fully understand the specific behaviours (*and* sets of behaviours) from each social agent, *and* their potential combinations, *and* the specific moments in which these behaviours should occur, in relation to the way they impact upon motivation - then more research is undoubtedly necessary.

One very salient benefit of the new vein of research being suggested is that, by examining the situational influences on athlete motivation in detail, there is increased potential to decrease the conceptual distance between theory and practice. Where theoretical relationships are well understood and well supported, such research would return a relatively comprehensive list of the ways in which these theoretical ideas can be conveyed or emphasised by coaches, parents and peers. This would facilitate the provision of specific advice to key protagonists involved in the development of motivated athletes. Indeed, without increased relevance and immediacy, research into motivation may be in danger of being left out of coach education programmes (and coaches' thoughts) entirely.

From an applied perspective, decreasing the conceptual distance between theory and practice would facilitate the following improvement to the advice which applied practitioners can offer (in *italics*): "Here is what [Theory A] says about motivating athletes. Here is some research supporting [Theory A]. *Here are some (carefully researched) pragmatic suggestions as to how you can implement this theory and research in your own practice [coaching/parenting].*" In addition, however, rather than prescribing a certain way of acting most of the time, the best advice that can be given in light of the 'complex interactivity' described in the Keegan *et al.* studies is for key social agents to keep in mind the following: what 'good' motivation looks like, how this varies in different circumstances, what actions and behaviours tend to precipitate 'good motivation', and how certain behaviours may take on a different light depending on recent, co-occurring and subsequent behaviours (perhaps these combinations might be termed *atmospheric complexes* – cf. Elliot, 1999). One of the most fruitful avenues for future research would be to try and begin understanding these complexities and interactions in the motivational atmosphere and the ways in which they combine to influence motivation. The literature is also beginning to recognise dual-roles for certain social agents, for example parent-coaches, sibling-team-mates, spouse-coaches etc. (Jowett & Meek, 2000). These may also offer interesting insights into the motivational atmosphere. If a single person is carrying out multiple roles in an athlete's motivational atmosphere - competitive roles, training roles, evaluative roles and supporting social and emotional needs - how might this impact upon the athlete?

Provided that the basic findings of Keegan et al. are substantiated in the future (either by research evidence, critical debate, or both), then the most pressing avenue for further research is in trying to 'solve,' or at least understand, the enigma of the complex interactions that occur in shaping athletes' immediate motivation. Future studies may wish to examine: a) interactions between 'atmospheric' variables/themes; b) interactions between a behaviour and the athlete's own predispositions/personality (e.g., momentary and/or 'socialisation'); c) the specific impact of behaviours in context (for example, is a relationship a direct influence on motivation or does it moderate the way that certain behaviours are perceived? Or is it both?); and d) how important is consistency in a motivational atmosphere? For example, if a single derogatory comment is made against a background of general praise, facilitative coaching and a positive relationship, is it simply ignored or is it even more detrimental? What about a single derogatory comment against a background of consistent criticism? And under what circumstance might one of these 'frames-of-reference' change from generally positive to generally negative, or vice-versa? This research could take the form of quantitative experiments, perhaps chipping away at one variable at a time, or qualitative action research attempting to ascertain *what* can each key protagonist do, *when* (i.e., what circumstances), and *how* do they go about it (cf. Smith, 1989)?

It is perhaps worth noting that all the above-suggested ideas for studies focus on the situational level: on immediate behaviours and on collections of behaviours. This is a marked departure from the general tendency in motivational research to focus on the most abstract of contextual levels and/or general perceptions. One of the most fruitful aspects of the Keegan et al. studies was the methodological decision that, rather than building a model influenced by, and derived from, theoretically prescribed ideas (e.g., task and ego climates), it may well be possible to construct models reflecting 'real-life' situational occurrences and behaviours, which could even be observed quite objectively. This might also reduce the requirement to 'short-circuit' the process-of-discovery by exclusively assessing athletes' subjective perceptions (often at a very general level), using questionnaire items derived from quite abstract theoretical tenets. If, by examining the situational level without any *a priori* commitment to current models of motivational regulation, future research were to progress in a way that allows coaches, parents and peers alike to become reflectively aware of their impact on athlete motivation, then this would arguably constitute significant progress in the field of motivation research in sport.

References

Adie, J., Duda, J.L., & Ntoumanis, N. (2008). Autonomy support, basic need satisfaction and the optimal functioning of adult male and female sport participants: A test of basic needs theory. *Motivation & Emotion,* 32, 189-199.

Ainsworth, M.D.S., Blehar, M.C., Waters, E., & Wall, S. (1978). *Patterns of attachment: A psychological study of the strange situation* .Hillsdale, NJ: Erlbaum.

Allen, J.B. (2003). Social motivation in youth sport. *Journal of Sport and Exercise Psychology*, 25, 551-567.

Allen, J.B. (2006). The perceived belonging in sport scale: Examining validity. *Psychology of Sport and Exercise*, 7, 387-405.

Allen, J.B. & Hodge, K. (2006). Fostering a learning environment: Coaches and the motivational climate. *International Journal of Sport Science and Coaching,* 1, 260-277.

Allen, J.B., & Howe, B. (1998). Player ability, coach feedback and female adolescent athletes' perceived competence and satisfaction. *Journal of Sport and Exercise Psychology,* 20, 280-299.

Allen, J.P., Marsh, P., McFarland, C., McElhaney, K.B., Land, D.J., Jodl, K.M., & Peck, S. (2002). Attachment and autonomy as predictors of the development of social skills and delinquency during mid-adolescence. *Journal of Consulting and Clinical Psychology,* 70, 56-66.

Ames, C. A. (1984a).Achievement attributions and self instruction under competitive and individualistic goal structures. Journal of Educational Psychology, 76, 478-487.

Ames, C. A. (1984b). Competitive, cooperative, and individual goal structures: A cognitive-motivational analysis. In R. Ames & C. Ames (Eds.), Research on motivation in education: Student motivation (pp. 177-207). New York: Academic Press.

Ames, C. (1992a). Classrooms: Goals, structures, and student motivation. Journal of Educational Psychology, 84, 261- 271.

Ames, C. (1992b). Achievement goals, motivational climate, and motivational processes. In G.C. Roberts (Ed.) *Advances In Motivation in Sport and Exercise.* pp. 161-176. Champaign, IL: Human Kinetics.

Ames, C. & Archer, J. (1988). Achievement goals in the classroom: Students' learning strategies and motivation processes. *Journal of Educational Psychology*, 80, 260- 267.

Ames, C. A., Ames, R., & Felker, D. (1977). Effects of competitive reward structure and valence of outcome on children's achievement attributions. *Journal of Educational Psychology*, 69, 1-8.

Amorose, A.J., & Anderson-Butcher, D. (2007). Autonomy-supportive coaching and self-determined motivation in high school and college athletes: A test of self-determination theory. *Psychology of Sport and Exercise,* 8, 654-670.

Amorose, A.J. & Horn, T.S. (2000). Intrinsic motivation: Relationships with collegiate athletes' gender, scholarship status, and perceptions of their coaches' behavior. *Journal of Sport and Exercise Psychology*, 22, 63-84.

Amorose, A. J., & Horn, T. S. (2001). Pre- and post-season changes in intrinsic motivation of first year college athletes: Relationships with coaching behavior and scholarship status. *Journal of Applied Sport Psychology,* 13, 355-373

Amorose, A.J., & Weiss, M.R. (1998). Coaching feedback as a source of information about perceptions of ability: A developmental examination. *Journal of Sport & Exercise Psychology,* 20, 395-420.

Anderson, R., Manoogian, S.T., & Reznick, J.S. (1976). The undermining and enhancing of intrinsic motivation in preschool children. *Journal of Personality and Social Psychology,* 34, 915-922.

Assor, A., Roth, G., & Deci, E.L. (2004). The emotional cost of parents' conditional regard: A self-determination theory analysis. *Journal of Personality*, 72, 47-88.

Atkinson, J. (1957). Motivational determinants of risk-taking behaviour. *Psychological Review*, 64, 359-372.

Atkinson, J. and Birch, D. (1970). *The dynamics of action*. John Wiley & Sons

Atkinson, J., & Birch, D. (1978). *An introduction to motivation* (2nd ed.). Cincinnati: D. Van Nostrand Company

Balaguer, I., Duda, J.L., & Crespo, M. (1999). Motivational climate and goal orientations as predictors of perceptions of improvement, satisfaction and coach ratings among tennis players. *Scandinavian Journal of Medicine and Science in Sport*, 9, 381-388.

Balaguer, I., Duda, J.L., Atienza, F.L., Mayo, C. (2002). Situational and dispositional goals as predictors of perceptions of individual and team improvement, satisfaction and coach ratings among elite female handball teams. *Psychology of Sport and Exercise,* 3, 293-308.

Bargh, J.A., Chartrand, T.L. (1999). The unbearable automaticity of being, *American Psychologist,* 54, 462-479.

Barkoukis, V., Thogersen-Ntoumani, C., Ntoumanis, N., & Nikitaras, N. (2007). Achievement goals in physical education: Examining the predictive ability of five different dimensions of motivational climate. *European Physical Education Review*, 13, 267-285.

Berlyne, D.E. (1975). Behaviourism? Cognitive theory? Humanistic psychology? To Hull with them all. *Canadian Psychological Review,* 16, 69-80.

Bernard, L.L. (1924). *Instinct: A study of social psychology*. New York: Holt.

Berndt, T.J., & Keefe, K. (1995). Friends influence on adolescents adjustment to school. *Child Development,* 66, 1312-1329.

Biddle, S., Cury, F., Goudas, M., Sarrazin, P., Famose, J.P. and Durand, M. (1995). Development of scales to measure perceived physical education class climate: A cross-national project. *British Journal of Educational Psychology*, 65, 341-358.

Biddle, S. J. H., Duda, J. L., Papaioannou, A., & Harwood, C. (2001). *Physical education,* positivism, and optimistic claims from achievement goal theorists: A response to Pringle. *Quest*, 53, 457-470.

Blank, P.D., Reis, H.T., & Jackson, L. (1984). The effects of verbal reinforcements on intrinsic motivation for sex-linked tasks. *Sex Roles*, 10, 369-387.

Blumenfeld, P.C. (1992). Classroom learning and motivation – clarifying and expanding goal theory. *Journal of Educational Psychology*, 84, 272-281.

Blanchard, C. M., Mask, L., Vallerand, R. J., De La Sablonniere, R., & Provencher, P. (2007). Reciprocal relationships between contextual and situational motivation in a sport setting. *Psychology of Sport and Exercise*, 8, 854-873.

Boaz, A., Ashby, D., & Young, K. (2002). Systematic reviews: what have they got to offer evidence based policy and practice. ESRC UK Centre for evidence based policy and practice: working paper 2.

Boixadós, M., Cruz, J., Torregrosa, M., & Valiente, L. (2004). Relationships among motivational climate, satisfaction, perceived ability and fair play attitudes in youth soccer players. Journal of Applied Sport Psychology, 16, 301-317.

Bolles, R. C. (1975). *Theory of* motivation (2nd ed.). New York: Harper & Row.

Brière, N.M., Vallerand, R.J., Blais, M.R., & Pelletier, L.G. (1995). Développement et validation d'une mesure de motivation intrinsèque, extrinsèque et d'amotivation en contexte sportif : L'Echelle de Motivation dans les Sports (EMS). *International Journal of Sport Psychology, 26,* 465-489.

Bukowski, W. M., & Hoza, B. (1989). Popularity and friendship: Issues in theory, measurement, and outcome. In T. J. Berndt & G. W. Ladd (Eds.) *Peer relationships and child development* (pp. 15-45). New York: Wiley

Cacioppo, J.T., von Hippel, W., & Ernst, J.M. (1997). Mapping cognitive structures and processes through verbal content: The thought-listing technique. *Journal of Consulting and Clinical Psychology,* 65, 928-940.

Cacioppo, J.T., Crites, S.L., & Gardner, W.L. (1996). Attitudes to the right: Evaluative processing is associated with lateralised late positive event-related brain potentials. *Personality and Social Psychology Bulletin,* 22, 1205-1219.

Carpenter, P. J., & Morgan, K. (1999). Motivational climate, personal goal perspectives, and cognitive and affective responses in physical education classes. *European Journal of Physical Education*, 4, 31–44.

Carr, S., & Weigand, D.A. (2001). Parental, peer, teacher and sporting hero influence on the goal orientations of children in physical education. *European Physical Education Review*, 7, 305-328.

Carstensen, L.L. (1993). Motivation for social contact across the lifespan. In J. Jacobs (Ed.) *Nebraska symposium on Motivation: Developmental Perspectives on Motivation* (Vol. 40, pp.209-254). Lincoln: University of Nebraska Press.

Chatzisarantis, N. Biddle, S. Hagger, M. & Smith, B (2003). A path analytic meta-analysis of the perceived locus of causality in sport, physical education and physical activity contexts. *Journal of Sport and Exercise Psychology,* 25, 284-306.

Church, M.A., Elliot, A.J., & Gable, S.L. (2001). Perceptions of classroom environment, achievement goals, and achievement outcomes. *Journal of Educational Psychology,* 93, 43-54.

Clark, L.A., & Watson, D. (1999). Personality, disorder, and personality disorder: Towards a more rational conceptualization. *Journal of Personality Disorders,* 13, 142-151.

Clifford, M.M. (1988). Failure tolerance and academic risk-taking in ten-to twelve-year-old students. *British Journal of Educational Psychology,* 58, 15-27.

Clifford, M.M. (1990). Students need challenge, not easy success. *Educational Leadership,* 48, 22-26.

Coatsworth, J.D., & Conroy, D.E. (2009). The Effects of Autonomy-Supportive Coaching, Need Satisfaction, and Self-Perceptions on Initiative and Identity in Youth Swimmers. *Developmental Psychology,* 45, 320-328.

Conroy, D. E., Elliot, A. J., & Hofer, S. M. (2003). A 2 X 2 achievement goals questionnaire for sport: Evidence for factorial invariance, temporal stability, and external validity. *Journal of Sport & Exercise Psychology*, 25, 456-476.

Costa, P.T., & McCrae, R.R. (1992). "Four ways five factors are not basic": Reply. *Personality and Individual Differences,* 13, 861-865.

Côté, J., Baker, J., & Abernathy, B. (2003). From play to practice: A developmental framework for the acquisition of expertise in team sport. In J. Starkes and K.A. Ericsson (Eds.), *Expert performance in sports: Advances in research on sport expertise,* (pp. 89-113). Champaign, IL: Human Kinetics.

Côté, J., & Hay, J. (2002a). Children's involvement in sport: A developmental perspective. In J.M. Silva & D.E. Stevens (Eds.) *Psychological foundations of sport* (pp. 484-502). Boston: Allyn & Bacon.

Côté, J., & Hay, J. (2002b). Family influences on youth sport performance and participation. In Silva, J. & Stevens, D. (Eds.). *Psychological foundations of sports* (pp. 503-519). Boston, MA: Allyn and Bacon.

Covington, M.V., & Omelich, C.L. (1979). It's best to be able and virtuous too: Student and teacher evaluative responses to successful effort. *Journal of Educational Psychology,* 71, 688-700.

Cresswell, S.L., & Eklund, R.C. (2005). Motivation and burnout in professional rugby players.
Research Quarterly for Exercise and Sport, 76, 370-376.

Cresswell, S.L. & Eklund, R.C. (2005). Changes in athlete burnout and motivation over a 12-week league tournament. *Medicine and Science in Sports and Exercise*, 37, 1957-1966.

Crowne, D.P., & Marlowe, D. (1960*).* A new scale of social desirability independent of psycho- pathology. *Journal of Consulting Psychology*, 24, 349–354.

Csikszentmihalyi, M., & Csikszentmihalyi, I. (1988). *Optimal experiences: Psychological studies of flow in consciousness.* New York: Cambridge University Press.

Csikszentmihalyi, M., Rathunde, K., & Whalen, S. (1993). *Talented teenagers: The roots of success and failure.* New York: Cambridge University Press.

Cumming, S.P., Smith, R.E., Smoll, F.L., Standage, M., & Grossbard, J.R. (2008). Development and validation of the Achievement Goal Scale for Youth Sports. *Psychology of Sport and Exercise,* 9, 686-703.

Cury, F., Da Fonseca, D., Rufo, M., & Sarrazin, P. (2002). Perceptions of competence, implicit theory of ability, perception of motivational climate, and achievement goals: A test of the trichotomous conceptualization of endorsement of achievement motivation in the physical education setting. *Perceptual and Motor Skills*, 95, 233-244.

Cury, F., Elliot, A., Sarrazin, P., Da Fonseca, D., & Rufo, M. (2002). The trichotomous achievement goal model and intrinsic motivation: A sequential mediational analysis. *Journal of Experimental Social Psychology*, 38, 473-481.

DeCharms, R. (1968). *Personal causation.* New York: Academic Press.

Deci, E. L. (1971). Effects of externally mediated rewards on intrinsic motivation. *Journal of Personality and Social Psychology,* 18, 105-115.

Deci, E. L. (1975). *Intrinsic motivation.* New York: Plenum Publishing Co.

Deci, E.L. (1995). Self determination theory and education. *Ceskoslovenska Psychologie*, 38, 420-426.

Deci, E.L., Betley, G., Kahle, J., Abrams, L., & Porac, J. (1981). When trying to win: Competition and intrinsic motivation. *Personality and Social Psychology Bulletin,* 7, 79–83.

Deci, E.L., Eghrari, H., Patrick, B.C., & Leone, D.R. (1994). Facilitating internalization: The self-determination theory perspective. *Journal of Personality,* 62, 119-142.

Deci, E. L., Koestner, R., & Ryan, R. M. (1999). A meta-analytic review of experiments examining the effects of extrinsic rewards on intrinsic motivation. *Psychological Bulletin*, 125, 627-668.

Deci, E. L., Koestner, R., & Ryan, R. M. (2001). Extrinsic rewards and intrinsic motivation in education: Reconsidered once again. *Review of Educational Research*, 71, 1-27.

Deci, E.L., & Ryan, R.M. (1985). *Intrinsic motivation and self-determination in human behav*ior. New York: Plenum.

Deci, E. L., & Ryan, R. M. (1987). The support of autonomy and the control of behavior. In E. T. Higgins & A. W. Kruglanski (Eds.), *Motivational science: Social and personality perspectives* (pp. 128-145). Philadelphia, PA: Psychology Press.

Deci, E. L., & Ryan, R. M. (1991). A motivational approach to self: Integration in personality. In R. Dienstbier (Ed.), *Nebraska symposium on motivation: Perspectives on motivation, vol. 38* (pp. 237-288). Lincoln, NE: University Of Nebraska Press.

Deci, E. L., & Ryan, R. M. (1995). Human autonomy: the basis for true self-esteem. In M.Kernos (Ed.) *Efficacy, agency and self-esteem* (pp. 31-49). New York: Plenum Press.

Deci, E.L., & Ryan, R.M. (2000). The "what" and "why" of goal pursuits: Human needs and the self-determination of behavior. *Psychological Enquiry*, 11, 227-268.

Deci, E. L., Ryan, R. M., Gagné, M., Leone, D. R., Usunov, J., & Kornazheva, B. P. (2001). Need satisfaction, motivation, and well-being in the work organizations of a former Eastern Bloc country. *Personality and Social Psychology Bulletin,* 27, 930-942.

Deci, E.L., Schwartz, A., Scheinman, L., & Ryan, R.M. (1981). An instrument to assess adult's orientations toward control versus autonomy in children: Reflections on intrinsic motivation and perceived competence. *Journal of Educational Psychology,* 73, 642-650.

Deci, E.L., Speigel, N.H., Ryan, R.M., Koestner, R., & Kauffman, M. (1982). Effects of performance standards on teaching styles: Behaviour of controlling teachers. *Journal of Educational Psychology,* 74, 852-859.

Deci, E.L., Vallerand, R.J., Pelletier, L.G., & Ryan, R.M. (1991). Motivation and education: The self-determination perspective. *The Educational Psychologist,* 26, 325-346.

Diener, C.I., & Dweck, C.S. (1978). Analysis of learned helplessness: Continuous changes in performance, strategy and achievement cognitions following failure. *Journal of Personality and Social Psychology*, 36, 451-462.

Diener, C.I., & Dweck, C.S. (1980). An analysis of learned helplessness 2: The processing of success. *Journal of Personality and Social Psychology*, 39, 940-952.

Digelidis, N., Papaioannou, A., Laparidis, K., & Christodoulidis, T. (2003). A one-year intervention in 7th grade physical education classes aiming to change motivational climate and attitudes towards exercise. *Psychology of Sport and Exercise*, 4, 195-210.

Dollinger, S.J., & Thelen, M.H. (1978). Over-justification and children's intrinsic motivation: Comparative effects of four rewards. *Journal of Personality and Social Psychology,* 36, 1259-1269.

Dorobantu, M., & Biddle, S.J.H. (1997). The influence of situational and individual goals on the intrinsic motivation of adolescents towards Physical Education. *The European Yearbook of Sport Psychology,* 1, 145-168.

Duda, J.L. (1992). Motivation in sport settings: A goal perspective approach .In G.C. Roberts (Ed.), *Motivation, and Sport and Exercise* (pp.57-91). Champaign, Illinois: Human Kinetics.

Duda, J.L. (1993). Goals: A social-cognitive approach to the study of achievement motivation in sport. In R. Singer, M. Murphey, & L.K. Tennant (Eds.), *Handbook of Research in Sport Psychology* (pp. 421-436). New York: Macmillan.

Duda, J. L. (2001). Achievement goal research in sport: Pushing the boundaries and clarifying some misunderstandings. In: G. C. Roberts (Ed.), *Advances in motivation in sport and exercise*. (pp. 129-183). Champaign: IL, Human Kinetics.

Duda, J.L. & Chi, L. (1989). The effect of task- and ego-involving conditions on perceived competence and causal attributions in basketball. Communication to the *Association for the Advancement of Applied Sport Psychology*, University of Washington, Seattle, WA, September.

Duda, J.L., Chi, L., Newton, M.L., Walling, M.D., & Catley, D. (1995). Task and ego orientation and intrinsic motivation in sport. *International Journal of Sport Psychology*, 26, 40-63.

Duda, J.L., & Hall, H.K. (2001). Achievement goal theory in sport: Recent extensions and future directions. In R. Singer, H. Hausenblas, & C. Janelle (Eds.), *Handbook of sport psychology* (pp. 417-443). New York: Wiley.

Duda, J. L., & Nicholls, J. G. (1992). Dimensions of achievement motivation in schoolwork and sport. *Journal of Educational Psychology*, 84, 290-299.

Duda, J.L., Olson, L., & Templin, T. (1991). The relationship of task and ego orientation to sportsmanship attitudes and the perceived legitimacy of injurious acts. *Research Quarterly for Exercise and Sport*, 62, 79-87.

Duda, J.L., & White, S.A. (1992). Goal orientations and beliefs about the causes of success among elite athletes. *The Sport Psychologist*, 6, 334-343.

Duda, J.L., & Whitehead, J. (1998). Measurement of goal perspectives in the physical domain. In J.L Duda (Ed.), *Advances in sport and exercise psychology measures*, (pp. 21-48). Morgantown, WV: Fitness Information Technology.

Dunlap, K. (1919). Are there any instincts? *Journal of Abnormal Psychology*, 14, 35-50.

Dweck, C.S. (1975). The role of expectations and attributions in the alleviation of learned helplessness. *Journal of Personality and Social Psychology*, 31, 674-685.

Dweck, C. S. (1986). Motivational processes affecting learning. *American Psychologist*, 41, 1040-1048.

Dweck, C. S. (1999). *Self theories: Their role in motivation, personality, and development.* Philadelphia, PA: Psychology Press.

Dweck, C. S., Chiu, C.-y., & Hong, Y.-y. (1995). Implicit theories and their role in judgments and reactions: A world from two perspectives. *Psychological Inquiry*, 6, 267-285.

Dweck, C. S., & Leggett, E. L. (1988). A social-cognitive approach to motivation and personality. *Psychological Review*, 95, 256-273.

Dwyer, J.J.M. (1995). Effect of perceived choice of music on exercise intrinsic motivation. *Health Values,* 19, 18-26.

Eccles, J., Adler, T.F., Futterman, R., Goff, S.B., Kaczala, C.M., Meece, J.L. & Midgley, C. (1983). Expectations, values and academic behaviours. In J.T. Spence (Ed), *Achievement and Achievement Motivation.* (pp. 75-146). San Francisco: W.H. Freeman.

Ekman, *P.* & Friesen, *W. V. (1975). Unmasking the face. A guide to recognizing emotions from facial clues.* Englewood Cliffs, New Jersey: Prentice-Hall.

Elliot, A. J. (1994). *Approach and avoidance achievement goals: An intrinsic motivation analysis.* Unpublished Doctoral Dissertation, University of Wisconsin, Madison.

Elliot, A. J. (1997). Integrating the "classic" and "contemporary" approaches to achievement motivation: A hierarchical model of approach and avoidance achievement motivation . In M. L. Maehr & P. R. Pintrich (Eds.), *Advances in motivation and achievement* (Vol. 10, pp. 143-179). Greenwich, CT: JAI Press.

Elliot, A. J. (1999). Approach and avoidance motivation and achievement goals. *Educational Psychologist*, 34, 169-189.

Elliot, A.J. (2005). A conceptual history of the achievement goal construct. In A. Elliot and C. Dweck (Eds.) *Handbook of Competence Motivation.* (pp. 52-72) NY: Guilford Press.

Elliot, A. J., & Church, M. A. (1997). A hierarchical model of approach and avoidance achievement motivation. *Journal of Personality and Social Psychology*, 72, 218-232.

Elliot, A. J., & McGregor, H. A. (2001). A 2 X 2 achievement goal framework. *Journal of Personality and Social Psychology*, 80, 501-519.

Elliot, A. J., & Conroy, D. E. (2005). Beyond the dichotomous model of achievement goals in sport and exercise psychology. *Sport & Exercise Psychology Review*, 1, 17-25.

Elliot, A. J., & Covington, M. V. (2001). Approach and avoidance motivation. *Educational Psychology Review,* 13, 73-92.

Elliot, A.J., & Dweck, C.S. (2005). Competence and Motivation: Competence as the core of achievement motivation. In A.J. Elliot and C.S. Dweck (Eds.) *Handbook of Competence and Motivation.* New York: Guildford.

Elliot, A. J., & Thrash, T. M. (2001). Achievement goals and the hierarchical model of achievement motivation. *Educational Psychology Review*, 13, 139-156.

Elliot, A.J., & Thrash, T.M. (2002). Approach-avoidance motivation in personality: Approach and avoidance temperaments and goals. *Journal of Personality and Social Psychology.* 82, 804-818.

Epstein, J.L. (1989). Family structures and student motivation: a developmental perspective. In: C. Ames & R. Ames (Eds.) *Research on motivation in education*: Vol. 3. (pp. 259-295). New York, Academic Press.

Escarti A., & Gutierrez, M. (2001). Influence of the Motivational Climate in Physical Education on the Intention to Practice Physical Activity or Sport. *European Journal of Sport Sciences*, 1, 1-12.

Feyerabend, P.K. (1975). Against method*: Outline of an anarchistic theory of knowledge*. Humanities Press, London.

Flink, C., Boggiano, A.K., & Barrett, M. (1990). Controlling teaching strategies: Undermining children's self-determination and performance. *Journal of Personality and Social Psychology,* 59, 916-924.

Flowerday, T., & Schraw, G. (2003).Effect of choice on cognitive and affective engagement. *Journal of Educational Research,* 96, 207-215.

Flowerday, T., Schraw, G. & Stevens, J. (2004). The role of choice and interest in reader engagement. *Journal of Experimental Education,* 72, 93-114.

Frederick-Recascino, C. M., & Ryan, R. M. (1993). Differences in motivation for sport and exercise and their relations with participation and mental health. *Journal of Sport Behavior*, *16*, 124-146.

Fredricks, J.A., & Eccles, J.S. (2002). Children's competence and value beliefs from childhood through adolescence. *Developmental Psychology*, 38, 519-553.

Fredricks, J.A., & Eccles, J.S. (2005). Family socialization, gender, and sport motivation and involvement." *Journal of Sport & Exercise Psychology*, 27, 3-31.

Fry, M. D. (2001). The development of motivation in children. In G.C. Roberts (Ed.), *Advances in Motivation in Sport and Exercise*. Champaign, IL; Human Kinetics.

Fry, M. D. & Duda, J. L. (1997). A developmental examination of children's understanding of effort and ability in the physical and academic domains. *Research Quarterly for Exercise and Sport*, 66, 331-344.

Fry, M.D., & Newton, M. (2003). Application of achievement goal theory in an urban youth tennis setting. Journal of Applied Sport Psychology, 15, 50-66.

Gable, S.L., Reis, H.T., & Elliot, A.J. (2003). Evidence for bivariate systems: An empirical test of appetition and aversion across domains. *Journal of Research in Personality*. 37, 349-372.

Gagné, M., Ryan, R. M., & Bargman, K. (2003). Autonomy support and need satisfaction in the motivation and well-being of gymnasts. *Journal of Applied Sport Psychology*, 15, 372–390.

Gano-Overway, L.A., & Ewing, M.E. (2004). A longitudinal perspective of the relationship between perceived motivational climate, goal orientations, and strategy use. *Research Quarterly for Exercise and Sport*, 75, 315-325.

Gano-Overway, L.A., Guivernau, M., Magyar, T.M., Waldron, J.J., & Ewing, M.E. (2005). Achievement goal perspectives, perceptions of the motivational climate, and sportspersonship: Individual and team effects. *Psychology of Sport and Exercise*, 6, 215-232.

Gazzaniga, M.S. (1998). *The Mind's Past*. Berkeley: University of California Press.

Giacobbi, P.R., Poczwardowski, A., & Hager, P. (2005). A pragmatic research philosophy for applied sport psychology. *The Sport Psychologist*, 19, 1-31.

Gillet, N., Berjot, S., & Gobance, L. (2009). A motivational model of performance in the sport domain. *European Journal of Sport Science*, 9, 151-158.

Gottfried, A.E., Fleming, J.S., & Gottfried, A.W. (1994). Role of parental motivational practices in academic intrinsic motivation and achievement. Journal of Educational Psychology, 86, 104-113.

Goudas, M. & Biddle, S. (1994). Perceived motivational climate and intrinsic motivation in school physical education classes. *European Journal of Psychology of Education*, 9, 241-250.

Goudas, M., Biddle, S., Fox, K., & Underwood, M. (1995). It ain't what you do, it's the way that you do it! Teaching style affects children's motivation in track and field lessons. *The Sport Psychologist*, 9, 254-264.

Gould, D., Lauer, L., Rolo, C., Jannes, C., & Pennisi, N. (2008). The role of parents in tennis success: Focus group interviews with junior coaches. *The Sport Psychologist,* 22, 18-37.

Gray, J.A. (1990) Brain systems that mediate both emotion and cognition. *Cognition and Emotion,* 4, 269-288.

Grolnick, W.S. (2003). *The psychology of parental control: How well-meant parenting backfires*. NJ: Erlbaum.

Grolnick, W.S., Ryan R.M., & Deci, E.L. (1991). Inner resources for school achievement: Motivational mediators of children's perceptions of their parents. *Journal of Educational Psychology,* 83, 508-517.

Guay, F., Vallerand, R.J., & Blanchard, C. (2000). On the assessment of situational intrinsic and extrinsic motivation: The situational Motivation Scales (SIMS). *Motivation and Emotion*, 24, 175-213.

Guiffrida, D.A., Gouveia, A., Wall, A., & Seward, D.X. (2008). Development and validation of the Need for Relatedness at College Questionnaire (NRC-Q). *Journal of Diversity in Higher Education, 1*, 251-261.

Hall, C., & Lindzey, G. (1985). *Introduction to Theories of Personality.* New York: John Wiley & Sons.

Harwood, C.G., & Hardy, L. (2001). Persistence and effort in moving achievement goal research forward: A response to Treasure and colleagues. *Journal of Sport and Exercise Psychology*, 23, 330-345.

Harwood, C.G., Hardy, L., & Swain, A.B. (2002). Achievement goals in sport: A critique of conceptual and measurement issues. *Journal of Sport & Exercise Psychology*, 22, 235 - 255.

Harwood, C.G., Spray, C.M., & Keegan, R.J. (2008). Achievement goal theories in sport. In T. Horn (Ed.), *Advances in sport psychology* (3rd Edition). (pp. 157-185). Champaign, Illinois: Human Kinetics.

Harwood, C.G., & Swain, A.B. (2001). The development and activation of achievement goals in tennis: 1. Understanding the underlying factors. *The Sports Psychologist*, 15, 319-341.

Harter, S. (1978). Effectance motivation reconsidered: Toward a developmental model. *Human Development*, 21, 34-64.

Harter, S. (1981). A new self-report scale of intrinsic verses extrinsic orientation in the classroom: motivational and informational components. *Developmental Psychology,* 17, 300-312.

Hastorf, A., & Cantril, H. (1954). They saw a game: A case study. *Journal of Abnormal and Social Psychology*, 49, 129-134.

Henderlong, J., & Lepper, M.R. (2002). The effect of praise on children's intrinsic motivation: A review and synthesis. *Psychological Bulletin,* 128, 774-795.

Henwood, K.L. and Pidgeon, N.F. (2003). Grounded theory in psychological research. In P. Camic, L. Yardley and J.E. Rhodes (Eds.) *Qualitative Research in Psychology: Expanding Perspectives in Methodology and Design.* Washington DC: APA publications.

Hess, R.D., & McDevitt, T.M. (1984). Some cognitive consequences of maternal intervention: A longitudinal study. *Child Development,* 55, 2017-2030.

Heyman, G. D., Gee, C. L., & Giles, J. W. (2003). Preschool children's reasoning about ability. *Child Development*, 74, 516-534.

Hodge, K., Lonsdale, C., & Ng, J. (2008). Burnout in elite rugby: Relationships with basic psychological needs fulfilment. *Journal of Sports Sciences*, 26, 835-844.

Hokoda, A., & Fincham, F.D. (1995). Origins of children's helpless and mastery achievement patterns in the family. *Journal of Educational Psychology,* 87, 375-385.

Hollembeak, J., & Amorose, A. J. (2005). Perceived coaching behaviors and college athletes' intrinsic motivation: A test of self-determination theory. *Journal of Applied Sport Psychology, 17,* 20-36.

Holt, N. L., Black, D. E., Tamminen, K. A., Mandigo, J. L., & Fox, K. R. (2008). Levels of social complexity and dimensions of peer experience in youth sport. Journal of Sport & Exercise Psychology, *30*, 411-43.

Holt, N.L., Tamminen, K.A., Black, D.E., Mandigo, J.L. & Fox, K.R. (2009). Youth sport parenting styles and practices. *Journal of Sport & Exercise Psychology*, 31, 37-59.

Holt, N. L., Tamminen, K. A., Black, D. E., Sehn, Z. L., & Wall, M. P. (2008). Parental involvement in competitive youth sport settings. *Psychology of Sport and Exercise, 9*, 663-685.

Howes, C., & James, J. (2002). Children's social development within the context of childcare and early childhood education. In: P. Smith & C. Hart (Eds.) *Blackwell Handbook of Social Development.* (pp. 137–155). Blackwell; Oxford.

Jackson, S.A & Roberts, G.C. (1992). Positive performance states of athletes: Toward a conceptual understanding of peak performance. *The Sport Psychologist*, 6, 156-171.

Jourden, F.J., Bandura, A., & Banfield, J.T., (1991). The impact of conceptions of ability on self-regulatory factors and motor-skill acquisition. *Journal of Sport and Exercise Psychology*, 13, 213-226.

Jowett, S. & Meek, G.A (2000). The coach–athlete relationship in married couples: An exploratory content analysis. *The Sport Psychologist*, 14, 157–175

Kamins, M.L., & Dweck, C.S. (1999). Person versus process praise and criticism: Implications for contingent self worth and coping. *Developmental Psychology*, 35, 835-847.

Kasser, V. G., & Ryan, R. M. (1999). The relation of psychological needs for autonomy and relatedness to vitality, well-being , and mortality in a nursing home. *Journal of Applied Social Psychology,* 29, 935-954.

Kast, A., & Connor, K. (1988). Sex and age differences in response to informational and controlling feedback. *Personality and Social Psychology Bulletin,* 14, 514-523.

Kavussanu, M., & Roberts, G.C. (1996). Motivation in physical activity contexts: The relationship of perceived motivational climate to intrinsic motivation and self-efficacy. *Journal of Sport and Exercise Psychology*, 18, 264-280.

Kavussanu, M. & Roberts, G.C. (2001). Moral functioning in sport: An achievement goal perspective. *Journal of Sport and Exercise Psychology*, 23, 37-54.

Keller, J., & Bless, H. (2008). Flow and regulatory compatibility: An experimental approach to the flow model of intrinsic motivation. *Personality and Social Psychology Bulletin*, 34, 196-209.

Keegan, R.J., Harwood, C.G., Spray, C.M., & Lavallee, D.E. (2009). A qualitative investigation exploring the motivational climate in early-career sports participants: Coach, parent and peer influences on sport motivation. *Psychology of Sport and Exercise*, 10, 361-372.

Keegan, R.J., Spray, C.M., Harwood, C.G., & Lavallee, D.E. (2010). The 'motivational atmosphere' in youth sport: Coach, parent and peer influences on motivation in specializing sport participants. *Journal of Applied Sport Psychology,* 22, 87-105.

Keegan, R.J., Spray, C.M., Harwood, C.G., & Lavallee, D.E. (in submission). A qualitative investigation of the broader motivational climate in elite sport participants: What (and who) makes elite performers tick?

Keith, T.Z., Keith, P.B., Troutman, C.G., Bickley, P.G., Trivette, P.S., & Singh, K. (1993). Does parent involvement affect eighth-grade students' achievement? Structural analysis of national development. *School Psychology Review,* 22, 474-496.

Kelley, S.A., Brownell, C.A., & Campbell, S.B. (2000). Mastery motivation and self-evaluative affect in toddlers: Longitudinal relations with maternal behavior. *School Psychology Review,* 71, 1061-1071.

Kempner, S., & Pomerantz, E.M. (2003). Mothers' use of praise in their everyday interactions with their children: The moderating role of children's gender. *Paper presented at the Society for Research on Child Development*, Tampa, FL.

Koestner, R., Ryan, R.M., Bernieri, F., & Holt, K. (1984). Setting limits on children's behaviour: The differential effects of controlling versus informational styles on intrinsic motivation and creativity. *Journal of Personality,* 52, 233-248.

Kowal, J., Fortier, M.S. (2000). Testing relationships from the hierarchical model of intrinsic and extrinsic motivation using flow as a motivational consequence. *Research Quarterly for Exercise and Sport,* 71, 171-181.

Krane, V., Greenleaf, C.A., & Snow, J. (1997). Reaching for gold and the price of glory: A motivational case study of an elite gymnast. *The Sport Psychologist*, 11, 53-71.

Kukla, A. (1972). Foundations of an attributional theory of performance, *Psychological Review,* 79, 454-470.

Ladd, G.W. (1990). Having Friends, Keeping Friends, Making Friends and Being Liked by Peers in the Classroom: Predictors of Children's Early School Adjustment. *Child Development,* 61, 1081-1100.

Lazarus, R.S. (1966). *Psychological stress and the coping process.* New York; McGraw-Hill

Lemyre, P.-N., Treasure, D.C., & Roberts, G.C. (2006). Influence of variability in motivation and affect on elite athlete burnout. *Journal of Sport and Exercise Psychology*, 28, 32-48.

Lloyd, J., & Fox, K. (1992). Achievement goals and motivation to exercise in adolescent girls: A preliminary intervention study. *British Journal of Physical Education: Research Supplement*, 11, 12-16.

Liukkonen, J., Telama, R., & Biddle, S.J.H. (1998). Enjoyment in youth sport: A goal perspectives approach. *European Yearbook of Sport Psychology*, 2, 55-75.

Locke, E.A., & Latham, G.P. (1984). *Goal setting: A motivational technique that works!* Englewood Cliffs, NJ: Prentice Hall.

Locke, E.A., & Latham, G.P. (1990). *A theory of goal setting and task performance.* Englewood Cliffs, NJ: Prentice Hall.

Lopez, D.F. (1999). Social cognitive influences on self regulated learning: The impact of action-control beliefs and academic goals on achievement related outcomes. *Learning and Individual Differences,* 11, 301-319.

Maehr, M.L. (1984). Meaning and motivation: toward a theory of personal investment. In R. Ames and C. Ames (Eds.) *Research on motivation in education (Volume 1): student motivation*. San Diego: Academic Press, Inc.

Maehr, M.L., & Braskamp, L.A. (1986). *The motivation factor: A theory of personal investment.* Lexington, MA: Lexington Books.

Maehr, M.L., & Midgley, C. (1991). Enhancing student motivation: A schoolwide approach. *Educational Psychologist*, 26, 399-427.

Maehr, M. L., & Nicholls, J.G. (1980). Culture and achievement motivation: A second look. In N. Warren (Ed.), Studies in cross-cultural psychology: Vol. 3, (pp. 221-267). New York: Academic Press.

Mageau, G.A., & Vallerand, R.J. (2003). The coach-athlete relationship: A motivational model. *Journal of Sport Sciences,* 21, 883-904.

Magyar, T.M., & Feltz, D.L. (2003). The influence of dispositional and situational tendencies on adolescent girls' sport confidence sources. *Psychology of Sport and Exercise*, 4, 175-190.

Mallet, C.J., & Hanrahan, S.J. (2004). Elite athletes: why does the 'fire' burn so brightly? *Psychology of Sport and Exercise*, 5, 183-200.

Markland, D., & Hardy, L. (1997). On the factorial and construct validity of the Intrinsic Motivation Inventory: Conceptual and operational concerns. *Research Quarterly for Exercise & Sport, 60,* 48–58.

Markland, D., & Vansteenkiste, M. (2008). Self-determination theory and motivational interviewing in exercise. In M. S. Hagger & N. L. D. Chatzisarantis (Eds.), *Intrinsic motivation and self-determination in exercise and sport* (pp. 87-100). Champaign, IL: Human Kinetics.

Marsh, H.W. & Peart, N.D. (1988). Competitive and cooperative physical fitness training programs for girls: Effects on physical fitness and multidimensional self concepts. *Journal of Sport and Exercise Psychology*, 10, 390-407.

Maslow, A.H. (1954). *Motivation and Personality*. New York: Harper & Row.

Mayer, J. D., Faber, M., & Xu, X. (2007). Seventy-five years of motivation measures (1930-2005): A descriptive analysis. *Motivation and Emotion,* 31, 83-103.

Mayo, R.J. (1977). The development and construct validation of a measure of intrinsic motivation. *Dissertation Abstracts International,* 37, 5417B.

McAuley, E., Duncan, T., & Tammen, V. V. (1989). Psychometric properties of the intrinsic motivation inventory in a competitive sport setting: A confirmatory factor analysis. *Research Quarterly for Exercise and Sport,* 60, 48-58

McClelland, D.C., Atkinson, J.W., Clarke, R.A., & Lowell, E.L. (1953). *The achievement motive.* New York: Appleton-Century-Crofts.

McCrae, R.R., & Costa, P.T. (1987). Validation of the five-factor model of personality across instruments and observers. *Journal of Personality and Social Psychology,* 52, 81-90.

McDougall, W. (1926). *Introduction to social psychology.* Boston: Luce and Co.

Meyer, W. (1987). Perceived ability and achievement related behavior. In F. Halisch & J. Kuhl (Eds.) *Motivation, intention and volition* (pp 72-86) New York: Springer-Verlag.

Miller, S.A., Manhal, M., & Mee, L.L. (1991). Parental beliefs, parental accuracy, and children's cognitive performance: A search for causal relations. *Developmental Psychology,* 37, 863-874.

Miller, B.W., Roberts, G.C., & Ommundsen, Y. (2004). Effect of motivational climate on sportspersonship among competitive youth male and female football players. *Scandinavian Journal of Medicine and Science in Sport,* 14, 193-202.

Mischel, W. (1968). *Personality and assessment.* New York: Wiley

Moller, A.C., Deci, E.L., & Ryan, R.M. (2006). Choice and ego-depletion: The moderating role of autonomy. *Personality and Social Psychology Bulletin,* 32, 1024-1036.

Morgan, K., Sproule, J., Weigand, D., & Carpenter, P. (2005). A computer-based observational assessment of the teaching behaviours that influence motivational climate in Physical Education. *Physical Education and Sport Pedagogy,* 10, 83–105.

Mueller, C. M., & Dweck, C. S. (1998). Praise for intelligence can undermine children's motivation and performance. Journal of Personality and Social Psychology, 75, 33-52.

Murray, H. A. (1938). *Explorations in personality*. New York: Oxford University Press.

Newby, T.J., (1991). Classroom motivation; Strategies of first-year teachers. *Journal of Educational Psychology,* 83, 195-200.

Newton, M. & Duda, J.L. (1993). Elite adolescent athletes achievement goals and beliefs concerning success in tennis. *Journal of Sport and Exercise Psychology,* 15, 437-448.

Newton, M. & Duda, J.L. (1995). Relations of goal orientations and expectations on multidimensional state anxiety. *Perceptual and Motor Skills*, 81, 1107-1112.

Newton, M., Duda, J.L., & Yin, Z.N. (2000). Examination of the psychometric properties of the Perceived Motivational Climate in Sport Questionnaire-2 in a sample of female athletes. *Journal of Sports Sciences*, 18, 275-290.

Nicholls, J. G. (1979). Quality and equality in intellectual development: The role of motivation in education. *American Psychologist*, 34, 1071-1084.

Nicholls, J.G. (1984). Achievement motivation: Conceptions of ability, subjective experience, task choice, and performance. *Psychological Review*, 91, 328-346.

Nicholls, J.G. (1989). *The competitive ethos and democratic education.* Cambridge, MA: Harvard University Press.

Nicholls, J. G., Cheung, P. C., Lauer, J., & Patashnick, M. (1989). Individual differences in academic motivation: Perceived ability, goals, beliefs, and values. *Learning & Individual Differences*, 1, 63-84.

Nicholls, J.G., & Miller, A.T. (1983). The differentiation of the concepts of difficulty and ability. *Child Development*, 54, 951–959.

Nicholls, J.G. & Miller, A.T. (1984). Development and its discontents: The differentiation of the concept of ability. In J.G. Nicholls (Ed.), *Advances in motivation and achievement, Vol. 3: The development of achievement motivation* (pp. 185-218). Greenwich, CT: JAI Press.

Niiya, Y., Crocker, J., & Bartmess, E.N. (2004). From vulnerability to resilience - Learning orientations buffer contingent self-esteem from failure. *Psychological Science,* 15, 801-805.

Ntoumanis, N. (2005). A prospective study of participation in optional school physical education using a self-determination theory framework. *Journal of Educational Psychology,* 97, 444-453.

Ntoumanis, N., and Biddle, S.J.H. (1998a). The relationship of coping and its perceived effectiveness to positive and negative affect in sport. *Personality and Individual Differences*, 24, 773-788.

Ntoumanis, N. & Biddle, S. (1998b). The relationship between competitive anxiety, achievement goals, and motivational climates. *Research Quarterly for Exercise and Sport*, 69, 176-187.

Ntoumanis, N., & Biddle, S. (1999). A review of motivational climate in physical activity. *Journal of Sports Sciences*, 17, 643-665.

Ntoumanis, N., Biddle, S. J. H., & Haddock, G. (1999). The mediating role of coping strategies on the relationship between achievement motivation and affect in sport. *Anxiety, Stress, and Coping*, 12, 299-327.

Ntoumanis, N., & Vazou, S. (2005). Peer motivational climate in youth sport: Measurement development and validation. *Journal of Sport & Exercise Psychology*, 27, 432-455.

Ommundsen, Y., & Roberts, G.C. (1999). Effect of motivational climate profiles on motivational indices in team sport. Scandinavian Journal of Medicine and Science in Sport, 9, 389-397.

Ommundsen, Y., Roberts, G.C., & Kavussanu, M. (1998). Perceived motivational climate and cognitive and affective correlates among Norwegian athletes. Journal of Sport Sciences, 16, 153-164.

Ommundsen, Y., Roberts, G.C., Lemyre, P.N., & Treasure, D. (2003). Perceived motivational climate in male youth soccer: relations to social-moral functioning, sportspersonship and team norm perceptions. Psychology of Sport and Exercise, 4, 397-413.

Pajares, F. & Miller, M.D. (1994). Role of self efficacy and self-concept beliefs in mathematical problem solving – A path analysis. *Journal of Educational Psychology,* 86, 193-203.

Parish, L.E., & Treasure, D.C. (2003). Physical activity and situational motivation in physical education: Influence of the motivational climate and perceived ability. *Research Quarterly for Exercise and Sport*, 74, 173-182.

Parkhurst, J.T., & Hopmeyer, A. (1998). Sociometric popularity and peer-perceived popularity: Two distinct dimensions of peer status. *Journal of Early Adolescence,* 18(2). 125-144.

Papaioannou, A. (1994). The development of a questionnaire to measure achievement orientations in Physical Education. *Research Quarterly for Exercise and Sport*, 65, 11-20

Papaioannou, A. (1995). Differential perceptual and motivational patterns when different goals are adopted. *Journal of Sport and Exercise Psychology*, 17, 18-34.

Papaioannou, A. (1997). Perceptions of motivational climate, perceived competence, and motivation of students of varying ages and sport experience. *Perceptual and Motor Skills*, 85, 419-430.

Papaioannou, A. (1998). Students' perceptions of the physical education class environment for boys and girls and the perceived motivational climate. *Research Quarterly for Exercise and Sport*, 69, 267-275.

Papaioannou, A., & Kouli, O. (1999). The effect of task structure, perceived motivational climate and goal orientations on students' task involvement and anxiety. *Journal of Applied Sport Psychology*, 11, 51-71.

Papaioannou, A., Marsh, H.W., & Theodorakis, Y. (2004). A multi-level approach to motivational climate in physical education and sport settings: An individual or group level construct? *Journal of Sport and Exercise Psychology,* 26, 90-118.

Papaioannou, A., Milosis, D., Kosmidou, E., & Tsigilis, N. (2007). Motivational climate and achievement goals at the situational level of generality. *Journal of Applied Sport Psychology,* 19, 38-66.

Patall, E.A., Cooper, H., & Robinson, J.C. (2008). The effects of choice on intrinsic motivation and related outcomes: A meta-analysis of research findings. *Psychological Bulletin,* 134, 270-300.

Peet, S.H., Powell, D.R., O'Donnel, B.K. (1997). Mother-teacher congruence in perceptions of the child's competence and school engagement: Links to academic achievement. *Journal of Applied Developmental Psychology,* 18, 373-393.

Pelletier, L. G., Fortier, M. S., Vallerand, R. J., Tuson, K. M., & Brière, N. M. (1995). Toward a new measure of intrinsic motivation, extrinsic motivation, and amotivation in sports: The sport motivation scale (SMS). *Journal of Sport and Exercise Psychology*, 17, 35-53.

Pensgaard, A.M., & Roberts, G.C. (2000). The relationship between motivational climate, perceived ability and sources of distress among elite athletes. *Journal of Sport Sciences*, 18, 191-200.

Pensgaard, A.M., & Roberts, G.C. (2002). Elite athletes' experiences of the motivational climate: The coach matters. *Scandanavian Journal of Medicine and Science in Sport,* 12, 54-59.

Pittman,T.S., Davey, M.E., Alafat, K.A., Wetherill, K.V., & Kramer, N.A. (1980). Informational versus controlling verbal rewards. *Personality and Social Psychology Bulletin,* 6, 228-233.

Pomerantz, E.M., Grolnick, W.S., & Price, C.E. (2005). The role of parents in how children approach achievement: A dynamic process perspective. In A.J. Elliot and C.S. Dweck (Eds.) *Handbook of Competence and Motivation.* (pp. 202-221). Guildford Press, NY: Spring Street.

Pomerantz, E.M., & Eaton, M.M. (2001). Maternal intrusive support in the academic context: Transactional socialization processes. *Developmental Psychology,* 37, 174-186.

Pringle, R. (2000). Physical education, positivism, and optimistic claims from *achievement goal* theorists. Quest, 52, 18-31.

Reeve, J. (2009). *Understanding motivation and emotion.* (5th Edition). New York: John Wiley & Sons.

Reeve, J., Bolt, E., & Cai, Y. (1999). Autonomy-supportive teachers: How they teach and motivate students. *Journal of Educational Psychology,* 91, 537-548.

Reeve, J., Jang, H., Hardre, P., & Omura, M. (2002). Providing a rationale in an autonomy-supportive way as a strategy to motivate others during an uninteresting activity. *Motivation and Emotion,* 26, 183-207.

Reeve, J., & Jang, H. (2006). What teachers say and do to support students' autonomy during learning activities. *Journal of Educational Psychology,* 98, 209-218.

Reeve, J., Nix, G., & Hamm, D. (2003). Testing models of the experience of self-determination in intrinsic motivation and the conundrum of choice. *Journal of Educational Psychology,* 95, 375-392.

Reeve, J., Jang, H., Hardre, P., & Omura, M. (2002). Providing a rationale in an autonomy supportive way as a strategy to motivate others during an uninteresting activity. *Motivation & Emotion,* 26, 183-207.

Reinboth, M., & Duda, J. L. (2006). Perceived motivational climate, need satisfaction and indices of well-being in team sports: A longitudinal perspective. *Psychology of Sport and Exercise*, 7, 269-286.

Reinboth, M., Duda, J.L., & Ntoumanis, N. (2004). Dimensions of coaching behavior, need satisfaction, and the psychological and physical welfare of young athletes. *Motivation and Emotion,* 28, 297-313.

Roberts, G.C. (1992). *Motivation in Sport and Exercise*. Champaign, IL: Human Kinetics.

Roberts, G.C. (1993). Understanding and enhancing the motivation and achievement of children. In R. N. Singer, M. Murphey, & L. K. Tennant (Eds.) *Handbook of research on sport psychology* (pp. 405-420). New York: Macmillan.

Roberts, G.C. (2001). Understanding the dynamics of motivation in physical activity: The influence of achievement goals on motivational processes. In G.C. Roberts (Ed.), *Advances in Motivation in Sport and Exercise*. (pp. 1-50) Champaign, IL; Human Kinetics.

Roberts, G.C., & Balague, G. (1989). *The development of a social-cognitive scale of motivation*. Paper presented at the Seventh World Congress of Sport Psychology. Singapore.

Roberts, G.C., & Balague, G. (1991). The development and validation of the Perception of Success Questionnaire. Paper presented at the *FEPSAC Congress*. Cologne: Germany.

Roberts, G.C. & Ommundsen, Y. (1996). Effect of goal orientations on achievement beliefs, cognitions, and strategies in team sport. *Scandinavian Journal of Medicine and Science in Sport*, 6, 46-56.

Roberts, G.C., & Treasure, D. C. (1992). Children in sport. *Sport Science Review*, 2, 46-64.

Roberts, G. C., Treasure, D. C., & Balague, G. (1998). Achievement goals in sport: The development and validation of the Perception of Success Questionnaire. Journal of Sport Sciences, 16, 337-347.

Roberts, G.C., Treasure, D.C., & Kavussanu, M. (1996). Orthogonality of achievement goals and its relationship to beliefs about success and satisfaction in sport. *The Sport Psychologist*, 10, 398-408.

Rogers, C.R. (1961). *On Becoming a Person: A therapist's view of psychotherapy*. London: Constable.

Rousson, V., Gasser, T., & Seifert, B. (2002). Assessing intra-rater, inter-rater and test-retest reliability of continuous measurements. *Statistical Medicine*, 21, 3431-3446.

Ryan, R.M. (1982). Control and information in the interpersonal sphere: An extension of cognitive evaluation theory. *Journal of Personality and Social Psychology*, 43, 450-461.

Ryan, R. M. (1993). Agency and organization: Intrinsic motivation, autonomy, and the self in psychological development. In R. Dienstbier & J. E. Jacobs (Eds.), Nebraska Symposium on Motivation: Vol. 40. Developmental Perspectives on Motivation (pp. 1-56). Lincoln: University of Nebraska.

Ryan, R. M., & Connell, J. P. (1989). Perceived locus of causality and internalization. *Journal of Personality and Social Psychology*, 57, 749-761.

Ryan, R. M., & Deci, E. L. (2002). An overview of self-determination theory. In E. L. Deci & R. M. Ryan (Eds.), *Handbook of self-determination research* (pp. 3-33). Rochester, NY: University of Rochester Press.

Ryan, R. M., & Deci, E. L. (2008). Active human nature: Self-determination theory and the promotion and maintenance of sport, exercise, and health. In M. S. Hagger & N. L. D. Chatzisarantis (Eds.), *Intrinsic motivation and self-determination in exercise and sport* (pp. 1-19). Champaign, IL: Human Kinetics.

Ryan, R.M., Mims, V., & Koestner, R. (1983). Relation of reward contingency and interpersonal context to intrinsic motivation: A reward and test using cognitive evaluation theory. *Journal of Personality and Social Psychology*, 45, 736-750.

Ryska, T.A., Yin, Z., & Boyd, M. (1999). The role of dispositional goal orientation and team climate on situational self-handicapping among young athletes. *Journal of Sport Behavior*, 22, 410-425.

Sansone, C., Wiebe, D. J., & Morgan, C. (1999). Self-regulating interest: The moderating role of hardiness and conscientiousness. *Journal of Personality*, 61, 701-733.

Sansone, C., Weir, C., Harpster, L., & Morgan, C. (1992). Once a boring task always a boring task?: Interest as a self-regulatory mechanism. *Journal of Personality and Social Psychology*, 63, 379-390.

Sarrazin, P., Vallerand, R., Guillet, E., Pelletier, L., & Cury, F. (2002). Motivation and dropout in female handballers: a 21-month prospective study. *European Journal of Sport Psychology,* 32, 395-418.

Scanlan, T.K., Carpenter, P.J., Lobel, M., & Simons, J.P. (1993). Sources of enjoyment for youth sport athletes. *Pediatric Exercise Science*, 5, 275-28.

Schunk, D.H. (1991). Self-efficacy and academic motivation. *Educational Psychologist*, 26, 207-231.

Seifriz, J.J., Duda, J.L. & Chi, L. (1992). The relationship of perceived motivational climate to intrinsic motivation and beliefs about success in basketball. *Journal of Sport & Exercise Psychology*, 14, 375-391.

Seligman, M.E.P. (1975). *Helplessness: On depression, development and death.* San Fransisco: W.H. Freeman.

Senechal, M., & LeFevre, J. (2002). Parental involvement in the development of children's reading skills: A five year longitudinal study. *Child Development,* 73, 445-460.

Skinner, B.F. (1953). *Science and Human Behavior*. New York: Macmillan.

Skinner, R.A., & Piek, J.P. (2001). Psychosocial implications of poor motor coordination in children and adolescents. *Human Movement Science*, 20, 73-94.

Smith, A.L. (1999). Perceptions of peer relationships and physical activity participation in early adolescence. *Journal of Sport and Exercise Psychology*, 21, 329-350.

Smith, R.E. (1989). Applied sport psychology in an age of accountability. *Journal of Applied Sport Psychology,* 1, 166-180.

Smith, A.L. (2003). Peer relationships in physical activity contexts: a road less travelled in youth sport and exercise psychology research. *Psychology of Sport and Exercise*, 4, 25-39.

Smith, R.E., Cumming, S.P., & Smoll, F.L. (2008). Measurement of motivational climate in youth sports: The Motivational Climate Scale for Youth Sports. *Journal of Applied Sport Psychology*, 11,116-136.

Smith, R.E., Smoll, F.L., & Cumming, S.P. (2007). Effects of a motivational climate intervention for coaches on young athletes' sport performance anxiety. *Journal of Sport and Exercise Psychology*, 29, 39-59.

Smith, R.E., Smoll, F.L., & Cumming, S.P. (2009). Motivational climate and changes in young athletes' achievement goal orientations. *Motivation and Emotion*, 3, 173-183.

Smith, A.L., Ullrich-French, S., Walker, E. & Hurley, K.S. (2006). Peer relationship profiles and motivation in youth sport. *Journal of Sport & Exercise Psychology*, 28, 362-382.

Soenens, B., Vansteenkiste, M., Duriez, B., Luyten, P., & Goosens, L. (2005). Maladaptive perfectionistic self-representations: The meditational link between psychosocial control and adjustment. *Personality and Individual Differences,* 28, 487-498.

Spray, C.M., & Keegan, R.J. (2005). Beyond the dichotomous model of achievement goals in sport and exercise psychology: Comment on Elliot and Conroy (2005). *Sport and Exercise Psychology Review*, 1, 2005, 47-49.

Standage, M., Duda, J.L., & Ntoumanis, N. (2003a). Predicting motivational regulations in physical education: the interplay between dispositional goal orientations, motivational climate and perceived competence. Journal of Sport Sciences, 21, 631-647.

Standage, M., Duda, J.L., & Ntoumanis, N. (2003b). A model of contextual motivation in physical education: Using constructs from self-determination and achievement goal theories to predict physical activity intentions. *Journal of Educational Psychology,* 95(1) 97-110.

Stuntz, C.P., & Weiss, M.R. (2003). Influence of social goal orientations and peers on unsportsmanlike play. *Research Quarterly for Exercise and Sport*, 74, 421-435.

Taleb, N. (2007). *The Black Swan: The Impact of the Highly Improbable.* New York: Random House.

Tauer, J. M., & Harackiewicz, J. M. (2004). The effects of cooperation and competition on intrinsic motivation and performance. *Journal of Personality and Social Psychology, 86,* 849-861.

Taylor, I., & Ntoumanis, N. (2007). Teacher motivational strategies and student self-determination in physical education. *Journal of Educational Psychology,* 99, 747-760.

Tellegen, A. (1985) Structure of mood and personality and their relevance to assessing anxiety, with an emphasis on self-report. In A. H. Tuma and J. D. Maser (eds.) *Anxiety and the Anxiety Disorders* (pp. 681-706). Hillsdale, NJ: Lawrence Erlbaum.

Theeboom, M., De Knop, P., & Weiss, M.R. (1995). Motivational climate, psychological responses, and motor skill development in children's sport: A field-based intervention study. *Journal of Sport and Exercise Psychology,* 17, 294-311.

Tolman, E.C. (1932). *Purposive Behavior in Animals and Men.* New York: Appleton-Century-Crofts.

Todorovich, J. R., & Curtner-Smith, M. D. (2002) Influence of the motivational climate in physical education on sixth grade pupils' goal orientations. *European Physical Education Review*, 8, 119-138.

Treasure, D.C., Duda, J.L., Hall, H.K., Roberts, G.C., Ames, C., & Maehr, M.L. (2001). Clarifying misconceptions and misrepresentations in achievement goal research in sport: A response to Harwood, Hardy, and Swain. *Journal of Sport and Exercise Psychology,* 23, 317-329.

Treasure, D.C., Lemyre, N., Kuczka, K.K., & Standage, M. (2008). Motivation in elite sport: A self-determination perspective. In M.S. Hagger & N. Chatzisarantis (Eds.) *Self-Determination Theory in Exercise and Sport.* (pp 153-166) Champaign, IL: Human Kinetics.

Treasure, D., & Roberts, G.C. (1995). Achievement goals, motivational climate and achievement strategies and behaviour in sport. *International Journal of Sport Psychology,* 26, 64-80.

Treasure, D., & Roberts, G.C. (1998). Relationship between female adolescents' achievement goal orientations, perceptions of the motivational climate, belief about success and sources of satisfaction in basketball. *International Journal of Sport Psychology*, 29, 211-230.

Treasure, D., & Roberts, G.C. (2001). Students' perceptions of the motivational climate, achievement beliefs, and satisfaction in physical education. *Research Quarterly for Exercise and Sport*, 72, 165-175.

Ullrich-French, S. & Smith, A.L. (2006). Perceptions of relationships with parents and peers in youth sport: Independent and combined prediction of motivational outcomes. *Psychology of Sport and Exercise,* 7, 193-214.

Urdan, T., & Maehr, M. L. (*1995*). Beyond a two-goal theory of motivation: A case for social goals. *Review of Educational Research*, 65, 213-244.

Valentini, N.C., & Rudisill, M.E. (2004a). An inclusive mastery climate intervention and the motor skill development of children with and without disabilities. *Adapted Physical Activity Quarterly*, 21, 330-347.

Valentini, N.C., & Rudisill, M.E. (2004b). Motivational climate, motor-skill development, and perceived competence: Two studies of developmentally delayed kindergarten children. *Journal of Teaching in Physical Education*, 23, 216-234.

Vallerand, R.J. (1993). La motivation intrinsèque et extrinsèque en context naturel. Implications pour les secteurs de l'éducation, du travail, des relations interpersonalles et des loisirs [Intrinsic and extrinsic motivation in natural setting: Implications for education, work, interpersonal relationships and leisure.] In R.J. Vallerand and E.E. Thill (Eds.) *Introduction à la psychologie de la motivation.* (pp. 533-581). Laval (Quebec): Edition Etudes Vivantes.

Vallerand, R.J. (1997). Toward a hierarchical model of intrinsic and extrinsic motivation. In M. Zanna (Ed.) *Advances in Experimental Social Psychology*, 271-360. New York: Academic Press.

Vallerand, R. J. (2007). Intrinsic and extrinsic motivation in sport and physical activity: A review and a look at the future. In G. Tenenbaum, & E. Eklund (Eds.), *Handbook of sport psychology* (3rd ed., pp. 49-83). New York: John Wiley.

Vallerand, R.J., & Fortier, M.S. (1998). Measures of intrinsic and extrinsic motivation in sport and physical activity: A review and critique. In J. Duda (Ed.) *Advances in Sport and Exercise Psychology Measurement.* (pp. 83-100) Morgantown WV: Fitness Information Technology.

Vallerand, R. J., Gauvin, L. I., & Halliwell, W. R. (*1986*). Negative effects of competition on children's intrinsic motivation. *Journal of Social Psychology,* 126, 649-657.

Vallerand, R. J., Pelletier, L. G., Blais, M. R., Briere, N. M., Senecal, C., & Valliéres, E. F. (1992). The academic motivation scale: A measure of intrinsic, extrinsic, and amotivation in education. *Educational and Psychological Measurement*, *52*, 1003-1017.

Vallerand, R. J., Pelletier, L. G., Blais, M. R., Briere, N. M., Senecal, C., & Valliéres, E. F. (1993). On the assessment of intrinsic, extrinsic, and amotivation in education: Evidence on the concurrent and construct validity of the academic motivation scale. *Educational & Psychological Measurement*, *53*, 159-172.

Vallerand, R. J., & Reid, G. (1984). On the causal effects of perceived competence on intrinsic motivation: A test of cognitive evaluation theory. *Journal of Sport Psychology*, *6*, 94-102.

Vallerand, R.J., & Thill, E.E. (1993). Introduction au concept du motivation [Introduction to the concept of motivation]. In R.J. Vallerand and E.E. Thill (Eds.) *Introduction à la psychologie de la motivation.* (pp. 3-39). Laval (Quebec): Edition Etudes Vivantes.

Vansteenkiste, M., Soenens, B., & Lens, W. (2008). Intrinsic versus extrinsic goal promotion in sport and exercise: Understanding their differential impact on performance and persistence. In M. S. Hagger and N. Chatzisarantis (Eds.) *Self-determination theory in exercise and sport.* Human Kinetics.

Vazou, S., Ntoumanis, N., & Duda J.L. (2005). Peer motivational climate in youth sport: A qualitative inquiry. *Psychology of Sport & Exercise*, 6, 497-516.

Walling, M.D., Duda, J.L. & Chi, L. (1993). The Perceived Motivational Climate in Sport Questionnaire: Construct and predictive validity. *Journal of Sport and Exercise Psychology*, 15, 172- 183.

Wason, P.C. (1960). On the failure to eliminate hypotheses in a conceptual task. *Quarterly Journal of Experimental. Psychology*, 12, 129-140.

Wason, P. C. (1966). Reasoning. In B. M. Foss (Ed.) *New horizons in psychology*. Harmondsworth: Penguin.

Watson, J. B. (1913). Psychology as the behaviorist views it. *Psychological Review*, 20, 158-177.

Watson, D., & Clark, L.A. (1993). Behavioral disinhibition versus constraint: A dispositional perspective. In D. M. Wegner & J. W. Pennebaker (Eds.), *Handbook of mental control* (pp. 506-527). New York: Prentice-Hall

Weinberg, R., & Ragan, J. (1979). Effects of competition, success failure and sex on intrinsic motivation. *Research Quarterly in Exercise and Sport,* 50, 505-510.

Weiner, B. (1979). A theory of motivation for some classroom experiences. *Journal of Educational Psychology, 71, 3-25.*

Weiner, B. (1985). An attributional theory of achievement motivation and emotion. *Psychological Review*, 92, 548-573.

Weiner, B. (1986). *An attributional theory of motivation and emotion*. New York: Springer-Verlag.

Weiner, B. (1990). History of motivational research in education. *Journal of Educational Psychology*. 82, 616–622.

Weiner, B. (1995). Judgments of responsibility: A foundation for a theory of social conduct. New York: Guilford

Weiss, M.R., & Amorose, AJ. (2008). Motivational orientations and sport behaviour. In T.S. Horn (Ed.), *Advances in sport psychology* (2nd ed., pp. 115-156). Champaign, IL: Human Kinetics.

Weiss, M.R., Bredemeier, B.J., & Shewchuk, R.M. (1985). An intrinsic/extrinsic motivation scale for the youth sport setting: a confirmatory factor analysis, *Journal of Sport Psychology,* **7**, 75–91.

Weiss, M.R., & Smith, A.L. (2002). Friendship quality in youth sport: Relationship to age, gender, and motivation variables. *Journal of Sport & Exercise Psychology, 24*, 420-437

Weiss, M.R., Smith, A.L., & Theeboom, M. (1996). "That's what friends are for": Children's and teenagers' perceptions of peer relationships in the sport domain. *Journal of Sport & Exercise Psychology,* 18, 347-379.

Weiss, M.R., & Ferrer-Caja, E. (2002). Motivational orientations and sport behavior. In T.S. Horn (Ed.), *Advances in sport psychology* (2nd ed., pp. 101-183). Champaign, IL: Human Kinetics.

Wentzel, K. R. (1993). Social and academic goals at school: Motivation and achievement in early adolescence. *Journal of Early Adolescence*, 13, 4-20.

Wentzel, K.R. (1999). Social-motivational processes and interpersonal relationships: Implications for understanding motivation at school. Journal of Educational Psychology 91, 76-97.

Wentzel, K.R. (2005). Peer relationships, motivation, and academic performance at school. . In A.J. Elliot and C.S. Dweck (Eds.) *Handbook of Competence and Motivation.* (pp. 279-297). Guildford Press, NY: Spring Street.

Wentzel, K. R., Barry, C. M., & Caldwell, K. A. (2004). Friendships in middle school: Influences on motivation and school adjustment. *Journal of Educational Psychology,* 96, 195-203.

Wentzel, K.R., & Caldwell, K. (1997). Friendships, peer acceptance, and group membership: Relations to academic achievement in middle school. *Child Development,* 68, 1198-1209.

Wheeler, L., Reis, H.T., & Nezlek, J. (1983). Loneliness, social interaction and sex roles. *Journal of Personality and Social Psychology*, 45, 943-953.

White, R.W. (1959). Motivation reconsidered: The concept of competence. *Psychological Review,* 66, 297-333.

White, S.A. (1996). Goal orientation and perceptions of the motivational climate initiated by parents. *Pediatric Exercise Science*, 8, 122- 129.

White, S.A. (1998). Adolescent goal profiles, perceptions of the parent initiated motivational climate and competitive trait anxiety. *The Sport Psychologist*, 12, 16-28.

White, S.A., Duda, J.L. & Hart, S. (1992). An exploratory examination of the parent-initiated motivational climate questionnaire. *Perceptual and Motor Skills*, 75, 875- 880.

Whitehead, J. Andrée, K. V., & Lee, M. J. (2004). Achievement perspectives and perceived ability: How far do interactions generalise in youth sport? *Psychology of Sport and Exercise*, 5, 291-317.

Wilko, A.M. (2004). *Influence of coaching behaviours and motivational climate on female adolescent athletes' psychosocial responses*. Unpublished master's thesis, University of West Virginia, Charlottesville.

Williams, L. (1998). Contextual influences and goal perspectives among female youth sport participants. *Research Quarterly for Exercise & Sport*, 69, 47-57.

Wilson, P. M, Rodgers, W.M, Hall, C.R, & Gammage, K.L. (2003). Do autonomous exercise regulations underpin different types of exercise imagery? *Journal of Applied Sport Psychology*, 15, 294-306.

Wigfield, A., & Eccles, J.S., (1992). The development of achievement task values: A theoretical analysis, *Developmental Review,* 12, 265-310.

Williams, L. (1998). Contextual influences and goal perspectives among female youth sport participants. *Research Quarterly for Exercise & Sport*, 69, 47-57.

Winsler, A., Diaz, R.M., McCarthy, E.M., Atencio, D.J., & Chabay, L.A. (1999). Mother-child interaction, private speech, and task performance in preschool children with behavior problems. *Journal of Psychology and Psychiatry and Allied Disciplines,* 40, 891-904.

Wylleman, P., Alfermann, D., Lavallee, D. (2004). Career transitions in sport: European perspectives. *Psychology of Sport and Exercise*, 5, 7-20.

Wylleman, P., De Knop, P., Ewing, M., & Cumming, S. (2000). Transitions in youth sport: a developmental perspective on parental involvement. In D. Lavallee, & P. Wylleman (Eds.), *Career transitions in sport: International perspectives* (pp. 143–160). Morgantown, WV: Fitness Information Technology.

Xiang, P., & Lee, A. (2002). Achievement goals, perceived motivational climate, and students' self-reported mastery behaviours. *Research Quarterly for Exercise and Sport*, 73, 58-65.

Yoo, J. (1999). Motivational-behavioral correlates of goal orientation and perceived motivational climate in physical education contexts. *Perceptual and Motor Skills*, 89, 262-274.

Zuckerman, M., Porac, J., Lathin, D., Smith, R., & Deci, E.L. (1978). On the importance of self-determination for intrinsically motivated behaviour. *Personality and Social Psychology Bulletin,* 4, 443-446.

In: Encyclopedia of Sports and Athletics
Editors: Jack L. Murray and Emily O. Watson

ISBN: 978-1-61209-959-0

Chapter XIX

Being Superstitious in Sports: Effect of Superstitious Beliefs on Athletes' Cognitive and Affective Responses

Vassilis Barkoukis[1*], *Stefanos Perkos*[2] *and Sotiris Kokkinopoulos*[1]
[1] Aristotle University of Thessaloniki, Greece
[2] University of Thessaly, Greece

Abstract

Superstition can be defined as a person's unrealistic perception of control over behavioral outcomes in different situations. Although it is assumed that superstitious beliefs may help athletes prepare for a competition, they represent a rather unexplored area in sport psychology. The aim of the present study was to investigate the influence of superstitious beliefs on several performance-related dispositions, such as achievement goals, locus of control, self-handicapping and trait anxiety, and then examine the moderating role of athletes' age and years of competitive experience. The sample of the study consisted of 297 male basketball athletes (M = 23.86, SD = 4.63) participating in Greek professional leagues. The athletes completed a questionnaire regarding measures of positive and negative superstitious beliefs, self-handicapping strategies, internal and external locus of control and luck, achievement goals and trait anxiety. The results of the regression analyses indicated that positive superstitious beliefs significantly predicted self-handicapping and external locus of control. Negative superstitious beliefs were significant predictors of somatic anxiety, worry, and performance avoidance goals. Moderation regression analysis further indicated that the effect of superstitious beliefs on worry was stronger among athletes with less sports experience. The present study provides valuable information regarding the role of superstitious beliefs in better understanding athletes' cognitive and affective responses, and sets the basis for future research in this rather unexplored area.

* Correspondence should be addressed to Vassilis Barkoukis,
Aristotle University of Thessaloniki, Greece
Email: bark@phed.auth.gr, telephone: +30 2310 992225

Paranormal beliefs reflect a person's belief in phenomena that contradict the basic principles of scientific thinking (Broad, 1953). Those beliefs include superstition (i.e., black cats and breaking mirrors cause bad luck), precognition (i.e., psychics and astrologers can predict the future), extra sensory perception and a range of similar phenomena (i.e., some people can move objects with the power of their mind) (Dudley, 1999). In other words, superstitious beliefs reflect people's tendency to make causal inferences and offer explanations for several phenomena without necessarily taking into account, or even sometimes by contradicting, scientific evidence pointing to alternative and more scientifically-grounded explanations (Zebb & Moore, 2003; see Lindeman & Aarnio, 2007 for a more detailed presentation of superstitious beliefs' definitions).

Past research has shown that superstitious beliefs are associated with adverse psychological outcomes, such as low self-efficacy (Tobacyk & Shrader, 1991), high trait anxiety and dissociative experiences (Wolfradt, 1997), irrational beliefs (Roig, Bridges, Renner, & Jackson, 1998) and external locus of control (Dag, 1999; Tobacyk, Nagot, & Miller, 1988). On the other hand, Dudley (1999) found that higher scores in superstitious beliefs can help improve performance in solving puzzles during instances of uncontrollability because they may prevent this lack of control. The evidenced effect of superstitious beliefs on task performance may have implications for the study of athletes' performance in sports.

Nevertheless, research in this area is scarce. An early study by Neil, Anderson, and Sheppard (1981) showed that highly competitive ice hockey athletes were keen on adopting superstitious behaviours, such as rituals. In another study, Buhrmann and Zaugg (1983) suggested that higher scores in religiosity led to stronger superstitious beliefs among basketball players. Van Raalte, Brewer, Nemeroff, and Linder (1991) further indicated that people who believed they could control chance events through their actions were more likely to adopt superstitious behaviors. Ciborowski (1997) suggested that athletes tend to adopt superstitious behaviors as a way to improve their performance, without necessarily admitting a direct connection between the adopted behavior and their actual sports performance. More interestingly, he reported that if an individual believed that a particular behavior could improve performance, that behavior should not be considered superstitious. Furthermore, Bleak and Frederick (1998) reported that the use of superstitious rituals varied across sports, and that the most frequently used superstitious behaviors were not necessarily the ones that were rated by the athletes to be most effective in improving sport performance. Finally, a more recent study (Foster, Weigand, & Baines, 2006) indicated that superstitious beliefs significantly affected performance in free-throw shot in basketball.

Uncertainty and lack of control have been proliferated as important determinants of superstitious beliefs, similar to the experience of anxiety (Martens, Vealey & Burton, 1990; Spielberger, 1972), In fact, superstitious beliefs may increase during periods of ambiguity, uncertainty, or uncontrollability (Dudley, 1999), and soothe people by providing an illusory sense of control, or at least an explanation of why events are uncontrollable. In simple words, in the face of uncertainty, individuals attempt to achieve control by investing in irrelevant objects or actions, resting on the assumption that there exists a causal link between those objects or actions and particular results (Ciborowski, 1997; Wright & Erdal 2008).

Despite anecdotal reports published in newspapers and magazines on the influence of superstitious beliefs on sport performance, there is only limited scientific evidence about sport-related superstitions (Foster et al., 2006). For instance, Ciborowski (1997) and Schippers and Van Lange (2006) found that elite athletes are more likely to employ superstitious rituals in high uncertainty and anxiety-provoking situations, as well as in important competitions. Additionally, anxiety was also associated with the use of rituals (Schippers & Van Lange, 2006). Athletes' skill level and task difficulty were also found to influence superstitious beliefs. Specifically, low skill athletes in an easy condition and high skill athletes in difficult condition had the higher scores in superstitious behavior (Wright & Erdal, 2008). Contrary to this evidence, Bleak and Frederick (1998) reported that the use of rituals was not associated with anxiety or perceived importance of success in collegiate athletes.

Trait Anxiety in Sport

Anxiety is an area of major concern that is heavily researched in sport psychology. Early work on anxiety distinguished between two important facets, namely state and trait anxiety (Spielberger, 1966). State anxiety was described as an unpleasant emotional state elicited by a nonspecific and nonconscious danger (May, 1977), or as the emotional reaction evoked by a stimulus that is perceived to be threatening (irrespectively of its objective nature) (Spielberger, 1972). State anxiety is characterized by arousal of the autonomic nervous system, which is accompanied by feelings of tension and apprehension, as well as unpleasant and negative thoughts (Martens et al., 1990). On the other hand, trait anxiety refers to 'differences in the disposition to perceive a wide range of stimulus situations as dangerous or threatening, and in the tendency to respond to such threats with state anxiety reactions' (Spielberger, 1972, p. 39).

Most research in sport psychology has focused on the effects of state anxiety on sport performance, where its negative effect has been well documented (Woodman & Hardy, 2001). Another venue in anxiety research concerns the effect of trait anxiety on state anxiety and performance. Research evidence suggested that athletes with higher trait anxiety scores were more likely to react with elevated levels of state anxiety in a threatening situation and, hence, perform poorly, as compared to athletes with lower scores in trait anxiety (Hanton, Mellalieu & Hall, 2002; Martinent & Ferrand, 2007). Similarly to state anxiety, there have been identified two dimensions of trait anxiety, somatic (i.e., physiological and affective elements of anxiety) and cognitive anxiety (worry; negative expectations about performance, cognitive concerns about oneself and negative self-evaluation, cognitive concerns about the situation at hand and the consequences of a potential failure) (Smith, Smoll, & Schutz, 1990).

Although there is some research linking trait anxiety with performance (Robazza & Bortoli, 2007) and situational and performance-related responses, such as attention (Hainaut, Monfort, & Bolmont, 2006), perfectionism (Martinent & Ferrand, 2007), and chocking (Wang, Marchant, Morris & Gibbs, 2004), there is limited evidence on the antecedents of competitive trait anxiety.

Achievement Goal Theory (AGT)

AGT states that the demonstration of competence is the main criterion defining success in achievement contexts. In the original achievement goal approach, two independent goal orientations, namely, task and ego goal orientations were identified (Ames, 1984; Dweck, 1986; Nicholls, 1989). Individuals adopting task orientation engage in an achievement activity in order to achieve personal development and master the tasks at hand. The criteria of success are self-referenced; that is, involvement is successful when the individual improves performance. On the other hand, individuals adopting ego orientation become involved in an activity to demonstrate superior ability compared to others (Nicholls, 1989). In this case the criteria are normative or comparative and outperforming others is defined as success. Substantial research provided evidence that task orientation is related to more adaptive motivational outcomes such as greater effort and persistence (Williams & Gill, 1995), fair play (Smith, Hall & Wilson, 1999), greater enjoyment (Duda, Chi, Newton, Walling & Catlin, 1995), and lower anxiety (Ommundsen & Pedersen, 1999) (see Duda & Hall, 2001, for a detailed review).

Elliot and his colleagues (Elliot, 1997; Elliot & Church, 1997; Elliot & Thrash, 2001) argued that the dichotomous approach to achievement goals (i.e., task and ego orientations) does not address adequately the valence of achievement goals in a specific context. They suggested that ego orientation should be divided into two distinct categories, reflecting approach and avoidance goals respectively. This model, labelled the hierarchical model of approach and avoidance achievement motivation, identified three goals: mastery goals, performance-approach, and performance-avoidance goals. Mastery goals are conceptually similar to task orientation (Barkoukis, Ntoumanis & Nikitaras, 2007) and reflect involvement with an activity for self-improvement and mastery. Performance-approach goals are similar to ego orientation (Barkoukis et al., 2007), and reflect engagement in an activity to demonstrate superior competence relative to others. Finally, performance-avoidance goals reflect the tendency to avoid demonstrating low competence and poor performance (Elliot, 1997; Elliot & Church, 1997). Research evidence has provided empirical support for the hierarchical model of approach and avoidance achievement motivation, and indicated that performance-approach and performance-avoidance goals have differential effect on several responses such as intrinsic motivation (Cury, Elliot, Sarrazin, Da Fonséca & Rufo, 2002; Elliot & Harackiewicz, 1996), competence valuation, state anxiety, and task absorption (Cury et al., 2002; Cury, Da Fonséca, Rufo, Peres & Sarrazin, 2003) and academic performance (Elliot & Church, 1997). These findings suggest that mastery and performance-approach goals construe an approach orientation and they are associated with adaptive responses. On the contrary, performance-avoidance goals construe an avoidance orientation that negatively affects involvement in an achievement context. Rawsthorne and Elliot's (1999) meta-analysis provided further support to these findings.

Elliot and McGregor (2001) further extended this approach by applying the approach-avoidance distinction to mastery goals. The so-called 2 X 2 achievement goal model includes four achievement goals: mastery-approach, mastery-avoidance, performance-approach, and performance-avoidance goals. The newly introduced concept of mastery-avoidance goals reflects an individual's emphasis on avoiding lack of improvement and task failure. Research evidence with the 2 X 2 model indicated that mastery-avoidance goals were associated with negative responses, thus suggesting that they construe an avoidance orientation (Cury, Elliot, Da Fonséca & Moller, 2006; Elliot & McGregor, 2001).

The 2 X 2 model is the current epitome of achievement goal literature with substantial research in educational settings (Elliot & McGregor, 2001; Finney, Pieper, & Barron, 2004, Chen, Wu, Kee, Lin, & Shui, 2009). However, it is a rather unexplored approach in sport psychology. Although Conroy, Elliot, and Hofer (2003) provided a psychometrically sound instrument to measure the four achievement goals in sport contexts, research with athletes did not endorse this approach. In their study Conroy et al. (2003) further showed that performance-approach, performance-avoidance and mastery-avoidance goals were positively related to fear of failure. Stoeber, Stoll, Pescheck and Otto (2008) showed that approach goals (mastery and performance) were positively associated with striving for perfection, whereas both avoidance goals were positively associated with negative reactions to imperfection. In addition, Mouratidou, Barkoukis and Rizos (in press) indicated that athletes adopting performance (approach and avoidance) goals showed lower moral competence. Recent research has investigated the antecedents of the four achievement goals. Conroy, Kaye and Coatsworth (2006) found that athletes were more likely to adopt avoidance goals when they perceived their coach to emphasize these goals, and Morris and Kavussanu (2008) indicated that each achievement goal was predicted by different aspects of parent and team motivational climate with mastery goals showing a more positive profile compared to performance goals. To the best of our knowledge, there is no research evidence linking the four achievement goals with superstitious beliefs.

Self-Handicapping Strategies

Self-handicapping has been defined as 'an individual's attempt to reduce a threat to esteem by actively seeking or creating inhibitory factors that interfere with performance and thus provide a persuasive causal explanation for failure' (Arkin & Baumgardner, 1985, p. 170). Several behaviors and dispositions have been proliferated as typical self-handicapping strategies, including procrastination, lack of effort or practice, illness, shyness, excuses, moodiness, drug or alcohol use, lack of sleep, and overinvolvement with friends or activities (Urdan & Midgley, 2001). The use of such strategies helps individuals to maintain a sense of control when confronted with social comparison (Ryska, 2002). In this sense, athletes attribute potential failure to other-referent and uncontrollable factors, whereas self-referent factors (i.e., ability or intelligence) are not blamed for performance failure. Conversely, athletes using self-handicapping strategies attribute success to high ability as it has been achieved despite the presence of performance-debilitating obstacles (Ryska 2002). Self-handicapping may be elicited by prior non-contingent successes, performance uncertainty, adoption of performance goals, and public self-consciousness (see Elliot & Church, 2003 for a more detailed review) or the individual's attempt to protect his self-worth (Martin, Marsh & Debus, 2003).

To date, self-handicapping in sport has been treated as a coping strategy that is likely to yield both costs and benefits to the athlete. For instance, Bailis (2001) suggested that self-handicapping was positively associated with performance besides the positive relationship with poorer practice and nutrition before important events during the competitive season. Yet, the vast majority of research in sport implied a negative association of self-handicapping with event-related preparatory factors such as emotion-oriented coping strategies (Prapavessis, Grove, Maddison, & Zillman, 2003), lowering practice effort prior to important events (Rhodewalt, Saltzman, & Wittmer, 1984), strong perceptions of team cohesion that posed a threat on the athlete to perform well (Hausenblas & Carron, 1996; Carron, Prapavessis, & Grove, 1994), lower levels of mastery and higher of performance goals (Ryska, Yin, & Boyd, 1999; Thill & Cury, 2000), lower levels of mastery-involving motivational climate, self-efficacy, and perceived event importance (Kuczka & Treasure (2005), negative precompetitive mood states such as anxiety (Prapavessis & Grove, 1994; Prapavessis et al., 2003; Ryska, Yin, & Cooley, 1998) and lower performance (Ryska, 2002). This research evidence led Kuczka and Treasure (2005) to conceptualize self-handicapping as a maladaptive coping strategy due to placing the self-handicapping athlete at-risk for motivational difficulties that may have a negative effect on long-term involvement and performance.

Locus of Control

Based on Rotter's (1966) original theory, locus of control can be defined as people's belief that outcomes are either internally controlled by personal agency and effort or externally controllable by chance factors or other outside forces. Locus of control is assumed to be a bipolar structure with internal (i.e., what happens in life is the outcome of personal efforts and abilities) and external (i.e., what happens in life is the result of chance or external forces uncontrolled by the person) locus of control being respectively placed at the two opposites of a continuum. People with internal locus of control, therefore, tend to perceive their life as internally controllable, whereas those with external locus of control are more likely to attribute their life outcomes to external forces, such as other people, luck, chance, or fate (Lefcourt, 1991).

Research in sport psychology has utilized locus of control in several domains, and the findings suggest that internal locus of control tends to be associated with positive outcomes. More specifically, Lambert, Moore and Dixon (1999) investigated the link between locus of control and self- or other-set goals in gymnastics. The findings indicated that gymnasts with a more internal locus of control spent relatively more time working with the task under the self-set goal condition while those with a more external locus of control spent more time working with the task when the coach set their goals. Similarly, high school athletes with an internal locus of control were more likely to meet their goals in a meeting camp and avoid injury during training (Labbe & Welsh, 1991). Furthermore, locus of control seems to be related to the athletes' age. Stewart and Meyers (2004) suggested that older and more experienced athletes demonstrated higher levels of internal locus of control compared to younger athletes, who were more likely to attribute control to luck and other external sources.

Brandwein (2003) investigated the association of locus of control with achievement goals and sportspersonship. The results from this study showed that mastery oriented athletes were more likely to have an internal locus of control and demonstrate a more moral profile. Finally, athletes with an internal locus of control were approaching their competitive activity in a more positive way, as compared to athletes with an external locus of control. Furthermore, after investigating the relationship of locus of control with psychological traits such as self-esteem and trait anxiety, Kerr and Goss (1997) found that external locus of control was negatively associated with self-esteem, and positively correlated with trait anxiety. Extending these findings, Ntoumanis and Jones (1998) suggested that the direction of the anxiety experience is more closely associated with locus of control. Sport performers with internal locus of control perceived their trait anxiety as more facilitative and less debilitative than those with an external locus of control, while no significant differences were found in the intensity of trait anxiety experience.

Contrary to these findings suggesting that internal locus of control is associated with more adaptive responses, Van Raalte et al., (1991) reported that internal locus of control was also associated with superstitious behaviour. They conducted an experiment to test whether chance orientation in golf can affect superstitious behavior. Interestingly, the results of this experiment indicated that sport participants with higher internal locus of control were more likely to use a "lucky ball" following a successful attempt. Similarly, Granito and Carlton (1993) did not find any differences between internals and externals in terms of satisfaction with the team and competitive level.

The Present Study

Superstitious beliefs are considered as a core personality characteristic, associated with religiosity and a deep view of the self and its position in the world, that can affect individual's dispositional and situational responses (Dudley, 1999; Lindeman & Aarnio, 2007). The effect of such beliefs is increased in situations of uncertainty and uncontrollability such as in competitive sport (Dudley, 1999). Hence, in the present study we investigated the effect of superstitious beliefs on elite athletes' cognitive and affective responses. More specifically, the aim of the present study was to examine the effect of positive and negative superstitious beliefs on competitive trait anxiety, locus of control, self-handicapping and achievement goal orientations in competitive basketball. Athletes that compete regularly under such conditions of uncertainty and uncontrollability may have developed dispositions characterized by elevated levels of competitive trait anxiety (Zebb & Moore, 2003; Schippers &Van Lange, 2006) and high tendency for using self-handicapping strategies. Therefore, superstitious athletes were assumed to report high levels of competitive trait anxiety and self-handicapping strategies (hypothesis 1).

Furthermore, situations of uncertainty and uncontrollability and, thus, the use of superstitious rituals are closely associated with external types of locus of control (Dag, 1999). It was expected that superstitious athletes would attribute success and/or failure to external reasons such as the effectiveness of the rituals, charms etc. Hence, although Van Raalte et al. (1991) suggested that the superstitious behaviors are positively related to internal locus of control, we assumed that athletes high in superstitious beliefs would attribute sport-related events on external sources such as others' behavior, fate or luck. Consequently, we hypothesized that high superstitious beliefs would have a positive effect on external locus of control and luck, and a negative or neutral effect on internal locus of control (hypothesis 2).

Achievement goal orientations could also be affected by superstitious beliefs as they represent perceptions of success and failure which can be attributed to the uncertainty and the lack of control of the situation. Conceptually, avoidance goals are expected to be elicited by maladaptive thoughts and beliefs (Elliot, 1997; Elliot & Church, 1997). Based on these theoretical predictions and research evidence we hypothesized that superstitious beliefs will have a positive effect on performance avoidance goals and a negative or neutral effect on mastery approach and performance approach ones (hypothesis 3). No hypothesis was set for mastery avoidance goals since there are no concrete research findings regarding the antecedents of this type of achievement goal.

A secondary purpose of the present study was to examine the moderating role of athletes' age and competitive experience in the superstitious beliefs – cognitive and affective responses relationships. Research evidence has indicated that as athletes grow older and gain more experience they change their views, thoughts and beliefs regarding their sport. For instance,

Kavussanu, Seal and Phillips (2006) and Mouratidou et al. (in press) provided evidence that older and more experienced athletes showed less moral competence compared to younger and less experienced ones. Based on these findings, which suggest that older and more experienced athletes form a more maladaptive profile of cognitions and affect, we hypothesized that athletes' age and years and experience would moderate the superstitious beliefs – cognitive and affective responses relationship with older and more experienced athletes showing the more maladaptive profile (hypothesis 4).

Method

Participants

Two hundred ninety seven (N=297) male basketball athletes participated in this study. Athletes' mean age was 23.86 years (SD = 4.63). The athletes were recruited from 27 teams participating in the Greek national leagues. All athletes were participating regularly to team's practices. Mean experience in national leagues was 12.72 years (SD = 6.45).

Measures

Superstitious Beliefs

The Paranormal Beliefs Scale (PBS) of Tobacyk (1988) was used to measure athletes' superstitious beliefs. PBS consists of six items measuring positive (3 items) and negative (3 items) beliefs. An example item of negatives superstitious beliefs was "*Do you avoid walking under a ladder because they say that it brings bad luck?*" while an example of positive ones was "*Do you say 'touch wood' or actually touch wood?*" Participant's responded on a 5-point Likert scale ranging from 1 (*definitely no*) to 5 (*definitely yes*).

Achievement Goals

Conroy's et al.'s (2003) Achievement Goals Questionnaire for Sport was used to assess the four goals in the 2 x 2 approach. The questionnaire consists of 12 items (3 items per each achievement goal). The original questionnaire was adapted according to Elliot and Murayama (2008) suggestions to more accurately estimate athletes' strivings during sport involvement. Example items are "*My goal is to perform as well as I possibly can*" for the mastery-approach goal, "*My objective is to perform better than the others athletes*" for the performance approach goal, "*My goal is to avoid not performing as well as I possibly can*" for the mastery avoidance goal and "*My aim is to avoid performing worst than the others athletes*" for the performance avoidance goal. Participants responses were anchored on a 7-point Likert scale ranging from 1 (*strongly disagree*) to 7 (*totally agree*). Mouratidou, et al. (in press) provided evidence on the factorial validity and reliability of the scale with Greek athletes.

Trait Anxiety

The 21 items Sport Anxiety Scale (SAS; Smith, et al., 1990) was used. This scale assesses three dimensions of competitive trait anxiety: somatic anxiety (9 items; example item "*My stomach feels tense*"), worry (7 items; example item "*I worry if I cannot stand the pressure of the game*") and concentration disruption (5 items; example item "*During games various thoughts about bad performance have a negative effect on my concentration*"). Participants responded on a 4-point Likert scale ranging from 1 (*not at all*) to 4 (*very much*). Grouios and Barkoukis (manuscript under preparation) provided support to the factorial validity (CFI = .90, SRMR = .056, RMSEA = .072) and reliability of the scale (aphas > .70) and suggested its use with Greek athletes.

Self-Handicapping Strategies

An adapted to competitive sport version of Midgley et al.'s (1996) scale was used to measure self-handicapping. The scale consists of six items measuring one single factor (example item: "*Some athletes do not try hard during practices so that if they don't do well on competitions, they can say that is the reason. How true is this of you?*" Participants responded on a 5-point Likert scale ranging from 1 (*not true for me*) to 5 (*very true for me*).

Locus of Control

An adaptation to competitive sport of the Exercise Objectives Locus of Control Scale developed by Doganis, Theodorakis and Bagiatis (1991) was used to measure locus of control in the athletes of the sample. This scale assesses two main orientations, internal and external locus of control. External locus of control is further divided into three categories, luck, coach and other people. The scale consists of 18 items (6 items for internal locus of control, 6 items for luck, 3 items for coach and 3 items for other people). The athletes responded to the stem "Performing according to my ability in competition depends ...". Example items include "*...on my own actions*" for internal locus of control, "*...on my coach's training program*" for coach, "*...on how lucky I will be*" for luck and "*...on other people mostly*" for other people. Responses were given on a 5-point Likert scale ranging from 1 (*definitely no*) to 5 (*definitely yes*).

Procedure

Team managers were contacted and permission was granted to administer the questionnaire to athletes. The questionnaire was administered to athletes in quiet conditions in locker rooms by the researchers prior to the evening practice. The training staff was not present. Both oral and written instructions were provided to athletes regarding questionnaire's completion. According to APA guidelines, athletes were reassured about the confidentiality of their responses and were informed on their right to withdraw from the study any time they wish. No one athlete withdrew from the study. The completion of the questionnaire lasted approximately 15 minutes.

Results

Psychometric Properties of the Scales

The confirmatory factor analysis (CFA) was used in order to test the factorial validity of the superstitious beliefs and locus of control scales. CFA was conducted via EQS, 6.1

structural equation modeling computer program (Bentler, 2004). Both absolute and incremental indices were used to examine the factorial validity of the scales. The Comparative Fit Index (CFI), the Standardized Root Mean-square Residual (SRMR) and Root Mean Square Error of Approximation (RMSEA) were used as more appropriate indices to evaluate the adequacy of models as, contrary to χ^2, they are not influenced by sample size (Fan, Thompson, & Wang, 1999). The comparative fit index (CFI) was used as a focal index of goodness-of-fit, as it has a standardized 0-1 range, small sample variability, and stability with various sample sizes (Bentler, 2004). CFI scores of .90 or above are considered acceptable for model fit with scores above .95 indicating excellent fit (Hu & Bentler, 1999). For SRMR and RMSEA scores close or below .05 and .08 respectively are considered appropriate for satisfactory model fit (Hu & Bentler, 1999).

Regarding the Paranormal Beliefs Scale, the results of the CFA supported the two-factor structure of the scale. Two models were tested, a measurement model assuming the factors to be uncorrelated and a 2-factor correlated model assuming the presence of positive and negative superstitious beliefs. The results regarding the measurement model provided low and unacceptable fit indices. Regarding the 2-factor correlated model the results indicated that although the χ^2 was statistically significant ($\chi^2(6) = 28.94$, $p < .001$) the absolute and incremental fit indices were at acceptable levels. The CFI exceeded the criterion of excellent model fit (CFI = .963) and the SRMR was accordingly low (SRMR = .03). The RMSEA was relatively high (RMSEA = .11) suggesting that the addition of further items would help the model achieve better fit. Nevertheless, these findings provide support to the factorial validity of the scale. The investigation of the internal consistency provided adequate and satisfactory values for both subscales (alpha > .70) (see Table 1).

To test for the factorial validity of the adapted version of the Exercise Objectives Locus of Control Scale three models were tested, a measurement model assuming that the factors are not correlated, a 2-factor correlated model including internal locus of control and external locus of control and a 4-factor correlated model assuming that external locus of control should be further divided on attributions to luck, coach and other people. The results of the CFA revealed low and unacceptable scores for the measurement and 2-factor correlated models. On the contrary, the results of the analysis provided support to the 4-factor correlated model. Although the χ^2 was significant ($\chi^2(115) = 464.04$, $p < .001$), the absolute and incremental fit indices were at borderline but acceptable levels. The CFI was above the .90 criterion of acceptable model fit (CFI = .912) and the SRMR and the RMSEA were also close to acceptable levels (SRMR = .07, RMSEA = .10). These findings provide support to the factorial validity of the scale. The internal consistency coefficients of the subscales were high and acceptable supporting scale's reliability (alpha > .70) (see Table 1).

Descriptive Statistics

Means, standard deviations, and normality statistics of the study's variables are presented in Table 1.

Table 1. Descriptive Statistics of the Study's Variables

	Mean	SD	Skewness	Kurtosis	Cronbach α
Negative beliefs	2.38	.98	.23	-.78	.70
Positive beliefs	2.98	1.08	-.05	-.91	.73
Self-handicapping	1.79	1.00	1.41	1.60	.87
Somatic anxiety	1.79	.48	.58	.57	.81
Worry	1.78	.52	.82	1.01	.81
Concentration Disruption	1.71	.54	.65	.43	.74
Internal LC	3.23	.97	.02	-1.15	.88
External LC	2.61	.67	.15	.83	.70
Luck	3.09	1.04	.02	-.99	.94
Mastery approach	5.09	1.71	-.43	-1.02	.89
Mastery avoidance	5.00	1.69	-.42	-1.07	.92
Performance approach	4.38	1.30	-.28	-.03	.76
Performance avoidance	3.97	1.32	-.11	-.02	.76

Note: LC = Locus of Control.

Linear regression analyses were performed to examine the effect of superstitious beliefs on sport-related cognitive and emotional responses. The results of the analyses indicated that positive superstitious beliefs were significant predictors of self-handicapping ($F(2,274) = 10.89$, $p < .001$, $R^2 = .07$, $b = .19$) and external locus of control on other people ($F(2,296) = 8.57$, $p < .001$, $R^2 = .05$, $b = .29$). Negative superstitious beliefs were significant predictors of somatic anxiety ($F(2,225) = 4.68$, $p < .05$, $R^2 = .02$, $b = .14$), worry ($F(2,296) = 5.11$, $p < .01$, $R^2 = .03$, $b = .16$), and performance avoidance goals ($F(2,296) = 5.92$, $p < .001$, $R^2 = .04$, $b = .17$). No significant effect of positive or negative superstitious beliefs was found on concentration disruption, internal locus of control, external locus of control on coach and luck, and mastery goals (approach and avoidance) and performance approach goals.

Moderating Effects of Age and Sport Experience

Moderated hierarchical regression analyses were performed to examine the superstitious beliefs-cognitive and affective responses relationship, and whether the athletes' age and years of experience act as moderators. According to Baron and Kenny (1986), to test for moderation effects a) predictors should have a unique effect on the dependent variable, b) both predictors and moderators should be mean centered, c) an interaction effect should be computed between each predictor and each moderator, and d) the interaction effect should have unique effect on the dependent variable.

To examine the moderating role of athletes' age and years of experience in the superstitions beliefs – cognitive and affective responses relationships the predictor variables included athletes' superstitious beliefs, age or years of experience and an interaction term denoting a multiplicative association between these variables (i.e., superstitious beliefs × age; Baron & Kenny, 1986). To explore the moderation effects all variables were mean-centered. A simple moderated effect emerges when either the variance explained by the interaction term is statistically significant, over and above the variance explained by the main effects of the predictor variables or, alternatively, if the Beta value of the interaction term is significant (Aiken & West, 1991; Baron & Kenny, 1986). The moderated regression analysis examines the hypothesis that the predictive effect of the interaction term will differ significantly from zero (null effect). Based on the findings of the linear regression analyses and the criteria posed by Baron and Kenny (1986) moderated regression analyses were performed for self-handicapping, somatic anxiety, worry, external locus of control on other people and performance avoidance goals.

The first moderation analysis was performed at three steps and assessed the interaction between positive superstitious beliefs and self-handicapping. Positive superstitious beliefs were entered at the first step and predicted 1.0% (Adj R^2) of the variance in self-handicapping. Years of experience were entered at the second step and did not have significant effect on the variance predicted. The interaction term (positive superstitious beliefs × years of experience) was entered at the final step of the analysis, and also did not produce a significant increase in predicted variance. Similarly, the second moderation analysis on the positive superstitious beliefs - self-handicapping relationship indicated that age had no moderating effect. The same procedure was followed for positive superstitious beliefs – external locus of control on other people relationship. The results of the moderated hierarchical regression analyses showed no moderating effect of age and years of experience in the positive superstitious beliefs – external locus of control on other people relationship.

The same procedure was followed with respect to negative superstitious beliefs. The first moderation analysis was performed to assess the interaction between negative superstitious beliefs and somatic anxiety. Negative superstitious beliefs were entered at the first step and predicted 0.2% (Adj R^2) of the variance in somatic anxiety. Years of experience were entered at the second step and had a significant effect on the variance predicted ($R^2_{change} = .20$, $p < .05$). The interaction term (negative superstitious beliefs × years of experience) was entered at the final step of the analysis, but did not produce a significant increase in predicted variance. Similarly, the second moderation analysis on the negative superstitious beliefs – somatic anxiety relationship indicated that age had no moderating effect.

The results of the moderated hierarchical analysis revealed significant moderating effect of years of experience on the negative superstitious beliefs – worry relationship. More specifically, negative superstitious beliefs predicted 0.5% (Adj R^2) of the variance in somatic anxiety. Years of experience were entered at the second step but did not have a significant effect on the variance predicted. The interaction term (negative superstitious beliefs × years of experience) was entered at the final step of the analysis, and produced a significant increase in predicted variance (Beta = -.19). On the contrary, the second moderation analysis on the negative superstitious beliefs – worry relationship indicated that age had no moderating effect.

Finally, the moderated hierarchical analyses on the negative superstitious beliefs – performance avoidance goals relationship revealed no moderating effect of years of experience and age.

Discussion

There is a great deal of anecdotal evidence suggesting that athletes use superstitious behaviors as a way to improve their sport performance. This is largely attributed to the belief that these behaviors can actually decrease uncertainty, provide a sense of control over the events, and protect the athletes' self-worth (Dag, 1999; Tobacyk et al., 1988). However, there is only limited evidence on the effect such beliefs have on several performance-related dispositions. The present study was designed to examine the effect of superstitious beliefs on self-handicapping and competitive trait anxiety, locus of control, achievement goals, as well as the moderating role of athletes' age and years of experience. The results of the regression analyses showed that positive superstitious beliefs were significant predictors of self-handicapping and external locus of control on other people. Negative superstitious beliefs were significant predictors of somatic anxiety, worry, and performance avoidance goals. The moderated regression analyses revealed a significant moderating effect of experience in negative superstitious beliefs – worry relationship.

More specifically, the results of the analyses provided partial support to our first hypothesis. Regarding competitive trait anxiety, the results indicated that negative superstitious beliefs positively predicted trait somatic anxiety and worry. These findings are consistent with theoretical predictions (Dudley, 1999) and previous research (Ciborowski, 1997; Schippers & Van Lange, 2006). According to Dudley, situations of ambiguity, uncertainty, or uncontrollability foster the development of superstitious beliefs. Similarly, these situations lead to the experience of anxiety (Speilberger, 1972). Hence, it could be assumed that athletes with high superstitious beliefs may experience ambiguity about their abilities, uncertainty about the outcome of their involvement in sports (i.e., participation in the team, winning or losing etc) and a lack of control over this outcome, which, in turn, results in the experience of elevated levels of competitive trait anxiety. Importantly, superstitious beliefs influenced both the bodily and cognitive symptoms of the anxiety experience. Although Ciborowski (1997) and Wright and Erdal (2008) argued that athletes adopt superstitious beliefs and behaviors in an attempt to achieve control over situations of ambiguity and uncertainty, it seems that these situations also trigger the experience of anxiety. This might imply that superstitious beliefs and anxiety can jointly act as an athlete's tendency to react in the sport context which is often characterized by high uncertainty and ambiguity. Future research should further investigate the effect of superstitious beliefs on various situations and different sports and the joint effect of superstitious beliefs and trait anxiety on sport-related outcomes, such as enjoyment and satisfaction from training and competitions, effort and persistence in difficulties and failures, and performance.

With respect to self-handicapping, positive superstitious beliefs significantly predicted the use of self-handicapping strategies. Congruent to Ryska (2002), these findings imply that superstitious athletes use self-handicapping as coping strategy in order to maintain control in situations characterized by uncertainty. In our study, only positive beliefs predicted self-handicapping. Although we measured self-reported strategies and not actual strategies, these findings may imply that both positive beliefs and self-handicapping are approach strategies. That is, superstitious athletes have a sense that did anything within their power (i.e., rituals and lucky charms) to control the environment and succeed, but there are other incidental reasons (i.e., lack of practice, illness, moodiness, lack of sleep, etc) that led to unsuccessful results. Future research should investigate the effect of superstitious beliefs on actual self-handicapping behavior (i.e., intentionally avoiding facilitative or engaging debilitative behaviours). Such research would provide important information regarding the effect of superstitious beliefs on a behavioral variable during sport involvement.

The results of the analyses partially supported our second hypothesis as well. Positive superstitious beliefs positively predicted external locus of control on other people. This finding is in support of Dag's (1999) theoretical predictions, but contradicts van Raalte et al's (1991) results, by suggesting that high superstitious athletes tend to attribute unsuccessful results to others. This seems to be an important mechanism to protect their self-worth. These athletes may believe that their ability or their rituals are not responsible for failure but they blame other people for this failure. Interestingly, neither making attributions to luck nor to the coach were predicted by superstitious beliefs. These beliefs represent, in fact, the belief that external forces can influence the person's behaviour and environment. Yet, they were not significant predictors of luck, although luck represents a similar concept regarding the effect of external forces on behavior. A plausible explanation might be that by attributing success or failure to luck, the athlete would invalidate his efforts to control luck via superstitious behaviours. Therefore, superstitious athletes may believe that they control luck with rituals and lucky charms, and, consequently, they don't attribute outcomes to luck and outside forces.

Furthermore, athletes do not ascribe outcomes to their coaches. No clear conceptual-based explanation can be provided for this finding. Perhaps, superstitious athletes believe that superstitious behaviors can help them control the sporting environment, including coach's behavior. Or, in conjunction with the significant effect on the external locus to other people, this could act as a protecting mechanism of the superstitious behavior. Neither the rituals and lucky charms, nor other event-related factors (i.e., the coach) were responsible for an unfortunate result. Instead the adverse outcomes were attributed to other people, whose roles could not be anticipated and controlled. In both cases, the lack of effect on external locus to coach implies a strong self-protecting mechanism. Clearly, future research should more thoroughly investigate superstitious beliefs and behaviors in conjunction with athletes' levels of self-esteem, self-worth and self-concept.

The results of the present study supported the third hypothesis regarding the effect of superstitious beliefs on achievement goals. Performance avoidance goals were predicted by negative superstitious beliefs, whereas no significant effect was found for approach goals (mastery and performance). Previous research has indicated that approach goals have an adaptive pattern of responses during sport involvement. Thus, it was expected to be negatively or neutrally associated with superstitious beliefs. Although there is some evidence that superstitious beliefs can positively influence performance (van Raalte et al., 1991), this may be considered to be a false way to achieve mastery and win a competition by approach-oriented athletes. With respect to mastery approach goals, this is further corroborated by the study of Mouratidou et al. (in press) who argued that mastery approach oriented athletes show more moral competence during sport involvement and use of legitimate ways to succeed. Interestingly, superstitious beliefs did not predict performance approach goals. On several occasions, performance approach goals have been associated with maladaptive responses, such as fear of failure (Conroy et al., 2003) and moral incompetence (Mouratidou et al., in press). However, it seems that performance approach oriented athletes striving to outperform their opponents do not value superstitious behaviors as important and, thus, do not endorse the respective beliefs.

On the other hand, superstitious beliefs significantly predicted performance avoidance goals. This finding is consistent with theory and previous research since this type of goals has shown the less adaptive profile of antecedents and consequences (Elliot, 1997; Elliot & Church, 1997; Rawsthorne & Elliot, 1999). Performance avoidance oriented athletes are characterized by high levels of fear of failure which are elicited in situations of uncertainty and lack of control. Thus, superstitious athletes are more prompt to adopt performance avoidance goals. With respect to mastery avoidance goals, no significant effect revealed. The antecedents and consequences of mastery avoidance goals in sport contexts have not been clearly articulated so far. Present findings indicated that mastery avoidance goals function as adaptive motivational orientations that are not associated with negative beliefs. Clearly, more research is needed to better comprehend the impact of superstitious and other beliefs on mastery avoidance goals.

A final objective of the present study was to examine the moderating role that athletes' ages and competitive experience can have on the superstitious beliefs – cognitive and affective responses relationships. The results of the analyses did not support our hypothesis that older and more experienced athletes would moderate these relationships with these athletes, showing the more maladaptive profile. In almost all of the cases no moderating effect was revealed. These findings imply that superstitious beliefs are not dependent on age and experience. It seems that, regardless of age and competitive experience, all athletes may endorse such beliefs. Further, the effect of these beliefs on cognitive and affective responses is identical. However, it should be noted that in the present study only basketball players were included. In basketball and other team sports, athletes can compete until their mid thirties. In individual sports, such as swimming, skiing etc, the athletes' age range is smaller and experience is gained earlier. Perhaps in these sports age and experience may play a more important role. Future research should extend these findings to more sports and larger age ranges.

Athletes' experience moderated only the superstitious beliefs – worry relationship. In this case, younger superstitious athletes showed higher levels of worry. Seemingly, younger athletes tend to respond to the uncertainty and lack of control experienced in sports with the development of high superstitious beliefs which, in turn, lead to negative thoughts, negative expectations and apprehension. In addition, it could be assumed that they have not developed effective coping strategies, besides superstitious rituals; thus, they experience elevated levels of competitive trait worry. If this is the case, it is suggested that coaches should teach younger athletes coping strategies such as relaxation, imagery, thought control, logical thinking, and disengagement (Gaudreau & Blondin, 2002). If athletes are taught these strategies they will be able to efficiently cope with uncertainty and uncontrollability and decrease the experience of anxiety.

In conclusion, the results of the present study indicated that superstitious beliefs significantly predicted several cognitive and affective responses, such as self-handicapping, somatic anxiety and worry, external locus of control and performance avoidance goals. Athletes' age and competitive experience did not moderate almost none of the relationships examined. Overall, superstitious beliefs were associated with negative cognitive and affective responses. The present study was correlational in nature and no cause and effect inferences can be made. Still, it provides interesting information regarding the impact of superstitious beliefs on athletes' cognitive and affective responses, and sets the basis for future research in this rather unexplored area. Future research should extend these findings to other sports too, and investigate the role of superstitious beliefs and behaviors to situational responses and actual performance.

References

Aiken, L. S., & West, S. G. (1991). *Multiple regression: Testing and interpreting interactions.* Newbury Park CA: Sage.

Ames, C. (1984). Competitive, cooperative and individualistic goal structures: A motivational analysis. In R. Ames & C. Ames (Eds.), *Research on motivation in education: Student motivation* (pp. 177-207). NY: Academic Press.

Arkin, R. M., & Baumgardner, A. H. (1985). Self-handicapping. In J. H. Harvey, W. Ickes, & R. F. Kidd (Eds.), *New Directions in attribution research* (Vol 3, pp. 169-202). Hillsdale NJ: Lawrence Erlbaum Associates.

Bailis, D. (2001). Benefits of self-handicapping in sport: A field study of university athletes. *Canadian Journal of Behavioral Science, 33*, 213–223.

Baron R. M., & Kenny D. A. (1986). The moderator–mediator variable distinction in social psychological research: Conceptual, strategic, and statistical considerations. *Journal of Personality and Social Psychology, 51,* 1173–1182.

Barkoukis, V., Ntoumanis, N., & Nikitaras, N. (2007). Comparing dichotomous and trichotomous approaches to achievement goal theory: An example using motivational regulations as outcome variables. *British Journal of Educational Psychology, 77, (3),* 683-702.

Bentler, P. M. (2004). *EQS structural equations modeling software* (Version 6.1). Encino, CA: Multivariate Software.

Bleak, J. L., & Frederick, C. M. (1998). Superstitious behavior in sport: Levels of effectiveness and determinants of use in three collegiate sports *Journal Sport Behavior, 21,* 1–15.

Brandwein, D. (2003). The role of achievement motivation and locus of control in shaping sportspersonship behaviors among competitive activity participants. *ETD Collection for Pace University.* Paper AAI3073664. http://digitalcommons.pace.edu/dissertations/AAI3073664.

Broad, C. D. (1953). *Religious, philosophy, and physical research.* NY: Harcourt & Brace.

Buhrmann, H. G., & Zaugg, M. K. (1983). Superstitions amongst basketball players: An investigation of various forms of superstitious beliefs and behavior amongst competitive basketballers at junior high to university level. *Journal of Sport Behavior, 4,* 163–174.

Carron, A. V., Prapavessis, H., & Grove, J. R. (1994). Group effects and self-handicapping. *Journal of Sport & Exercise Psychology, 16,* 246-257.

Chen, L. H., Wu, C. H., Kee, Y. H., Lin, M. S., & Shui, S. H. (2009). Fear of failure, 2 × 2 achievement goal and self-handicapping: An examination of the hierarchical model of achievement motivation in physical education. *Contemporary Educational Psychology, 34,* 298-305.

Ciborowski, T. (1997). "Superstition" in the collegiate baseball player. *The Sport Psychologist, 11,* 305-317.

Conroy, D. E., Elliot, A. J., & Hofer, S. M. (2003). A 2 x 2 Achievement Goals Questionnaire for Sport: Evidence for Factorial Invariance, Temporal Stability, and External Validity. *Journal of Sport & Exercise Psychology, 25(4),* 456-476.

Conroy, D. E., Kaye, M. P., & Coatsworth, J. D. (2006). Coaching climates and the destructive effects of mastery-avoidance achievement goals on situational motivation.

Journal of Sport & Exercise Psychology, 28(1), 69-92.

Cury, F., Da Fonséca, D., Rufo, M., Peres, C., & Sarrazin, P. (2003). The trichotomous model and investment in learning to prepare for a sport test: A mediational analysis. *British Journal of Educational Psychology, 73,* 529–543.

Cury, F., Elliot, A. J., Da Fonséca, D., & Moller, A. (2006). The social–cognitive model of achievement motivation and the 2 X 2 achievement goal framework. *Journal of Personality and Social Psychology, 90 (4),* 666-679.

Cury, F., Elliot, A., Sarrazin, P., Da Fonséca , D., & Rufo, M. (2002). The trichotomous achievement goal model and intrinsic motivation: A sequential mediational analysis. *Journal of Experimental Social Psychology, 38,* 473–481.

Dag, I. (1999). The relationships among paranormal beliefs, locus of control and psychopathology in a Turkish college sample. *Personality and Individual Differences, 26,* 723–737.

Dweck, C. S. (1986). Motivational processes affecting learning. *American Psychologist, 41,* 1040-1048.

Doganis, G., Theodorakis, Y., & Bagiatis, K. (1991). Self-esteem and locus of control in adult female fitness program participants. *International Journal of Sport Psychology, 22 (2),* 154-164.

Duda, J., Chi, L., Newton, M., Walling, M., & Catley, D. (1995). Task and ego orientation and intrinsic motivation in sport. *International Journal of Sport Psychology, 26,* 40–63.

Duda, J. L., & Hall, H. (2001). Achievement goal theory in sport: Recent extensions and future directions. In R. N. Singer, H. A. Hausenblas, & C. M. Janelle (Eds.), *Handbook of sport psychology* (2nd ed., pp. 417–443). NY: Wiley.

Dudley, T. R. (1999). The effect of superstitious belief on performance following an unsolvable problem. *Personality and Individual Differences, 26,* 1057-1064.

Elliot, A. J. (1997). Integrating "classic" and "contemporary" approaches to achievement motivation: A hierarchical model of approach and avoidance achievement motivation. In P. Pintrich & M. Maehr (Eds.), *Advances in motivation and achievemen*t (Vol. 10, pp. 143–179). Greenwich, CT: JAI Press.

Elliot, A. J., & Church, M. (1997). A hierarchical model of approach and avoidance achievement motivation. *Journal of Personality and Social Psychology, 72,* 218–232.

Elliot A. J. & Church, M. A. (2003). A motivational analysis of defensive pessimism and self-handicapping, *Journal of Personality, 71* (3), 369–396.

Elliot, A. J., & Harackiewicz, J. (1996). Approach and avoidance achievement goals and intrinsic motivation: A mediational analysis. *Journal of Personality and Social Psychology, 70,* 461–475.

Elliot, A. J., & McGregor, H. A. (2001). A 2 x 2 achievement goal framework. *Journal of Personality and Social Psychology, 80,* 501–519.

Elliot, A. J., & Murayama, K. (2008). On the measurement of achievement goals: Critique, illustration, and application. *Journal of Educational Psychology, 100,* 613–628.

Elliot, A. J., & Thrash, T. (2001). Achievement goals and the hierarchical model of achievement motivation. *Educational Psychology Review, 13,* 139–156.

Fan, X., Thompson, B., & Wang, L. (1999). Effects of sample size, estimation methods, and model specification on structural equation modeling fit indexes. *Structural Equation Modeling, 6(1),* 56-83.

Finney, S. J., Pieper, S. L., & Barron, K. E. (2004). Examining the psychometric properties of the Achievement Goal Questionnaire in a general academic context. *Educational and Psychological Measurement, 64, (2)*, 365-382.

Foster, D. J., Weigand, D. A., & Baines, D. (2006). The effect of removing superstitious behavior and introducing a pre-performance routine in basketball free throw performance. *Journal of Applied Sport Psychology, 18,* 167–171.

Granito, V. J., & Carlton, E. B. (1993). Relationship between locus of control and satisfaction with intercollegiate volleyball teams at different levels of competition. *Journal of Sport Behavior, 16 (4),* 221-228.

Grouios, G. & Barkoukis, V. (manuscript under preparation). Handedness and trait anxiety in sport. Aristotle University of Thessaloniki, Greece.

Hanton, S., Mellalieu, S. D., & Hall, R. (2002). Re-examining the competitive anxiety trait-state relationship. *Personality and Individual Differences*, *33*, 1125-1136.

Hainaut, J. P., Monfort, V., & Bolmont, B. (2006). Trait-anxiety dependence of movement time performance in a bimodal choice task in subjects exposed to moderate anxiogenic conditions. *Neuroscience Letters, 409, (3),* 196-199.

Hausenblas H. A., & Carron, A. V. (1996). Group cohesion and self-handicapping in females and male athletes. *Journal of Sport and Exercise Psychology, 18,* 132-143.

Hu, L., & Bentler, P. M. (1999). Cutoff criteria for fit indexes in covariance structure analysis: Conventional criteria versus new alternatives. *Structural Equation Modeling, 6(1),* 1-55.

Kavussanu, M., Seal, A. R., & Phillips, D. R. (2006). Observed prosocial and antisocial behaviors in male soccer teams: Age differences across adolescence and the role of motivational variables. *Journal of Applied Sport Psychology, 18,* 326–344.

Kerr, G. A., & Goss, J. D. (1997). Personal control in elite gymnasts: the relationships between locus of control, self-esteem and trait anxiety. *Journal of Sport Behavior, 20 (1),* 69-82.

Kuczka, K. K. & Treasure, D. C. (2005). Self-handicapping in competitive sport: influence of the motivational climate, self-efficacy, and perceived importance. *Psychology of Sport and Exercise, 6, (5),* 539-550.

Labbe, A. E., Welsh, C. (1993). Children and running: Changes in physical fitness, self-efficacy, and health locus of control. *Journal of Sport Behavior, 16,* 85-98.

Lambert, S. M., Moore, D. W., & Dixon, R. S. (1999). Gymnasts in training: The differential effects of self-and coach-set goals as a function of locus of control. *Journal of Applied Sport Psychology, 11 (1),* 72-82.

Lefcourt, H. M. (1991). Locus of control. In Robinson, J. P., Shaver, P. R. & Wrightsman, L. S. (Eds), *Measures ofpersonality and social psychological atrirudes* (pp. 413-499). NY: Academic Press.

Linderman, M., & Aarnio, K. (2007). Superstitious, magical, and paranormal beliefs: An integrative model. *Journal of Research in Personality, 41,* 731-744.

Martens, R., Vealey, R., & Burton, D. (1990). *Competitive Anxiety in Sport.* Champaign Illinois: Human Kinetics.

Martin, A., Marsh, H., & Debus, R. (2001). Self-handicapping and defensive pessimism: A model of self-protection from a longitudinal perspective. *Contemporary Educational Psychology, 28*, 1–36.

Martinent, G., & Ferrand, C. (2007). A cluster analysis of precompetitive anxiety: Relationship with perfectionism and trait anxiety. *Personality & Individual Differences,*

43, (7), 1676-1686.

May, R. (1977). *The meaning of anxiety.* NY: Norton.

Midgley, C., Arunkumar, R., & Urdan, T. (1996). "If I don't do well tomorrow, there's a reason": Predictors of adolescents' use of academic self-handicapping strategies. *Journal of Educational Psychology, 88,* 423-434.

Morris, R. L., & Kavussanu, M. (2008). Antecedents of approach-avoidance goals in sport. *Journal of Sports Sciences, 26(5),* 465-476.

Mouratidou, K., Barkoukis, V., & Rizos, S. (in press). Achievement goals and moral competence in sport: Examining the moderating role of demographic characteristics. *European Psychologist.*

Neil, G., Anderson, B., & Sheppard, W. (1981). Superstitions among male and female athletes of various levels of involvement. *Journal of Sport Behavior, 4*, 137–148.

Nicholls, J. G. (1989). *The competitive ethos and democratic education.* Cambridge. MA: Harvard University Press.

Ntoumanis, N., & Jones, G. (1997). Interpretation of competitive trait anxiety symptoms as a function of locus of control beliefs. *International Journal of Sport Psychology, 29,* 99-114.

Ommundsen, Y., & Pedersen, B. H. (1999). The role of achievement goal orientations and perceived ability upon somatic and cognitive indices of sport competition trait anxiety: A study of young athletes. *Scandinavian Journal of Medicine & Science in Sports, 9 (6),* 333-343.

Prapavessis, H., & Grove, J. R. (1994). Personality variables as antecedents of precompetitive mood state temporal patterning. *International Journal of Sport Psychology, 22,* 347-365.

Prapavessis, H., Grove, J.R., Maddison, R., & Zillmann, N. (2003). Self-handicapping tendencies, coping, and anxiety responses among athletes. *Psychology of Sport and Exercise*, *4*, 357-375.

Rawsthorne, L. J., & Elliot, A. J. (1999). Achievement goals and intrinsic motivation: A metaanalytic review. *Personality and Social Psychology Review, 3*, 326–344.

Rhodewalt, F., Saltzman, A. T., & Wittmer, J. (1984). Self-handicapping among competitive athletes: The role of practice in self-esteem protection. *Basic and Applied Social Psychology*, *5, (3),* 197–209.

Robazza, C., & Bortoli, L. (2007). Perceived impact of anger and anxiety on sporting performance in rugby players. *Psychology of Sport and Exercise, 8,* 875-896.

Roig, M., Bridges, K. R., Renner, C. H., & Jackson, C. R. (1998). Belief in the paranormal and its association with irrational thinking controlled for context effects. *Personality and Individual Differences, 24,* 229–236.

Rotter, J. B. (1966). Generalized expectancies for internal versus external control of reinforcement. *Psychological Monographs, 80,* 1-28.

Ryska, T. A. (2002). Effects of situational self-handicapping and state self-confidence on the physical performance of young participants. *The Psychological Record*, *52,* 461-478.

Ryska, T. A., Yin, Z., Boyd, M. (1999). The role of dispositional goal orientation and team climate on situational self-handicapping among young athletes. *Journal of Sport Behavior, 22,* 410-425.

Ryska, T. A., Yin, Z. N., & Cooley, D. (1998). Effects of trait and situational self-handicapping on competitive anxiety among athletes. *Current Psychology*, *17,* 48-56.

Schippers, M. C., & Van Lange, P. A. M. (2006). The psychological benefits of superstitious rituals in top sport: A study among top sportspersons. *Journal of Applied Social Psychology, 36 (10),* 2532-2553.

Smith, M., Hall, H., & Wilson, P. (1999). The relationship of goal orientation and competitive climate to sportsmanship attitudes and the perceived legitimacy of intentionally injuries acts. *Proceedings of the 10th European Congress of Sport Psychology.* Prague, Czech Republic.

Smith. R. E., Smoll, F. L., & Schultz, R. W. (1990). Measurement and correlates of sponspecific cognitive and somatic trait anxiety: The Sport Anxiety Scale. *Anxiety Research, 2,* 263-280.

Spielberger, C. D. (1966). Theory and research on anxiety. In C. D. Spielberger (Ed.), *Anxiety and behaviour* (pp. 3-22). NY: Academic Press.

Spielberger, C. D. (1972). Anxiety as an emotional state. In C. D. Spielberger (Ed.), *Anxiety: Current trends in theory and research* (Vol 1, pp. 24-54). NY: Academic Press.

Stewart, C., & Meyers, M. (2004). Motivational traits of elite young soccer players. *Physical Educator, 61,* 213-218.

Stoeber, J., Stoll, O., Pescheck, E., & Otto, K. (2008). Perfectionism and achievement goals in athletes: Relations with approach and avoidance orientations in mastery and performance goals. *Psychology of Sport and Exercise, 9, (2),* 102-121.

Thill, E. E., & Cury, F. (2000). Learning to play golf under different goal conditions: their effects on irrelevant thoughts and on subsequent control strategies. *European Journal of Social Psychology, 30 (1),* 101-122.

Tobacyk, J. (1988). A revised paranormal belief scale. Unpublished manuscript, Louisiana Tech University, Rushton, LA.

Tobacyk, J., Nagot, E., & Miller, M. (1988). Paranormal beliefs and locus of control: A multidimensional examination. *Journal of Personality Assessment, 52,* 241–246.

Tobacyk, J., & Shrader, D. (1991). Superstition and self-efficacy. *Psychological Reports, 68,* 1387–1388.

Urdan, T., & Midgley, C. (2001). Academic self-handicapping: What we know, what more there is to learn. *Educational Psychology Review, 13,* 115–138.

Van Raalte, J. L., Brewer, B. W., Nemeroff, C. J., & Linder, D. E. (1991). Chance orientation and superstitious behavior on the putting green. *Journal of Sport Behavior, 14,* 41–50.

Wang, J., Marchant, D., Morris, T., & Gibbs, P. (2004). Self-consciousness and trait anxiety as predictors of choking in sport. *Journal of Science and Medicine in Sport, 7, (2),* 174-185.

Williams, L., & Gill, D. L. (1995). The role of perceived competence in the motivation of physical activity. *Journal of Sport and Exercise Psychology, 17,* 363-378.

Wolfradt, U. (1997). Dissociative experiences, trait anxiety and paranormal beliefs. *Personality and Individual Differences, 23,* 15–19.

Woodman, T. & Hardy, L. (2001). A case study of organisational stress in elite sport. *Journal of Applied Sport Psychology, 13,* 207-238.

Wright, P. B., & Erdal, K. J. (2008). Superstition as a function of skill level and task difficulty. *Journal of Sport Behavior, 31, (2),* 187-201.

Zebb, B. J., & Moore, M. C. (2003). Superstitiousness in perceived anxiety control as predictors of psychological distress. *Anxiety Disorders, 17,* 115-130.

In: Encyclopedia of Sports and Athletics
Editors: Jack L. Murray and Emily O. Watson

ISBN: 978-1-61209-959-0

Chapter XX

A Developmental Risk Research Model: Overcoming Socio Psychological Risk among At-Risk Student Athletes

***Thomas W. Miller*[1] *and Douglas Wolf*[2]**
[1]University of Kentucky, US
[2]Nationwide Children's Hospital
Columbus Ohio, US

Introduction

Developmental risk researchers has made it possible to identify youth who are significantly more likely than their peers to succumb to at-risk and high risk behaviors often leading to emotional or social disturbances (Kalichman, Simbayi, Vermaakk, Jooste, Cain. 2008; Yoon & Barton 2008; Miller, Kraus, Veltkamp, 2008; Beane, Miller, & Spurling 2008;Lin, Neafsey, & Strickler,2008; Clayton, Grant-Harrington, Turner, Miller, Durden 2006; Neafsey, Jarrin, Luciano, & Coffman,2007;Norton, Amico, Copenhaver, Cornman, Fisher, Fisher, Kozal, & Friedland,2008; Miller, 2006; Park, C. L. 2008). Two forms of risk are recognized by these researchers. The first involves youth with demographic risk are those with multiple environmental at risk experiences that increase the likelihood of disturbance, including poverty, exposure to violence, or familial disruptions. The second focuses on youth with what is commonly referred to as "functional risk.' Functional risk experiences are those who do not meet recognized criteria for a clinical or psychiatric disorder but do offer evidence of early dysfunctional behaviors that may represent the early stages of such disorders. Both functional and demographic risk has become the basis for selected preventive interventions. This chapter addresses an approach for intervention specialists that offer a case illustration involving student athletes and their use of over the counter pain medications.

Available research suggests that at risk youth are predisposed to drug abuse. Prior to the turn of the century, the NIDA Resiliency and Risk Workgroup convened a group of experienced clinical researchers with expertise in areas of drug abuse and related research to determine how the further application of available research based data can advance prevention effectiveness beyond current levels. Dr. Alan Leshner, Director of the National Institute on Drug Abuse is a psychologist and behavioral scientist and provided the leadership for this team. The research team generated several key recommendations that should be a model for prevention science research. The major recommendations of the group included advocated the development of prevention interventions which target: youth within the family setting and encouraged family functioning and communication as critical buffer against problematic personality characteristics and at risk behaviors among youth.

Among the recommendations of this NIDA Resiliency and Risk Work group panel of senior researchers with expertise in areas of drug abuse and related research was a definitive endorsement for the further development and expansion of prevention programs which focus on the communication and behaviors that are influenced by family functioning. Drawing on a variety of research findings showing the strong drug abuse resilience and risk influence of the family on youth and adolescents, the panel strongly encouraged the development of preventive interventions which respond to the individual in the context of their particular family unit. In other words, a significant part of the origin of drug abuse is often the abusers' families' dysfunctions and inadequacies and a significant factor in resistance is often the positive characteristics and influences of the family (Glantz 1995).

The NIDA Resiliency and Risk Workgroup further suggested that research to date indicates that a range of potentially problematic early childhood characteristics often preclude and may present as a diathesis to drug experimentation, use and abuse. This includes not only numerous early diagnosable psychopathological disorders but also, pre-morbid conditions, sub-threshold conditions and components of psychopathologies. Research (Glantz 1995; Clayton, Grant-Harrington, Turner, Miller, Durden, 2000) indicates that these types of early childhood characteristics are often associated with individuals who progress to more severe levels of drug involvement. The panel felt that youth with such characteristics could often be identified early in their lives, prior to the exacerbation of their conditions and prior to their drug involvement.

Another major recommendation of the NIDA Resiliency and Risk Workgroup was the development of prevention programs which identify and ameliorate these early childhood characteristics. The panel further stressed the need to recognize the common occurrence of multiple problem behaviors and the inter relationship of these behaviors, and the importance of not conceptualizing or targeting drug abuse as an isolated behavior (Glantz 1995). The major recommendation derives from research findings which indicate that deficits or impairments in certain abilities are commonly characteristic of and probable predisposition to drug experimentation, use and abuse and secondary forms of drug involvement.

In their model, the recommendation of the "skill areas group" proposed that as intervention targets need to focus on executive and cognitive functions of youth in the at risk setting. More specifically the intervention targets needed to include goal setting, analysis, planning, organization and problem solving. They further contended that "affect regulation, " including both impulse control and techniques for adaptively coping with and controlling strong negative at risk and high risk behaviors be complimented by positive reinforcement (Glantz 1995).

Finally, the skills area group noted that drug experimenters, users and abusers' coping skills and defenses are oriented around escape from problems and negative affects rather than being based on active positive coping involvement approach. A point raised by the panel was that some of the naturally occurring transitions in society and developmental characteristics of children and adolescents are not taken into account in many cases. For example, having youth go to the same school for eight years and then transferring to high school for four years rather then having them make the typical additional transition to middle or junior high schools seems to facilitate better function in a number of ways. Keeping the first eight years of students together seems to foster protection of the younger students by the older ones and not having school transitions co-occur with critical developmental transitions seems to avoid exacerbation of some potential difficulties. Recognition of and accommodation to these types of developmental factors could facilitate better function and greater resistance to drug experimentation, use, abuse and involvement.

The NIDA Resiliency and Risk Workgroup also recommended that there be further development of prevention programs which facilitate youth bonding with critical adult models in their lives and with peer groups who provide pro-social encouragement, self acceptance, healthy self esteem, and positive self standards, self regulation and expectations. Glantz (1995) also noted in his report that the importance of peers as influences on drug involvement and the potential of peer based interventions for prevention, particularly interventions where peers themselves are the interveners. A logical extension of these concepts is the need for attractive alternative activities, organizations and opportunities and the importance of ensuring that children and adolescents who wish to change their associations and join prosaically interpersonal networks and groups be accepted. The home and the schools were identified as important foci for prevention intervention strategies.

Combining and extending some of the general concepts of the above recommendations, the panel supported the concept of interventions which promote adult liaisons and which help to organize parents and others into supportive groups. Taking this concept further, communities might be aided to function as active empowered social communities which have a sense of identity, cohesion and responsibility, which act for the protection, well-being and betterment of the community, and which guide, protect and ensure the conduct of the members of the community including all of the adults, adolescents and children. An idealized concept of a village was the model for this recommendation and the suggestion was made that these types of efforts already "naturally" occur and should be studied to determine how they function and how their principles can be extended to other groups and areas.

The last set of recommendations related to the science and research of prevention intervention strategies. The NIDA Resiliency and Risk Workgroup strongly encouraged the development of better measures of drug involvement liability, drug use, and drug use patterns and the development of measurements sensitive to change. They encouraged a meta-study of prevention and the principles of preventive intervention. The group called for more etiological research to extend and validate current findings and hypotheses and endorsed efforts to distill identified protective and risk influences into a limited number of functional patterns with principles describing the interaction of the factors within the patterns (Glantz 1995).

Practice Applications in Developmental Risk Research

Intervention specialists have recognized the importance of character education in the school and family environment. Character education was recently endorsed by the Office of Rural Health Policy (2004), the National Advisory Committee on Rural Health Policy (2004) and the U.S. Department of Health and Human Services (2007). There has for some time been support for "character education" in local and state governments, state departments of education, and educational organizations. Successful programs include the process of building community consensus and commitment helping different religions and cultures realize common values. Several state and federal court decisions refer to the obligation educators have to teach the values upon which democracy and social order depend. In Board of Education v. Pico (1982) Justice Brennan wrote that local schools must be permitted "to establish and apply their curriculum in such a way as to transmit community values." Since 1971 in Lemon v. Kurtzman, the court found that laws and actions are constitutional under the Establishment Clause if they (a) have a secular or civic purpose, (b) have the primary effect of neither advancing nor inhibiting religion, and (c) avoid excessive entanglement with religion.

For prevention research purposes, character education does not provide a challenge due to moral, civic or positive social values. Character, refers to those aspects of personality that are learned through experience, through training, and through a socialization process. One's "character" refers primarily to things a person learns about how he or she should conduct him- or herself or behave in social or interpersonal situations. Part of this shaping of our behavior is based on the need to be seen in a positive way, as moral or virtuous (i.e., as having a good reputation), but another part relates to how people want to see and feel about themselves. A primary characteristic, noted by virtually all theorists who have carefully studied this concept over time, is consistency in behavior across time as reflected in ethical and moral development. The cocept of "character" is a quality that is enduring, not transient like an interest, emotion, or attitude**.** Character is defined through the Josephson Institute (2008) as six core ethical values including such qualities as Trustworthiness, Respect, Responsibility, Fairness, Caring and Citizenship. Each are discussed and defined elsewhere at the Josephson Institute web site.

Prevention researchers such as Benninga & Wynne (1998) Miller, Kraus, Veltkamp, (2008) Beane, Miller, Spurling, (2008) have reported that document the record-breaking rates of distress afflicting American youth and form an essential backdrop for character development. The annual rates of death of young (15 to 19 year-old) white males by homicide and suicide are at their highest points since national record keeping began. The rates of out-of-wedlock births to young (15 to 19 years-old) white females are also at or near their highest points since national record keeping began Benninga & Wynne (1998). Bennigan and Wynne (1998) argue that character educators want children and adolescents to learn to feel a sense of belonging, bonding to and responsibility for others. They believe that instability and individual feelings of anxiety and dissatisfaction sometimes resulting in depression, suicidal ideation, and other forms of disorder. They believe that youth need age-appropriate responsibilities, in order to feel socially integrated and respected. They believe that adults with authority should feel comfortable disciplining youngsters who fail to carry out those significant duties. In this configuration, the responsibility of adult models for youth is to critically examine their social environments and to design and manage them to those environments that help youth grow into mature and moral adults (Bennigan & Wynne, 1998). Moral development is critical in this model.

Intervention specialists are often involved in a spectrum of dysfunctional or antisocial behaviors. According to Walker, Horner, Sugai, Bullis Sprague, Bricker and Kaufman (1996) well developed antisocial behavior patterns and high levels of aggression evidenced early in a child's life are among the best predictors of delinquent and violent behavior years later. Poor moral development and a lack of bonding with others is often core to this problem. These behavior patterns become elaborated and more destructive over time; they negatively effect the school environment and lower the quality of life for students and staff alike. (Hawkins & Catalalano, 1992; Patterson, Reid, & Dishion, 1992). In an effort to assess at risk youth in rural communities, the Rural Education Achievement Project (REAP) which is summarized elsewhere (Clayton, Grant Harrington, Turner, Miller, Durden, 2000; Miller, Veltkamp, & Kraus, 2005) was designed to evaluate the effectiveness of a universal, protocol-driven, school-based character education and problem behavior prevention program; a selective, comprehensive, protocol-driven, school-based summer program designed to reduce risk factors and strengthen protective factors related to drug use/problem behaviors among youth; and a selective, protocol-driven family program for parents/guardians of at risk students often seen by intervention specialists. All 4th grade students in nine of the 11 elementary schools in a predominantly rural southeastern county, predominantly rural, and with the highest percentage African American population were selected for study (Clayton., Grant Harrington, Turner, Miller, Durden.2000) Students in 3 schools were in the no treatment control condition. Students in the remaining 6 schools received a school-based curriculum driven character education program. Students in two of these six schools not only received the curriculum, but 1/3 (chosen on the basis of poor academic achievement and externalizing behavior (youth self report and teacher appraisals) also received a six week, protocol driven, summer academic (4 weeks) and experiential education program for two weeks. In the final two schools, all 4th grade students received the curriculum, 1/3 (chosen on the basis of poor academic achievement and externalizing behaviors) received the six-week intervention, and the parents of these students received an eight-session version of the *Duke Family Coping Power* program. The summer camp intervention was delivered by the teachers with these students who they were scheduled to have in the 5th grade. The *Gearing up to Success* (GUTS) program which employed the combined experimental curriculum and summer camp experience wherein high risk students were able to utilize skills learned through the character education program involving both experiential and didactic components. Teacher and counselors utilized the involvement of the GUTS program with their fourth and fifth grades to assess the effectiveness of the prevention intervention on academic performance and social competence.

The results obtained in this prevention education research project led to the predictor variable of academic achievement for children aged 9 to 11 years of age and yielded a Chi-Square of 8.21 (p=.76) with 12 degrees of freedom. A key dimension of the targeted predictor variable, Academic Achievement, was school bonding. Here it is shown that the summer program participants had stronger gains in bonding to school personnel and school activities then did those students who did not receive the intervention. There were no significant differences between the participants in summer camp whose parents received the family program and those who just received the summer program. However, this result is not surprising given that the family program was targeted more toward the direct effect of strengthening interactions among family members rather than strengthening the academic performance of students.

In considering the critical conditions in the study, the curriculum on character education offered during the school year, the family intervention involving training in parenting skills, and the camp experience involving school bonding through teacher-student interaction in a social and educational setting. A one-way ANOVA which addresses the factors by each condition yields a significant result ($F=3.056$, $df=167$, $p<.30$), suggesting that of the conditions considered, the summer camp experience makes the greatest difference in these students participating in this study. A dose response relationship was observed among the intervention conditions for social competence. Here students who received the most comprehensive intervention (summer program, curriculum, and the family component) had the highest increases in social competence, followed by those who received both the curriculum and the summer program. The lowest increase in social competence was observed among those who only received the curriculum program.

The findings for parental investment show that the family program was effective at increasing the amount of parent and child interactions. These data show that students in the other two intervention conditions had fewer interactions with parents over the study period. In a developmental perspective, one would expect to find a decreasing amount of parental investment over time. As the child begins to assert independence and develop peer networks, they are drawn them away from family activities and more toward those with peers. Thus, the family component was efficacious at slowing the natural progression of detachment that occurs during adolescence.

At Risk Student Athletes and Prevention Science: A Case for Prevention Research

In the highly competitive environment of college sports, about twenty percent of student-athletes use nonprescription analgesics to allow them to play with injury (Tricker, 2000). It is likely that NSAID use following injury is thought to improve performance (Warner, Schnepf, Barrett, Dian, Swigonski. (2002). Other researchers found that over long periods of NSAID use, the muscles ability to heal is significantly suppressed (Berstein, Stovitz, & Kuffner, 2003). This has led research clinicians to suggest that NSAIDs may "mask" pain, an important indicator to alter activity, putting athletes at risk for more serious injuries (Berstein, Stovitz, & Kuffner, 2003). Student-athletes may well be unaware of the dangers of nonprescription analgesic use, as 22% of NCAA division I athletes have no knowledge of side effects of analgesic medication (Tricker, 2000). Medications known as non-steroidal anti-inflammatory drugs (NSAIDs), have analgesic (pain killing) and anti-inflammatory actions and are used to alleviate problems associated with pain and swelling of injuries. NSAIDS that have been used for the treatment of sports injuries include diclofenac (Voltaren), ibuprofen (Advil, Aleve,Motrin), ketoprofen (Orudis), naproxen (Anaprox), etc. and compounds such as Indomethacin (Indocin) and sulindac (Clinoril), Vioxyl, Celebrex. Laster-Bradley (1991) have concluded that the practice of trainers administering and sometimes prescribing drugs is widespread. Her study of youth using and abusing pain related drugs found that prescription medications were being distributed to student athletes by people other than doctors. The report also found that access to medication was not monitored, and that Federal regulations regarding packaging and labeling were frequently overlooked.

For the prevention intervention scientist, it becomes critical to understand the access channels for drug experimentation, use and abuse among our youth. Because of the potential for overuse of nonprescription analgesics and the associated ill health effects more information on the use of nonprescription analgesics in youth athletes and factors related to nonprescription analgesic use is warranted. Characteristics of those who are most likely to use nonprescription analgesics and their reasons for doing so must be identified. Many of the practices employed by athletic coaches, training staffs and other in the athletics field that often focus on empowering youth athletes to use over the counter and prescription medications must be addressed more closely. Also, the enabling of experimentation,, use and abuse should be better defined. So what is the scope of the problem as we have come to know it today? To answer this question we must know and understand the demographic characteristics of student athletes who misuse nonprescription analgesics. We also need to know the reasons student athletes may misuse nonprescription analgesics including lack of knowledge of active ingredients and proper instructions for use, neglecting to read and follow label directions, and misuse facilitated by athletic personnel. Critical is the communication behaviors between student athletes, athletic personnel and physicians and how these communication behaviors affect the use of nonprescription analgesics by student athletes. Finally, what are the sources by which student athletes obtain nonprescription analgesics and how this source of supply may facilitate misuse of nonprescription analgesics?

Essential to the prevention scientist's understanding of a unique study involving use and abuse of medications for pain among youth athletes, are key definitions associated with such use and abuse. Here are a few critical definitions.

- Adverse drug effect: a harmful, unintended reaction to a drug administered at normal dosage ("Mosby's", 1998)
- Nonsteroidal anti-inflammatory drugs (NSAIDs): any group of drugs having antipyretic, analgesic, and anti-inflammatory effects ("Mosby's", 1998)
- Nonprescription: available to the consumer without a prescription (over-the-counter) ("Mosby's", 1998)
- Analgesic: relieving pain or a drug that relieves pain ("Mosby's", 1998)
- Dispensation: the selection, acquisition, control, storage, delivery, packaging, labeling, dispensing, and administration of medication (Kahanov et al., 2003)
- Distribution: giving a drug in a quantity greater than would be used in a single dose (Prentice, 1999)
- Administration: giving a single dose of a particular medication (Prentice, 1999)
- Drug misuse: the unintentional inappropriate use of a medication
- Drug abuse: the overuse of a drug for a non-therapeutic effect ("Mosby's", 1998)

Sample, Analysis and Procedures

Sample size is critical in addressing an area of prevention research on this topic. Again this study is summarized elsewhere in much greater detail (Wolf 2006). Examined in this sample of student athletes (n = 1155). The independent variables are demographic characteristics; reasons for use; communication and interaction with ATC, physicians, and pharmacists; source of supply; and knowledge and attitudes about nonprescription analgesics. Frequencies were obtained for all data. Mean and standard deviation were obtained for age. Chi-square was also used to determine if significant differences exist in the dose of nonprescription analgesic taken between football players who use nonprescription analgesics for football related reasons and those that do not. Chi-square was used to determine if significant differences exist in the consecutive days taken between football players who use nonprescription analgesics for football related reasons and those that do not. Alpha level was set at $p < 0.05$.

Answers to our critical questions yielded the following results. Clearly 72.7% participants reported having used a nonprescription analgesic for football related pain in the previous season. Student athletes who primarily play on offense are more likely to use nonprescription analgesics (85.3%) compared to special teams, kickers, and punters (75%) or defensive players (58.7%) ($p = .05$). Student athletes with more years of football experience are also more likely to use nonprescription analgesics than those with less experience as shown in table 3 ($p = .101$).

About 75% of white football players and 69.% of black student athletes used nonprescription analgesics. More than 8 in 10 (83.3%) who are of ethnicity other than white or black used nonprescription analgesics. Most reported use of ibuprofen (80.1%) followed by aspirin (70.6%), acetaminophen (29.4%), naproxen sodium (20.2%), and ketoprofen (2.8%). A small number (7.1%) of youth in this survey reported having used some other nonprescription analgesic. Of those who used other nonprescription analgesics, 98.6% did not list the names of the other nonprescription analgesic. Atletes who responded to this survey demonstrated a low level of awareness of the active ingredient in nonprescription analgesics. When asked what brand of nonprescription analgesic they used most players report Tylenol, a brand of the active ingredient acetaminophen. In contrast, when asked what active ingredient they used most reported having used ibuprofen not acetaminophen.

Reasons for Nonprescription Analgesic Use

Fewer than half of those studied reported having used a nonprescription analgesic in anticipation of pain (41%), while less than one-third reported having used a nonprescription analgesic to avoid missing a practice or game (31.3). Starters at their primary position were also more likely to have taken a nonprescription analgesic to avoid missing a practice or game. One-third (32.9%) of the subjects studied in this survey who are starters at their primary position reported taking a nonprescription analgesics to avoid missing a practice or game compared to 29.7% of non-starters who took a nonprescription analgesics to avoid missing a practice or game.

Greater than 6 in 10 (62.7%) who took a nonprescription analgesic in anticipation of pain and 66.7% who took an nonprescription analgesic to avoid missing a practice or game reported there was nothing wrong with taking a nonprescription analgesic to play with an injury. More than one-third (37.3%) of survey respondents who took a nonprescription analgesic in anticipation of pain agreed a nonprescription analgesic can prevent a decrease in performance while almost half (48.9%) of subjects who took a nonprescription analgesic to avoid missing a practice or game agreed with that statement.

Communication Among Youth, their Teachers, Coaches & Mentors

Earlier in this chapter we noted the importance of communication. More than half of the student athletes (60.8%) stated they were instructed on proper use of nonprescription analgesics every time they obtained nonprescription analgesics from a team coach or physician. Of the subjects that stated they were not instructed on proper use of nonprescription analgesics every time, 14.7% were instructed on proper use sometimes, 13.3 were never instructed on proper use and 11.2% were instructed on proper use the first time only. Youth athletes who were not instructed on proper use of nonprescription analgesics every time were more likely to use more than the recommended dose (35.5%) than those who are instructed on the proper use of nonprescription analgesics every time (27.3%) thus leading to misuse and abuse.

More than three-fourths (75.7%) of student athletes in this survey stated they did not have a team physician or athletics staff member recommend more than the recommended dose of a nonprescription analgesic. It should be noted however that 7.6% stated a team physician or coach has recommended more than the recommended dose of a nonprescription analgesic, while 6.3% did not know the recommended dose of a nonprescription analgesic. These subjects who were recommended to take more than the recommended dose were more likely to use more than the recommended dose (45.5%) than those who were not recommended more than the recommended dose (31%) (p = .28). However, student athletes who did not know the recommended dose were more likely to use more than the recommended dose (55.6%). Thus again, the illustration of use, misuse and abuse based on communication or the lack thereof by athletics' personnel.

The majority of the subjects in our sample (Wolf 2006)(67.1%) sought advice regarding nonprescription analgesics. Most of the youth studied sought advice regarding nonprescription analgesics from a team staff (49.3%), team physician (27.9%), or staff (14.3%). This is the character formation effect at work. Student athletes who did not seek advice regarding nonprescription analgesics were somewhat more likely to use more than the recommended dose (39%) compared to those who do not seek advice (33.3%).

In terms of frequency, more student athletes failed to notify a team physician or staff when they were using a nonprescription analgesic "sometimes" (38.2%) than "never" (22.2%), "not too often" (20.8%), and "always" (18.8%). Subjects who used nonprescription analgesics for football related pain were more likely to "always" (84.6%) or "sometimes" (86.8%) not notify a team physician or athletic personnel, they are using a nonprescription analgesic compared to "not too often" (71.4%) and "not at all" (40.6%) (p = .00). Those who took a nonprescription analgesic in anticipation of pain were more likely to "always" (63%) not notify a team physician or athletic trainer about nonprescription analgesic use than "sometimes" (41.8%), "not too often" (30%), or "never" (31.3%) (p = .04). In fact, student athletes who used more than the recommended dose were increasingly more likely to not notify a team physician or staff of nonprescription analgesic use (p = .01)). Survey respondents who reported use of nonprescription analgesics to avoid missing a practice or game (p = .01) or agreed nonprescription analgesics were safer than prescription medications (p = .07) were also increasingly more likely to not notify a team physician or athletic staff of nonprescription analgesic use.

The Case for Prevention Intervention Strategies

The results of this study indicate student athletes use nonprescription analgesics at a rate greater than the general population and other student athletes. Seventy-three percent of the youth studied used nonprescription analgesics for athletic competition, while only 58% of all athletes use nonprescription analgesics regularly during their sports season (Tricker, 2000). In contrast, 47% of Americans over the age 18 have used a nonprescription analgesic in the past 6 months (Attitudes, 2001). Use of nonprescription analgesics among youth athletes is similar, however, to that of high school football players. Three-fourths of high school football players reported having used NSAIDs in the previous 3 months (Warner et al., 2002).

Most student athletes are using nonprescription analgesic properly. Only 6% of players report using nonprescription analgesics for longer than 10 consecutive days or everyday. Half of high school football players who use NSAIDs report using nonprescription analgesics everyday (Warner et al., 2002). One in three student athletes use more than the recommended dose of nonprescription analgesics, the same rate as the general population (Attitudes, 2001). Four percent of athletes report not knowing the recommended dose of nonprescription analgesics. Researchers suggest that unintentional overuse results from a misconception of the recommended dose (Ellen et al, 1998). According to this study over half (55.6%) of student atholetes who reported not knowing the recommended dose also reported having used more than the recommended dose.

Most (89%) of the sample believe football players require more of a nonprescription analgesic because football players are larger than the general population. This belief provides evidence why over half (56.7%) of offensive linemen and over one-third (37.5%) of defensive linemen, generally very large athletes, use more than the recommended dose of a nonprescription analgesic. However, doses based on body weight should only be used for children with a body weight less than a normal adult weight, otherwise the normal adult dose must be used (Kuffner, 2003).

Communication between Athletes and Athletic Personnel

Results suggest that poor instruction by athletic personnel or physician increases the likelihood that student athletes will use more than the recommended dose of a nonprescription analgesic. Student athletes who are not instructed on proper use every time they receive nonprescription analgesics from a team physician or athletic personnel are more likely to use more than the recommended dose. Despite over half (54%) of the staff allowing athletes to take more than the recommended dose (Tricker, 2000), only 8% of players state they have been told to use more than the recommended dose of a nonprescription analgesic. Those that stated they did not know the recommended dose were more likely to use the recommended dose than those who were told to take more than the recommended dose or to take only the recommended dose of a nonprescription analgesic.

Prevention researchers must realize that student athletes do not notify a team physician or coaches about nonprescription analgesic use more often than they notify a team physician or coaches. Student athletes who use more than the recommended dose and those that use nonprescription analgesics to avoid missing a practice or game are both more likely to fail to inform a team physician or athletic trainer about their nonprescription analgesic use.

Prevention Strategies in Drug use among Student Athletes

There are several prevention strategies cited by athletic staff that focuses on team-building exercises or programs for athletes that incorporate alcohol-free recreational activities. In addition, coordinating community service and volunteer opportunities for student athletes may be beneficial. It is important to promote a healthy environment through the recruitment and admissions procedures for student athletes. Oversee prospective student athlete placement for weekend visits with responsible athletes. Explicitly state to interested applicants that alcohol and other drug use is not tolerated. The making available substance-free residence options and encourages student athletes to use them. Educating faculty and staff about behavioral indicators, student norms, and cultural attitudes related to high-risk or illegal alcohol use. Furthermore, encouraging faculty and athletics personnel to engage in monitoring and mentoring of students is critical. Finally, communicate campus alcohol and drug policies clearly and frequently to athletes, including consequences for violations.

Student athletes who use nonprescription analgesics for athletic competition do not significantly misuse nonprescription analgesic more often than student athletes who do not use nonprescription analgesics for athletic competition. The majority of student athletes use nonprescription analgesics and many misuse nonprescription analgesics. Student athletes who decide on their own and purchase their own nonprescription analgesics; those with poor communication regarding nonprescription analgesic use; those with poor knowledge/beliefs about nonprescription analgesics; and those using nonprescription analgesics in anticipation of pain or to avoid missing a practice or game are associated with misuse of nonprescription analgesic.

Lessons Learned

Based on the results obtained, improving communication between student athletes, physicians and coaching staff should have a significant impact of the misuse of nonprescription analgesic among student athletes. Increased communication should begin with inclusion of a question regarding nonprescription analgesic use on pre-participation physical exams. Student athletes who use more than the recommended dose of a nonprescription analgesic more frequently fail to inform staff or physician regarding nonprescription analgesic use. Perhaps youth who are involved in competitive sports are not notifying team personnel because they are not being asked. Although the accuracy of response would be questionable, inquiring about nonprescription analgesic use on pre-participation physical exams would provide a ground work for increased communication regarding nonprescription analgesics.

Intervention specialists should take the following steps based on this study and that is to identify at-risk youth and provide proven interventions that include a combination of curriculum, parent or significant others, intervention and experiential opportunities for students to utilize the skills they learn from these programs offer primary, secondary and tertiary prevention strategies for at risk youth at all levels of prevention. At the primary prevention level, strategies should include:

- Programs that focus on communication strategies and effective interaction with youth often generate improved risk reduction patterns between athletes and athletic personnel. . Programs that interrupt the at-risk behavior, that often includes such things as bullying and peer victimization and pressure deter effective communication between students and the bully.
- Programs that increase understanding of enhancing protective factors in the home, school and community improve bonding with parents, family, school personnel and athletic staff and peers. Programs that maximize helping networks like peer counseling and proactive counseling services for at-risk youth who have poor socialization and need peer social competency skills

Secondary Prevention Strategies often include:

- Identifying youth and families at risk and provide referral to school and/or community services to promote bonding
- Monitoring high risk students through peer counseling programs and risk assessment models
- Providing education and counseling strategies for students who need to develop social competency and self regulation skills through mentoring.

Tertiary Prevention Strategies may include:

- Reducing the incidence and prevalence of at-risk behaviors and promoting protective factors
- In the home, family and school networks through effective open communication and modeling.

- Multiple strategies involving character education components in the curriculum, school bonding experiences, active involvement of teachers, counselors and parents facilitate school and family bonding.

Prevention Intervention Strategies for School based at Risk Student Athletes

Intervention specialists need to be aware of the risk and protective factors among peers, schoo land athletics personnel, family and community members. These include the following: peer group risk factors include emotional problems and an inability to delay gratification. Aggressive behavior and sensation seeking are major risk factors and lead to alcohol and substance abuse. Protective factors among peers often involve respect authority, responsible behavior and effective independent thinking skills and good communication skills permit social competence and self regulation.

School based risk factors often include little or no home support, low achievement expectations, family dysfunction and lack of school commitment. Protective school factors include caring school personnel, social skills encouraged in the classroom and cooperative learning and an effective teacher/child relationship are encouraged.

Risk factors in the family include distress/low stability; marital/family conflict; parental abuse/neglect and lack of discipline. Protective family factors include a positive child/parent relationship; support and affection from family, high expectations regarding behavior and discipline and rule enforcement in the home.

Community risk factors often include concentrated poverty, schools with high failure/dropout rates and firearms and crime. Often there is a lack of positive role models. Protective factors in the community include trustworthy role models, adults helping students, responsibility and relationship and respect for both self and others.

Delivering Prevention Interventions for At Risk Youth in Rural Communities

The question remains as to how to delivery intervention services for rural and underserved populations and communities. New directions in education, health care and clinical practice have led to applications for clinical consultation that enhance the quality of patient care through telehealth. Miller, Burton, Hill, Lutfman, Veltkamp, Swope (2005) Whitten, Cook Shaw et al (1998) Sargent (1999), Miller, Miller, Kraus, Sprang (2003) Shaw, Boodwin, Whitten, Doolittle (1999) and Whitten and Cook (1999) Young & Irenson (2003) have all addressed the use of school based telemedicine applications. Through this medium, youth in need of specialized care that might not readily be available to them can have the specialty consultation of experts using telehealth technology. Summarized in Table 1 are some of the emerging trends in each of these categories. Most notable among these changes are the multiple uses of telehealth in the administrative and clinical models of health care delivery.

Prevention Through a Telehealth Intervention Model

Telehealth is the use of telecommunications technology to provide clinical consultation across distances and has recently reemerged as a potentially clinically appropriate, cost-effective means of meeting the needs of some students in the changing health care system. Telehealth has been considered a partial solution to the problems of delivering health care to remote areas, as well as to areas underserved by health care professionals. Various projects have demonstrated a wide variety of clinical tasks that can successfully be accomplished by a interactive television, and voice communication systems. The need for such systems is obvious in the face of the major obstacles clinicians face in providing a high standard of health care delivery in a time efficient and cost-effective manner. (Bashshur & Armstrong, 1996; Forkner, Reardon, Carson, 1996; Miller, 1998; Miller, Elliott, Long, Marzenac, Moder 2006; Mahue, Whitten Allen, 2001). The first author of this chapter is a child psychologist in a consulting practice, wherein a rural school system asked for clinical evaluations of several students and student athletes who had been presenting a spectrum of behavioral disorders described as seriously disruptive in the school setting. Realizing the complexity of problems and no board certified child psychiatrists in the area, it was proposed that through the use of an innovative telecommunications approach, needed clinical services could be provided to this school system with a multidisciplinary consultation that would include a child clinical psychologist on site working with a school psychologist, an advanced practice nurse, clinical social worker, special education specialist and the consultation of a child psychiatrist by video link to a university based department of psychiatry through an inexpensive and cost effective model of telehealth. Through the use of specialized telemetric link, the provision of needed interdisciplinary clinical consultation and service would be provided to school officials and support staff in a cost effective and timely manner. The service ranged from consultation about each of the referred youth to a clinical diagnostic evaluation, a multidisciplinary team treatment plan and subsequent implementation of clinical services.

Youth with special needs in rural settings are seen in their community setting through the rural school system. The clinician may wish the consultation of a local or regional specialist and may use Internet video technology through a community clinic. In some cases, the need to have specialized psychiatric consultation services from a medical center based child psychiatric clinic linked to a community clinic or school district may be offered through telehealth technology. In this case, clinical records can be shared through electronic medical records to consulting clinicians, school personnel and provide them with an opportunity to review information individually and respond to relevant clinical issues. The clinical staffing of the youth can involve the referring clinician in the rural setting, the community consulting specialists and the university based specialist can be achieved through interactive video. Using secure two way interactive technology, a spectrum of services can be provided in a more cost effective and time efficient manner resulting in various levels of prevention interventions including consultation, clinical management, patient education, family education, continuing education for school personnel and direct services to the troubled youth(Miller, 2005, Miller & Holcomb 2007) .

Issues in the Technology of Telehealth

The technology of telehealth involves a spectrum of interactive video transmission modes. Currently, transmission modes include analog and digital. The analog mode, transmitted in the form of waves, is the technology of broadcast television. Among its advantages are the high resolution of the images transmitted and its familiarity. There are disadvantages with interactive video transmission, the most prominent of which is the expense associated with transmission and the size and complexity of the hardware that is required for such efforts. The digital mode, on the other hand, takes advantage of developments in computer science and transmits in the form of a digital byte-stream of zero's and ones. Its advantages are lower transmission costs, reduced equipment size, simplicity of operation and easy interface with computers and with computerized systems. The relative disadvantages of the digital system appear to include the so called echoes of motion that appear at slow transmission speeds (Sanders and Bashshur, 1995;Miller, 2006).

A prevention intervention service to rural school districts for school personnel and for students with special needs is among the options for telehealth services can offer. Telehealth services through the schools offers a visionary method of providing access for students, teachers and administrators to a spectrum of services not often easily available. Standardized and universal coverage to all children by linking metropolitan and flagship university medical centers and specialist services with rural school districts can be accomplished through this technology. The impact and cost on the provision of standard-based clinical services must be evaluated through clinical research and outcome studies to assess the effectiveness of the use of telehealth in the provision of such clinical services (Ghosh, McLaren, Watson, 1997, Stamm, Friedman, Schnurr, Hsieh, Rudolph, & Millman, 1998). Telehealth and its adaptability to clinical services offer new avenues for provision of clinical care in the areas of consultation, diagnosis and treatment services to underserved populations. Herein described has been another model where telehealth can provide innovation in assessing human factors in the delivery of comprehensive standards of care to populations in need of such services.

Table 1. Patterns in Telehealth Consultation and Care

	Past Patterns	**Contemporary Patterns**
Administrative Paradigms	Time consuming referrals and long, delayed consultations to medical centers, independent clinical practices and community expertise. Travel time and expense of travel for at risk youth	Quick, efficient, confidential and secure networks and alliances; contracting through integrated services delivery system of service providers using teleconferencing.
Clinical Models	Provider-focused, clinicians and individual providers/specialists. They provide services on an independent basis to school, courts.	Patient-focused, clinical models, clinician, and team of providers and specialists provide easy and secure access to care
Information Models	Paper records, provider developed record systems, local accessibility in the schools, health care and court systems to records. Long delays in transfer of information	Internet and interactive television consultation, electronic health records, online support systems, electronic files and e-mail electronic information exchange for comprehensive and integrated network of services.

Take Home Messages for Prevention Researchers

In summary, it is essential that developmental risk researchers carefully re-examine critical elements in design and methodology addressed earlier. Consistent with the results of the most consensual of the NIDA Resiliency and Risk Workgroup recommendations was a definitive endorsement for the further development and expansion of prevention programs which focus on the family (Glantz 1995). Drawing on the discussion in this chapter along with a variety of research findings showing the strong drug abuse resilience and risk influence of the family on children and adolescents, the panel strongly encouraged the development of preventive interventions which respond to the individual in the context of their particular family. Therefore a significant part of the origin of drug abuse is often the abusers' families' dysfunctions and inadequacies and a significant factor in resistance is often the positive characteristics and influences of the family. Therefore, the panel's first major recommendation was that interventions should be directed at mitigating these family problems and/or enhancing family strengths. This would necessitate, more often than not, intervening with and probably "treating," not just the individual but the family. The family would not merely be the medium for intervention but would be a direct target of the intervention. The "family" would include extended, non-traditional and surrogate families. Strengthening family identity and long term activities was suggested as an integral part of this goal (Glantz 1995).

Glantz (1995) notes that the major recommendation of the NIDA Resiliency and Risk Workgroup derives from multiple research findings which indicate that deficits or impairments in certain abilities are commonly characteristic of and probably predisposition to drug use and abuse. The skill areas proposed as intervention targets should include executive/cognitive function including goal setting, analysis, planning, organization and problem solving; affect regulation including both impulse control and techniques for adaptively coping with and controlling strong negative feelings and positive reinforcement approach skills. This last skill area refers to the observation that many drug abusers' coping skills and defenses are oriented around escape from problems and negative affects rather than being based on active positive coping involving approach. What is clear for development risk researchers at this time is we have benefited from the guidance of such panels as the NIDA Resiliency and Risk Workgroup and several of the prevention scientists noted in this chapter. It is to the next generation of prevention scientists that this chapter is intended in an effort to provide them with some direction for the future of the science and practice of a developmental risk research model for overcoming socio psychological risk among at-risk youth.

Acknowledgments

Thomas W. Miller, Ph.D., ABPP is a Professor, Department of Psychiatry University of Kentucky, College of Medicine, Lexington, Kentucky. Douglas F. Wolf, MS, ATC, CSCS is Program Coordinator, Community Health Initiative, Athletic Trainer, Sports Medicine, Nationwide Children's Hospital, Sports Medicine & Orthopedic Center, Nationwide Children's Hospital, Columbus , Ohio. The authors wish to acknowledge the support and assistance of. Professors Linda Pescatello Ph.D. and Christopher Barnes Ph.D. University of Connecticut, Will French, M.D., Lane J. Veltkamp MSW, Charles Lowe Ph.D., and Brenda Frommer in the preparation of this manuscript. In addition, the assistance of Jill Livingston MLS, Tag Heister MLS library services is appreciated.

References

Anderson, K and Anderson L.E. (1998) *Mosby's Pocket Dictionary of Medicine, Nursing & Allied Health*. New York: Mosby Publishers Incorporated.

Bashshur, R., & Armstrong, P. (1996). Telemedicine: a new mode for the delivery of health care. *Inquiry* 113: 233-244

Beane, A, Miller, T. W. & Spurling, R. (2008) The Bully Free Program: A Profile for Prevention in the School Setting. In: Miller, T. W. (ed) School *Violence and Primary Prevention*. New York: Springer Publisher, Inc.

Benninga, G. and Wynne, A.B. Trends in Youth Character Development. *The Construction of Children's Character*. Chicago Illinois: The National Society for the Study of Education.

Bernstein J, Stovitz S, Kuffner E. (2003) Analgesia in sports medicine: integral issues for the sports-related injury. Proceedings of the 54th Annual Meeting & Clinical Symposia of the National Athletic Trainers' Association; 2003 June 26; St. Louis, Missouri. SynerMed Communications

Board Of Education v. Pico, 457 U.S. 853 (1982), Legal Decision available at: http://www.oyez.org/cases/1980-1989/1981/1981_80_2043/

Clayton, Richard R., Nancy Grant Harrington, William Turner, Thomas Miller, Donna Durden. (2000). *Rural Educational Achievement Project (REAP)* Unpublished executive summary. Lexington, Ky.: University of Kentucky, Center for Prevention Research.

Ellen Scholder P, Fitzgerald Bone P, Stuart EW. How well do young people follow the label? An investigation of four classes of over-the-counter drugs. *Journal of Public Policy & Marketing. 1998*;17(1):70-85.

Ghosh, G.J., McLaren, P.M., & Watson, J.P. (1997). Evaluating the alliance in video-link teletherapy. *Journal of Telehealth, 3* (suppl. 1), 33-35.

Glantz, M. (1995) The Application of Resiliency and Risk Research to the Development of Preventive Interventions. Rockville, Maryland: NIDA Resiliency and Risk Workgroup. Retrieved April 08, 2008 at NIDA Resiliency and Risk Workgroup website http://www.nida.nih.gov/ResilandRiskWG/ResilandRiskWG.html

Josephson Institute (2008) Defining Character: *The Six Pillars of Character*. Retrieved at web site: http://josephsoninstitute.org/sixpillars.html

Kalichman, S.C., Simbayi, L.C., Vermaakk, R., Jooste, S., and Cain, D. (2008). HIV/AIDS Risk among Men and Women Who Drink at Informal Alcohol Serving Establishments (Shebeens) Cape Town, South Africa. *Prevention Science, 9,* 55-62.

Kuffner E.(2003) Over-the-counter analgesics: what athletic trainers need to know. Analgesia in sports medicine: integral issues for the sports-related injury. Proceedings of the 54th Annual Meeting & Clinical Symposia of the National Athletic Trainers' Association; 2003 June 26; St. Louis, Missouri. SynerMed Communications; 2003

Lester-Bradley, J (1991) Schools struggling to enforce drug rules. Unpublished Manuscript, Washington State University, Department of Athletics.

Lin, C.A., Neafsey, P.J., & Strickler, Z. (2008). Usability Testing by Older Adults of a Computer-Mediated Health Communication Program. *Journal of Health Communication,* 14(2) 167-179.

Mahue, M., Whitten, P., & Allen, A. (2001). *E-health, telehealth, and telemedicine: A practical guide to start-up and success.* San Francisco: Jossey-Bass.

Miller, T.W. (2005) School related violence and primary prevention. Guest Editorial. *Journal of Primary Prevention* 26 (5) 381-382.

Miller, T.W., Burton, D. Hill, K., Luftman, S. Veltkamp, L. J. & M. Swope (2005) Telepsychiatry: Critical Dimensions for Forensic Services *Journal of the Academy of Psychiatry and the Law.* 33: (4) 539-546.

Miller, T.W., Elliott, B., Long, K. Marzenac, C., Moder, M. (2006) Telehealth Home Health Applications for Adults with Developmental Disabilities. *Telemedicine & e-Health 12 (2) 56-64.*

Miller, T. W. (2006). Telehealth issues in consulting psychology practice. *Consulting Psychology Journal: Practice and Research,* 58, 82-90.

Miller, T.W. & Holcomb, T.F. (2007) Telehealth Applications for Counselors in the Schools. *Kentucky Counseling Association Journal* 26 (1) 6-13.

Miller, T. W., Miller, J.M., & Kraus, O.F, Sprang, R. (2003). Telehealth a clinical Application model for rural consultation. *Consulting Psychology Journal, 55(2),* 119-127.

Miller, T. W., Kraus, R. F. and Veltkamp, L. J. (2008) Character Education as a Prevention Strategy for School-related Violence. In: Miller, T. W. (ed) *School Violenceand Primary Prevention.* New York: Springer Publisher, Inc.

Miller, T.W. & Holcomb, T.F. (2007) Telehealth Applications for Counselors in the Schools. *Kentucky Counseling Association Journal* 26 (1) 6-13.

Nickelson, D. W. (1998). Telehealth and the evolving health care system: Strategic opportunities for professional psychology. *Professional Psychology: Research and Practice, 29,* 527-534.

National Advisory Committee on Rural Health and Human Services (2004).The 2004 Report to the Secretary: Rural Health and Human Services. Available at: ftp://ftp.hrsa.gov/ruralhealth/NAC04web.pdf

Neafsey, P.J., Jarrin, O., Luciano, S. & Coffman, M. (2007). Self-medication practices of Spanish-speakingolder adults in Hartford, Connecticut. *Hispanic Health Care International, 5*(4), 169-179.

Nickelson, D. (1996). Behavioral telehealth: Emerging practice, research, and policy opportunities. *Behavioral Sciences and the Law*, 14, 443-457

Norton, W.E. (g), Amico, K.R., Copenhaver, M., Cornman, D.H., Fisher, J.D., Fisher, W.A., Kozal, M., & Friedland,G. (2008). Attitudinal correlates of needle sharing in a sample of HIV+ patients in clinical care. *AIDS Care, 20(4)*, 462-469.

Office of Rural Health Policy, Health Resources and Services Administration. (1994). *Reaching: Rural health travel in the telecommunications highway.* Rockville, MD: Federal Office of Rural Health Policy.

Park, C. L. (2008). Estimated longevity and changes in spirituality in the context of advanced congestive heart failure. *Journal of Supportive and Palliative Care, 6,* 3-11.

Sanders, J.H., & Bashshur, R.L. (1995) Perspective: Challenges to the implementation of telemedicine. *Telemedicine Journal*, 1, 115-123.

Sargent, I. (1999). School based mental health in rural Kansas: A novel use for telepsychiatry. abstract]. *Telemedicine Journal*, 5(1), 55-58.

Shaw, P., Goodwin, J., Whitten, P., & Doolittle, G., (1999). Tele-Kid Care: An urban telemedicine service for an underserved pediatric population. [abstract]. *Telemedicine Journal, 5* (1), 25-26.

Stamm, B.H., Friedman, M.J., Schnurr, P., Hsieh, F., Rudolph, J.M., & Millman, A. (1998, April). Using telemedicine tools for the administration of a multi-site clinical trail. Poster session presented at the annual meeting of the American Telemedicine Association, Orlando, FL.

Tricker R. (2000) Painkilling drugs in collegiate athletics: knowledge, attitudes, and use of student athletes. *Journal of Drug Education*, 30(3):313-24.

U.S. Department of Health and Human Services. (1997). Exploratory evaluation of rural applications of telemedicine [Online]. Available: www.ntia.doc.gov

Walker, H.M., Horner, R.H., Sugai, G., Bullis, M., Sprague, J.R., Bricker, D., & Kaufman, M.J. (1996). Integrated approaches to preventing antisocial behavior patterns among school-age children and youth. *Journal of Emotional and Behavioral Disorders,* 4(4), 194-209.

Warner DC, Schnepf G, Barrett MS, Dian D, Swigonski NL. (2002) Prevalence, attitudes, and behaviors related to the use of non-steroidal anti-inflammatory drugs (NSAIDs) in student athletes. *Journal of Adolescent Health*. 2002 Mar;30(3):150-6.

Whitten, B., Cook, D.J., Shaw, P., Ermer, D., & Goodwin, J. (1998). Telekid Care: Bringing health care into schools. *Telemedicine Journal*, 4(4), 335-43.

Whitten, P.S., & Cook, D.J. (1999). School-based telemedicine: Using technology to bring healthcare to inner-city children. [abstract]. *Journal of Telemedicine and Telecare,* 5, (Suppl 1), S23-5.

Wolf, D. F. (2005) Nonprescription Analgesic Use Among Division 1-A Football Players Pilot Research Project to assess the Use of Over the Counter Drugs Used by Athletes. Columbus Children's Hospital & Ohio State University. Unpublished Manuscript.

Yoon, J.S. & Barton, E. (2008) The Role of Teachers in School Violence and Bullying Prevention In: Miller, T. W. (ed) *School Violence and Primary Prevention.* New York: Springer Publisher, Inc.

Young, T & Irenson, C (2003) Effectiveness of School based Telehealth Care in Rural Elementary Schools. *Pediatrics* 112 (5) 1088-1096.

In: Encyclopedia of Sports and Athletics
Editors: Jack L. Murray and Emily O. Watson
ISBN: 978-1-61209-959-0

Chapter XXI

Understanding the Basis for Sport Friendships in Adapted Sport Athletes: Does Fulfilling Basic Psychological Needs Matter?

Philip M. Wilson*[*,1] Diane E. Mack[1], Enrique García Bengoechea,[2] Xie Bin,[3] Susanna Cheung[1], and Benjamin D. Sylvester[1]

[1] Faculty of Applied Health Sciences, Brock University, Canada
[2] Department of Kinesiology & Physical Education, McGill University, Canada
[3] Xi'An Physical Education University, Peoples Republic of China

Abstract

Objective

Characteristics of social relationships such as friendship quality have important motivational implications within the context of sport (c.f., McDonough & Crocker, 2005). The purpose of this study was to examine the utility of Basic Psychological Needs Theory (BPNT; Deci & Ryan, 2002) as a framework for understanding friendship quality amongst athletes competing in adapted sport.

Methods

Participants (N = 51; 55.80% male) drawn from cohorts reporting either a congenital or acquired disability completed a self-report instrument on a single occasion assessing perceived competence, autonomy and relatedness experienced when engaged in adapted

[*] Correspondence concerning this article should be addressed to Philip M. Wilson, PhD,
Behavioural Health Sciences Research Lab,
Department of Physical Education & Kinesiology, Faculty of Applied Health Sciences,
500 Glenridge Avenue, Brock University, St Catharines, Ontario, L2S 3A1
Tel: (905) 699-5550 Ext. 4997, Fax: (905) 688-8364, e-mail: pwilson4@brocku.ca

sport. The instrument also contained the Sport Friendship Quality Scale (SFQS; Weiss & Smith, 1999) to assess perceived friendship quality in sport.

Results: Bivariate correlations revealed a pattern of moderate-to-strong correlations between the five SFQS dimensions and a weak-to-moderate pattern of associations between indices of psychological need satisfaction. Simultaneous multiple regression models indicated that perceptions of psychological need satisfaction accounted for small-to-moderate amounts of the variance in the five SFQS constructs. Perceived relatedness was the dominant predictor of sport friendship quality irrespective of the SFSQ dimension investigated with the strongest association evident with SFSQ-Companionship and Pleasant Play and the weakest with SFSQ-Conflict.

Conclusion

Overall, this study offers initial support for the role of BPNT's psychological needs within the realm of adapted sport as a vehicle for understanding sport friendships. It appears that perceived relatedness with fellow athletes in adapted sport contexts is a plausible route for developing secure friendships within the realm of adapted sport. The extent to which perceptions of autonomy and competence matter in relation to friendship experiences within adapted sport contexts beyond perceived relatedness warrants further inquiry.

Introduction

Social relationships can play an integral role in shaping the experiences derived from participation in competitive sport (Smith & McDonough, 2008). Evidence to substantiate the importance of social relationships for understanding a broad range of issues germane to continued youth sport involvement has emerged. Embedded within qualitative frameworks, social relationships have been found to be complex yet salient to youth sport participants with reference to both parents and peers (Garcia Bengoechea & Strean, 2007; Holt, Black, Tamminen, Fox, Mandigo, 2008; Holt, Tamminen, Black, Sehn, & Wall, 2008). Additional evidence substantiates the notion that social relationships in the form of sport friendships appear essential for understanding youth sport motivation (Ullrich-French & Smith, 2006), indicators of well-being (McDonough & Crocker, 2007), and behavioral participation (Ullrich-French & Smith, 2009). With growing consensus that social relationships play an important role in youth sport, understanding 'how' and 'why' social relationships form emerges as a key avenue for sport psychology research.

One theory that holds promise in terms of understanding the dynamics of 'how' and 'why' social relationships develop within applied contexts such as sport is Self-Determination Theory (SDT; Deci & Ryan, 2002). SDT is a macro-level theory of human motivation and development that is comprised of five 'mini-theories' which collectively account for the nature and function of human motivation and development. The central organizing principle that integrates SDT's 'mini-theories' concerns the ongoing interaction between organisms with aspects of their social world that facilitate (or hinder) assimilation, growth, and optimal human development (Deci & Ryan, 2002). Although the SDT-based approach posits that humans are naturally endowed with the capacity for growth and development, Deci and Ryan (2002) argue that these innate tendencies flourish (or flounder) as a function of fulfilling basic psychological needs for competence, autonomy, and relatedness.

Basic Psychological Needs Theory (BPNT; Deci & Ryan, 2002; 2008) is the sub-component of SDT that outlines the nature and function of psychological needs. The psychological needs for competence, autonomy, and relatedness are central to BPNT. Each psychological need, when satisfied authentically, enhances social functioning, promotes adaptation, integrates functioning, and optimizes well-being (Deci & Ryan, 2002; 2008). Competence refers to the feeling of mastery (or effectance; White, 1959) that accompanies engaging in tasks that challenge us in optimal ways. Autonomy concerns feeling volitional in one's actions such that behavior is undertaken willingly as opposed to under the duress of an external cause (deCharms, 1968). Finally, relatedness is concerned with establishing and maintaining secure bonds or meaningful attachments with others who occupy our social world (La Guardia & Patrick, 2008). While not without controversy (Iyengar & Lepper, 1999), an emerging body of evidence across domains (including sport) illustrates the positive effects stemming from the fulfillment of competence, autonomy, and to a lesser extent relatedness needs, in terms of motivational development, behavioral persistence, and enhanced well-being (Deci & Ryan, 2008, Hagger & Chatzisarantis, 2007).

Although the role of social relationships in domains outside of sport has been examined using SDT (Grolnick & Apostoleris, 2002) and BPNT (La Guardia & Patrick, 2008), limited attention has been afforded the role of BPNT in terms of understanding the dynamic nature of social relationships amongst athletes. Isolated studies (Ullrich-French & Smith, 2006; 2009) have examined perceptions of competence in soccer. For example, Ullrich-French and Smith (2006) note stronger associations between feelings of acceptance by peers than sport friendships with perceived competence in youth soccer players (M_{age} < 12 years) although interactive effects were noted between social relationship constructs and competence. As the integration of SDT-based constructs with dimension of social relationships could be informative (Ullrich-French & Smith, 2006) to sport psychologists this area seems ripe for further research for a number of reasons. First, previous sport-based studies have used only 'select' psychological needs drawn from Deci and Ryan's (2002) BPNT. Outside the realm of competitive sport, compelling evidence has been demonstrated that all three psychological needs central to BPNT have relevance to understanding social relationships (La Guardia, Ryan, Couchman, & Deci, 2000; La Guardia & Patrick, 2008). Second, Ullrich-French and Smith (2006) combined dimensions of friendship quality into a unitary index which is consistent with the broader literature concerning social relationships (c.f., Sharabany, 1994) yet may obfuscate the nature of the basic psychological need-friendship quality relationship. Third, the role afforded BPNT in terms of social relationship issues and processes has been examined predominantly in youth sport athletes ergo excluding adults where the mechanisms influencing social dynamics within relationships remains an important research issue (La Guardia & Patrick, 2008). Finally, social relationships have been conceptualized as a 'determinant' of either perceived competence or relatedness in previous sport psychology research (Ullrich-French & Smith, 2006; 2009). Drawing from the literature concerning BPNT (c.f., Deci & Ryan, 2002; La Guardia & Patrick, 2008), it seems likely that fulfilling the psychological needs for competence, autonomy, and relatedness via sport provides an avenue through which social relationships 'develop' rather than 'emerge' (La Gaurdia et al., 2000).

In an effort to address Deci and Ryan's (2002) contentions, the main aim of this investigation was to examine the utility of BPNT as a framework for understanding the quality of social relationships in athletes competing across Canada in adapted sport leagues. A secondary purpose concerned testing the degree of interdependency amongst perceived competence, autonomy, and relatedness needs fulfilled via adapted sport participation. The quality of sport friendships served as the indicator of social relationships in the present investigation because 1) limited data concerning the nature or function of friendship quality outside of the realm of youth sport contexts exists (c.f., Weiss & Smith, 1999), and 2) advances in relationship science (La Guardia & Patrick, 2008) contend that friendships (alongside romantic partners) provide the greatest insight into relationship dynamics given the "reciprocal, mutual exchange" (p. 201) inherent in such relationships.

The hypotheses for this study were drawn from previous theorizing pertaining to the nature and function of basic psychological needs within the BPNT approach (Deci & Ryan, 2002), and SDT-based research that has linked fulfillment of basic psychological needs with adaptive elements of social relationships (La Guardia & Patrick, 2008). First, it was hypothesized that experiences of competence, autonomy, and relatedness would be positively associated with one another given that they form the cornerstone for optimal functioning within SDT's organismic-dialectical approach to human functioning (Deci & Ryan, 2002). Second, it was hypothesized that fulfillment of all three psychological needs inherent within BPNT would be positively associated with adaptive elements (e.g., having common interests) of sport friendships and negatively associated with dysfunctional elements (e.g., conflict) based on the work of La Guardia and Patrick (2008). Third, consistent with La Guardia et al. (2000), it was hypothesized that perceived relatedness would be more strongly linked with elements of sport friendships than either perceived competence or autonomy.

Methods

Participants

Participants were male (n = 29; M_{age} = 35.50 years; SD = 12.09 years; 67.90 % full-time employed; 92.90% Caucasian/White) and female (n = 14; M_{age} = 35.31 years; SD = 16.64 years; 28.63% full-time employed; 85.70% Caucasian/White) athletes competing at the time of data collection in adapted sport leagues throughout Canada. Nine athletes providing data for this project did not disclose their gender. The average length of time involved in adapted sport competition for this sample was 21.76 years (SD = 13.73 years) for males and 18.21 years (SD = 9.50 years) for females. The majority of participants reported living with a disability that was acquired (58.50%) as opposed to congenital (41.50%). The prevalence of various disabilities within the sample was as follows: (a) Spinal Cord Injury (31.00%); (b) Cerebral Palsy (11.90%); (c) Amputee (11.90%); (d) Spina Bifida (9.50%); (e) Visual Impairments (4.80%); (f) Polio (4.80%); (g) Other (2.40%). On average, these athletes reported living with their disability for 23.42 years although considerable variability was evident in participant responses (SD = 13.78 years; values ranged from 2.00 to 65.00 years inclusive). Greater variability was evident in the female compared to the male data pertaining to the different competitive levels of sport undertaken by participants, yet 83.70 percent of the sample reported competing at the national level. Self-reported training history varied across in-season (M = 14.19 hours/week; SD = 9.25 hours/week), off-season (M = 7.96 hours/week; SD = 5.89 hours/week), and pre-season (M = 10.62 hours/week; SD = 6.73 hours/week) time periods but did not differ as a function of athlete's gender (Wilk's $\Lambda = 0.97$, $F_{3,34} = 0.39$, partial $\eta^2 = 0.03$). Most of the athletes providing data indicated that they competed in a competitive adapted sport league (35.70%) or a competitive league that integrated adapted sport athletes with able-bodied athletes (52.40%). For those indicating participation in recreational leagues, 7.10% were exclusive to adapted sport athletes and 4.80% indicated they competed with able-bodied athletes.

Instruments

Perceived Competence

Participants completed the 6-item Perceived Competence subscale of the Intrinsic Motivation Inventory (IMI-PC; Ryan, 1982) as an index of their feelings of competence in adapted sports. The set of IMI-PC items was preceded by a stem that contextualized participant responses within the realm of adapted sport ("The following questions represent different feelings people have when they are engaged in sport. Please answer the following questions by considering how you typically feel when participating in sport using the scale provided."). A sample IMI-PC item used in this study is as follows: "I think I am pretty good at sport". Using a Likert-type format, each response was anchored at the extremes with (1) = "Not at all true" and (7) = "Very true". Previous research using variants of these IMI-PC items indicate that participant responses in a sample of competitive athletes contained minimal error variance (Cronbach's $\alpha = 0.80$) and correlated positively with a proxy index of intrinsic motivation (McAuley, Duncan, & Tammen, 1989).

Perceived Autonomy

Participants completed 7 items modified from the Basic Need Satisfaction in General (BNSG) instrument (c.f., Gagné, 2003) to assess perceived autonomy (BNSG-A) experienced by athletes participating in adapted sport. The BNSG is a family of instruments designed to capture feelings of competence, autonomy, and relatedness experienced globally in one's life that have been used extensively in SDT-based research to assess feelings of psychological need satisfaction. The original BNSG-A items were modified slightly to be specific to adapted sport (e.g., the original BNSG-A item "I feel like I can pretty much be myself in my daily situations" was modified to "I feel like I can pretty much be myself in sport"). The full set of 7 modified BNSG-A items used in this study was preceded by an instructional stem designed to situate participant responses in the context of their typical experiences within adapted sport ("The following statements represent different feelings people have when they are engaged in adapted sport. Please answer the following questions by considering how you typically feel when participating in your sport using the scale provided."). Each item was responded to across a 7-point Likert-scale anchored by (1) = Not at all true and (7) = Very true). Previous research using adaptations of the BNSG-A items within sport indicate responses to these items present minimal problems in terms of error variance (Cronbach $\alpha > 0.83$) and correlate positively with more self-determined motivation and negatively with one facet of athlete burnout (Lonsdale, Hodge, & Rose, 2009).

Perceived Relatedness

Participants completed 6 items modified from the Relatedness to Others in Physical Activity Scale (ROPAS; Wilson & García Bengoechea, under review) to be sport specific for adapted sport athletes. The original items comprising the ROPAS were developed using an iterative approach to construct validation in order to capture feelings of connection and belongingness within the broad spectrum of physical activities people engage in their leisure time (Sample item: "I feel like I have a close bond with others"). The instructional stem used to orientate participant responses to the BNSG-A was also used with the ROPAS. Each ROPAS item was anchored on a 6-point Likert rating scale with verbal descriptors ranging from 1 (False) and 6 (True). Previous studies using the ROPAS indicate that scores derived from this instrument represent a single latent factor that appears invariant across gender and contains minimal error variance (Cronbach α's = 0.89-0.93 across gender-specific subsamples; Wilson & García Bengoechea, under review). Use of the ROPAS in the present study represents the first attempt to employ the instrument in a sport setting or with adapted sport athletes.

Sport Friendships

Weiss and Smith's (1999) Sport Friendship Quality Scale (SFSQ) was used to assess the quality of sport friendships felt by adapted sport athletes in relation to their best friend within adapted sport. The SFSQ is comprised of 22 items that assess the following 6 dimensions of sport friendships quality: (a) Self-Esteem Enhancement and Supportiveness; (b) Loyalty and Intimacy; (c) Things in Common; (d) Companionship and Pleasant Play; (e) Conflict Resolution; and (f) Conflict. An instructional stem developed by Weiss and Smith (1999) for use with young athletes was included in this study that requested participants to list the name of their best friend in adapted sport and respond to each SFSQ item in relation to their experiences with that person. Each SFSQ item was anchored on a 5-point Likert rating scale with verbal descriptors affixed to response options 1 (Not at all true) and 5 (Really true). Previous research using youth sport athletes from the United States of America (Weiss & Smith, 1999) and Canada (McDonough & Crocker, 2005) provide support for the internal consistency reliability of responses to the items comprising the SFSQ (Cronbach α's ranged from 0.70-0.92 across samples) and mixed support for the structural validity of the measurement model posited to underpin SFSQ responses. Dimensions of sport friendship quality indexed by the SFSQ have been linked with peer acceptance (Weiss & Smith, 2002) and to a lesser extent sport commitment (McDonough & Crocker, 2005) in a logical manner.

Data Collection Procedures & Data Analyses

Adapted sport athletes were contacted initially using a variety of approaches designed to capture an assortment of adapted sport athletes for the purposes of this study. Initial recruitment strategies included electronic advertisements posted to internet websites, dissemination of recruitment information via relevant listserv's, and personal contact with sport-specific organizations (e.g., Ontario Cerebral Palsy Sports Association) who subsequently advertised the study to their membership. Initial recruitment strategies were then followed by snowball sampling. All participants who expressed an interest in being involved in the study received a Letter of Invitation (LOI) via e-mail outlining the nature of the study, the benefits (and costs) of the study, and provided all potential participants with an opportunity to address questions or raise concerns they had regarding their involvement. After receiving the LOI, interested participants selected a weblink that sent them to a secure internet site where they completed an informed consent protocol before starting the study. After the provision of informed consent, each athlete completed a multi-section instrument on a single occasion. This study protocol was reviewed and received clearance by a university research ethics committee prior to any participant recruitment or data collection.

Data analysis proceeded in sequential stages. First, the data were screened for patterns of missing values, identification of statistical outliers, and examined for conformity with relevant statistical assumptions. Second, internal consistency estimates (Cronbach's α; Cronbach, 1951) and descriptive statistics were calculated across study variables. Subscale scores were subsequently computed by taking the average of the relevant items/construct. Third, bivariate correlations (Pearson *r*'s) were computed to examine associations between perceived psychological need satisfaction and the dimensions of sport friendship quality measured by the SFSQ. Finally, a series of multiple regression models were specified and tested to examine the contributions of perceived competence, autonomy, and relatedness to predicting dimensions of sport friendship quality in adapted sport athletes. The order of variable entry in the regression models was simultaneous in each of the six models tested where SFSQ dimensions served as the criterion and indices of psychological need satisfaction experienced within adapted sport were denoted as the predictors.

Results

Preliminary Data Analysis

Examination of participant responses indicated no out-of-range data for any manifest IMI-PC, BNSG-A, ROPAS, or SFQS items. Missing data varied considerably across individual items comprising the questionnaire used in this study. Items comprising the IMI-PC demonstrated the least missing data (22.60-24.50%) whilst the largest amount of missing data was evident across the SFSQ items (32.10-37.70%). Little's (1988) test implied that these non-response data was missing completely at random ($\chi^2 = 337.53$, $df = 457$, $p = 0.99$). Considering the absence of any visual or statistical pattern of missing data in the sample, all missing values were replaced using an expectation maximization algorithm that used available data within the sample to estimate missing values.

Estimates of internal consistency reliability (Cronbach's α; Cronbach, 1951) were computed for scores derived from the IMI-PC, BNSG-A, ROPAS, and SFSQ items. Internal consistency reliability coefficients ranged from 0.56 to 0.92 in this sample (see Table 1 for specific values). Closer inspection of the reliability coefficients indicated that greater error variance was evident amongst the BNSG-A scores than either the IMI-PC or the ROPAS scores in this sample. The reliability estimate for the Conflict Resolution items comprising the SFSQ exhibited the most error variance. Further examination indicated that one of the three SFSQ-Conflict Resolution items ("My friend and I make up easily when we have a fight") was weakly correlated with one other item comprising this subscale of the SFSQ ("When we have an argument, my friend and I talk about how to reach a solution"). Item-level analyses indicated that removal of this item would have reduced the amount of error variance in responses to the SFSQ-Conflict Resolution items ($\alpha_{\text{2-item SFSQ.CR}} = 0.60$) but the improvement in reliability was considered trivial therefore all SFSQ-Conflict Resolution items were retained in subsequent analyses.

Table 1. Descriptive statistics and internal consistency estimates of reliability

	M	*SD*	*Skew.*	*Kurt.*	α
1. Competence	5.75	1.26	-0.69	0.49	0.81
2. Autonomy	5.35	0.10	0.18	-0.30	0.63
3. Relatedness	5.22	0.09	-0.83	0.49	0.92
4. SFQS-Things in Common	4.02	0.11	-1.38	3.46	0.90
5. SFQS-Self-Esteem Enhancement & Supportiveness	4.62	0.06	-1.58	2.61	0.81
6. SFQS-Loyalty & Intimacy	4.17	0.09	-1.08	2.35	0.81
7. SFQS-Things in Common	4.02	0.11	-1.38	3.46	0.90
8. SFQS-Companionship & Pleasant Play	4.38	0.09	-2.89	12.51	0.92
9. SFQS-Conflict Resolution	4.00	0.10	-0.71	1.27	0.56
10. SFQS-Conflict	1.81	0.10	1.18	1.26	0.88

Note: *M* = Mean. *SD* = Standard Deviation. *Skew.* = Univariate Skewness. *Kurt.* = Univariate Kurtosis. α = Internal consistency reliability estimate (Cronbach, 1951). SFQS = Sport friendship Quality Scale (Weiss & Smith, 1999).

Descriptive Statistics and Bivariate Correlations

Inspection of descriptive statistics (see Table 1) revealed several interesting patterns in the data. Perceived competence was the most satisfied psychological need reported by these adapted sport athletes followed by perceptions of autonomy then relatedness. A more distinct pattern was evident in terms of dimensions of sport friendship quality assessed by the SFSQ. Notably, adapted sport athletes reported minimal endorsement of Conflict with their best friend in sport that constitutes feeling mad, getting embroiled in arguments, or fighting (Weiss & Smith, 1999). Contemporaneously, the most strongly endorsed dimension of the SFSQ concerned Self-Esteem Enhancement and Supportiveness indicating that these athletes experienced a considerable degree of praise, encouragement and support from their best friend in sport (Weis & Smith, 1999).

Bivariate correlations between indices of psychological need satisfaction experienced in adapted sport measured with scores from the IMI-PC, BNSG-A, and ROPAS displayed an interesting pattern of relationships. These correlations suggested overlap between scores across these psychological need satisfaction indicators varied considerably ($|r_{12}|$ = 0.18 to 0.57). Perceived competence was most strongly correlated with perceived autonomy (r_{12} = 0.57; $p < .01$) and to a lesser extent with perceived relatedness (r_{12} = 0.38; $p < .01$). The bivariate relationship between perceived autonomy and relatedness was positive albeit modest in magnitude (r_{12} = 0.18; p = .22).

Results of the correlational analyses concerning the relationship between psychological need satisfaction and sport friendship quality dimensions are presented in Table 2. Bivariate correlations between perceptions of competence and autonomy with dimensions of sport friendship quality measured by the SFSQ observed in this sample were generally in the hypothesized direction, although largely weak in magnitude (Cohen, 1992). One notable exception was the relationship between perceived competence with SFSQ-Self-Esteem Enhancement and Supportiveness. Bivariate associations between perceived competence and SFSQ-Loyalty and Intimacy and perceived autonomy with SFSQ-Self-Esteem Enhancement and Supportiveness approached conventional levels of statistical significance (p = 0.10). In contrast, the pattern of bivariate correlations concerning perceived relatedness with dimensions of sport friendship quality were uniformly positive (with the exception of the SFSQ-Conflict) and ranged in magnitude from weak-to-moderate (Mean $|r_{12}|$ = 0.30; Cohen, 1992).

Multiple Regression Analyses Predicting Sport Friendship Quality from Psychological Need Satisfaction

Six separate multiple regression models examined the predictive relationship between indices of psychological need satisfaction (the predictor variables) experienced in adapted sport and each dimension of sport friendship quality assessed with the SFSQ (the criterion variables). Joint consideration of the Variance Inflation Factor (1.15-1.71) and Tolerance (0.58-0.87) values implied the presence of collinearity in the data. Further consideration of the Variance Proportion Values (Range = 0.14 to 0.56) when the Condition Index (CI) exceeded 10.00 (CI's ranged from 1.00 to 27.63 across regression models) indicated that no two VPV's exceeded 0.50 in any regression model suggesting little concern with collinearity in this sample's data (Pedhazur, 1997).

Summary observations from the regression analyses are presented in Table 3 and yield several interesting observations. First, examination of the variance accounted for within each dimension of sport friendship quality by markers of psychological need satisfaction suggests considerable variability in this sample (Adjusted R^2 values ranged from 0.01 to 0.26). Second, it is evident from an inspection of the standardized beta-coefficients and structure coefficients that perceived relatedness was the dominant predictor of each adaptive dimension of sport friendship quality assessed with the SFSQ. Perceived autonomy made the strongest contribution to the regression model concerning SFSQ-Conflict with the direction of the beta and structure coefficients indicating greater feelings of volition and choice were associated with less conflict with friends in sport. Despite this observation, only four of the six regression models were significantly different from zero (F-values ranged from 3.31 to 6.61; all p's < .05). When SFSQ-Conflict (F = 1.21; df = 3,47; p = 0.32) and SFSQ-Things in Common (F = 2.48; df = 3,44; p = 0.07) served as criterion variables, conventional levels of statistical significance were not attained.

Table 2. Bivariate correlations between indices of psychological need satisfaction and sport friendship quality

	SFSQ-Self-Esteem Enhancement & Supportiveness	SFSQ-Loyalty & Intimacy	SFSQ-Things in Common	SFSQ-Companionship & Pleasant Play	SFSQ-Conflict Resolution	SFSQ-Conflict
1. Competence	0.36	0.24	0.13	0.15	-0.11	0.01
2. Autonomy	0.24	0.05	0.03	0.10	-0.17	-0.20
3. Relatedness	0.49	0.43	0.29	0.38	0.25	-0.06

Note. SFSQ = Sport Friendship Quality Scale (Weiss & Smith, 1999). Correlation matrix ix based on pairwise comparisons. Sample size is consistent across each element of the *r*-matrix used in the pairwise comparisons ($N = 52$). All *r*-values in the matrix greater than or equal to 0.26 are statistically significant in this sample ($p < .05$; two-tailed significance).

Supplemental Analyses: Identification of Best Friends within Sport

Table 3. Simultaneous multiple regression analysis predicting sport friendship quality from psychological need satisfaction

Criterion Variables	R^2_{adj}	*B*	*SE*	*β*	*t-values*	$r_{y,x1(x2)}$	r_s
SFQS-Self-Esteem Enhancement & Supportiveness	0.24						
Competence		0.08	0.08	0.16	1.02	0.02	0.68
Autonomy		0.05	0.10	0.07	0.49	0.00	0.45
Relatedness		0.29	0.09	0.42	3.12	0.15	0.92
SFQS-Loyalty & Intimacy	0.17						
Competence		0.16	0.11	0.25	1.48	0.04	0.54
Autonomy		-0.19	0.13	-0.24	-1.48	0.04	-0.08
Relatedness		0.32	0.12	0.36	2.54	0.11	0.89
SFQS-Things in Common	0.03						
Competence		0.11	0.13	0.16	0.85	0.01	0.53
Autonomy		-0.13	0.16	-0.14	-0.84	0.01	-0.24
Relatedness		0.27	0.15	0.27	1.80	0.02	0.92
SFQS-Companionship & Pleasant Play	0.26						
Competence		0.09	0.08	0.18	1.13	0.02	0.51
Autonomy		-0.08	0.09	-0.13	-0.85	0.01	0.07
Relatedness		0.32	0.09	0.49	3.64	0.20	0.97
SFQS-Conflict Resolution	0.12						
Competence		-0.09	0.12	-0.13	-0.76	0.01	-0.10
Autonomy		-0.11	0.14	-0.12	-0.76	0.01	-0.31
Relatedness		0.41	0.14	0.43	2.99	0.16	0.86
SFQS-Conflict	0.01						
Competence		0.18	0.15	0.23	1.24	0.03	0.04
Autonomy		-0.33	0.18	-0.32	-1.84	0.07	-0.75
Relatedness		-0.10	0.17	-0.09	-0.58	0.01	-0.21

Note. R^2_{adj} = Adjusted R-squared value from each regression model. *B* = Unstandardized Beta Coefficients. *SE* = Standard Error for each Unstandardized Beta Coefficients. *β* = Standardized Beta Coefficients. *t-values* = Observed *t*-statistic for each predictor variables included per model in the regression analyses. $r_{y,x1(x2)}$ = Estimate of unique variance per predictor variable in the regression models where values represent the square of the part-correlation coefficients for each predictor (Hair et al., 2006). r_s = Structure coefficients for each predictor variable included in the regression models estimated with the following formula: r/R (where r is the bivariate correlation and R is the Multiple Regression Coefficient per predictor in the model).

Responses to the prompt "Who is your best friend in the sport you are currently playing?" that prefaced the SFSQ items in accordance with the recommendations of Weiss and Smith (1999) were analyzed to determine participant compliance with the instructional format used in this study. Over one third of the participants did not provide a response to this question (32.70%) while the majority of respondents provided either a name or initials of a person they considered their best friend in the sport they currently played (57.70%). The remaining participants provided an irrelevant response (1.90% of the sample indicated a professional English football team as his/her best friend), noted they competed in a sport they considered to be individualized in nature (1.90%), or stated they had more than one best friends in sport or many friends but none they considered a best friend in sport (5.80%). For example, one participant indicated, "I have many good friends – no one I would consider my best friend" while another noted "No one I would consider best friend – I see below you need one so I'll pick my 65 instructor who I interact most consistently with in terms of play…I'm 38 he is 65…play is relative."

Discussion

The main aim of this study was to examine the tenability of BPNT (Deci & Ryan, 2002) as a framework for understanding the quality of friendships experienced amongst athletes engaged in adapted sport competition. Specifically, this study tested the relationship between perceived competence, autonomy, and relatedness derived from competitive sport in association with indices of friendship quality experienced in adapted sport contexts. The results of this preliminary investigation make it apparent that feeling isolated from others as opposed to socially enmeshed (or related) in meaningful ways is linked with indices of friendship quality amongst athletes competing in adapted sport in a manner concordant with Deci and Ryan's (2002) assertions. The absence of hypothesized links between perceived competence and perceived autonomy with most indicators of sport friendship quality is not wholly in line with our hypotheses or the fundamental tenets of BPNT (Deci & Ryan, 2002). Perhaps of greater theoretical interest is the observation that fulfilling basic psychological needs for competence, autonomy, and relatedness were positively inter-related—a finding consistent with the corpus of research using BPNT as a guiding framework (Deci & Ryan, 2002; Wilson & Rodgers, 2007). Overall, only partial support for the *a priori* hypotheses was noted in this study. Yet it seems apparent that feeling related to others is intertwined with the social networks that formulate as friendships develop within adapted sport.

BPNT and Adapted Sport: What Do We Know? What Do We 'Need' to Know?

The observed pattern of uniformly positive relationships between perceptions of competence, autonomy, and relatedness was congruent with our *a priori* hypothesis and the underlying theory guiding this study (Deci & Ryan, 2002). While the magnitude of these relationships is less troubling and likely attributable to sampling variability, it is interesting to speculate on the extraneous factors (e.g., age, gender, type of sport, competitive level, etc.) that could impact the overall strength and potential interplay between these needs within cohorts of competitive athletes. Deci and Ryan (2002) have generally restricted their arguments concerning basic psychological needs to the direction of the relationships anticipated between feeling competent, autonomous, and related presumably on the basis of the functional role theorized to stem from psychological need fulfillment within BPNT. Closer inspection of previous studies using young gymnasts in America (Gagné et al., 2003; Mean $|r_{12}|$ = 0.64, Range = 0.51 to 0.83) and elite Canadian athletes (Lonsdale et al., 2009; Mean $|r_{12}|$ = 0.36, Range = 0.29 to 0.45) substantiate the observation that the strength of association between experiences fulfilling each psychological need embedded in BPNT varies considerably within and across samples of athletes. The underlying cause for this variability remains unknown yet worthy of additional scrutiny to advance our understanding of basic psychological needs within sport further using BPNT.

Several possible explanations could account for the observed variability in strength of association between perceived competence, autonomy, and relatedness needs in this sample that deserve attention. First, it is conceivable that the modified (i.e., IMI-PC or BNSG-A) or novel (i.e., ROPAS) instruments used to assess BPNT's constructs attenuated (or magnified) these relationships. Partial support for this speculative explanation is evident in the reliability analyses where it is clear that scores indexing perceived autonomy with the BNSG-A subscale displayed a level of error variance that is concerning and could account for the weak correlation between perceived autonomy and relatedness noted in this study. None of the instruments used in this study to measure BPNT's constructs considered nuances of adapted sport athletes in their development and presently no instrument has been 'established' in the sport domain to measure these psychological constructs. It is plausible that the items embedded within each instrument used in this study failed to fully represent each psychological need as fulfilled within the realm of adapted sport, which poses interpretational concerns (Messick, 1995). Construct validation remains a pervasive yet overlooked aspect of the literature concerning BPNT within physical activity contexts (c.f., Wilson & Rodgers, 2007) so it seems reasonable to assert that future research attend to the development of sport-specific instruments to measure BPNT's central constructs preferably using a construct validation framework (see Messick, 1995, for further details on this approach).

Beyond construct validation issues, it seems reasonable to speculate about other explanations that could account for the variability in strength of association demonstrated between psychological needs in this study. Nuances particular to athletes that compete in adapted sport venues remain inadequately understood and could influence the association between perceived competence, autonomy, and relatedness needs. Few investigations to date (e.g., Farrell, Crocker, McDonough, & Sedgwick, 2004; Perreault & Vallerand, 2007) have examined issues germane to athletes who compete in adapted sport using the BPNT framework set forth by Deci and Ryan (2002). This sample had a disproportionally lower representation of female athletes than previous studies (26.90 percent compared with 43.10 and 44.70 percent; Farrell et al., 2004; Perreault & Vallerand, 2007). Further comparisons with published studies make it apparent that self-reported weekly training history and length of sport involvement noted in this sample were considerably longer than comparable indices reported in previous investigations (M = 7.70 years and M = 8.60 years; Perreault & Vallerand, 2007; Farrell et al., 2004). The extent to which such sampling idiosyncrasies impact 'what' contributes to fulfilling basic psychological needs and perhaps 'how' these psychological needs function together in cohorts of adapted sport athletes remains unknown yet ripe for further inquiry. Such ventures may wish to consider using qualitative techniques comparable to those employed by Farrell et al. (2004) that do not suffer from the same limitations as modifying instruments designed for use primarily in other populations.

Friendship Quality in Adapted Sport: Do Perceived Competence, Relatedness, and Autonomy Matter to Athletes?

The main aim of this study was to examine the role of fulfilling basic psychological needs advocated by SDT proponents (Deci & Ryan, 2002; La Guardia & Patrick, 2008) in relation to dimensions of sport friendship quality. Observations from both the bivariate correlation and multiple regression analyses lend credence to the notion that feeling a genuine sense of relatedness to others within adapted sport contexts is linked more with adaptive elements of sport friendships such as loyalty and intimacy rather than dysfunctional conflict. Such findings are wholly consistent with *a priori* hypotheses and the broader corpus of literature concerning attachment and social relationships grounded in BPNT (La Guardia et al., 2000; La Guardia & Patrick, 2008; Patrick, Knee, Canevello, & Lonsbary, 2007).

It seems likely that feeling a sense of relatedness to others by adapted sport athletes was associated with more adaptive dimensions of sport friendships for at least two reasons. First, it seems likely that social contacts that develop into friendships within adapted sport do so because athletes share common goals and values. Deci and Ryan (2002) have extolled the importance of perceived relatedness in terms of facilitating the internalization of salient beliefs or value structures shared within and between social networks. Second, it seems equally likely that adapted sport athletes who feel related to others when they compete are less prone to social isolation that can alienate people from one another based on personal characteristics. In other words, feeling a secure and meaningful connection with other people when competing in adapted sport encourages a sense of 'fit' with the broader community involved in adapted sport. One recent investigation of British exercisers has forwarded the notion that perceived relatedness concerns the degree of interpersonal connection with target referents (or personal relatedness) and the feeling of being socially enmeshed rather than isolated within the broader group environment (Markland & Tobin, 2010). Inspection of the ROPAS items used to measure perceived relatedness in this study implies both feelings of personal relatedness (Sample ROPAS item: "I feel like I am supported by others in this activity") and assimilation within a broader community (Sample ROPAS item: "I feel like I fit in well with others") seem to be represented within the instrument.

It is interesting to conjecture on the lack of supportive evidence in this study for the hypothesized links between perceived competence and autonomy with dimensions of sport friendship quality measured by the SFSQ. Previous studies identifying a social agent have demonstrated links between competence and autonomy needs with indices of relationship quality (La Guardia et al., 2000). For example, La Guardia and colleagues assessed autonomy (Sample item: "When I am with my mother, I feel free to be who I am") and competence (Sample item: "When I am with my best friend, I feel very capable and effective") by specifying another person as the reference point for each psychological need. In contrast, the present study targeted perceptions of effectiveness in executing particular skill-based tasks germane to sport along with feelings of self-governance as the focal sources for competence and autonomy in adapted sport athletes. It seems plausible that the focal point of the assessment method may be responsible for the aberrant findings pertaining to both competence and autonomy in relation to dimensions of sport friendships (i.e., best friend) in this study and warrants investigation with sport-specific social referents (e.g., coach, trainer, team mate, etc.).

Summary, Limitations and Future Directions

While the results of this study are informative and insightful with reference to BPNT, (Deci & Ryan, 2002), a number of study limitations warrant recognition alongside directions for future research. First, the study is limited to a cross-sectional design using purposive sampling techniques that restrict the external validity of the interpretations derived from this study of adapted sport athletes. The cross-sectional study design offers limited insight into the dynamics of causal flow between concepts central to Deci and Ryan's (2002) BPNT approach and social development issues such as sport friendships. Future studies would do well to consider assessing the variables central to BPNT across multiple test administrations to provide evidence informing the nature and rate of change for each psychological need, as well as, the dynamics of changing feelings of competence, autonomy, and relatedness in relation to the ebb and flow of friendship quality markers. A second limitation was the relatively small sample size providing data for this investigation that was collected using purposive sampling techniques. The sampling method employed combined with the absolute sample size questions the degree of external validity attributable to the data prior to replication studies that use probability-based sampling techniques to more fully represent the population of adapted sport athletes competing in Canada and other countries. Finally, this investigation employed concepts drawn from Deci and Ryan's (2002) BPNT to the exclusion of other concepts that have yet received scant empirical attention at best. Future studies could examine the roles of perceived structure and involvement alongside feelings of autonomy support as foundations that contribute to the fulfillment of basic psychological needs in adapted sport athletes (Markland & Tobin, 2010).

In summary, this study represents an initial attempt to frame issues of friendship quality within the broader context of motivational processes embedded within BPNT in athletes competing in adapted sport contexts. Partial support for the utility of BPNT is evident in the results of this study with particular relevance to the role afforded perceived relatedness in relation to indices of friendship quality. Consistent with our original hypotheses and previous literature (La Guardia & Patrick, 2008), athletes competing in adapted sport contexts who felt a stronger social bond with others were likely to experience more adaptive dimensions of friendship quality than dysfunctional components in the form of conflict. The limitations of this study notwithstanding, it seems reasonable to assert that these initial findings implicate perceived relatedness to others amongst adapted sport athletes as an important process that could play a transformative role in building adaptive friendship dimensions amongst sport competitors. The evidence favoring the role of perceived autonomy and competence in relation to the quality of friendships that can be generated as a function of adapted sport involvement is less convincing and worthy of additional scrutiny. Despite the obvious necessity of replicating and extending this study to address the aforementioned limitations, the results of this study represent a useful stepping stone for advancing the study of issues within adapted sport contexts using the fundamental tenets set forth by Deci and Ryan (2002) within BPNT as a guiding framework.

Authors' Notes

The authors' gratefully acknowledge the role of the participants who freely provided data for this study. This research was supported by funds from the Social Sciences and Humanities Research Council of Canada (SSHRC) awarded to Drs. Wilson and García Bengoechea. Dr. Mack's research program was supported by separate SSHRC grants at the time of data collection and manuscript preparation. Dr. Xie Bin was a visiting international scholar under the mentorship of Dr. Wilson. Dr. Xie Bin was supported by funds from the China Scholarship Council (Ministry of Education for the People's Republic of China) to support her tenure as a visiting scholar at Brock University during the 2009-2010 academic year.

References

Cohen, J. (1992). A power primer. *Psychological Bulletin, 112*, 155-159.

Cronbach, L. J. (1952). Coefficient alpha and the internal structure of tests. *Psychometrika, 16*, 297-234.

deCharms, R. (1968). *Personal causation: The internal affective determinants of behaviour*. New York, NY: Academic Press.

Deci, E. L., & Ryan, R. M. (2002). *Handbook of Self-Determination Research*. Rochester, NY: University of Rochester Press.

Deci, E. L., & Ryan, R. M. (2008). Facilitating optimal motivation and psychological well-being across life's domains. *Canadian Psychology*, *49*, 14-23.

Farrell, R. J., Crocker, P. R. E., McDonough, M. H., & Sedgwick, W. A. (2004). The driving force: Motivation in special Olympians. *Adapted Physical Activity Quarterly*, *21*, 153-166.

Gagné, M. (2003). The role of autonomy support and autonomy orientation in prosocial behaviour engagement. *Motivation & Emotion*, *27*, 199-223.

Gagné, M., Ryan, R. M., & Bargmann, K. (2003). Autonomy support and need satisfaction in the motivation and well-being of gymnasts. *Journal of Applied Sport Psychology*, *15*, 372-390.

García Bengoechea, E., & Strean, W. B. (2007). On the Interpersonal Context of Adolescents' Sport Motivation. *Psychology of Sport & Exercise*, *8*, 195-217.

Grolnick, W. S., & Aposoleris, N. H. (2002). What makes parents controlling? In E. L. Deci, & R. M. Ryan (Eds.), *Handbook of self-determination research* (pp. 161-181). Rochester, NY: University of Rochester Press.

Hagger, M. S., & Chatzisarantis, N. L. (2007). *Intrinsic motivation and self-determination in exercise and sport*. Champaign, IL: Human Kinetics.

Hair, J. F., Black, W. C., Babin, B. J., Anderson, R. E., & Tatham, R. L. (2006). *Multivariate data analysis (6th Edition)*. Upper Saddle River, NJ: Prentice Hall.

Holt, N. L., Black, D. E., Tamminen, K. A., Fox, K. R., & Mandigo, J. L. (2008). Levels of social complexity and dimensions of peer experiences in youth sport. *Journal of Sport & Exercise Psychology*, *30*, 411-431.

Holt, N. L., Tamminen, K. A., Black, D. E., Sehn, Z. L., & Wall, M. P. (2008). Parental involvement in competitive youth sport settings. *Psychology of Sport & Exercise*, *9*, 663-685.

Iyengar, S. S., & Lepper, M. (1999). Rethinking the value of choice: A cultural perspective on intrinsic motivation. *Journal of Personality & Social Psychology*, *76*, 349-366.

La Guardia, J. G., & Patrick, H. (2008). Self-determination theory as a fundamental theory of close relationships. *Canadian Psychology*, *49*, 201-209.

La Guardia, J. G., Ryan, R. M., Couchman, C. E., & Deci, E. L. (2000). Within-person variation in security of attachment: A self-determination theory perspective on attachment, need fulfillment, and well-being. *Journal of Personality & Social Psychology*, *79*, 367-384.

Little, R. J. A. (1988). A test of missing completely at random for multivariate data with missing values. *Journal of the American Statistical Association, 83*, 1198-1202.

Lonsdale, C., Hodge, K., & Rose, E. (2009). Athlete burnout in elite sport: A self-determination perspective. *Journal of Sport Sciences*, *27*, 785-795.

Markland, D., & Tobin, V. J. (2010). Need support and behavioural regulations for exercise among exercise referral scheme clients: The mediating role of psychological need satisfaction. *Psychology of Sport & Exercise*, *11*, 91-99.

McAuley, E., Duncan, T., & Tammen, V. V. (1989). Psychometric properties of the Intrinsic Motivation Inventory in competitive sport setting: A confirmatory factor analysis. *Research Quarterly for Exercise & Sport*, *60*, 48-58.

McDonough, M. & Crocker, P. R. E. (2005). Sport participants motivation in young adolescent girls: The role of friendship quality and self-concept. *Research Quarterly for Exercise & Sport*, *76*, 456-467.

McDonough, M., & Crocker, P. R. E. (2007). Testing self-determined motivation as a mediator of the relationship between psychological needs and affective and behavioural outcomes. *Journal of Sport & Exercise Psychology*, *29*, 645-663.

Messick, S. (1995). Validity of psychological assessment: Validation of inferences from persons' responses and performances as scientific inquiry into score meaning. *American Psychologist, 50*, 741-749.

Morris, J. D. (1979). A comparison of regression prediction accuracy on several types of factor scores. *American Educational Research Journal*, *16*, 17-24.

Patrick, H., Knee, C. R., Canevello, A., & Lonsbary, C. (2007). The role of need fulfillment in relationship functioning and well-being: A self-determination theory perspective. *Journal of Personality & Social Psychology*, *92*, 434-457.

Perreault, S., & Vallerand, R. J. (2007). A test of self-determination theory with wheelchair basketball players with and without a disability. *Adapted Physical Activity Quarterly*, *24*, 305-316.

Pedhazur, E. J. (1997). *Multiple regression in behavioural research: Explanation and prediction*. Orlando, FL: Harcourt Brace.

Ryan, R. M. (1982). Control and information in the interpersonal sphere: An extension of cognitive evaluation theory. *Journal of Personality & Social Psychology*, *43*, 450-461.

Sharabany, R. (1994). Intimate friendship scale: Conceptual underpinnings, psychometric properties and construct validity. *Journal of Social & Personal Relationships*, *11*, 449-469.

Smith, A. L., & McDonough, M. H. (2008). Peers. In A. L. Smith, & S. J. H., Biddle (Eds.), *Youth physical activity and sedentary behaviou*r (pp. 295-320). Champaign, IL: Human Kinetics.

Ullrich-French, S., & Smith, A. L. (2006). Perceptions of relationships with parents and peers in youth sport: Independent and combined prediction of motivational outcomes. *Psychology of Sport & Exercise*, *7*, 193-214.

Ullrich-French, S., & Smith, A. L. (2009). Social and motivational predictors of continued youth sport participation. *Psychology of Sport & Exercise*, *10*, 81-95.

Weiss, M. R., & Smith, A. L. (1999). Quality of youth sport friendships: Measurement development and validation. *Journal of Sport & Exercise Psychology, 21*, 145-166.

Weiss, M. R., & Smith, A. L. (2002). Friendship quality in youth sport: Relationship to age, gender, and motivation variables. *Journal of Sport & Exercise Psychology*, *24*, 420-437.

White, R. W. (1959). Motivation reconsidered: The concept of competence. *Psychological Review*, *66*, 297-333.

Wilson, P. M., & García Bengoechea, E. (under review). The Relatedness to Others in Physical Activity Scale I: Instrument development and gender invariance. *Journal of Applied Biobehavioural Research.*

Wilson, P. M., & Rodgers, W. M. (2007). Self-determination theory, exercise, and well-being. In M. S. Hagger & N. L. D. Chatzisarantis (Eds.), *Intrinsic Motivation and Self-Determination in Exercise and Sport* (pp. 101-112). Champaign, IL: Human Kinetics.

In: Encyclopedia of Sports and Athletics
Editors: Jack L. Murray and Emily O. Watson
ISBN: 978-1-61209-959-0

Chapter XXII

Mental Toughness – A Critical Review of Recent Developments and Future Directions

Simon G. D. Crampton and Changiz Mohiyeddini
Roehampton University, London, United Kingdom

Introduction

Mental toughness is a term frequently used in the sporting community by athletes, coaches and psychologists alike to differentiate the "good" from the "great" in their pursuit for sporting excellence (Sheard, 2010). When physical, technical and tactical skills are evenly matched, which so often is the case at the highest levels of competition, it is often the 'mentally toughest' of the two that is thought to prevail (Gucciardi, Gordon & Dimmock, 2009a). In recent years, momentum has gathered and significant developments in the mental toughness literature have been made which has led to growing understanding of the construct. Nevertheless, concurrence concerning its conceptualisation, definition and how it is developed is yet to be established. The aim of this review is to present the current emerging definitions and conceptualisations of mental toughness, to examine the developments in measuring mental toughness and explore recent findings in the literature. Future research directions will then be discussed.

Defining and Conceptualising Mental Toughness

Early perspectives of mental toughness have varied, depicting the construct as anything from a personality-trait (Cattell, 1957; Kroll, 1967), a defence mechanism against adversity (Loehr, 1982; 1986), to a constellation of mental skills (Goldberg, 1998; Bull, Albinson & Shambrook, 1996) to even simply a state of mind (Gibson, 1998). Despite their insight, these approaches (which were based mainly on anecdotal evidence) have simply fuelled further conceptual confusion surrounding mental toughness. As a result, at one time or another, virtually every positive or desirable psychological characteristic typically associated with success has been labelled as mental toughness (Jones, Hanton, & Connaughton, 2002). More recently however, a number of studies have contributed to better understanding and conceptualisation of mental toughness by adopting more rigorous approaches to investigating the construct (Clough, Earle & Sewell, 2002; Gucciardi, et al, 2008; Jones, et al., 2002, 2007).

Within the context of Kelly's (1955) Personal Construct Psychology (PCP) theory, Jones et al. (2002) investigated mental toughness by adopting a qualitative approach, conducting focus group and individual interviews with ten elite international sportsmen. As a result, Jones et al. (2002) defined mental toughness as; "having the natural and developed psychological edge that enables you to: generally, cope better than your opponents with the many demands (competition, training, lifestyle) that sport places on a performer; specifically, be more consistent and better than your opponents in remaining determined, focused, confident and in control under pressure" (p. 209). Twelve distinct attributes that were considered fundamental to mental toughness were also identified and ranked in order of their importance (see Table 1.). These related to self-belief, desire and motivation, controlling performance and lifestyle-related focus, dealing with competition-related pressure and anxiety as well as dealing with hardship (physical and emotional).

Table 1. Mental toughness attributes and importance ranking

Rank	Attribute
1	Having an unshakable self-belief in your ability to achieve your competition goals
2	Bouncing back from performance setbacks as a result of increased determination to succeed
3	Having an unshakable self-belief that you posses unique qualities and abilities
=4	Having an insatiable desire and internalised motives to succeed
=4	Remaining fully-focused on the task at hand in the face of competition specific distractions
6	Regaining psychological control following unexpected, uncontrollable events (competition-specific)
7	Pushing back the boundaries of physical and emotional pain, while still maintaining technique and effort under distress (in training and competition)
8	Accepting that competition anxiety is inevitable and knowing that you can cope with it
=9	Thriving on the pressure of competition
=9	Not being adversely affected by others' good and bad performances
11	Remaining fully-focused in the face of personal life distractions
12	Switching a sport focus on and off as required

Adapted from Jones et al. (2002, p. 211).

In a follow-up study adopting similar investigative techniques, Jones et al. (2007) triangulated perceptions of mental toughness taken from a sample of super-elite sports performers (i.e. Olympic/World Champions) as well as coaches and sport psychologists who have coached and consulted with such performers. In doing so, Jones et al. (2007) verified their earlier definition of mental toughness and extended the list of attributes considered essential to the make-up of mental toughness to 30. These were subsequently categorised into 13 sub-components of mental toughness, which developed a framework of mental toughness (see Figure 1.) comprising four dimensions; a general dimension (attitude/mindset) and three time-specific dimensions (training competition and post-competition). The *attitude/mindset* dimension was divided in two subcomponents, belief and focus, which were purported to enable mentally tough performers to remain on course in achieving their ultimate goal, regardless of obstacles and circumstances. Likewise the subcomponents with the three time-specific dimensions identified the psychological constructs and strategies used to achieve and maintain mental toughness levels across three training and performance contexts.

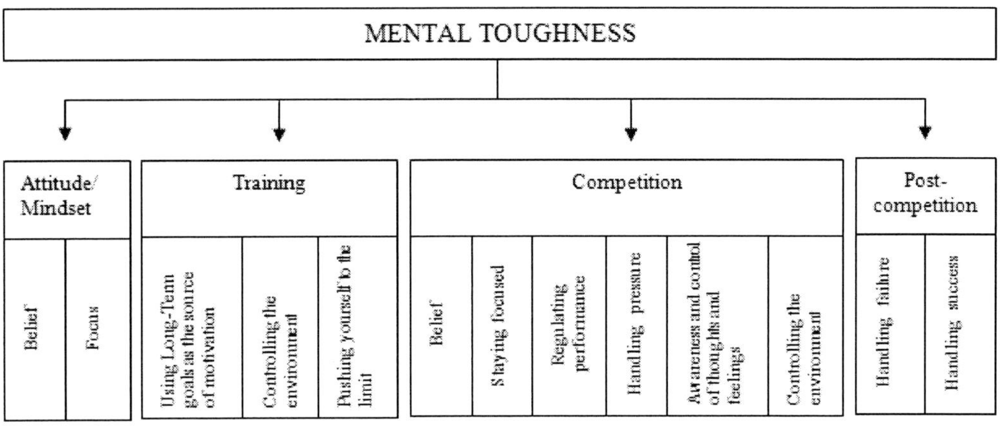

Jones et al.'s (2007).

Figure 1. Mental toughness framework (p. 249).

In two independent studies, support was provided for Jones et al.'s (2002) conceptual definition of mental toughness by Bull, Shambrook, James and Brooks (2005) and Thelwell, Weston and Greenlees (2005), who conducted single sport, context-specific approaches to investigating the mental toughness phenomenon. Bull et al. (2005) investigated the systematic development of mental toughness in elite English cricketers and presented 20 global themes of mentally tough characteristics that were organised around five general dimensions; Developmental factors, Personal responsibility, Dedication and commitment, Belief and Coping with pressure. A framework of mental toughness that further highlighted the interaction of a performer's environment, character, attitudes and thinking, in the mental toughness development process was also constructed. On the other hand, Thelwell et al. (2005) investigated the perceptions of mental toughness with respect to professional soccer. In this instance, Thelwell et al. (2005) also highlighted considerable overlap between the Jones et al. (2002) definition but with one main discrepancy. The sample of soccer players postulated that mental toughness enabled soccer players to *always* cope better than their opponents as opposed to *generally* coping better. Thelwell et al. (2002) also only identified ten essential attributes of mental toughness which varied from those prescribed by Jones et al. (2002), however this supports the contention that mental toughness may be contextual. Bull et al. (2005) suggested that different types of mental toughness may exist in that the mental toughness required for a golfer will differ from that needed by a racing driver or a marathon runner. Based on this assertion, it could then be argued that a generalised conceptualisation of mental toughness that does not consider these discrepancies may be limited as a result.

Another sport-specific investigation of mental toughness, that also adopted a PCP framework, was conducted by Gucciardi et al., (2008). They defined mental toughness in Australian-rules football as; " a collection of values, attitudes, behaviours, and emotions that enable you to persevere and overcome any obstacle, adversity or pressure experienced, but also to maintain concentration and motivation when things are going well to consistently achieve your goals" (p. 278). Interviews of eleven elite Australian-rules football coaches also resulted in the construction of a grounded theory conceptual model of mental toughness (see Figure 2.) which highlighted the interaction between three central components of mental toughness in Australian-rules football; *characteristics*, *situations* and *behaviours*. Thirty-two characteristics that were identified were categorised under 11 key bipolar constructs (i.e. self belief vs. self-doubt; work ethic vs. lazy); the situations identified represented the events (internal and external) which demanded degrees of mental toughness; likewise, behaviours referred to the overt behavioural indicators that would be displayed in such situations (e.g. superior decision-making). Importantly, this framework represents a significant development in the understanding of mental toughness as it offers the first insight into both the processes and outcomes of mental toughness, albeit centred in the context of Australian football.

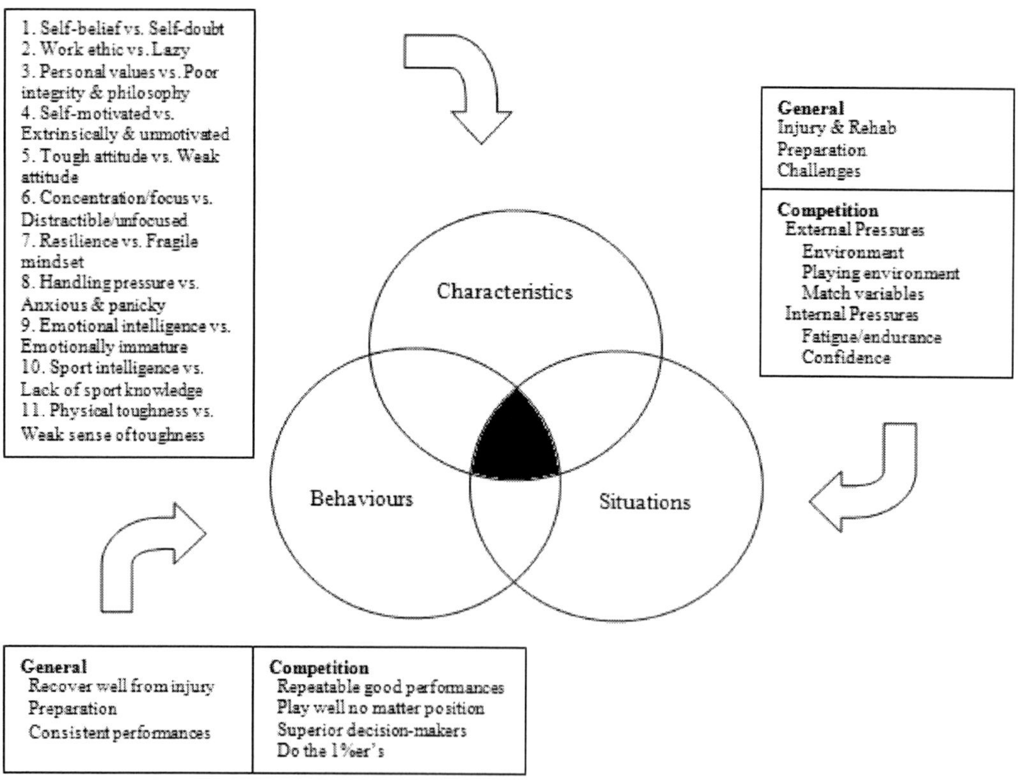

Adapted from Gucciardi et al., 2008.

Figure 2. A model of mental toughness in Australian football.

A third conceptualisation, which is prevalent in the mental toughness literature, is that proposed by Clough et al. (2002) that sought to bridge the gap between theoretical research and applied practice. To do so, Clough et al. (2002) incorporated the ecologically valid views and experiences of athletes and coaches with underlining theories drawn from an existing psychology framework from health psychology, namely Kobasa's (1979) model of hardiness, and one prominent study on physiological adaptation to stress (Dienstbier, 1989). As a result, Clough et al. (2002) proposed a multidimensional, 4C's model of mental toughness and offered the following definition; "mentally tough individuals tend to be sociable and outgoing; as they are able to remain calm and relaxed, they are competitive in many situation and have lower anxiety levels than others. With a high sense of self-belief and an unshakable faith that they can control their own destiny, these individuals remain relatively unaffected by competition or adversity" (p.38).

Given that both hardiness and mental toughness are characterised by; resiliency, perseverance, effectively coping with pressure or adversity, motives to achieve success (predominantly intrinsic) and a deep sense of purpose and thus involvement in activities and personal encounters; Clough et al. (2002) conceptualised hardiness and mental toughness as similar but distinct constructs. According to Clough et al., hardiness failed to capture the unique nature of the physical and mental demands of competitive sport and therefore Kobasa's (1979) model of hardiness is restricted to stress and health related contexts only. Consequently, it was proposed that confidence, also viewed as an integral part of mental toughness, could reflect the transposition of the related construct of hardiness into the more sport-specific concept of mental toughness. As a result, Clough et al. (2002) proposed that commitment, control, challenge (all components of hardiness) and confidence represent the 4C's model of mental toughness and defined it in terms of a trait-like characteristic that individual's posses.

In summary, the recent approaches aforementioned demonstrate the greater understanding, conceptual clarity and consistency currently developing within the mental toughness literature. Despite the differing approaches and theoretical frameworks to base or guide these conceptualisations, collectively they appear to support the contention that mental toughness can be defined in a similar fashion, irrespective of sport (Connaughton & Hanton, 2009). Support for this is evident in the consistency of several characteristics identified across various studies, including; an unshakable self-belief, control of focus, an insatiable desire and motivation to succeed, an ability to handle pressure and anxiety, as well as dealing with emotional or physical pain, and the overriding conception that mental toughness is multidimensional (Clough et al, 2002; Jones et al., 2002, 2007; Guccairdi at al., 2008). Importantly however, mental toughness has also been shown to be more than just the perception of control and an ability to perform under pressure, which suggests mental toughness is not exclusive to adverse situations. Mental toughness also concerns the mindset and approach that individuals have with respect to lifestyle, training, competition success as well as failure. Although mental toughness may vary slightly between specific sports and contexts, it appears there are a core set of attributes inherent to the general make-up of mental toughness that significantly contribute to an individual's ability to consistently achieve their goals. Given the developments in the conceptualisation of the concept of mental toughness, efforts have been subsequently directed towards the development of reliable and valid measures of mental toughness in order to assess mental toughness levels in individuals.

Mental Toughness Measurement

Recent developments in sport-specific as well as sport-general measures has lead to a surge in quantitative investigations into mental toughness designed to further our understanding of the construct as well as assess its potential to predict future performance and success in athletes. Establishing a valid and reliable measure of mental toughness is important because it may also provide valuable insight for practitioners by helping them to identify key components of mental toughness that individuals may be lacking which will consequently guide and tailor interventions. In this line of research, it has been suggested to differ between sport-general as well as sport-specific approaches to investigating mental toughness.

Sport-General Measures

The Psychological Performance Inventory (PPI; Loehr, 1986) is a 42-item measure of mental toughness developed to operationalise Loehr's (1982) definition of mental toughness. According to Loehr (1982, 1986), mentally tough athletes possess a learned or developed ability to increase the flow of positive energy when faced with adversity or a crisis and have the skill to think in ways that promote the right attitudes to solve problems, or deal with pressure, mistakes or competition. The PPI assesses these abilities via seven, 6-item subscales of Self-confidence, Negative energy, Attention Control, Visualisation and Imagery control, Motivation, Positive energy and Attitude control. Several studies have employed the PPI as a measure of mental toughness (Golby & Sheard, 2006; Golby, Sheard & Lavallee, 2003; Lee, Shin, Han & Lee, 1994; Shin, & Lee, 1994), however, following two independent psychometric assessments of the PPI (Golby, Sheard & van Wersch, 2007; Middleton et al, 2004), neither found support for its psychometric validity.

In a follow-up investigation into the alternative five-factor structure of the PPI proposed in Middleton et al.'s (2004) study, Golby et al., (2007) constructed a four-factor measure of mental toughness designed specifically for the athletic domain, the alternative-PPI (PPI-A). The PPI-A is a 14-item scale which yields an overall mental toughness score as well as scores for four subscales; Determination, Self-belief, Positive cognition and Visualisation. To date the only study reported to use the PPI-A is an investigation by Sheard (2009) which compared levels of mental toughness and hardiness in elite university rugby players. Results identified weak to moderate correlations among the mental toughness and hardiness subscales which supports its discriminant validity however further validation is require to enhance the efficacy in the scale as a valid and reliable measure of mental toughness.

The most commonly used measure within the current literature is the Mental Toughness Questionniare-48 (MTQ48; Clough e al., 2002) which was developed to operationalise Clough et al.'s (2002) 4C's model of mental toughness. Consisting of 48-items, the MTQ48 yields a total mental toughness score as well as six subscale scores related to the four key components (two of which are sub-divided) that includes; Commitment, Emotional Control, Life Control, Challenge, Interpersonal Confidence and Confidence in Abilities. In the development of the MTQ48, Clough et al. (2002) reported establishing its construct validity having found significant relationships with optimism, self-image, life satisfaction, self-efficacy as well as trait anxiety and also reported an overall test-retest coefficient of 0.9 with adequate internal consistencies for all the subscales. Criterion validity was purported by Clough et al. (2002) following lower reported ratings of exertion during a 30-minute cycle ride at 30% VO_2^{max} by those rating higher in mental toughness compared to their less mentally tough counterparts.

The fourth sport-general self-report measure of mental toughness currently reported in the literature is the Sports Mental Toughness Questionnaire (SMTQ; Sheard, Golby & van Wersch, 2009). In acknowledgement of the potential limitation of the PPI-A which failed to include a measure of control, a characteristic consistently cited across the mental toughness literature (Clough et al., 2002; Jones et al., 2002; Thelwell et al, 2005), Sheard et al., (2009) sought to address this issue. Consequently, the resultant SMTQ consists of 14-items encompassing three factors; Confidence, Constancy and Control. Initial reports suggest that the SMTQ possesses adequate psychometric properties and suitable discriminative power having demonstrated weak to moderate correlations with the subscales of key correlates including hardiness, dispositional optimism and affect (Sheard et al., 2009).

Despite the developments in these sport-general measures of mental toughness, it is important to acknowledge that whilst these measures may assess key components which are general across all sports (i.e. self-belief, motivation and control), they may not effectively capture the context-specific components of mental toughness that differs across sports (Gucciardi, Gordon & Dimmck, 2009b). As a result, the production of sport-specific measures of mental toughness instigated. Taken together, further construct validation and examination of the psychometric properties of mental toughness measurements would contribute to a better understanding of this construct.

Sport-Specific Measures

Based on the grounded theory conceptualisation of mental toughness in Australian-rules football (Gucciardi et al., 2008), Gucciardi, et al. (2009b) sought to construct a self-report measure that would capture the 11 key components of mental toughness specifically identified for Australian football developing the Australian football Mental Toughness Inventory (AfMTI; Gucciardi et al., 2009b). The AfMTI consists of 24-items but only supports four factors including; Thrive through challenge, Sport Awareness, Tough Attitude and Desire success. Although this model is substantially different to the initial 11-factor model that was proposed, the items within the AfMTI still reflect each of the 11 key components of Australian football mental toughness depicted by Gucciardi et al., (2008). Although further construct validation and examination of the psychometric properties of the AfMTI are encouraged, the results provide preliminary support for the factor structure, reliability and validity of the AfMTI. The development of the first sport-specific self report measure also represents a significant development in the examination of the antecedents and consequences of mental toughness which will assist researchers, coaches and practitioners in developing and assessing mental toughness development programmes in the future.

Consistent with the methods and procedures used by Gucciardi et al. (2008) in the development of a model of mental toughness for Australian-rules football and Gucciardi et al.'s (2009b) construction of a sport-specific measure to operationalise this model, a similar approach was adopted for cricket. Firstly, Gucciardi and Gordon (2009) conducted semi-structured interviews with 16 past and present national or international coaches and players to generate an understanding of mental toughness in cricket. This yielded six overarching categories including; Affective intelligence, Attention control, Self-belief, Resilience, Desire to achieve, and Cricket smarts. As a result, this conceptualisation provided the foundation upon which a 15-item self-report measure was developed, namely the Cricket Mental Toughness Questionnaire (CMTI). The CMTI comprises a five-factor model encompassing Affective intelligence, Attention control, Self-belief, Resilience, Desire to achieve and initial findings provide support for the assertion that mental toughness is conceptually related but distinct from psychological constructs such as flow, resilience and hardiness as well as burnout.

Given the ongoing advances in the development and validation of both sport-general as well as sport-specific measures of mental toughness, a more accurate assessment and a greater understanding of how mental toughness operates in relation to other psychological constructs is more feasible. Despite the differing approaches, general or context-specific, the assertion is not that one approach is superior to the other. Instead, it is suggested that moving forward, the complementary use of both specific and sport-general measures of mental toughness represents the most fruitful direction for future research which in turn may provide greater insight into the roles played by both the core attributes of general mental toughness as well as key contextually specific aspects.

Recent Findings

Currently, the most frequently used measure of mental toughness in the literature to date is the MTQ48 which has investigated the relationships between mental toughness and a number of key variables. These include; dispositional optimism and pessimism (Nicholls, Polman, Levy & Backhouse, 2008), injury rehabilitation (Levy, Polman, Clough, Marchant & Earle, 2006), affect intensity (Crust, 2009), leadership preference (Crust & Azadi, 2009) and psychological skill use (Crust & Azadi, 20010). Differences in mental toughness have also been explored in relation to gender, age and sport experience (Nicholls, Polman, Levy & Backhouse, 2009) as well as in managerial position and experience (Marchant et al., 2009). Two other areas of interest include the relationships between mental toughness and personality and mental toughness and coping.

Mental Toughness and Personality/Genetics

As previously mentioned, Clough et al.'s (2002) 4C's conceptualisation depicts mental toughness as a trait that individual's posses in varying degrees. In accordance with this trait approach, Horsburg, Schermer, Veselka and Vernon (2009) adopted a behavioural genetic approach to determine the extent to which genetic and environmental factors influence individual differences in mental toughness as well as examining its relationship with personality dimensions. Results from a sample of 219 pairs of adult monozygotic and dizygotic twins indicated that individual differences in mental toughness (as well as in personality) were largely attributable to genetic and non-shared environmental factors.

Support for the original hypothesis that mental toughness would correlate positively with extraversion, openness to experience, agreeableness and conscientiousness but negatively with neuroticism were also found. Findings also suggested mental toughness is in fact quite heritable and therefore indicated it may be more difficult to strengthen and modify than first suggested. These results have important implications for practitioners as it indicates that in order to strengthen mental toughness, individuals must focus on certain elements with the lowest heritabilities such as commitment or control.

Mental Toughness, Emotion and Coping

In all the conceptualisations of mental toughness aforementioned (Bull et al., 2005; Clough et al. 2002; Jones et al. 2002, 2007; Gucciardi et al. 2008; Thelwell et al., 2005), the notion of coping features prominently within the literature. Whether via the control of one's emotions, the ability to manage or cope with the demands, obstacles, challenges or adversities that one faces, the underlying conception is that individuals who are mentally tough, possess a superior ability to cope with the challenges they face compared to their less mentally tough counterparts, be it in training, competition or in general. Two related studies have recently investigated the relationships between mental toughness and coping (Nicholls et al., 2008) and the appraisal of a self-selected stressor (stressor intensity and perceived control over the stressor), coping strategies and coping effectiveness in sport (Kaiseler, Polman and Nicholls, 2009). Both found mental toughness to positively correlate with problem-focused or approach coping strategies (mental imagery, effort expenditure, thought control, relaxation and logical analysis) and negatively correlate with emotion-focused and avoidance coping strategies (distancing, mental distraction and resignation).

According to Kaiseler et al. (2009), mental toughness was associated with lower levels of stress and higher levels of perceived control. These findings suggest that mental toughness might moderate the link between perceived control (as coping skill) and stress, probably through influencing the appraisals of a situation as challenging rather threatening. Hence, it seems to be crucial for future research to explore the impact of mental toughness on stress (Fletcher, 2005) and that by following a transactional understanding of stress (Lazarus & Folkman, 1984) on can speculate that mental toughness may affect stress directly or trough perceived control or self-efficacy (Bandura, 1997).

Mental Toughness Development

Early perspectives on mental toughness development have been either based on learning, practice, and experience (Loehr, 1986), or focused simply on the development of superior mental techniques and skills (Bull et al., 1996; Goldberg, 1998). Although these approaches are intuitively appealing, they appear to lack any theoretical underpinning or systematic research to support their methods and fail to originate from any sound theoretical conceptualisation of mental toughness. More recently however, studies investigating the perceptions of elite athletes and coaches have identified the pivotal roles played by the environment (Bull et al., 2005; Connaughton, Hanton, Jones, & Wadey, 2008) and significant individuals (i.e. the coach) in the mental toughness development process (Gucciardi, Gordon, Dimmock & Mallett, 2009).

In this line of research, Bull et al. (2005) proposed that the performer's environment provides the foundation of all mental toughness development and presented a pyramid framework that highlights its influence in developing mental toughness through installing 'tough characters', 'tough attitudes' and 'tough thinking' at its pinnacle. Key components of the environmental influence identified were the importance of childhood experiences (including parental influence) as well as secondary influences such as an exposure to tough environments and being provided with opportunities to survive early setbacks. Whilst Bull et al. (2005), provide rich insight into an integral component of mental toughness development, little explanation on how these factors exert their influence is offered. Neither are the processes, strategies and mechanisms, through which they operate, disclosed.

Connaughton et al., (2008) however, proposed that the development of mental toughness "is a long-term process that encompasses a multitude of underlying mechanisms that operate in a combined, rather than independent fashion" (p. 83) thought to develop within three distinct career phases (early, middle and later). Like Bull et al. (2005), Connaughton et al.'s (2008) findings also emphasised the need for an appropriate environment or motivational climate, one that is firmly based on challenge, reward and enjoyment. Nevertheless, they also emphasized the role of various significant others (i.e. coaches, parents, peers, sport psychologists and team-mates), the experience of critical incidents (Hanton, Cropely, Neil, Mellalieu & Miles, 2007; Khoshaba & Maddi, 1999) in and outside of their sport, the development of psychological skills and strategies, as well as the possession of an insatiable desire and internalised motivation to succeed. It was also proposed that once mental toughness had been developed, important mechanisms where required to maintain the construct (i.e. an enriched motivation and desire, an effective and established support network and basic and advance psychological skills).

Most recently however, an alternative approach to mental toughness development was undertaken by Gucciardi, Gordon, Dimmock & Mallett, (2009) that explored elite coaches' perceptions of how *they* themselves could both facilitate, as well as impede, the developmental process. What emerged was a framework of which four central categories (Coach-athlete relationship, Coaching philosophy, Training environments and Specific strategies) were purported to nurture a "generalised form" of mental toughness and cultivate or facilitate this development into a more "sport-specific form". Consistent with Connaughton et al. (2008), this model also highlighted the importance of strategies and mechanisms related to motivational climates (creating training environments that continuously challenge and expose players to various challenges), relationships with significant others (positive coach-athlete relationships) and the development of psychological skills. However, unlike the other approaches, it placed most emphasis on the developmental role played by the coach and highlighted them as the key driver in the process. An interesting finding was the notion that the coach could also hinder the development of mental toughness through negative influences and experiences, notably by creating an easy unchallenging environment for the players. This has important considerations for practitioners and coaches alike when devising interventions or mental toughness development programmes in the future.

A number of practical implications have emerged from these few initial developmental studies which indicate that the development and maintenance of mental toughness is an extensive process and warrants further investigation from both a sport specific as well as sport general perspective to uncover other mechanisms underpinning mental toughness development. Encouragingly, early findings suggest that with the appropriate planning to create the right environment or motivational climate, having the right support network in place, and encouraging the development of the necessary basic and advanced mental skills, as well as fostering the right attitudes, philosophies, values and beliefs, the possibility of enhancing mental toughness appears fertile. In relation to findings from Horsburg et al. (2009), which indicated that certain characteristics of mental toughness may be more malleable than others, these findings offer some insight into how these can be enhanced in individual performers.

Future Directions for Research

Having considered the dominant conceptualisations and definitions that currently preside in the mental toughness literature (Clough et al., 2002; Jones et al., 2002, 2007; Gucciardi et al., 2008), it is encouraging that despite the different approaches, there appears to be some commonalities and consistency unfolding which may indicate greater conceptual clarity developing in the area. Collectively speaking, it would appear that mental toughness is a multidimensional construct, made up of multiple key components broadly encompassing a range of values, attitudes, cognitions, emotions and behaviours. It is also apparent that several characteristics appear common across all sports for example; self-belief/confidence, concentration and focus, self-motivation and resilience, yet others are more specific to the sport that they occupy. Nevertheless, moving forward, it is important that the contrasting foundations of these conceptualisation such as those based on athlete, coach and practitioner experiences (Jones et al, 2002, 2007; Gucciardi et al, 2008) and those adopted from pre-existing psychological theory (Clough et al., 2002), do not contradict each other and create future conceptual confusion.

Despite the advances in sport-general and -specific measures of mental toughness, inherent limitations of solely using self-report measures for assessing cognitive or psychological constructs (such as biased or socially desirable responding) suggest that ratings are frequently inaccurate, and consequently caution should be taken when interpreting their findings. It is therefore encouraged that researchers should look to use multi-source measures of mental toughness (i.e. self-report, coach-report, peer report measures) or more objective methods of measurement (i.e. physiological or biological parameters), so to provide more detailed and accurate insights into the construct as well as the individual (Crust, 2007, 2008). In order to do so, there is a need to establish accurate behavioural indicators related to mental toughness that accommodate both generalised and context-specific aspects of mental toughness so that it is more easily and accurately observable. Equally, key physiological (i.e. heart rate, peripheral resistance) and biological parameters (i.e. cortisol, adrenaline) may be used to assess mental toughness which may provide greater insight into the operational mechanisms underpinning mental toughness.

Despite the current surge of quantitative studies into mental toughness using the MTQ48, due to the ambiguity surrounding the development of the measure, the findings could appear to be somewhat misleading and potentially problematic. Although the findings are supportive of Clough et al.'s (2002) original trait-like 4C's conceptualisation and have unearthed a number of similarities with other conceptualisations (Jones et al., 2002, 2007; Gucciardi et al, 2008), until further clarity of the systemic, statistical procedures used to construct and develop this conceptualisation and subsequent inventory are reported, these findings will remain open to dispute.

With respects to mental toughness development, the initial findings of the sport-general approach by Connaughton et al. (2008) along with the context-specific approaches of Bull et al. (2005), Thelwell et al. (2005), and Gucciardi et al. (2009b), represent a fruitful avenue for future research. Accompanied with the mental toughness framework proposed by Jones et al. (2007) which may provide a structure to guide other single-sport approaches, it may also provide the foundation for the development of a more conceptually accurate and psychometrically valid and reliable measure of mental toughness (Connaughton & Hanton, 2009). This has important implications for development likewise the evaluation of intervention strategies on levels of mental toughness.

Conclusion

In summary, a number of recent developments in the conceptualisation, the definition and the identification of key attributes and characteristics of mental toughness has led to greater understanding of what mental toughness is which is leading towards greater conceptual clarity in the area. The development of a framework of mental toughness and the identification of other key factors involved in the development of mental toughness has also led to further understanding of the mechanisms that underpin this process, which in turn will help guide practitioners and training programmes moving forward. The development and validation of various self-report measures has led to a surge in quantitative assessments of mental toughness, which may assist in increasing the understanding of mental toughness in relation to other key constructs whilst also providing a basis for assessing longitudinal development and assessing the efficacy of interventions. Nevertheless, it is encouraged that further validation procedures on these measures continue in order to establish a comprehensively sound measure of mental toughness. This along with more objective measures of mental toughness and may in turn provide richer insight into the construct and its underlying mechanisms moving forward.

References

Bandura, A. (1997). Self-efficacy: The exercise of control. New York: Freeman.

Bull, S. J., Albinson, J. G., & Shambrook, C. J. (1996). *The mental game plan: Getting psyched for sport*. Eastbourne, England: Sports Dynamics.

Bull, S. J., Shambrook, C. J., James, W., & Brookes, J. E. (2005). Towards an understanding of mental toughness in elite English cricketers. *Journal of Applied Sport Psychology*, 17, 209-227.

Cattell, R. B. (1957). *Personality and motivation structure and measurement*. New York: Harcourt, Brace and World.

Clough, P. J., Earle, K., & Sewell, D. (2002). Mental toughness: the concept and its measurement. In I. Cockerill (Ed.). *Solutions in sport psychology* (pp. 32-43). London: Thomson Publishing.

Connaughton, D., & Hanton, S. (2009). Mental toughness in sport: Conceptual and practical issues. In S. D. Mellalieu & S. Hanton (Eds.). (2008) *Advances in applied sport psychology: A review* (pp. 317-346). London: Routledge.

Connaughton, D., Wadey, R., Hanton, S., & Jones, G. (2008). The development and maintenance of mental toughness: perceptions of elite performers. *Journal of Sports Sciences*, 26, 83-95.

Crust, L. (2007). Mental toughness in sport: A review. *International Journal of Sport and Exercise Psychology*, 5(3), 270-290.

Crust, L. (2008). A review and conceptual re-examination of mental toughness: Implications for future researchers. *Personality and Individual Differences*, 45, 576-583.

Crust, L. & Azadi, K. (2009). Leadership preferences of mentally tough athletes. *Personality and Individual Differences*, 47(4), 326-330.

Crust, L. & Azadi, K. (2010). Mental toughness and athletes' use of psychology strategies. *European Journal of Sport Science*, 10(1), 43-51.

Crust, L., & Clough, P. J., (2005). Relationship between mental toughness and physical endurance. *Perceptual & Motor Skills*, 100, 192-194.

Dienstbier, R. A. (1989). Arousal and physiological toughness: Implications for mental and physical health. *Psychological Review*, 96(1), 84-100.

Fletcher, D. (2005). "Mental toughness" and human performance: Definitional, conceptual and theoretical issues. *Journal of Sports Sciences*, 23, 1246-1247.

Fourie, S., & Potgieter, J. R. (2001). The nature of mental toughness in sport. *South African Journal for Research in Sport, Physical Education and Recreation*, 23, 63-72.

Gibson, A. (1998). *Mental toughness*. New York: Vantage Press.

Golby, J., & Sheard, M. (2004). Mental toughness and hardiness at different levels of rugby league. *Personality and Individual Differences*, 37, 933-942.

Golby, J., & Sheard, M. (2006). The relationship between genotype and positive psychological development in national-level swimmers. *European Psychologist* , 11(2), 143-148.

Golby, J., Sheard, M., & Lavellee, D. (2003). A cognitive-behavioural analysis of mental toughness in national league rugby teams. *Perceptual and Motor Skills*, 96, 455-462.

Golby, J., Sheard, M., & van Wersch, A. (2007). Evaluating the factor structure of the Psychological Performance Inventory. *Perceptual and Motor Skills*, 105, 309-325.

Goldberg, A. S. (1998). *Sports slump busting: 10 steps to mental toughness and peak performance.* Champaign, IL: Human Kinetics.

Gucciardi, D. F., & Gordon, S. (2009). Development and preliminary validation of the Cricket Mental Toughness Inventory (CMTI). *Journal of Sports Sciences*, 27 (12), 1293-1310.

Gucciardi, D. F., Gordon, S., & Dimmock, J. A. (2008). Towards an understanding of mental toughness in Australian football. *Journal of Applied Sport Psychology*, 20, 261-281.

Gucciardi, D. F., Gordon, S., & Dimmock, J. A. (2009a). Advancing mental toughness research and theory using personal construct psychology. *International Review of Sport and Exercise Psychology*, 2(1), 54-72.

Gucciardi, D. F., Gordon, S., & Dimmock, J. A. (2009b). Development and preliminary validation of a mental toughness inventory for Australian football. *Psychology of Sport and Exercise*, 10, 201-209.

Gucciardi, D. F., Gordon, S., Dimmock, J. A. & Mallett, C. J. (2009). Understanding the coach's role in the development of mental toughness: Perspectives of elite Australian football coaches. *Journal of Sports Sciences*, 27(13), 1483-1496.

Hanton, S., Cropley, B., Miles, A., Mellalieu, S. D., & Neil, R. (2007). An in-depth examination of experience in sport: Competitive experience and the relationship with competitive anxiety. *International Journal of Sport and Exercise Psychology*, 5, 28-53.

Horsburgh, V. A., Schermer, J. A., Veselka, L., & Vernon, P. A. (2009). A behavioural genetic study of mental toughness and personality. *Personality and Individual Differences,* 46, 100-105.

Jones, G., Hanton, S., & Connaughton, D. (2002). What is thing called mental toughness? An investigation of elite sport performers. *Journal of Applied Sport Psychology*, 14, 20-28.

Jones, G., Hanton, S., & Connaughton, D. (2007). A framework of mental toughness in the world's best performers. *The Sport Psychologist*, 21, 243-264.

Kaisler, M., Polman, R. C. J., & Nicholls, A. R. (2009). Mental toughness, stress, stress appraisal, coping and coping effectiveness in sport. *Personality and Individual Differences*, 47(7), 728-733.

Kelly, G. A. (1955). *The psychology of personal constructs*. New York: Norton.

Khoshaba, D. M., & Maddi, S. R. (1999). Early experiences in hardiness development. *Consulting Psychology Journal: Practice and Research*, 51, 106-116.

Kroll, W. (1967). Sixteen personality factor profiles of collegiate wrestlers. *Research Quarterly*, 38, 49-57.

Kobasa, S. C. (1979). Stressful life events, personality and health: An enquiry into hardiness. *Journal of Personality and Social Psychology*, 37, 1-11.

Lazarus, R. S., & Folkman, S. (1984). *Stress, appraisal and coping*. New York: Springer.

Lee, K. H., Shin, D. S., Han, M. W., & Lee, E. (1994) Developing the norm of Korean table tennis players' mental toughness. *Korean Journal of Sport Science*, 6, 103-120.

Levy, A., Polman, R. C. J., Clough, P. J., Marchant, D., & Earle, K. (2006). Mental toughness as a determinant of beliefs, pain and adherence in sport injury rehabilitation. *Journal of Sport Rehabilitation*,15, 246-254.

Loehr, J. E. (1982). *Athletic excellence: Mental toughness training for sports.* New York: Forum.

Loehr, J. E. (1986). *Mental toughness training for sports: Achieving athletic excellence.* Lexington, MA: Stephen Greene.

Marchant, D. C., Polman, R. C. J., Clough, P. J., Jackson, J. G., Levy, A. R., & Nicholls, A. R. (2009) Mental toughness: Managerial and age differences. *Journal of Managerial Psychology*, 24(5), 42-437.

Middleton, S. C., Marsh, H. W., Martin, A. J., Richards, G. E., & Perry, C. (2004a). Mental Toughness: Is the mental toughness test tough enough? *International Journal of Sport & Exercise Psychology,* 35, 91-108

Nicholls, A. R., Polman, R. C. J., Levy, A. R., & Backhouse, S. H. (2008). Mental toughness, optimism, pessimism and coping among athletes. *Personality and Individual Differences*, 44, 1182-1192.

Nicholls, A. R., Polman, R. C. J., Levy, A. R., & Backhouse, S. H. (2009) Mental toughness in sport: Achievement level, gender, age, experience, and sport type differences. *Personality and Individual Differences*, 47, 73-75.

Sheard., M. (2010). *Mental toughness: The mindset behind sporting achievement.* New York: Routledge

Sheard, M. (2009). A cross-national analysis of mental toughness and hardiness in elite university rugby league teams. *Perceptual and Motor Skills*, 109, 213-223.

Sheard, M., Golby, J., & van Wersch, A. (2009). Progress toward construct validation of the Sports Mental Toughness Questionnaire (SMTQ). *European Journal of Psychological Assessment*, 25, 186-193.

Shin, D. S. & Lee, K. H. (1994). A comparative study of mental toughness between elite and non-elite female athletes. *Korean Journal of Sport Science*, 6, 85-102.

Thelwell, R., Weston, N., & Greenless, I. (2005). Defining and understanding mental toughness within soccer. *Journal of Applied Sport Psychology*, 17, 326-332.

In: Encyclopedia of Sports and Athletics
Editors: Jack L. Murray and Emily O. Watson
ISBN: 978-1-61209-959-0

Chapter XXIII

Self-Talk in Sport

***Changiz Mohiyeddini*[1], *Sara LeBlanc*[1] *and Stephanie Bauer*[2]**
[1] Roehampton University, London, UK
[2] University of Heidelberg, Germany

The Evolving Definition of Self-Talk

Self-talk (similar terms: inner speech, private speech, egocentric speech, internal dialogue, internal monologue, verbal rehearsal and self-statements) includes all intentional and automatic self-focused thoughts that run through an individual's mind (Duncan & Cheyne, 2002; Mohiyeddin & Essau, 2010). The notion of automatic self-talk implies individuals are not always aware they are engaging in private inner speech (Winsler & Naglieri, 2003); yet, self-talk is a robust phenomenon that is one of the most frequent cognitive activities in human life. Almost every minute of our waking life we talk to ourselves (Morin, 1993). According to Morin (1993) the frequency, duration and intensity of self-talk increases when conflicting perspectives within the self or between the self and others occurs.

A workable definition of self-talk is still evolving as no universal definition has been agreed upon with the extant literature (Hardy, Hall & Hardy, 2005a). To date, different definitions have been posited that vary in the emphasis they place on both the behavioural and cognitive aspects of self-talk (Hardy, 2006).

Theodorakis, Chroni, Laparidis, Bebestos, and Douma (2001) define self-talk as both a non-verbal and verbal articulation that can be manifested in the form of a smile, thought or word. This definition highlights an important aspect of self-talk, as it implies that self-talk can be either overt or covert. However, it blurs the line between the behavioural consequences (i.e. smiling) of self-talk with the construct itself (Hardy, 2006). A commonly cited definition that highlights the cognitive aspects of self-talk was offered by Bunker and colleagues (1993) who conceptualized this construct as any internal cognitions a person has which plays a role in cognitive control. However, it should be noted that the indeterminate nature of this definition, as it refers to thoughts in general terms, makes self-talk difficult to quantify and measure (Hardy, 2006).

An alternate definition was posited by Hackfort and Schwenkmezger (1993) who conceptualize self-talk as a "dialogue [through which] the individual interprets feelings and perceptions, regulates and changes evaluations and convictions, and gives him/herself instructions and reinforcement" (p. 355). This functional definition alludes to the cardinal features of this construct, as it highlights the fact that self-talk is addressed to oneself and not others, with the primary purpose of self-regulation instead of communication (Hardy, 2006). Hardy and Hardy (2004) expanded this definition further viewing self-talk as a multi-dimensional construct centered on athlete's self-statements which can be either motivational or instructional in nature. A critical review by Hard (2006) attempted to resolve the semantic confusion surrounding self-talk, offering the following guidelines to be used by researchers when defining or investigating this construct: 1) verbal or non-verbal statements directed to the self 2) fundamentally multidimensional 3) content contains interpretive aspects 4) dynamic in nature and 5) has a functional purpose which is either motivational or instructional.

Functions of Self-Talk

A growing body of empirical evidence has helped to expose the role of self-talk as an important strategy in reasoning (Harris, 1986), problem solving (Depape, Hakim-Larson, Voelker, Page & Jackson, 2006) and in planning (Morin, & Everett, 1990). A burgeoning literature has shown that self-talk is closely related to self-awareness (Morin, 1993), self-efficacy (e.g., Vargas-Tonsing, Myers, & Feltz, 2004) and that it plays a crucial role in self-regulation (Meichenbaum, 1977; Duncan, & Cheyne, 2002). According to Depape, et al (2006), self-talk is a prerequisite of personal intelligence (Gardner, 1983, 1999) and of emotional intelligence (Salovey & Mayer, 1990) since it helps to integrate perspectives of others in one's own private speech and viewpoints. Segrist (1995) maintains that self-talk fosters both private self-consciousness and public self-consciousness because it facilitates acquiring information about the self.

Following the common sense that emotions and behavior can be generated through multiple cognitive processes, it is plausible to assume self-talk may provide a direct impetus for generating human emotion and behavior (Eysenck & Keane, 2005; Mohiyeddini, Pauli & Bauer, 2009). Alternatively, it could be theorized that emotional states activated by self-talk may intensify the relative impact of internal speech itself, thereby exacerbating behavior (Mohiyeddini, Pauli & Bauer, 2009). Accordingly, Morin and Everett (1990) maintain that the valence of accompanied emotions are decisive of whether or not self-talk constricts self-awareness (in the case of negative emotion) or fosters self-awareness (in the case of positive emotions). Apart from the valence of accompanied emotions, it is crucial to differentiate between self-talk with positive (e.g. you can do it!) or negative (e.g. you are a loser) connotations, as negative self-talk has been linked to psychopathology in both children and adults.

Self-Talk and Psychopathology

A key line of inquiry in self-talk research has focused on both the antecedents and consequences of self-talk in abnormal behavior and psychological disorders (e.g. Burns, 1980; Girodo & Roehl, 1978; Padesky, 1995; Zarb, 1992). It has been shown that negative self-talk in adults is related to the onset and progression of depression (Beck, Brown, Steer, Eidelson & Riskind, 1987), agoraphobia (Chambless, Caputo, Bright & Gallagher, 1984), binge drinking (Oei & Youn, 1987) and pathological gambling (Gaboury and Ladouceur, 1989). These findings seem to be somewhat universal, as similar trends have emerged in the adolescent literature (Kimberli, Treadwell and Kendall 1996). Hence, a cornerstone of cognitive-behavioral therapy for emotional disorders is the reduction and replacement of automatic negative self-talk with aware neutral or positive self-talk (e.g., Kendall & Choudhury, 2003).

Measuring Self-Talk

From both a theoretical and applied perspective, psychological research has posited that self-talk is a crucial component of regulatory and cognitive functioning (Hardy, 2006; Diaz & Berk, 1992; MacKay, 1992). Thus, a cardinal issue in self-talk research is how best to categorize and assess this construct. In both the counseling and clinical domains, practitioners have primarily focused on the affective and irrational component of self-talk in psychopathology (Ellis, 1962; Beck 1976), often measuring the frequency of specific maladaptive self-statements such as negative, distorted or hostile automatic self-talk (Snyder, Crowson, Houston, Kurylo, & Poirier, 1997; Kendall, Howard, & Hays, 1989). This approach provides a one-sided view of self-talk as it neglects to quantify the use of general or positive self-talk which may serve a mood repair (Salovey, Mayer, Goldman, Turvey, & Palfai, 1995) or self-regulatory function (Zinsser, Bunker and Williams, 2006; Finn 1985; Meichenbaum, 1977; Duncan, & Cheyne, 2002). However, a limited number of self-talk questionnaires have investigated one's general tendency to engage in inner speech. Duncan and Cheyne (1999) developed a 27-item questionnaire of overt self-talk (The Self-Verbalization Questionnaire) which measures the use of self-statements during various scenarios such as searching for a missing item or while trying to remember a phone number. This measure is primarily focused on the use of overt self-talk during mnemonic, cognitive and attentional situations which fails to measure the frequency of covert self-statements (a crucial form of self-talk), which may exert a strong impact on both self-regulation and behaviour. Similarily, Siegrist (1995) created an 18-item self-talk questionnaire which measures the use of self-talk in specific situations (ex. "I talk over with myself personal problems"), however this scale appears to chiefly measure maladaptive self-talk and the internal consistency and validity of this scale has not been demonstrated empirically. Hollon & Kendall's (1980) created the Automatic Thoughts Questionnaire (ATQ) which measures positive and negative self-statements that are generated automatically. Although this questionnaire has demonstrated adequate internal consistency in an adolescent population (Jolly & Wiesner, 1996), it fails to address the divergent functions of self-talk which may vary according to personality and individual differences (Brinthaupt, Hein and Kramer, 2009).

The importance of self-talk has been widely recognized and well researched in contemporary psychology. Yet the psychometric measurement of self-talk is a key feature that has received limited attention in the extant literature. Although various self-talk questionnaires have been created (for ex. the self-verbalization questionnaire and the ATQ) which measure different aspects of self-talk, a comprehensive measure that quantifies individual differences in self-talk frequency, while also encapsulating both the self-regulatory and behavioural functions of self-talk, is still required. Recently, Brinthaupt, Hein and Kramer (2009) addressed this issue, developing and validating, the self-talk scale (STS), a 16-item psychometric questionnaire measuring the individual frequency and function of self-talk in non-clinical populations. Factor analysis has indicated this psychometric tool measures five distinct domains of self-talk: Self-Criticism (ex. “I'm really upset with myself”), Social Assessment (ex. “I want to replay something that I've said to another person”) Self-Management (ex. “I want to remind myself of what I need to do”) and Self-Reinforcement (ex.” I want to reinforce myself for doing well”). This multi-dimensional questionnaire employs a 5-point Likert scale anchored at 1 = never and 5 = very often, with four items measuring each of the four distinct sub-scales. The STS varies from alternative self-talk measures in a variety of ways. First, it encapsulates both overt and covert self-talk which is a significant feature, as research shows the frequency of covert speech is substantially lower than that of internal speech (Brinthaupt, Boling, & Wilson, 2000). Secondly, the STS focuses on the frequency and function of self-talk opposed to merely the content (which is subjective as what may be viewed as negative self-talk to one person may be perceived to be challenging and motivational to another). This is a key feature of the STS because by investigating both when and why people use self-talk we may begin to shed some light on the ways in which people employ self-talk as a self-regulatory mechanism. However, a potential weakness of the STS is that it is a generalized measure, thus the frequency and function of self-talk, which may vary significantly according to situational demands (ex. Relaxing at home opposed to taking the game winning shot) is not addressed.

Identifying specific functions of the different types of self-talk in varying situations is a key research area that warrants further investigation: do people use self-talk for different purposes (i.e. reward or punishment), in what situations do people utilize self-talk for motivational purposes to achieve future goals or as an instructional tool? One of the key questions that currently remains unanswered is how self-talk influences self-regulation; research suggests that general self-talk may play a crucial role in managing emotions, attention and behaviour (Brinthaupt et al., 2009) however this pivotal research area requires further research.

To determine the similarities between objective and subjective self-talk measures, future research should utilize a mixed-method approach combining the results from self-reported measures (such as the STS) with overt recordings of self-talk obtained in either laboratory or naturalistic settings (Duncan & Cheyne, 1999). From a clinical perspective, it is paramount to determine how to enhance the level of self-awareness regarding self-talk, as self-talk frequency has been linked to obsessive compulsive tendencies and has been theorized to impact the depletion of ego resources (Muraven, Tice, & Baumeister, 1998). The STS can facilitate a deeper understanding of the interaction between the frequency of self-talk and a myriad of mental illnesses such as obsessive compulsive disorder, anxiety and depression which will aid in the development and cultivation of appropriate intervention and treatment strategies.

Self-Talk in Athletics

The investigation of self-talk in athletics has employed two main research strategies. The first focuses on inter-individual variability, comparing the psychological characteristics of successful athletes to their less successful counterparts (e.g. Highlen & Bennett, 1979). The second line of research has investigated intra-individual variances using self-reported psychological characteristics of athletes comparing their psychological profiles during optimal, moderate and poor performances (e.g., Eklund, 1996; Gould, Eklund, & Jackson, 1992b).

A qualitative study by Hardy, Gammage and Hall (2001) reported that self-talk served both a motivational and instructional role within an athletic sample. This finding was supported by the work of Theodorakis, Weinberg, Natsis, Douma and Kazkas (2000) and Hatzigeorgiadis, Theodorakis and Zourbanos (2004) who determined that the performance of detailed motor tasks was enhanced by instructional self-talk, whereas the performance of gross motor tasks was enhanced by motivational self-talk. In a similar vein, Zinsser, Bunker and Williams (2006) and Finn (1985) propose that self-talk serves a regulatory function, enhancing both effort and self-confidence, whilst Hardy (1996) suggests self-talk triggers suitable action thereby controlling anxiety levels. However, Nideffer (1993) and Landin (1994) posit an alternative function of self-talk, citing it as an effective strategy for attention control to task-related cues. A recent study by Theodorakis, Hatzigeorgiadis, and Chroni (2008) lends support to the multipurpose functions of self-talk posited in the extant literature. They suggest self-talk initiates automatic execution, enhances self-confidence, improves attention focus and regulates effort while also controlling both cognitive and emotional responses.

Efficacy of Self-Talk

The reinforcement of athletes to use positive self-talk and avoid negative self-talk is perceived to be one of the most strongly advocated and frequently applied coaching strategies within an athletic setting (Gould, Hodge, Peterson, & Giannini, 1989; Park, 2000). There is convincing evidence to support this practice, as positive self-talk has been positively correlated with enhanced performance in a myriad of sports such as basketball (Hamilton & Fremour, 1985), golf (Johnson-O'Connor & Kirschenbaum 1982; Kirschenbaum, Owens, & O'Connor, 1998; Thomas & Fogarty, 1997), figure skating (Ming & Martin, 1996), tennis (Defrancesco & Burke, 1997; Mamassis & Doganis, 2004; McPherson, 2000), soccer (Papaioannou et al., 2004), dart throwing (Van Raalte, Brewer, Lewis, Linder, Wildman, & Kozimor, 1995) and skiing (Rushall, Hall, Roux, Sasseville, & Rushall, 1988). A study by Van Raalte, Brewer, Rivera, and Petipas (1994) determined that positive self-talk improved concentration while also increasing motivation. In line with these findings, Landin and Hebert (1999) conducted a self-talk intervention study with collegiate tennis players in which they determined that positive self-talk served a facultative function increasing both confidence and attention control. Further support for the efficacy of self-talk was garnered by the work of Perkos, Theodorakis, and Chroni (2002) who implemented a 12-week instructional self-talk intervention program for youth basketball players. They determined that the increased use of self-talk improved both dribbling and overall athletic performance. Furthermore, a retrospective questionnaire revealed that athletes believed their increased use of self-talk had improved both their self-confidence and concentration. Similar results were obtained from a psychological intervention study by Thelwell and Greenlees (2003) conducted on recreational athletes completing a triathalon which revealed participants attributed an increase in motivation, attention focus and self-confidence to the use of positive self-talk. In a related vein, a single subject, multiple baseline designed study by Johnson, Hrycaiko Johnson, Hallas (2004) tested the efficacy of a self-talk training program in relation to performance for female football players. This study determined an increase in performance for two of the three athletes sampled with a relative increase in self-confidence for all three athletes who participated in the study.

Self-talk has also been investigated via direct observation, a research design that involves asking participants to verbalize their self-talk which is then recorded by the experimenter using the self-talk and gestures rating scale. A study by Van Raalte and colleagues (1994) utilized this technique while studying young tennis players participating in competitive matches. Their findings revealed match winners utilized less negative self-talk than match losers; however, the use of positive self-talk by both the winners and the losers did not vary significantly. Van Raalte and colleagues (1994) suggest that positive self-talk was not significantly correlated with performance in this study because positive self-talk is more likely to be internalized than negative self-talk and therefore was not made audible to the researchers.

The majority of studies have determined that positive self-talk has the ability to enhance various performance-related factors; conversely, some studies have shown performance increases when negative self-talk is utilized (Highlen & Bennett, 1983) or that the same type of self talk was utilized during both best and worst performances (Dagrou, Gauvin, & Halliwell, 1991). A study by Van Raalte Cornelius Brewer & Hatten (2000) investigating self-talk in youth tennis players determined negative self-talk was not related to losing. In line with these findings, a study by Rotella, Gansneder, Ojala and Billing (1980) did not find a significant difference between the negative self-talk used by elite skiers when compared to their less successful counterparts. Furthermore, a study by Highlen and Bennett (1983: Study 1) which investigated the use of self-talk within elite divers, determined non-qualifiers utilized positive self-talk more frequently than qualifiers competing to attend the Pan Am games. However, these findings should be interpreted with caution as this study was conducted on a small sample of athletes competing in a close-skilled, individual sport and these results were not repeated when a group of elite wrestlers were sampled (Highlen & Bennett, 1983: Study 2).

The unequivocal results discussed above highlight the convolution of the self-talk construct, as individual differences and interpretations seem to affect the impact self-talk has on performance. Therefore, the type of self-talk used (positive or negative) may not be as important as the meaning one attaches to the content (negative, positive or challenging). Take, for example, the following hypothetical situation: Athlete A tells himself to 'push harder' every time he makes a mistake thereby tying negative connotations to this phrase; whereas, athlete B tells himself to 'push harder' to psych himself up before competition as a motivational strategy. These two athletes are saying the same thing but their interpretation of the phrase is entirely different. In the latter example, what could be phrased as negative self-talk is interpreted to be challenging and motivational and could in fact lead to performance improvements. Thus, the impact self-talk has on performance may depend more on the athletes interpretation of their self-talk statements rather than on the content itself.

Pitfalls of Self-Talk

Although the advantages of self-talk are robust, several disadvantages may emerge in certain situations. For example, highly detailed, instructional self-talk may foster 'paralysis by analysis' whereby an athlete's performance is negatively impacted due to over-analysis which causes a failure to respond to the situational demands (Hardy, 2006). Furthermore, the use of elaborate rules, which shares many similarities with instructional self-talk, has been linked to performance detriments when performing motor skills under pressure (Masters, 2000). In addition, a study by Jackson and Wilson (1999) found that too much instructional self-talk can be damaging to performance in golf which led them to recommend the utilization of one primary self-statement instead of three. However, this may be the case primarily for instructional self-talk, as no evidence has emerged to prove this relationship exists for motivational self-talk. Future research should investigate this issue in greater detail to determine if there are disadvantages to motivational self-talk and if there is an optimal amount of instructional self-talk that should be implemented.

Self-Talk and Self-Efficacy

Self-efficacy is a key construct that is linked to self-talk. Bandura (1997) posits that influential self-statements may be an effective complimentary efficacy source. This supposition garners support from recent research as Weinberg, Grove, and Jackson (1992) found tennis coaches frequently endorsed the use of positive self-talk as an effective self-efficacy building strategy. This finding was supported by the work of Hardy Hall, Gibbs & Greenslade (2005b) who identified a link between the self-efficacy to perform a sit-up as well as the perception and valence of the relative dimensions of self-talk. A study by Hardy, Hall, Gibbs, and Greenslade (2005) determined that self-efficacy was positively correlated with self-talk in an experimental task which led them to suggest that the relationship between self-talk and performance may be mediated by self-efficacy. However, further research is required to determine the interaction between these two constructs. Does positive self-talk predict an increase in self-efficacy? Does self-efficacy mediate or moderate the relationship between performance and self-talk? Perhaps the most salient question that arises in an applied setting is how athletes can optimize their use of self-talk to enhance their level of self-efficacy? These are key questions that currently remain unanswered.

Conceptual and Empirical Issues

To date, self-talk literature has been strongly criticized for its lack of theory-driven research, which may be a contributing factor to the lack of semantic clarity (Hard, 2006). Furthermore, self-talk research is largely reliant on self report (using interviews or questionnaires) which requires the ability to accurately reflect on and report one's self-talk behavior which is problematic as recall is susceptible to inaccurate memory recall and may reflect a unique pattern of reporting biases (e.g., Primacy and recency effects, Murdock, 1962) and social desirability (e.g. The incorrect report of the frequency of negative self-talk). Considering the potential pitfalls of self-reported measures and the crucial role of self-talk in human functioning, future research should consider objective measurements of actual self-talk behavior.

A further issue highlighted by Peters and Williams (2006) is the fact that self-talk research has mainly neglected the impact of cultural background. The results of Heine and colleagues (Heine, 2001; Heine, Lehman, Markus, & Kitayama, 1999) study has shown that while positive self-perception is a key characteristic of individuals from an individualistic culture (e.g., European and Americans), self-critical orientation is a cardinal characteristic of individuals from collectivist cultures (e.g., Japanese and Chinese). Hence, the aforementioned results regarding the link between positive and negative self-talk in both the health and performance literature, may have limited generalizability due to significant cultural differences.

Finally, previous research has neglected to investigate the role of self-talk as an emotion regulation strategy. From a theoretical viewpoint, it seems plausible to assume that negative emotional states enhance self-talk with negative content (mood-dependent retrieval, Bower, 1981) and that negative self-talk in turn will maintain and intensify negative emotional states (distress-augmenting emotion regulation, Mohiyeddini, in prep). In contrast, self-talk with positive content may intensify or maintain positive emotional states (hedonistic emotion regulation, Larsen, 2000; Mohiyeddini, in prep) and serve as a mood repair emotion regulation strategy (Salovey, Mayer, Goldman, Turvey, & Palfai, 1995) that moderates or changes negative emotional states into positively valenced emotional states. In a related vein, it is crucial to investigate the link between rumination (Nolen-Hoeksema, 2000) emotional suppression (Gross, 2002) and self-talk. It could be hypothesized that individuals high in rumination or emotional suppression will utilize (automatic) negative self-talk more frequently. This suggestion may contribute to a better understanding of the antecedents and consequences of self-talk.

Future Directions

In the athletic domain, positive self-talk interventions are commonly conducted in an applied setting (Park, 2000) and a link between positive self-talk and enhanced performance has been demonstrated (Johnson-O'Connor & Kirschenbaum 1982; Kirschenbaum, Owens, & O'Connor, 1998; Thomas & Fogarty, 1997); however, conflicting results have been obtained as in some cases negative self-talk has facilitated enhanced performance levels (Highlen & Bennett, 1983). This illuminates both the complexity and ambiguity of the self-talk construct and the relative impact that individual differences and interpretations can exert on this construct. In moving forward, future research should not accept the utility of positive self-talk at face value but instead should begin to investigate the link between athletes' perceptions of self-talk and performance so that interventions can be developed that are tailored towards individual preferences instead of utilizing a 'one size fits all' approach which may be damaging to performance in certain situations.

Self-efficacy is a key construct that has been linked to self-talk (Bandura, 1997). Although a relationship has been established between these two variables, the majority of research has been correlational in nature; therefore, causality cannot be inferred. Future research should implement longitudinal research designs so that the relationship between self-efficacy and self-talk can be explained in greater detail in order to determine the directionality of this relationship (i.e. does self-talk predict self-efficacy, does self-efficacy predict self-talk or does a reciprocal relationship exist?) and whether or not self-efficacy serves as a mediator or moderator between self-talk and performance.

An additional area that warrants future research is the efficacy of motivational vs. instructional self-talk and its relative impact in both a training and competitive environment. Instructional self-talk has been found to have a deleterious impact on performance when used in excess by eliciting 'paralysis by analysis' (Hardy, 2006); however, little research has explored the potential weaknesses of motivational self-talk. Perhaps motivational self-talk is more effective in training whereas instructional self-talk is a more efficient tool during competition? Perhaps the efficacy of motivational vs. instructional self-talk is sport-specific? Perhaps individual differences play a crucial role in determining what type of self-talk should be utilized? By investigating both the advantages and disadvantages of motivational and instructional self-talk in greater detail we can begin to answer these questions and create guidelines for the appropriate use of self-statements with either instructional or motivational content so that the use of self-talk can be optimized.

References

Bandura, A. (1997). Self-efficacy: the exercise of control. New York: Freeman.

Beck, A. T. (1976). Cognitive therapy and the emotional disorders. New York:
New American Library.

Beck, A.T., Brown, G., Steer, R.A., Eidelson, I., & Riskind, J.H. (1987). Differentiating anxiety and depression utilizing the Cognition Checklist. Journal of Abnormal Psychology, 96, 179-183.

Bower, G.H. (1981). Mood and memory. American Psychologist, 36, 129-148.

Bunker, L., Williams, J. M., & Zinsser, N. (1993). Cognitive techniques for improving performance and building confidence. In J. M. Willaims (Ed.), Applied sport psychology: Personal growth to peak performance 2nd ed. Mountain View, CA: Mayfield.

Burns, D. (1980). Feeling good: The new mood therapy. New York: William Morrow.

Brinthaupt, T. M., Boling, J. S., & Wilson, C. (2000). Situational and individual differences in the self-talk of adults. Unpublished manuscript, Middle Tennessee State University, Murfreesboro.

Brinthaupt T.M. Hein M.B. Kramer T. (2009). The Self-Talk Scale: Development, factor analysis, and validation. Journal of Personality Assessment, 91, 82-92.

Chambless, D.L., Caputo, G.C., Bright, P., & Gallagher, R. (1984). Assessment of fear in agoraphobics: The Body Sensations Questionnaire and the Agoraphobic Cognitions Questionnaire. Journal of Consulting and Clinical Psychology, 52, 1090-1097.

Dagrou, E., Gauvin, L., & Halliwell, W. (1991). Mental preparation of Ivory Coast athletes: Current practice and research perspective. International Journal of Sport Psychology, 22, 15-34.

Defrancesco, C., & Burke, K.L. (1997) Performance enhancement strategies used in a professional tennis tournament. International Journal of Sport Psychology, 28, 185-195.

Depape, A.M.R., Hakim-Larson, J., Voelker, S., Page, S., & Jackson, D.L. (2006). Self-Talk and Emotional Intelligence in University Students. Canadian Journal of Behavioural Science, 38, 250-260.

Diaz, R. M., & Berk, L. E. (Eds.). (1992). Private speech: From social interaction to self-regulation. Hillsdale, NJ: Lawrence Erlbaum Associates.

Duncan, R. M., & Cheyne, J. A. (1999). Incidence and functions of self-reported private speech in young adults: A self-verbalization questionnaire. Canadian Journal of Behavioural Science, 31, 133-136.

Duncan, R. M., & Cheyne, J. A. (2002). Private speech in young adults: Task difficulty, self-regulation, and psychological predication. Cognitive Development, 16, 889-906.

Ellis, A. (1962). Reason and emotion in psychotherapy. New York: Lyle Stuart. Fenigstein, A., Scheier, M. F., & Buss, A. (1975). Public and private self- consciousness. Journal of Consulting and Clinical Psychology, 43, 522-527.

Eysenck, M.W., & Keane, M.T. (2005). Cognitive Psychology. Taylor & Francis Group.

Finn, J.A. (1985). Competitive excellence: it's a matter of mind and body. The Physician and Sport medicine, 13, 61-75.

Gaboury, A., & Ladouceur, R. (1989). Erroneous perceptions and gambling. Journal of Social Behavior and Personality, 4, 411-420.

Gardner, H. (1983). Frames of mind: The theory of multiple intelligences. New York: Basic Books.

Gardner, H. (1999). Intelligence reframed: Multiple intelligences for the 21st century. New York: Basic Books.

Gaboury, A., & Ladouceur, R. (1989). Erroneous perceptions and gambling. Journal of Social Behavior and Personality, 4, 411-420.

Gardner, H. (1983). Frames of mind: The theory of multiple intelligences. New York: Basic Books.

Gardner, H. (1999). Intelligence reframed: Multiple intelligences for the 21st century. New York: Basic Books.

Hackfort, D., & Schwenkmezger, P. (1993). Anxiety In R.N. Singer, M. Murphey, & L.K. Tennant, (Eds.). Handbook of research on sport psychology (pp. 328-364). New York: Macmillan.

Hamilton, S. A., & Fremour, W. J. (1985). Cognitive behavioral training for college basketball free-throw performance. Cognitive Therapy and Research, 9, 479-483.

Hardy, L. Jones G., & Gould, D. (1996). Understanding psychological preparation for sport: Theory and practice of elite performers, Jones Wiley & Sons, Chichester, UK.

Hardy, J., Hall, C. R., & Hardy, L. (2004). A note on athletes' use of self-talk. Journal of Applied Sport Psychology, 16, 251-257.

Hardy J. Hall C.R. Hardy L. (2005a). Quantifying athlete self-talk. Journal of Sports Psychology, 23, 905-917.

Hardy, J., Hall, C.R., C. Gibbs, & C. Greenslade (2005b). Self-talk and gross motor skill performance. Athletic Insight: The Online Journal of Sport Psychology, 7(2).

Hardy J. (2006). Speaking clearly: A critical review of the self-talk literature. Psychology of Sport and Exercise, 7, 81-97.

Harris, K.R. (1986). The effects of cognitive-behavior modification on private speech and task performance during problem solving among learning-disabled and normally achieving children. Journal of Abnormal Child Psychology, 14, 63-67.

Hatzigeorgiadis, A., Theodorkis, Y., & Zourbanos, N. (2004). Self-talk in the swimming pool: The effects of self-talk on though content and performance on water-polo tasks. Journal of Applied Sport Psychology, 16, 138-150.

Highlen, P. S., & Bennett, B. B. (1983). Elite divers and wrestlers: A comparison between open- and closed-skill athletes. Journal of Sport Psychology, 5, 390-409.

Heine, S. J., Lehman, D. R., Markus, H. R., & Kitayama, S. (1999). Is there a universal need for positive self-regard? Psychological Review, 106, 766-794.

Heine, S. J. (2001). Self as cultural product: An examination of East Asian and North American selves. Journal of Personality, 69, 881-906.

Highlen, P. S., & Bennett, B. B. (1979). Psychological characteristics of successful and nonsuccessful elite wrestlers: An exploratory study. Journal of Sport Psychology, 1, 123-137.

Hollon S.D. & P. Kendall P. (1980). Cognitive self-statements in depression: Development of an automatic thoughts questionnaire. Cognitive Therapy and Research, 4, 383-395.

Jackson, R.C., & Wilson, R. (1999). Using 'swing thoughts' to prevent paradoxical performance effects in golf putting In M.R. Farrally & A.J. Cochran (Eds.), Science and golf III: Proceedings of the world scientific congress of golf London: E & F.N.

Johnson-O'Connor, E. J., & Kirschenbaum, D. S. (1982). Something succeeds like success: Positive self-monitoring for unskilled golfers. Cognitive Therapy and Research, 10, 123-136.

Johnson, J. J. M., Hrycaiko, D. W., Johnson, G. V., & Hallas, J. M. (2004). Self-talk and female youth soccer performance. The Sport Psychologist, 18, 44-59.

Jolly, J. B., & Wiesner, D. C. (1996). Psychometric properties of the Automatic Thoughts Questionnaire–Positive with inpatient adolescents. Cognitive Therapy and Research, 20, 481-498.

Kendall, P. C., Howard, B. L., & Hays, R. C. (1989). Self-referent speech and psychopathology: The balance of positive and negative thinking. Cognitive Therapy and Research, 13, 583-598.

Kendall, P C., & Choudhury, M. S. (2003). Children and adolescents in cognitive-behavioral therapy: Some past efforts and current advances, and the challenges in our future. Cognitive Therapy and Research, 27, 89-104.

Kirschenbaum, D. S., Owens, D., & O'Connor, E. A. (1998). Smart golf: Preliminary evaluation of a simple, yet comprehensive, approach to improving and scoring the mental game. The Sport Psychologist, 12, 271-282.

Landin, D., & Hebert, E. P. (1999). The influence of self-talk on the performance of skilled female tennis players. Journal of Applied Sport Psychology, 11, 263-282.

Larsen, R. J. (2000). Toward a science of mood regulation. Psychological Inquiry, 11, 129-141.

MacKay, D. G. (1992). Constraints on theories of inner speech. In D. Reisberg (Ed.), Auditory imagery (pp. 121-149). Hillsdale, NJ: Lawrence Erlbaum Associates.

Mamassis G., & Doganis, G. (2004). The effects of a mental training program on juniors pre-competitive anxiety, self-confidence, and tennis performance. Journal of Applied Sport Psychology, 16, 118-137.

Masters, R. S. W. (2000). Theoretical aspects of implicit learning in sport. International Journal of Sport Psychology, 31, 530-541.

McPherson, S.L. (2000). Expert- novice differences in planning strategies during collegiate singles tennis competition. Journal of Sport and Exercise Psychology, 22, 39-62.

Meichenbaum, D. (1977). Cognitive-behavior modification: An integrative approach. New York: Plenum Press.

Ming, S., & Martin, G.L. (1996). Single-subject evaluation of a self-talk package for improving figure skating performance. The Sport Psychologist, 10, 227-238.

Mohiyeddini, C. & Essau, C. (2010). Self-talk. In S. Goldstein & J.A. Naglieri (eds.), Encyclopedia of Child Behavior and Development.

Mohiyeddini, C., Pauli, G. & Bauer, S. (2009). The role of emotion in bridging the intention–behaviour gap: The case of sports participation. Psychology of Sport & Exercise. 10, 226-234.

Mohiyeddini, C. (in prep.). Three dimensional emotion regulation.

Morin, A., & Everett, J. (1990). Inner speech as a mediator of self-awareness, self-consciousness, and self-knowledge: A hypothesis. New Ideas in Psychology, 8, 337-356.

Morin, A. (1993). Self-talk and self-awareness: On the nature of the relation. The Journal of Mind and Behavior, 14, 223-234.

Muraven, M., Tice, D. M., & Baumeister, R. F. (1998). Self-control as limited resource: Regulatory depletion patterns. Journal of Personality and Social Psychology, 74, 774-778.

Murdock, B. B. (1962). Direction of recall in short-term memory. Journal of Verbal Learning & Verbal Behavior, 1, 119-124.

Nideffer, (1993). Attention control training. In: R.N. Singer, M. Murphey and I.K. Tennant, Editors, Handbook of research on sport psychology. Macmillan: New York, 127-170.

Nolen-Hoeksema, S. (2000). The role of rumination in depressive disorders and mixed anxiety/depressive symptoms. Journal of Abnormal Psychology, 109, 504- 511.

Oei, T.P., & Young, R.M. (1987). The roles of alcohol-related self-statements in social drinking. International Journal of The Addiction, 22, 905-915.

Padesky, C. A. (with Greenberger, D.) (1995). Clinicians guide to mind over mood. New York: Guilford.

Papaioannou, A., Ballon, F., Theodorakis, Y., & Auwelle, Y. V. (2004). Combined effect of goal setting and self-talk in performance of a soccer-shooting task. Perceptual and Motor Skills, 98, 89-99.

Park, J. K. (2000). Coping strategies used by Korean national athletes. The Sport Psychologist, 14, 63-80.

Perkos, S., Theodorakis, Y., & Chroni, S. (2002). Enhancing performance and skill acquisition in novice basketball players with instructional self-talk. The Sport Psychologist, 16, 368-383.

Peters, H.J. & Williams, J.M. (2006). Moving Cultural Background to the Foreground: An Investigation of Self-Talk, Performance, and Persistence Following Feedback. Journal of Applied Sport Psychology, 18, 240-253.

Rotella, R. J., Gansneder, B., Ojala, D., & Billings, J. (1980). Cognitions and coping strategies of elite skiers: An exploratory study on young developing athletes. Journal of Sport Psychology, 2, 350-354.

Rushall, B. S., Hall, M., Roux, L., Sasseville, J., & Rushall, A. C. (1988). Effects of three types of thought content instructions on skiing performance. The Sport Psychologist, 2, 283-297.

Salovey, P., & Mayer, J. D. (1990). Emotional intelligence. Imagination, Cognition and Personality, 9, 185-211.

Salovey, P., Mayer, J., Goldman, S., Turvey, C., & Palfai, T. (1995). Emotional attention, clarity and repair: Exploring emotional intelligence using the Trait Meta-Mood Scale. In J.W. Pennebaker (Ed.), Emotion, disclosure, and health (pp. 125-154) Washington, DC: American Psychological Association.

Siegrist, M. (1995). Inner speech as a cognitive process mediating self-consciousness and inhibiting self-deception. Psychological Reports, 76, 259-265.

Snyder, C. R., Crowson, J. J. Jr., Houston, B. K., Kurylo, M., & Poirier, J. (1997). Assessing hostile automatic thoughts: Development and validation of the HAT scale. Cognitive Therapy and Research, 21, 477-492.

Thelwell, R. C., & Greenlees, I. A. (2003). Developing competitive endurance performance using mental skills training. The Sport Psychologist, 17, 318-337.

Theodorakis, Y., Weinberg, R., Natsis, P., Douma, I., & Kazakas, P. (2000). The effects of motivational and instructional self-talk on improving motor performance. The Sport Psychologist, 14, 253-271.

Theodorakis, Y., Chroni, S., Laparidis, K., Bebestos, V., & Douma, I. (2001). Self-talk in a basketball-shooting task. Perceptual and Motor Skills, 92, 309-315.

Theodorakis, Y. Hatzigeorgiadis, A. & Chroni, S. (2008). Self-Talk: it works, but how? Development and preliminary validation of the functions of Self-Talk Questionnaire. Measurement in Physical Education and Exercise Science, 12, 10-30.

Thomas, P.R. and Fogarty, G.J. (1997). Psychological skills training in golf: The role of individual differences in cognitive preference. The Sport Psychologist, 11, 86-106.

Treadwell, K.H., & Kendall, P.C. (1996). Self-Talk in Youth With Anxiety Disorders: States of Mind, Content Specificity, and Treatment Outcome. Journal of Consulting and Clinical Psychology, 64, 941-950.

Van Raalte, J. L., Brewer, B. W., Rivera, P. M., & Petitpas, A. J. (1994). The relationship between observable self-talk and competitive junior players' match performances. Journal of Sport and Exercise Psychology, 16, 400-415.

Van Raalte, J. L., Brewer, B. W., Lewis, B. P., Linder, D. E., Wildman, G., & Kozimor, J. (1995). Cork! The effects of positive and negative self-talk on dart performance. Journal of Sport Behavior, 3, 50-57.

Van Raalte, J. L., Cornelius, A. E., Brewer, B. W., & Hatten, S. J. (2000). The antecedents and consequences of self-talk in competitive tennis. Journal of Sport & Exercise Psychology, 22, 345-356.

Vargas-Tonsing, T. M., Myers, N. D., & Feltz, D. L. (2004). Coaches' and athletes' perceptions of efficacy-enhancing techniques. The Sport Psychologist, 18, 397-414.

Weinberg, R., Grove, R., & Jackson, A. (1992). Strategies for building self-efficacy in tennis players: A comparative analysis of Australian and American coaches. The Sport Psychologist, 6, 3-13.

Winsler, A., & Naglieri, J. (2003). Overt and covert verbal problem-solving strategies: Developmental trends in use, awareness, and relations with task performance in children aged 5 to 17. Child Development, 74, 659-678.

Zinsser, N., Bunker L., &Williams, J.M. (2006). Cognitive techniques for building confidence and enhancing performance. In: J.M. Williams, Editor, Applied sport psychology: Personal growth to peak performance (5th ed.), McGraw-Hill Companies, New York, 346-378.

In: Encyclopedia of Sports and Athletics
Editors: Jack L. Murray and Emily O. Watson

ISBN: 978-1-61209-959-0

Chapter XXIV

What Would you Do for a Championship? Willingness to Consider Acts of Desperation among Major League Baseball Fans

***Daniel L. Wann*[1*]*, Frederick G. Grieve*[2]*, Ryan K. Zapalac*[3]*, Jason R. Lanter*[4]*, Julie A. Partridge*[5]*, Sandra E. Short*[6]*, Paula M. Parker*[7]*, and Martin Short*[8]**

[1]Murray State University, US
[2]Western Kentucky University, US
[3]Sam Houston State University, US
[4]Kutztown University, US
[5]Southern Illinois University, US
[6]University of North Dakota, US
[7]East Stroudsburg University, US
[8]University of North Dakota, US

Abstract

Previous research found that highly identified fans report a willingness to engage in a variety of behaviors designed to assist their team, including instrumental aggression, illegal/unethical acts, and superstitious behaviors. The current investigation extended past research by investigating a willingness to engage in acts of desperation (e.g., giving up all drinks except water) if doing so would guarantee a championship. It was hypothesized that higher levels of team identification and rooting for a team that had failed to win a recent championship would predict willingness to consider the acts of desperation.

* Address correspondence to Daniel L. Wann,
Department of Psychology, Murray State University,
Murray, KY 42071 or to
dan.wann@murraystate.edu via Internet.

Participants (n = 655) completed a questionnaire packet assessing demographics, team identification with one's favorite Major League Baseball team, and willingness to consider 22 acts of desperation. Regression analysis confirmed both hypotheses and also indicated that men were more likely than women to consider the acts of desperation.

Over the course of the last few decades, sport science researchers from a variety of disciplines (e.g., sport psychology, sport sociology, sport marketing) have extended our understanding of the actions and attitudes of sport fans (Wann, Melnick, Russell, & Pease, 2001). Many lines of investigation have been undertaken including work examining fan violence (Giulianotti, Bonney, & Hepworth, 1994; Russell, 2008), attendance decisions (Fisher & Wakefield, 1998; Williamson, Zhang, Pease, & Gaa, 2003), motivation (James & Ross, 2004; Wann, Grieve, Zapalac, & Pease, 2008), and social connections among fans (Clopton, 2008; Crawford, 2004).

One of the most successful lines of investigation has examined the antecedents and consequences of sport team identification (Dietz-Uhler & Lanter, 2008; Wann, 2006). Team identification concerns the extent to which a fan feels a psychological connection to a team (Wann & Branscombe, 1993). A large body of literature indicates that highly identified fans (i.e., those with a strong psychological attachment to the team) tend to exhibit intense reactions to their team's competitions (Wann, Melnick, et al., 2001). In essence, for these fans, the team's successes are felt as their own successes and the team's failures are perceived as their own failures. As a result, these fans highly value team championships and often report that they would be willing to do almost anything to help their team win a championship.

For instance, these fans often engage in a variety of superstitions designed to help their team win (Wann et al., 2009). Wann and colleagues surveyed over 1,500 sport fans from a number of colleges and universities and found many common superstitions among the fans, including superstitions involving apparel (e.g., a lucky shirt), good luck charms, good luck gestures (e.g., crossing one's fingers), and lucky seats. The fans reported high levels of belief in the importance of the superstitions and in perceptions of the impact of the superstitions. Level of team identification was positively associated with perceptions of both the importance and impact of the superstitions as well as the number of superstitions listed.

Fans also report that they would be willing to cheat to help their favorite team win. Wann, Hunter, Ryan, and Wright (2001) assessed the level of team identification of a group of college student basketball fans. They then asked the participants to report their willingness to engage in several illegal or unethical behaviors designed to assist the team if the fan were guaranteed anonymity and there would be no negative consequences of their actions. The authors found that many of the fans were willing to consider the acts. For instance, 41% of the respondents reported a willingness to let a player cheat off of them in class, while 27% were willing to consider writing a class paper for a player. Further, 14% were willing to steal a test for a player and 13% admitted a willingness to consider bribing a referee. Most importantly for the current research, levels of willingness to consider the illegal/unethical acts were positively correlated with levels of team identification.

A different line of research investigated the extent to which fans are willing to consider injuring opposing players/coaches to help the team if their actions would remain anonymous. In their investigation of instrumental fan aggression, Wann, Peterson, Cothran, and Dykes (1999) assessed the team identification of college student basketball fans as well as the extent that they were willing to consider anonymously injuring a rival team's player and coach prior to a contest involving their team and the rival team, thereby eliminating the player and coach from participating. Participants were asked about their willingness to consider tripping the player/coach and breaking the leg of the player/coach. A sizeable minority of fans admitted a willingness to consider the anonymous acts of instrumental aggression. Specifically, 48% were willing to consider tripping the opposing player while 42% would consider tripping the coach. Further, 34% and 32% admitted a willingness to consider breaking a player's and coach's leg, respectively. Again, most important to the current line of research, Wann, Peterson, et al. (1999) found significant positive correlations between level of team identification and degree of willingness to consider the anonymous acts of aggression.

Each of the aforementioned studies indicates that highly identified fans report a willingness to consider a variety of acts in an attempt to assist their team. In the current work, we were interested in extending this line of investigation by examining the extent to which Major League Baseball fans were willing to consider various acts of desperation (e.g., give up all drinks except water) if doing so would guarantee their favorite team a championship. It was hypothesized that two variables would significantly predict willingness to consider acts of desperation: level of identification with the team and whether or not the team has recently won a World Series. With respect to team identification, based on the previously reviewed literature (e.g., Wann et al., 2009; Wann, Hunter, et al., 2001; Wann, Peterson, et al., 1999), it was expected that persons with higher levels of team identification would be particularly likely to report they would be willing to consider the acts of desperation.

In terms of whether or not a team had recently won a championship, we imagined that longer suffering fans would place a greater amount of importance on their team winning a championship, relative to fans of a team who had recently won a championship. Therefore, longer suffering fans would be particularly likely to consider the acts of desperation. This line of reasoning is based on research in the area of object/event scarcity. Objects and events that are perceived as scarce are often viewed as particularly valuable and important and, as a result, individuals often have a greater desire for them (Lynn, 1992). The scarcity effect has strong research support (e.g., Williams, Radefeld, Binning, & Sudak, 1993) and this includes work among sport fans (Wann, Bayens, & Driver, 2004).

Method

Participants

The original sample contained 705 students from one of seven universities (some participants received extra course credit in a college class in exchange for participation). However, 50 participants returned unusable questionnaires (e.g., did not list a favorite Major League Baseball team, listed a Football Team, left items blank) and were dropped from the sample. The final sample contained 655 persons (336 males; 319 females) with a mean age of 20.86 years (SD = 3.70).

Materials and Procedure

Upon entering the testing session and providing their consent, participants were handed a questionnaire packet containing three sections. The first section contained demographic items assessing age and gender. The second section contained the Sport Spectator Identification Scale (SSIS; Wann & Branscombe, 1993). Participants were asked to list their favorite Major League Baseball team and then to target this team when completing the scale. The SSIS has been used in a number of studies involving sport fans and has strong reliability and validity (Wann & Branscombe, 1993; Wann, Melnick, et al., 2001). The SSIS contains 7 Likert-type items with response options ranging from 1 (*low identification*) to 8 (*high identification*). Thus, higher numbers represent greater levels of identification. A sample item on the SSIS reads, "How strongly do you see yourself as a fan of (the Major League team listed above)?"

The third section of the packet contained 22 items assessing a willingness to engage in various acts of desperation if doing so would guarantee a championship for the Major League team listed previously. Participants read:

> Sports fans often talk about how they would "do anything" to guarantee their favorite team a championship. We are interested in what, exactly, they would be willing to do. Below, you will find a list of several hypothetical scenarios. We would like you to think about your favorite Major League Baseball team – the team you listed on the previous page. Please answer each of the following items involving actions you might consider doing to guarantee your favorite Major League Baseball team a championship. Please take your time as you work through these items, thinking carefully about each one before answering. Please be honest in your response, there are no "right" or "wrong" answers. Simply circle the item that best represents your response.

The first 17 items asked how long participants would be willing to engage in certain acts if doing so would guarantee a World Series Championship for their favorite Major League Baseball team (for a list of items, see Table 1). For instance, one of these items read, "How long would you be willing to wear the same underwear if doing so would guarantee a World Series Championship for your favorite Major League Baseball team?" Response options to these 17 items were *Not at All* (coded as 1), *One Day* (2), *One Week* (3), *Two Weeks* (4), *One Month* (5), *Two Months*, (6), *Six Months* (7), *A Year* (8). The final five items asked participants to indicate how willing they would be to consider various acts of desperation (for a list of items, see Table 1). These items were rated on a scale ranging from 1 (*I would never consider doing this*) to 8 (*I would definitely consider doing this*). For example, one of these items read, "How willing would you be to destroy your favorite keepsake (e.g., vase, picture, piece of jewelry, etc.) if doing so would guarantee a World Series Championship for your favorite Major League Baseball team?"

Table 1. Frequency Distributions (Percentages) of Responses to the 22 Items Assessing Acts of Desperation

	Response							
Item	1	2	3	4	5	6	7	8
How long would you be willing to…								
Wear same underwear	20	30	23	10	7	3	2	5
Give up all drinks except water	12	9	12	10	13	8	8	29
Give up all sweets	12	9	13	9	13	10	10	24
Stop talking to your best friend	45	15	14	8	7	4	2	5
Avoid all physical contact with others	50	18	15	6	6	2	2	2
Go without talking	40	32	13	7	3	2	1	2
Go without riding in a car	31	22	20	10	7	3	2	5
Go without bathing/showering	38	30	21	7	2	1	1	1
Go without shaving	14	6	15	12	14	11	6	21
Have your entire body/head shaved	64	4	4	3	4	3	4	14
Go without watching television	16	15	22	12	14	7	4	10
Wear only clothing of the opposite sex	44	21	13	6	6	2	2	6
Go without sex	20	7	14	8	12	11	8	20
Attend all of team's game in person	19	7	13	9	10	4	4	34
Stop using your cell phone	39	21	17	8	7	3	2	4
Stop checking social networking sites	20	11	15	8	12	8	5	21
Attend church daily	14	7	15	10	11	6	3	35
Never consider…definitely consider								
Cut off one of your fingers	90	3	2	2	2	1	0	1
Destroy your favorite keepsake	69	8	6	4	4	3	2	5
Get a permanent team-oriented tattoo	51	8	5	5	6	5	4	16
Donate an organ	53	10	7	7	6	4	4	10
Donate a paycheck to charity	25	10	9	8	8	10	7	25

Notes: For the "How long" items, 1 = *not at all*, 2 = *one day*, 3 = *one week*, 4 = *two weeks*, 5 = *one month*, 6 = *two months*, 7 = *six months*, and 8 = *one year*. For the five other items, responses ranged from 1 (*I would never consider doing this*) to 8 (*I would definitely consider doing this*). Percentages for each item may not sum to 100 due to rounding.

After the completion of the questionnaire packet (approximately 15 minutes), the participants were debriefed and excused from the testing session.

Results

The first series of analyses examined frequency distributions (percentages) of responses to the 22 items assessing willingness to consider the acts of desperation. These results appear in Table 1. As revealed in the table, a sizeable number of persons were willing to consider the various acts of desperation. For instance, over half of the sample was willing to give up all drinks except water, refrain from eating sweets, go without shaving and sex, attend all of the team's games and church daily, and stop checking social networking sites for at least one month. Almost half of the sample was willing to consider (i.e., listed a response of at least 2 on the 1-8 scale) getting a permanent team-oriented tattoo and donating an organ. Fully 75% of participants were willing to consider donating a paycheck to charity.

The next series of analyses involved examinations of the relationships among level of team identification (i.e., SSIS scores), gender, age, recent success (i.e., World Series Championship) of favorite Major League Baseball team, and willingness to engage in the acts of desperation. The seven items comprising the SSIS were combined to form a single index of team identification (Cronbach's alpha = .95). Similarly, the 22 items targeting the various acts of desperation were combined to form a single index of fan desperation (alpha = .93). The impact of gender on SSIS and desperation indices was assessed via a pair of one-way analyses of variance (ANOVA). These analyses revealed significant gender differences for both the SSIS, $F(1, 653) = 45.50, p < .001$, and the desperation index, $F(1, 653) = 56.26, p < .001$. Males scored higher on the SSIS ($M = 39.53$; $SD = 13.20$) than did females ($M = 32.55$; $SD = 13.30$) and males ($M = 82.10$; $SD = 31.92$) reported higher scores on the desperation index relative to female participants ($M = 64.61$; $SD = 27.45$). Because of the significant impact of gender, this variable was included in the regression analyses described below.

We also created a variable labeled "recent team championship" to place participants into two groups: those whose favorite team had recently won a World Series Championship and those whose team had not. Although a variety of options were considered for creating this variable, we chose to separate the teams into two groups based on whether or not the team had won a World Series Championship since 1994. Our logic here was that, given that a) the average age of the participants was about 21 and b) most fans probably don't truly begin to follow a team until they are at least 5 years old, it seemed reasonable to go back 15 years from the most recent season, 2009. Further, due to the players' strike, there was no World Series played in 1994, giving the data a clean break. Consequently, participants who reported that their favorite team was either the Atlanta Braves, New York Yankees, Florida Marlins, Arizona Diamondbacks, California Angles, Boston Red Sox, Chicago White Sox, St. Louis Cardinals, or Philadelphia Phillies were placed into the group of persons whose team had won a recent championship ($n = 388$). Fans ($n = 267$) selecting any other team as a favorite were placed into the other group (i.e., team had not won a recent championship). An ANOVA was used to compare the levels of team identification (SSIS scores) for persons in the two groups. This analysis failed to reveal a statistically significant difference [$F(1, 653) = 0.58, p > .40$] in identification between persons whose team had won a recent championship ($M = 35.78$; $SD = 13.92$) and those who team had not ($M = 36.62$; $SD = 13.35$). Additionally, an ANOVA was used to examine desperation index scores by recent team championship group. This analysis did reveal a significant relationship, $F(1, 653) = 6.70, p < .01$, as participants with a favorite team who had not won a recent championship reported higher desperation index scores ($M =$

77.35; *SD* = 32.48) than those whose favorite team had won a recent championship (M = 70.99; *SD* = 29.81). Because of this significant difference, recent team championship was used as a variable in the regression analyses described below.

Pearson correlations were used to examine the relationship between age, team identification, and desperation index scores. These correlations appear in Table 2. Because participant age was significantly correlated with scores on the desperation index, age was included as a predictor variable in the regression analyses below.

Table 2. Simple Correlations among the Variables

	1	2	3
Age (1)	--		
Identification (SSIS) (2)	0.06	--	
Desperation Index (3)	.09*	.71**	--

Note: * $p < .05$; ** $p < .01$.

The data were analyzed through a standard regression in which age, gender, recent team championship, and team identification served as the four predictor variables and scores on the desperation index were employed as the dependent variable (see Table 3). The combined effect of the four predictor variables on desperation index scores was significant, $F(4, 650) = 174.85$, $p < .0001$. With respect to independent contributions to desperation index scores, gender ($t = -3.48$, $p < .001$), recent team championship ($t = 2.52$, $p < .02$), and team identification ($t = 24.13$, $p < .0001$) accounted for a significant proportion of the unique variance. Specifically, higher desperation index scores were reported by males, persons with high levels of team identification, and persons whose favorite team had not won a recent World Series Championship. Age did not account for a significant proportion of the unique variance in desperation index scores, ($t = 0.85$, $p > .35$).

Table 3. Regression Equation with Age, Gender, Recent Championship, and Team Identification as Predictors of Desperation Index

Predictor variable	*B*	*SE B*	*Beta*	*t*	sig.
Age	0.198	0.232	0.024	0.85	0.394
Gender	-6.148	1.766	-0.099	-3.48	0.001
Recent Championship	4.369	1.736	0.069	2.52	0.012
Team Identification	1.542	0.064	0.68	24.13	0.001
Overall R	0.72				
Overall R^2	0.518				
Adjusted R^2	0.515				
Overall F (4, 650)	174.85*				

Note: * = $p < .0001$.

Discussion

Previous research had found that sport fans report a willingness to consider engaging in a variety of extreme behaviors if doing so will enhance their favorite team's chances of success. For instance, fans have reported engaging in a number of superstitious behaviors (Wann et al., 2009), have considered acts of cheating to assist their team (Wann, Hunter, et al., 2001), and have considered injuring a rival coach or player to increase their team's chances (Wann, Peterson, et al., 1999). Further, this literature reveals that these tendencies are most pronounced among fans with a high level of identification with the team, that is, those with a strong psychological connection to the team. In the current investigation, we expanded on this research by investigating the extent to which fans would consider engaging in acts of desperation, if doing so would guarantee a championship for their team. In particular, we examined the impact of two variables: level of team identification and whether or not the fan's favorite team had recently won a championship.

With respect to frequency data, inspection of the responses to the desperation items revealed that many of the participants were willing to consider the behaviors or believed they would be willing to engage in the behaviors for an extended period of time. For instance, at least half of the sample reported they would be willing to give up all drinks except water, give up sweets, go without shaving and sex, and attend church daily for at least a month if doing so would result in their favorite Major League Baseball team winning a World Series. Similarly, over 40% were willing to consider getting a permanent team-oriented tattoo, donating an organ, and donating a paycheck to assist the team. However, consistent with previous research (Wann, Haynes, McLean, & Pullen, 2003; Wann, Hunter, et al., 2001; Wann, Peterson, et al., 1999), fewer numbers of persons were willing to consider the more extreme behaviors. For instance, 50 percent of the participants were not willing to avoid all physical contact with others for any length of time while 64 percent were not willing to have their entire body shaved. Similarly, only 10% reported any level of willingness to consider having a finger cut off to guarantee their team a World Series Championship.

One subject variable of interest was the participant's level of team identification. Our prediction that identification would be a significant predictor of willingness to consider the acts of desperation was confirmed. For persons with a high level of team identification, the role of team follower is a central component of their overall social identity (Wann, Royalty, & Roberts, 2000). Consequently, the team's performances take on increased importance and, as a result, fans often attempt to impact the outcome of the game in order to give their team a competitive advantage. These attempts include superstitious actions (Wann et al., 2009) and instrumentally aggressive behaviors (Wann, Carlson, & Schrader, 1999), and highly identified fans do feel they can influence a competition (Wann, Dolan, McGeorge, & Allison, 1994). Humans have a strong desire to control their environments (Burger & Cooper, 1979; White, 1959) and the aforementioned fan behaviors reflect a desire to gain a sense of control in a situation where little exists. That is, although highly identified fans place a great deal of importance on the successful performance of their chosen team, in reality there is little they can do to bring about that performance. Therefore, they attempt a variety of actions, often in vain, to exercise control over the environment and assist their team.

A second variable of interest concerned a team's recent championship, or lack thereof. We hypothesized that fans would be more likely to express a willingness to consider the acts of desperation if their team had failed to win a championship in recent history (operationalized as the previous 15 seasons). The regression analyses revealed a pattern of effects confirming our expectations. Such a finding is consistent with work on the scarcity effect indicating that rare (scarce) events and objects are often viewed as more valuable and important (Lynn, 1992; Wann et al., 2004). Future researchers may want to add the "time since last championship" variable to previous investigations of fan actions, such as those targeting fan superstitions and cheating. Given the data reported above, one could predict that fans supporting teams without a recent championship may be particularly likely to engage in superstitious behaviors and illegal/unethical actions in order to assist their team. Similarly, this variable could be added to the research on anonymous fan aggression. Researchers have studied a number of variables that impact a fan's willingness to consider anonymous acts of spectator aggression including team identification (Wann et al., 2003), hostile and instrumental motives (Wann et al., 2003; Wann, Peterson, et al., 1999), and game outcome (Wann et al., 2005). However, researchers have yet to examine the impact of recent team championships. Given the current investigation, one would predict that fans (particularly those with high levels of identification) would be more likely to consider anonymous acts of instrumental aggression if their team had failed to win a recent championship.

An additional significant finding involved the relationship between gender and endorsement of the acts of desperation as males reported greater interest in the acts than females. Although unexpected, this finding is perhaps not that surprising given its consistency with previous, and perhaps related, research. For example, males have been found to be more impulsive than females (Thorell & Rydell, 2008) and men tend to score higher in sensation seeking than women (Kalichman & Rompa, 1995). These results likely explain, at least in part, the higher scores among males in the current sample. That is, given that men are, in general, more impulsive and tend to seek sensation (e.g., novel and exciting experiences), it seems logical to expect them to be more likely to endorse the acts of desperation targeted here.

In conclusion, it is important to note that we examined reports of consideration of the various acts of desperation, not actual behavior (e.g., no one in the current investigation actually performed the behaviors in question). Although an individual may report that he or she would engage in a specific act, this does not insure that the person would (or has) in fact done so. Thus, one may be tempted to question the validity of the results presented here. Although it is highly unlikely that there would be an exact correspondence between willingness to consider an act and the actual performance of the act, researchers have justified the use of methodologies such as this that utilize estimates of behavior (Russell & Baenninger, 1996). For example, investigators have found strong relationship between self-reported criminal activities and official police records (Elliott & Ageton, 1980). Further, given that fewer persons were willing to consider the more extreme acts of desperation (e.g., cutting off a finger), it is clear that the participants were carefully considering each action rather than simply reporting that they would be willing to do anything and everything. Thus, it is likely that the data described above are valid. Further, the current investigation was limited to only one sport, Major League Baseball. Further researchers should attempt to replicate our findings with other sports (e.g., football, basketball) at other levels of competition (e.g., Olympic, collegiate) to extend the generalizability of the data reported here.

References

Burger, J. M. & Cooper, H. M. (1979). The desirability of control. *Motivation and Emotion, 3,* 381-393.

Clopton, A. W. (2008). College sports on campus: Uncovering the link between fan identification and sense of community. *International Journal of Sport Management, 9,* 343-362.

Crawford, G. (2004). *Consuming sport: Fans, sport, and culture*. Routledge: London.

Dietz-Uhler, B., & Lanter, J. R. (2008). The consequences of sports fan identification. In L. W. Hugenberg, P. M. Haridakis, & A. C. Earnheardt (Eds.), *Sports mania: Essays on fandom and the media in the 21st century* (pp. 103-113). Jefferson, NC: McFarland.

Elliott, D. S., & Ageton, S. S. (1980). Reconciling race and class differences in self-reported and official estimates of delinquency. *American Sociological Review, 45*, 95-110.

Fisher, R. J., & Wakefield, K. (1998). Factors leading to group identification: A field study of winners and losers. *Psychology & Marketing, 15,* 23-40.

Giulianotti, R., Bonney, N., & Hepworth, M. (Eds.) (1994). *Football, violence, and social identity*. Routledge: London.

James, J. D. & Ross, S. D. (2004). Comparing sport consumer motivations across multiple sports. *Sport Marketing Quarterly, 13,* 17-25.

Kalichman, S., & Rompa, D. (1995). Sexual sensation seeking and sexual compulsivityscales: Reliability, validity, and predicting HIV risk behavior. *Journal of Personality Assessment, 65*, 586–601.

Lynn, M. (1992). Scarcity's enhancement of desirability: The role of naïve economics. *Basic and Applied Social Psychology, 13,* 67-78.

Russell, G. W. (2008). *Aggression in the sports world: A social psychological perspective.* New York: Oxford.

Russell, G. W., & Baenninger, R. (1996). Murder most foul: Predictors of an affirmative response to an outrageous question. *Aggressive Behavior, 22*, 175-181.

Thorell, L. B., & Rydell, A.-M. (2008). Behaviour problems and social competence deficits associated with symptoms of attention-deficit/hyperactivity disorder: Effects of age and gender. *Child: Care, Health & Development, 34*, 584-595.

Wann, D. L. (2006). The causes and consequences of sport team identification. In A. A. Raney & J. Bryant (Eds.,) *Handbook of sports and media* (pp. 331-352). Mahwah, NJ: Erlbaum.

Wann, D. L., Bayens, C., & Driver, A. K. (2004). Likelihood of attending a sporting event as a function of ticket scarcity and team identification. *Sport Marketing Quarterly, 13*, 209-215.

Wann, D. L., & Branscombe, N. R. (1993). Sports fans: Measuring degree of identification with the team. *International Journal of Sport Psychology, 24*, 1-17.

Wann, D. L., Carlson, J. D., & Schrader, M. P. (1999). The impact of team identification on the hostile and instrumental verbal aggression of sport spectators. *Journal of Social Behavior and Personality, 14,* 279-286.

Wann, D. L., Culver, Z., Akanda, R., Daglar, M., De Divitiis, C., & Smith, A. (2005). The effects of team identification and game outcome on willingness to consider anonymous acts of hostile aggression. *Journal of Sport Behavior, 28,* 282-294.

Wann, D. L., Dolan, T. J., McGeorge, K. K., & Allison, J. A. (1994). Relationships between spectator identification and spectators' perceptions of influence, spectators' emotions, and competition outcome. *Journal of Sport and Exercise Psychology, 16,* 347-364.

Wann, D. L., Grieve, F. G., End, C., Zapalac, R. K., Lanter, J. R., & Pease, D. G. (2009, September). Examining the superstitious behaviors of sport fans: Types of superstitions, perceptions of impact, and relationship with team identification. In F. G. Grieve (Chair) *Research involving sport fans: Identification and cognition.* Symposium paper presented at the meeting of the Association for Applied Sport Psychology, Salt Lake City.

Wann, D. L., Grieve, F. G., Zapalac, R. K., & Pease, D. G. (2008). Motivational profiles of sport fans of different sports. *Sports Marketing Quarterly, 17,* 6-19.

Wann, D. L., Haynes, G., McLean, B., & Pullen, P. (2003). Sport team identification and willingness to consider anonymous acts of hostile aggression. *Aggressive Behavior, 29,* 406-413.

Wann, D. L., Hunter, J. L., Ryan, J. A., & Wright, L. A. (2001). The relationship between team identification and willingness of sport fans to illegally assist their team. *Social Behavior and Personality: An International Journal, 29,* 531-536.

Wann, D. L., Melnick, M. J., Russell, G. W., & Pease, D. G. (2001). *Sport fans: The psychology and social impact of spectators.* New York: Routledge Press.

Wann, D. L., Peterson, R. R., Cothran, C., & Dykes, M. (1999). Sport fan aggression and anonymity: The importance of team identification. *Social Behavior and Personality: An International Journal, 27,* 597-602.

Wann, D. L., Royalty, J., & Roberts, A. (2000). The self-presentation of sport fans: Investigating the importance of team identification and self-esteem. *Journal of Sport Behavior, 23,* 198-206.

White, R. W. (1959). Motivation reconsidered: The concept of competence. *Psychological Review, 66,* 297-333.

Williams, K. B., Radefeld, P. S., Binning, J. F., & Sudak, J. R. (1993). When job candidates are "hard" versus "easy-to-get": Effects of candidate availability on employee decisions. *Journal of Applied Social Psychology, 23,* 169-198.

Williamson, D. P., Zhang, J. J., Pease, D. G., & Gaa, J. P. (2003). Dimensions of spectator identification associated with women's professional basketball game attendance. *International Journal of Sport Management, 4,* 59-91.

In: Encyclopedia of Sports and Athletics
Editors: Jack L. Murray and Emily O. Watson

ISBN: 978-1-61209-959-0

Chapter XXV

Spectators' Involvement in Sports and Suicidal Behaviour: Review of Current Evidence*

Karl Andriessen and Karolina Krysinska
Suicide Prevention Program, Flemish Mental Health Centres,
Martelaarslaan, Gent, Belgium

Introduction

Engagement in physical activity and sports, either actively as an athlete or in a passive way as a spectator is of great importance in many people's lives across countries and throughout history (e.g., Weber, 1971). Many studies have dealt with the outcomes of active engagement in sports and there has also been research on the impact of sport events on spectators, i.e. individuals who witness a sports event in person or via the media (Wann, Melnick, Russel et al., 2001). Attending sports events or watching them on television can impact individual functioning on many levels, including interpersonal behaviour (e.g., violence) and physical and mental health. Sports-related violence usually refers to aggression and riots by sports fans, and includes soccer hooliganism (Wann, Melnick, Russel et al., 2001), but watching sports events might also increase the risk of domestic violence against women by legitimizing and reinforcing violent behaviour (White, Katz, & Scarborough, 1992). Some major sports events, such as international championships and Olympic Games have been found to change patterns of mortality from coronary heart disease and stroke (Witte, Bots, Hoes et al., 2000) and to have an impact on the number of presentations to Accident and Emergency Departments (e.g., Jorm, Thackway, Churches et al., 2003; Moody, Hendry and Muscatello, 2007). However, this relationship cannot be generalised to all sports events and all groups of spectators (O'Donnell, 2003; Toubiana, Hanslik, & Letrilliart, 2001).

In regards to mental health and wellbeing, watching games might increase a sense of belonging, allow for release of tension, induce positive mood (Pringle, 2004) and reduce the

* Based on Andriessen & Krysinska (2009).

number of psychiatric presentations (Masterton & Mander, 1990). However, the defeat of the favoured team may lead to high psychological distress, in some cases reaching clinically significant levels similar to the impact of traumatic events, such as physical threats and natural disasters (Banyard & Shevlin, 2001). Being involved in sports as a spectator might also have an impact on suicidal behaviour, either increasing the risk or being a protective factor, and this chapter reviews the existing evidence regarding this relationship.

A systematic review of the literature published in English in peer-reviewed journals on the impact of sport events on suicidal behaviour (Andriessen & Krysinska, 2009) identified nine studies published between 1986 and 2009 on the relationship between sports events and suicidal behaviour. Three of these studies focused on completed suicide as the outcome (Curtis, Loy, & Karnilowicz, 1986; Trovato, 1998; Joiner, Hollar, & Van Orden, 2006), four studies on suicide and homicide (Fernquist, 2000, 2001, 2002; Lester, 1988), and two on suicide attempts (Masterton & Strachan, 1987; Steels, 1994). The sports studied were American football (Super Bowl), baseball, soccer, hockey, and basketball. The sport events identified in the studies, included single matches or games: Super Bowl (Curtis, Loy, & Kanilowicz, 1986; Joiner, Hollar, & Van Orden, 2006; Lester, 1988), last game of the baseball World Series (Curtis, Loy, & Kanilowicz, 1986; Lester, 1988), hockey "Miracle on Ice" at the Winter Olympics in Lake Placid, New York (Joiner, Hollar, & Van Orden, 2006), soccer Cup Final (Steels, 1994); and tournaments: soccer World Cup (Masterton & Strachan, 1987), and ice hockey Stanley Cup playoffs in Canada (Trovato, 1998). Two studies on the impact of other sports-related major events on suicide, such as geographical relocation of teams (Fernquist, 2001) and strikes of professional teams (Fernquist, 2002) were also included in the review. Details of the studies and the results are presented in Table 1.

In summary, the current evidence, based on data on national or local suicide rates, shows that sport events can have an impact on suicide mortality and morbidity. This relationship seems to be mediated by age, gender, marital status and alcohol consumption, as well as the process and outcome of the game, such as victory versus defeat of the favoured team. The following paragraphs present the possible explanations regarding the relationship between sports spectatorship and fatal and non-fatal suicidal behaviour.

Possible Links between Sports Spectatorship and Suicidal Behaviour

Social Rituals, Integration and Anomie

Durkheim's theories of suicide, rituals, ceremonies and religion (Durkheim, 1897; 1912/1965) suggest certain links between sports events and suicidal behaviour (Birrell, 1981; Fernquist, 2000; 2001; 2002; Pope, 2008). Fernquist (2001) applied the notion of anomie associated with sudden changes in social environment to the sport-suicide relationship in the context of the geographical relocation of professional sports teams, and suggested that such a change can lead to anomie and heightened risk of suicide among fans deeply identified with the team who are bereaved by the relocation and no longer can support their team in their area. His analysis of suicide rates in geographical areas affected by such moves supported this hypothesis.

Table 1. Sports events and fatal and non-fatal suicidal behavior

Study	Country	Sport event	Time range	Background theory	Type of study	Outcome focus	Results
Curtis, Loy & Karnilowicz (1986)	US	Super Bowl Sunday (football) and last game of World Series (baseball)	1972-1978	Theory of social integration (Durkheim, 1897) and theory of religion and ceremonies (Durkheim, 1912/1965)	Quasi-experimental comparison of observed versus expected suicide frequencies around sports events	Suicide	No significant decrease in suicide
Lester (1988)	US	Super Bowl Sunday (football) and last game of World Series (baseball)	1972-1984	Not specified	Comparison of observed versus expected suicide frequencies around sports events	Suicide (and homicide)	No significant decrease in suicide (and homicide)
Masterton & Strachan (1987)	Scotland (UK)	World Cup Soccer	1974, 1978, 1982, 1986	Not specified	Comparison of number of hospital admissions for deliberate self-harm before, during and after sport events and during control years	Non-fatal suicidal behavior	Significant reduction in deliberate self-harm hospital admissions
Steels (1994)	England (UK)	Soccer Cup Final	1991, 1992	Sudden disappointment, otherwise not specified	Comparison of number of hospital admissions for deliberate self-harm before, during and after sport events	Non-fatal suicidal behavior	Significant increase in deliberate self-harm hospital admissions after team defeat in 1991 and a non-significant increase after a less important team defeat in 1992
Trovato (1998)	Canada (Quebec)	Hockey Stanley Cup	1951-1992	Theory of social integration (Durkheim, 1897) and routine activities theory (Cohen & Felson, 1979)	Time trends analysis and comparison of incidence of suicide before and after a playoff game	Suicide	No significant impact of sport events on overall suicide rates and mixed findings regarding incidence of suicide in different age, gender and marital status groups during the sport event

Table 1 (Continued)

Fernquist (2000)	US (30 metropolitan areas)	Baseball, basketball, football, and hockey	1971-1990	Broken promise effect (Gabennesch, 1988), anomie (Durkheim, 1897), and theory of religion and ceremonies (Durkheim, 1912/1965)	Comparison of suicide and homicide rates when sports teams reach playoffs and win championship	Suicide (and homicide)	Significant inverse relation between championship status and suicide rates, and inverse relation between suicide (and homicide) rates and playoff status
Fernquist (2001)	US (3 areas)	Baseball, and football	1957, 1995-1996 and 1997-1998	Broken promise effect (Gabennesch, 1988) and anomie (Durkheim, 1897)	Comparison of suicide and homicide rates before, during, and after geographical relocation of sports teams	Suicide (and homicide)	A significant impact of geographical relocation of teams on suicide rates (no impact on homicide rates)
Fernquist (2002)	US	Baseball and hockey	1993-1996	Broken promise effect (Gabennesch, 1988) and theory of religion and ceremonies (Durkheim, 1912/1965)	Comparison of suicide and homicide rates before, during and after strikes of professional sports teams	Suicide (and homicide)	No significant impact of professional teams strikes on suicide rates (and significant impact on homicide rates)
Joiner, Hollar & Van Orden (2006)	US	College football (Study 1), Olympic hockey "Miracle on ice" (22 February 1980; Study 2) and Super Bowl Sunday (football; Study 3)	1990-2000 (Study 1), 1972-1989 (Study 2) and 1984-1994 (Study 3)	Interpersonal-psychological theory of suicide (Joiner, 2005)	Comparison of ranking of county college teams and county suicide rates (Study 1), comparison of number of suicides on 22 February 1980 and any other February 22 between 1972 and1989 (Study 2) and comparison of number of suicides on Super Bowl Sundays and other Sundays (Study 3)	Suicide	Significant correlation between college team ranking and county suicide rates (Study 1), significantly reduction in suicide on 22 February 1980 (Study 2), and significant reduction in suicide on Super Bowl Sundays (Study 3)

In regards to social rituals and ceremonies, there is empirical evidence showing that presidential elections, national holidays, and religious holidays are linked to lower suicide and overall mortality rates (i.e., a "death dip") and lower rates of attempted suicide (e.g., Bergen & Hawton, 2007; Boor, 1981; Jessen, Jensen, Arensman, et al., 1999; Masterton & Platt, 1989; Phillips & Feldman, 1973). However; the studies presented in Table 1 yielded mixed results regarding the occurrence of death dips around sportive occasions understood as social ceremonies; for example, Curtis et al. (1986) and Lester (1988) did not find significant drops in suicide numbers on sport-related occasions, albeit in the former study the death dip was observed around national holidays (July 4th and Thanksgiving Day). The absence of a death dip around sport events, in contrast to national holidays could be explained in several ways. Sport event may have smaller integrative effects, either in the intensity of social integration or in its scope (i.e., the actual numbers of people who participate in the event) than do national holidays, and thus have less impact on suicide (Curtis, Loy, & Karnilowicz, 1986). This could be related to the fact that public holidays involve people in a more direct and physical manner, including parties and gift giving, while involvement in sports events has a more vicarious character, mostly through the mass media (particularly television). Public holidays involve face-to-face interpersonal interaction usually concentrated on one particular day, while sports spectatorship is more impersonal - focusing on the game - and its impact may be smaller if it involves a series of games spread across time. In addition, public holidays are observed by practically everyone, while sports events usually engage only certain groups (such as young males) and thus have an impact on suicide only in certain subpopulations. Although the aggregated data that Curtis et al. (1986) used in their study did not allow testing this hypothesis, the results of Trovato's (1998) analysis seem to support this assumption.

Routine Activities Theory

According to the routine activities theory, people who share similar social backgrounds tend to share interests and lifestyles, and therefore are prone to participate together in social activities (Cohen & Felson, 1979; Trovato, 1998). Spending time with friends and significant others watching sports events on television might discourage or impede people considering suicide and taking action, while being in the proximity of others increases the chances of being found and rescued if a suicide attempt has taken place. Consequently, early defeat of the team and "an earlier than usual disbandment of the socially integrative context" (Trovato, 1998; p. 119) might lead to increased suicidality. Results of Trovato's (1998) study supported this hypothesis: early elimination of the local hockey team from the Stanley Cup was associated with increased suicide rates among young single males.

The Broken Promise Effect

According to the original formulation of the broken promise effect, "an event which generally induces positive anticipation may itself cause the suicidal individual's outlook to worsen by virtue of the unfavorable contrast between raised expectancy and stubborn reality. (….) A dysphoric mood is the result of the negative discrepancy between how one feels and how one expects (hopes) to feel" (Gabennesch, 1988; p. 138). In relation to sports events, failures of teams, particularly if repeated and in relation to important outcomes (e.g., not winning a championship versus not making the playoffs), might constitute a "broken promise" leading to dysphoric and suicidal moods in individuals deeply identifying with the teams (Fernquist, 2000). An analysis of suicide (and homicide) rates after strikes in sports (Fernquist, 2002) and geographical relocation of professional teams (Fernquist, 2001) showed a more complex picture of the broken promise effect in sports. Apparently, the source of the disappointment should be taken into consideration. If external, such as cancellation of the game related to a strike, it might result in negative emotions, including anger, being turned outwards and leading to externalized aggression (i.e., homicide) instead of suicide. In contrast, loss of the team due to its geographical relocation, might lead to feelings of loss and grief in faithful fans, and thus be seen as a "broken promise" and increase suicidality.

The Interpersonal-Psychological Theory of Suicide

The interpersonal-psychological theory of serious suicidal behaviour (Joiner, 2005) identifies the need to belong as one of the core human needs, and its fulfilment or frustration can have serious impact on risk of suicide of an individual. If met, it can be a very powerful protective factor; however, its frustration caused by lack of meaningful social relationships, social isolation or a lack of connectedness, might increase the risk of suicide. Being a sports fan creates camaraderie, a sense of belongingness and being cared for and can result in sports-related "pulling together" which might protect against suicide. Sports events increase social contact by bringing people together and, especially under condition of success of the favoured team, increase positive interpersonal interactions, including positive face-to-face social contact. All this may lower the individual risk of suicide and decrease suicide rates on local and national levels (Joiner, 2005). Results of Joiner et al.'s (2006) studies summarized in Table 1 support this theory.

Other Possible Links

Other explanations regarding potential drops in suicide around sport events have been proposed, but they have not been empirically tested: reduced incidence of media-related imitative ("copycat") suicides, sports gambling, decreased levels of family contact and increased sense of patriotism (Curtis, Loy, & Karnilowicz, 1986; Masterton & Strachan, 1987).

It has been established that media reports of suicide cases are linked to "copycat" suicides (Westerlund, Scaller, & Schmidtke, 2009), and it has been hypothesised (Curtis, Loy, & Karnilowicz; 1986) that major sport events shift the media focus to sport outcomes and related news instead of reporting negative events, such as suicides, and thus lead to the decreased incidence in "copycat" suicides. On the other hand, losing at gambling on sports could be a risk factor for suicide, but it is not certain whether this could cause a measurable and significant effect (Curtis, Loy, & Karnilowicz; 1986).

Also, watching sports events can provide distraction from personal problems and decrease the levels of negative interpersonal interactions, for example, in couples living together, thus preventing conflicts leading to suicidal ideation and behaviour. According to

Masterton and Strachan (1987), the media have suggested that the decreased level of interpersonal contact in couples and disruption of family life might increase the risk of suicide among female partners of sport fans (so called "football widows"), but the results of their study did not support this suggestion. In addition, referring to the soccer "tartan army", Masterton and Stachan (1987) suggested that the climate of "patriotism as during war" (p. 368) could have a preventive effect against suicide. However, this suggestion necessitates some caution as recent literature on the effect of war on suicide rates presents a mixed picture and specifically in Scotland the suicide rate of young males increased dramatically during the 2nd World War (Henderson, Stark, Humphry et al., 2006).

Sport Spectatorship and Suicide Prevention

Encouragement of active engagement in sports is a component of some suicide prevention programs for adolescents and young adults (e.g., Tester, Watkins, & Rouse, 1999), prisoners (e.g., Cooper & Berwick, 2001) and Australian Indigenous communities with a high risk of suicide (Cunningham & Beneforti, 2005). Interest in sports as a spectator can also become a vehicle for mental health promotion and suicide prevention programs. One of such programs is a "It's a Goal!", a community-based project in the UK run in collaboration between local health authorities and the soccer team Macclesfield Town (Pringle & Sayers, 2004). This program aims to help men to address issues related to self-esteem, depression and inclusion through group interventions and using football as a metaphor. The program's initial evaluation shows that "the power of football as a both motive and method for engaging this group [i.e., young males] is evident even in these early stages of the project, and it may well be that the experience at Macclesfield Town can be developed not only by other football clubs but also by other sports such as rugby and cricket where young men make up a large proportion of the attendance" (Pringle & Sayers, 2004; p. 238).

Similar initiatives have been developed in other counties. In Scotland, the National Strategy and Action Plan to Prevent Suicide (Scottish Government, 2002) issued a special suicide prevention postcard. The front side of the card shows a discarded football shirt with the slogan "There is no substitute for life"; while its back contains information on suicide warning signs, helpline telephone numbers and basic advice on how to help a person in a crisis. In Belgium, the Flemish Working Group on Suicide Survivors (De fauw & Andriessen, 2003) established the Sports Division which supports an indoor soccer team and participates in sports events aiming to increase public awareness of suicide prevention and support for people bereaved by suicide.

Conclusions and Suggested Areas for Future Research

On the basis of the review it can be concluded that although some studies did not detect a change in incidence of suicide in relation to major sport events, other research indicated that sport events can have an impact on non-fatal and fatal suicidal behaviour acting either as a protective or a risk factor. Such impact seems to depend on mediating variables such as characteristics of the spectator, including gender, age, and marital status, and characteristics of the sport event, such as an outcome (victory versus defeat) and importance of the game (playoff versus championship). Also, excessive use of alcohol during or after the game may be a triggering factor for auto-aggressive behaviours (Steels, 1994; Trovato, 1998).

The reviewed studies have provided a valuable insight into the impact of sport spectatorship on suicide behaviour and its prevention. Still, there are significant gaps in our knowledge and future studies may further clarify this relationship and help to translate research findings into suicide prevention practice. Table 2 presents research trends identified in studies conducted to-date and a number of suggestions for future research.

Table 2. Summary of current research trends and suggested future research areas

Current Research	Suggested Research Areas
• Studies conducted in English-speaking countries (UK and USA) and one study (Trovato, 1998) in predominantly French-speaking province Quebec, Canada. • Studies conducted on a limited range of sports, predominantly soccer, American football, hockey, baseball and basketball. • Studies based on diverse methodologies and theoretical frameworks which might account for inconsistent research findings and difficulties in comparing the results. • Studies based on aggregated data on national or local suicide rates focused predominantly on the impact of sports event on the societal level. • Lack of studies using individual, case-based data regarding the relationship between sport spectatorship and suicide risk on individual level.	• Studies on the impact of a wide range of sports events on suicidal behaviour in a variety of countries and cultures. • Studies on mediating variables which may have a significant effect on suicide risk or its prevention, including characteristics of sport spectators and sport events. • Integration of ecological studies, individual case studies, psychological studies on fanship and psychological autopsies. • Multi-centre studies on epidemiology of attempted suicide and psychological studies of individuals who engage in non-fatal suicidal behaviour. • Studies on the effectiveness of suicide prevention and mental health promotion programs based on spectator engagement in sports.

One of the biggest gaps (as well as challenges for the future) is the lack of research on how sport spectatorship might influence levels of suicide risk on *the individual level* and how mediating variables might operate on that level. Studies in sport psychology show that sport spectators are a heterogeneous group and differ in regards to the levels of sport involvement (Shank & Beasley, 1998), types of motivation in attendance of sport events (Bernthal & Graham, 2003), identification with the sport team (Wann, 2006a; 2006b) and other factors. It is possible that even die-hard fans suffering from depression and in suicidal crisis lose their interest in sports as much as in other aspects of their lives (Shneidman, 1993) and are not affected by successes and failures of "their teams". These mechanisms could account for the protective or negative impact (or lack of any impact) of sports engagement on suicide risk in a particular person.

Many of the theories applied to the relationship between sports and suicide are related to social integration, social ceremonies and activities, as well as interpersonal "pulling together".

According to Shneidman (2001) and Joiner (2005), the frustration of vital psychological needs, such as the need for affiliation or belonging, is the common stressor in suicide. The song "You'll never walk alone", originally from the musical "Carousel" by Richard Rodgers and Oscar Hammerstein, is a popular sports hymn[1]. Since it was adopted in the 1960s by fans of the Liverpool FC, it has become a popular soccer anthem across the world. The song lyrics aim to comfort a person recently bereaved by suicide of a spouse, and encourage her not to give up, continue with life and maintain hope (De fauw & Andriessen, 2008). Could the phrase "you'll never walk alone", so popular among the sport fans be an expression of social integration and affiliation?

References

Andriessen, K. & Krysinska, K. (2009). Can sport events affect suicidal behaviour? A review of the literature and implications for prevention. *Crisis, 30*, 144-152.

Banyard, P. & Shevlin, M. (2001). Responses of football fans to relegation of their team from the English Premier League: PTS? *Irish Journal of Psychological Medicine, 18*, 66-67.

Bergen, H. & Hawton, K. (2007). Variation in deliberate self-harm around Christmas and New Year. *Social Science and Medicine, 65*, 855-867.

Bernthal, M.J., & Graham, P.J. (2003). The effect of sport setting on fan attendance motivation: The case of minor league vs. collegiate baseball. *Journal of Sport Behavior, 26*, 223-239.

Birrell, S. (1981). Sport as ritual: Interpretations from Durkheim to Goffman. *Social Forces, 60*, 354-376.

Boor, M. (1981). Effects of United States presidential elections on suicide and other causes of death. *American Sociological Review, 46*, 616-618.

Cohen, L.E. & Felson, M. (1979). Social change and crime rate trends: A routine activity approach. *American Sociological Review, 44*, 588-608.

Cooper, C. & Berwick, S. (2001). Factors affecting psychological well-being of three groups of suicide-prone prisoners. *Current Psychology, 20*, 169-182.

Cunningham, J. & Beneforti, M. (2005). Investigating indicators for measuring the health and social impact of sport and recreation programs in Australian Indigenous communities. *International Review for the Sociology of Sport, 40,* 89-98.

Curtis, J., Loy, J., & Karnilowicz, W. (1986). A comparison of suicide–dip effects of major sport events and civil holidays. *Sociology of Sport Journal, 3*, 1-14.

De fauw, N. & Andriessen, K. (2003). Networking to support suicide survivors. *Crisis, 24*, 29-31.

De fauw, N. & Andriessen, K. (2008). "You'll never walk alone": een hymne voor nabestaanden na zelfdoding [a hymn for the bereaved by suicide]. In R. Van Nuffel (Ed.), *Geestelijke gezondheid: Zorg voor velen, door velen [Mental health: care for many, by many]* (pp. 134). Gent: Vlaamse Vereniging voor Psychiatrie [Flemish Psychiatric Association].

Durkheim, É. (1897). *Le Suicide. Étude de sociologie*. Paris: Presses Universitaires de France.

[1] This information was obtained from http://en.wikipedia.org/wiki/You'll_Never_Walk_Alone_(song) accessed 15 February, 2010.

Durkheim, É. (1965). *The elementary forms of the religious life [Transl. by J.W. Swain. Orig.: Les formes élémentaires de la vie religieuse: Le système totémique en Australie. Paris, 1912]*. New York: Free Press.

Fernquist, R. M. (2000). An aggregate analysis of professional sports, suicide and homicide rates: 30 U.S. metropolitan areas. *Aggression and Violent Behavior*, *5*, 329-341.

Fernquist, R. M. (2001). Geographical relocation, suicide and homicide: An exploratory analysis of the geographic relocation of professional sports teams in three U.S. areas and the impact on suicide and homicide rates. *Sociology of Sport Online, 4*. Retrieved June 2, 2008 from http://physed.otago.ac.nz/sosol/v4i2/v4i2Fernquist.htm

Fernquist, R. M. (2002). The 1994-1995 baseball and hockey strikes and their impact on suicide and homicide rates in the United States. *Archives of Suicide Research*, *6*, 103-110.

Gabennesch, H. (1988). When promises fail: A theory of temporal fluctuations in suicide. *Social Forces*, *67*, 129-145.

Henderson, R., Stark, C., Humphry, R.W et al. (2006). Changes in Scottish suicide rates during the Second World War. *BMC Public Health, 6*, 167.

Jessen, G., Jensen, B.F., Arensman, E. et al. (1999). Attempted suicide and major public holidays in Europe: Findings from the WHO/ERO Multicentre Study on Parasuicide. *Acta Psychiatrica Scandinavica*, *99*, 412-418.

Joiner, T. (2005). *Why people die by suicide?* Cambridge: Harvard University Press.

Joiner, T.E., Hollar, D., & van Orden, K. (2006). On Buckeyes, Gators, Super Bowl Sunday, and the Miracle on Ice: "Pulling together" is associated with lower suicide rates. *Journal of Social and Clinical Psychology*, *25*, 179-195.

Jorm, L.R., Thackway, S.V., Churches, T.R. et al. (2003). Watching the games: Public health surveyance for the Sydney 2000 Olympic Games. *Journal of Epidemiology and Community Health, 57*, 102-108.

Lester, D. (1988). Suicide and homicide during major sports events 1972-1984: Comment on Curtis, Loy, and Karnilowicz. *Sociology of Sport Journal*, *5*, 285.

Masterton, G. & Mander, A.J. (1990). Psychiatric emergencies and the World Cup Finals. *British Journal of Psychiatry*, *156*, 475-478.

Masterton, G. & Platt, S. (1989). Parasuicide and general elections. *British Medical Journal, 298*, 803-804.

Masterton, G. & Strachan, J.A. (1987). Parasuicide, Scotland, and the World Cup. *British Medical Journal, 295*, 368.

Moody, W.E., Hendry, R.G., & Muscatello, D. (2007). Were attendances to accident and emergency departments in England and Australia influenced by the Rugby World Cup Final 2003? *European Journal of Emergency Medicine*, *14*, 68-71.

O'Donnell, J.J. (2003). The Football World Cup 2002: Analysis of related attendances to an Irish Emergency Department. *Irish Medical Journal*, *96*, 90-91.

Phillips, D.P. & Feldman, K.A. (1973). A dip in deaths before ceremonial occasions: Some new relationships between social integration and mortality. *American Sociological Review*, *38*, 678-696.

Pope, W. (2008). Emile Durkheim. In Stones, R. (Ed), *Key sociological thinkers* (pp. 76-89). New York: Palgrave Macmillan.

Pringle, A. (2004). Can watching football be a component of developing a state of mental health for men? *Journal of the Royal Society for the Promotion of Health*, *124*, 122-128.

Pringle, A. & Sayers, P. (2004). It's a Goal!: Basing a community psychiatric nursing service in a local football stadium. *Journal of the Royal Society for the Promotion of Health, 124*, 234-238.

Scottish Government (2002). *Choose Life: A National Strategy and Action Plan to Prevent Suicide in Scotland.* Retrieved February 10, 2010 from http://www.chooselife.net/web /FILES/Choose_Life.pdf

Shank, M.D., & Beasley, F.M. (1998). Fan or fanatic: Refining a measure of sports involvement. *Journal of Sport Behavior,* 21, 435-443.

Shneidman, E. (1993). *Suicide as psychache: A clinical approach to self-destructive behavior.* Northvale, NJ: Jason Aronson.

Shneidman, E. (2001). Epilogue: This I believe. In *Comprehending suicide: Landmarks in 20th century suicidology* (pp. 197-203). Washington: American Psychological Association.

Steels, M.D. (1994). Deliberate self-poisoning: Nottingham Forest Football Club and F.A. Cup defeat. *Irish Journal of Psychological Medicine, 11*, 76-78.

Tester, G.J., Watkins, G.G., & Rouse, I. (1999). The Sports Challenge International programme for identified "at risk" children and adolescents: A Singapore study. *Asia-Pacific Journal of Public Health, 11*, 34-38.

Toubiana, L., Hanslik, T., & Letrilliart, L. (2001). French cardiovascular mortality did not increase during 1996 European football championship. *British Medical Journal, 322*, 1306.

Trovato, F. (1998). The Stanley Cup of Hockey and suicide in Quebec, 1951-1992. *Social Forces, 77*, 105-127.

Wann, D.L. (2006a). Understanding the positive social psychological benefits of sport team identification: The team identification-social psychological health model. *Group Dynamics: Theory, Research, and Practice, 10,* 272-296.

Wann, D.L. (2006b). Examining the potential causal relationship between sport team identification and psychological well-being. *Journal of Sport Behavior, 29*, 79-95.

Wann, D.L., Melnick, M.J., Russell, G.W. et al. (2001). *Sport fans: The psychology and social impact of spectators.* New York: Routlegde.

Weber, E. (1971). Gymnastics and sports in *fin-de-siècle* France: Opium for the classes? *American Historical Review, 76*, 70-98.

Westerlund, M., Schaller, S., & Schmidtke, A. (2009). The role of mass media in suicide prevention. In D. Wasserman, & C. Wasserman (Eds.), *Oxford textbook of suicidology and suicide prevention. A global perspective* (pp. 515-523). Oxford: Oxford University Press.

White, G.F., Katz, J., & Scarborough, K.E. (1992). The impact of professional football games upon violent assaults on women. *Violence and Victims, 7*, 157-171.

Witte, D.R., Bots, M.L., Hoes, A.W. et al. (2000). Cardiovascular mortality in Dutch men during 1996 European football championship: Longitudinal population study. *British Medical Journal, 321*, 1552-1554.

In: Encyclopedia of Sports and Athletics
Editors: Jack L. Murray and Emily O. Watson
ISBN: 978-1-61209-959-0

Chapter XXVI

Predictors of Collective Efficacy in Elite Female Athletes: A Multilevel Analysis

Heidi Wilkinson, Richard B. Fletcher* and Mieke Sachsenweger
Massey University, Albany, US

Abstract

This study investigated predictors of collective efficacy in elite female athletes using Hierarchical Linear Modeling (HLM). HLM analyses both individual and team level effects simultaneously and addresses a perennial issues in collective efficacy research, namely the unit of analysis and the cross-level effects. The participants were 318 elite female netball players from 31 teams. Participants completed a questionnaire within 24 hours of the start of either of two national level competitions. The questionnaire included a demographic section and questions relating to team functioning as well as four measures (i.e., Perceptions of Success (POS) (Roberts & Balague, 1991), Sources of Sport Confidence (SSCQ) (Vealey, Hayashi, Garner-Holman, & Giacobbi, 1998), Group Environment Questionnaire (GEQ) (Carron, Widmeyer, & Brawley, 1985), and a Collective Efficacy measure developed for the present study). Using the procedure suggested by Bryk and Raudenbush (1992), the results suggest that the team level predictors accounted for approximately 73 % of the variance in collective efficacy at the team level. Overall, mastery orientations of the POS (at the player level), length of time spent in team meetings and team cohesion (Group Integration-Task subscale of the GEQ) (at the team level) were found to be significant predictors of collective efficacy. The results do not support those of Spink (1990a) who noted social aspects of team cohesion to be related to collective efficacy. Results concur with previous research by Paskevich, Brawley, Dorsch and Widmeyer (1999) who noted task related aspects of team cohesion to be related to collective efficacy.

* Correspondence concerning this article should be addressed to Richard Fletcher, School of Psychology, Massey University Albany, Private Bag 102 904, North Shore Mail Centre, Aotearoa, New Zealand.
e-mail: R.B.Fletcher@massey.ac.nz

Over the last decade, researchers have investigated a group phenomenon known as collective efficacy, which are the beliefs teams/groups have about their combined capabilities in coordinating and performing specific tasks or abilities. Researchers have found collective efficacy to be related to other variables, such as group performance (e.g. Feltz & Lirgg, 1998; Prussia & Kinicki, 1996). The relationship with group performance is of particular interest to psychologists in the sports domain. As many sports become professional, and athletes are paid for their ability to perform, high performance and factors that lead to increases in performance become particularly important to coaches, managers, and athletes. Poor performance of a team can result in financial loss to the many people involved within that team/organization, so it is very important for coaches and athletes to understand what factors can hinder or enhance team performance. Additionally, if teams with a high sense of collective efficacy perform better, then understanding what factors contribute to collective efficacy will have implications for development and training for all levels of team sports.

Bandura proposed the concept of collective efficacy as an extension of self-efficacy theory, which concerns peoples' beliefs about their capabilities to exercise control over events that affect their lives (Bandura, 1990). Collective efficacy is a group attribute and can be defined as "a group's shared belief in its conjoint capabilities to organize and execute the courses of action required to produce given levels of attainments" (Bandura, 1997, p. 477). Collective efficacy, as it suggests, requires a significant degree of interdependence among team members' judgments regarding certain tasks and abilities (Zaccaro, Blair, Peterson & Zazanis, 1995). Measurement of collective efficacy requires researchers to provide evidence that individual collective efficacy beliefs can be used as a proxy for the group level construct and thus the focus is on shared beliefs (Feltz & Lirgg, 1998, Moritz & Watson, 1998).

There are a few studies that have attempted to measure collective efficacy from a theoretical perspective (Kozub & McDonnell, 2000, Paskevich et al., 1999). The Paskevich et al. study is noteworthy in that it provided a well articulated approach to measuring collective efficacy based on Bandura's (1997) suggestions. Paskevich et al. provided preliminary psychometric data for a multidimensional scale of collective efficacy that assesses players' perceptions of their team's confidence in relation to offence, defense, motivation, obstacles in general practice and competition situations, and communication with teammates and coaches. The results showed the two task measures of the Group Environment Questionnaire (the Group Integration (GI-Task), and Individual Attractions to Group (ATG-Task) measures) had the greatest number of significant bivariate relationships with the various aspects of collective efficacy, thus providing support for the predictive validity of the collective efficacy measure.

The brief literature concerning collective efficacy in sport settings has identified several predictors related to collective efficacy. For example, collective efficacy has been shown to be related to prior group performance/performance outcome and vicarious experiences (i.e. observing others achieve success) (Hodges & Carron, 1992; Prussia & Kinicki, 1996), level of interdependence and quality of teamwork (Bandura, 1997), positive and negative team feedback (Prussia & Kinicki, 1996), goal setting (Spink, 1990a), leadership behaviours (Weldon & Weingart, 1993), goal commitment (Bandura, 1997), prior performance (Zaccaro et al., 1995) and team cohesion and performance (Kozub & McDonnell, 2000; Paskevich et al., 1999; Spink, 1990a, 1990b).

The interest in group related constructs, such as team cohesion (Widmeyer, Brawley, & Carron, 1985) and collective efficacy (Paskevich, et al., 1999), has raised questions regarding the most appropriate method for analyzing data that is hierarchically structured (Moritz &

Watson, 1998). As individuals are nested within groups and groups nested within organizations and so on, then the data are *multilevel* and therefore statistical analyses need to address this issue. Generally, however, research has not done this; many analyses either focus on individual-level variables or group-level variables (Moritz & Watson, 1998). There are difficulties with each of these narrow approaches. A focus on individual-level variables violates the assumption independence and fails to take into the group-level effects. Conversely, a focus on team-level variables ignores important variation between individuals and reasons for this variation. A focus on team-level variables may also result in an over-reliance on averages or trends which may result in exaggerating relationships that would not otherwise be apparent (de Leeuw, 1992). The important issue to note here is that both levels of the data need to be considered simultaneously.

In response to the aggregation problems, Kenny and LaVoie (1985) suggested a method to assess individual and team level effects by estimating correlations at the both levels and then testing these correlations for evidence of non-independence. If independence is observed, then group level effects are not observed. Thus, correlations should be computed and analysed at the individual level, and vice versa for situations where non-independence is indicated (Kenny & LaVoie, 1985). There are several limitations of this technique. One limitation is the assumption of random assignment to groups, and the ability to control other variables (Moritz & Watson, 1998). It is not always possible to randomly assign players to teams and thus this technique violates this assumption. Another limitation is that this approach does not deal with the cross-level effects by treating the levels as being mutually exclusive. In essence, the structure of the data are overridden as the cross level effects are ignored.

A more appropriate statistical method for analysing group data is multilevel modeling or Hierarchical Linear Modeling (HLM; Bryk & Raudenbush, 1992; Moritz & Watson, 1998). Multilevel models can distinguish between the individual and group levels of data, and account for the possibility of aggregation bias by analysing the two levels (individual and group) simultaneously (Novy & Francis, 1989). HLM is therefore suited to analyzing collective efficacy data, once the issue of within group agreement (homogeneity of responses) has been dealt with (Moritz & Watson, 1998). HLM analyses data by effectively performing regressions of regressions (Arnold, 1992). At the first level (Level 1), regression equations for each team predict player outcomes as a function of other player characteristics within each team, and the equations are called 'within-unit' models (Arnold, 1992). There is one such equation for each team. The intercepts and coefficients from these analyses are then used as the dependent variables in the second-level (Level 2) regression equations with teams as the unit of analysis. Team characteristics are the independent variables in the Level 2 equations, which are called 'between-unit' models. In HLM the variance around each parameter from Level 1 is also taken into account in the regression analyses at Level 2 (Arnold, 1992). In more simple terms, the relationships between outcome variables and explanatory variables are examined within the groups (Level 1), and then each groups' regression slopes become outcome variables modeled as a function of group explanatory variables (Level 2) (Zhu, 1997). The strength of this approach is that both levels of the analysis are computed simultaneously to account for both individual and group level effects.

Given the brief literature on collective efficacy and the methodological issues surrounding group measurement, especially in the sport related area, this study had two main aims. The first was to develop a theory-driven measure of collective efficacy that was specific to the current sample (elite netball players) based on the theoretical framework suggested by Paskevich et al. (1999). Few measures have been developed to investigate collective efficacy (Feltz & Chase, 1998), and thus more research is needed to validate this construct, including the development of more specific measures to enhance our understanding of this construct.

Table 1. Predictors of collective efficacy

1	Vicarious experiences	(e.g. Bandura, 1997; Hodges & Carron, 1992; Prussia & Kinicki, 1996)
2.	Leadership behaviours	(Weldon & Weingart, 1993)
3.	Prior performance (mastery experiences)	(e.g. Bandura, 1997; Zaccaro et al., 1995)
4.	Feedback	(e.g. Bandura, 1997; Greenlees et al., 1999; Prussia & Kinicki, 1996)
5.	Social influences	(Spink, 1990a)
6.	Focus of athletes (e.g. goal orientations)	(Spink, 1990a)
7.	Past history of the team (e.g. how long the team has been together)	(Spink, 1990a)
8.	Team cohesion	(e.g. Paskevich et al., 1999; Spink, 1990a)

The second aim of this study is to investigate potential predictors of collective efficacy using the HLM framework. Thus, we were interested in examining theoretically driven predictors of collective efficacy derived from the literature, as well as some exploratory variables (see Table 1). These included both individual level and team level variables derived from several existing measures. The Perceptions Of Success measure and its two subscales (Mastery and Competitive) were included as a representation of players' goal orientation, and focus of the athletes and player motivation, all of which are suggested to be linked to collective efficacy (e.g. Roberts, Treasure, & Balague, 1998; Spink 1990b). Roberts et al. state that there is considerable data to show that the goal orientations are relevant to individuals' achievement behaviour, and impact on the motivation process, therefore impacting the efficacy of the individual and team. The Sources of Sport Confidence Questionnaire was used at the individual level because the source of players' sport confidence seems to represent the individuals' self-efficacy in terms of affect, behaviour, and cognition (Vealey, 1986, 1988). However, only certain subscales were used in the analyses. The subscales were selected by sources of collective efficacy previously found in the literature (see Table 1). The subscales consequently included in the modeling were the Mastery, Vicarious Experiences, Coach's Leadership and Social Support subscales. The length of time spent in team meetings was included as a team level variable as it appeared to represent feedback from coaches and teammates, which has been found to be a source of collective efficacy in previous research (e.g. Bandura, 1997; Greenlees, Graydon, & Maynard,1999; Prussia & Kinicki, 1996). Team cohesion was included as a level two variable, through the use of the Group Environment Questionnaire subscales, due to previous research which suggests a close link with collective efficacy (e.g. Paskevich et al., 1999; Spink, 1990a. Also see Paskevich, Estabrooks, Brawley, & Carron, 2001 for a review of the cohesion performance relationship). It should be noted however, that prior team performance outcome was not included as a predictor in the present study. This was due to teams participating in this study being formed approximately two months before the competitions and most had not played any competitive games together prior to the competition.

Method

Participants

Data were collected on 318 elite female netball players aged 14-37 (mean = 20.34, SD = 4.29), in 31 teams (range = 9-12 players per team) at the two highest level national netball competitions in New Zealand (i.e., national under-21's (17 teams) and national senior level (14 teams)). The National New Zealand netball team are world ranked and the players at these competitions represent the very highest performing athletes in their respective groups. Approximately 50% of the teams competing in the two competitions agreed to participate in the study.

For accurate estimation of multilevel parameters it is preferable to have more level-2 observations (teams) with fewer level-1 observations (players), than to have fewer teams and more players per team (Hox & Maas, 2001). Consequently, to increase the power of the HLM analyses, both sets of data were combined to increase the level-2 units, thus enhancing generalisability of the results to elite level netball players.

Measures

Four measures were employed: Perceptions of Success Questionnaire (Roberts & Balague, 1991), Group Environment Questionnaire (Carron et al., 1985), Sources of Sport Confidence Questionnaire (Vealey et al.,1998), and a collective efficacy measure developed for this study. Demographic information was obtained on age, playing status, years spent playing netball, years at elite level. Other information was collected on the length of time a team had been together, practices (e.g. length of practices, focus on team or individual skills during practice), amount of time spent on team building and amount of time spent socialising with teammates.

Perceptions of Success Questionnaire (POS)

The POS is a sport-specific measure of task and ego goal motivations (Roberts & Balague, 1991). The measure consists of 12 items that represent two factors, namely task and ego orientations. The task or mastery subscale includes items such as “I work hard” and “I reach a goal”. The ego or competitiveness subscale includes items such as “I am the best” and “I outperform my opponents”. Participants respond to each item using a five point scale using the stem “When playing sport, I feel most successful when...”. Psychometric data on the POS support a two factor model as well as high test-retest reliability (Roberts, Treasure & Balague, 1998). Concurrent validity evidence was demonstrated by correlating POS with the Task and Ego Orientation in Sport Questionnaire (TEOSQ), where ego orientation on the POS correlated $r = 0.80$ and the task orientation correlated $r = 0.71$ to ego and task orientations of the TEOSQ respectively (Roberts et al., 1998). Roberts et al. (1998) reported that the use of the questionnaire so far has shown that it is a reliable and valid instrument to measure ego and task orientations in sport.

Group Environment Questionnaire (Geq)

The GEQ is a measure of team cohesion that assesses the task and social aspects of an individual's perceptions of their team as a whole, as well as the individual's attraction to the team that is related to the development and maintenance of team cohesion (Carron et al., 1985). The GEQ is an 18 item measure with four subscales: Individual Attractions to Group-Social (ATG-Social, 5 items); Individual Attractions to Group-Task (ATG-Task, 4 items); Group Integration-Task (GI-Task, 5 items); and Group Integration-Social (GI-Social, 4 items). Participants respond on a nine point Likert scale (strongly disagree to strongly agree). Psychometric evidence for the GEQ largely supports a four-factor structure (Carron et al., 1985; Li & Harmer, 1996; Widmeyer et al., 1985), however others have not supported this (Schutz, Eom, Smoll, & Smith, 1994). Such results highlight the need to confirm the factor structure of the current data set. Carron et al. (1985) reported adequate reliability estimates for the ATG-Task (α = 0.75), ATG-Social (α = 0.64), GI-Task (α = 0.70), and GI-Social (α = 0.76) subscales.

Sources of Sport Confidence Questionnaire (SSCQ)

The SSCQ was developed to measure the sources of sport confidence in athletes, using the sport-confidence framework of Vealey (1986,1988, Vealey et al.,1998). The SSCQ is a multidimensional measure consisting of 43 items representing nine subscales: mastery (five items), vicarious experience (five items) demonstration of ability (six items), physical/mental preparation (six items), physical self-presentation (three items), social support (six items), coach's leadership (five items), environmental comfort (four items), and situational favourableness (three items). Participants respond using a Likert scale (1 = not at all important, 4 = moderately important, 7 = of highest importance). All items are preceded by a common stem "I usually gain self-confidence in my sport when I (stem)" (e.g. master a new skill in my sport). A confirmatory factor analysis suggests adequate support for the hypothesized nine factor structure (Vealey et al., 1998). Internal reliability estimates for the subscales are high ranging from α =.71 through α = .93 (Vealey et al., 1998).

Collective Efficacy Questionnaire

Following the suggestions by Bandura (1996), Paskevich et al. (1999) noted that measurement of collective efficacy is situation/sport specific. With this in mind, four experts in the area of netball (a current netball coach, and three ex-netball players) were asked about their views and opinions concerning skill areas in netball. From this information, 42 items were developed to make up four of the six netball skills subscales (i.e. communication, obstacles, motivation and general). A total of 72 items representing many different skill areas in netball were written such that they reflected: (1) offense (e.g. "feed the goal circle effectively"; n = 16); (2) defense (e.g. "obtain possession by forcing a turnover"; n = 14); (3) motivation (e.g., "remain motivated after losing the previous game"; n = 7); (4) obstacles in general practice and competition situations (e.g. "play at the same level when our team is behind in a game"; $n = 17$); (5) communication with teammates and coaches (e.g. "use feedback from the coach to increase our performance"; $n = 7$); and (6) general everyday functions (e.g. "use our practices effectively"; $n = 11$). All items were preceded with the stem, "Our team's confidence that we can...", in order to focus on the team level. Participants were asked to rate their team's confidence in relation to specific collective netball skills on a 11 point Likert scale from 0% (no confidence at all) to 100% (complete confidence). This type of scale measures the strength of the confidence, as suggested by Bandura (1997) and follows the method used in previous studies (e.g. Feltz & Lirgg, 1997; Paskevich et al., 1999).

The high stakes associated with the two national level netball competitions meant access to the players was limited, and coaches only agreed to participate in the study prior to the start of competition. Thus, participants were administered the questionnaire containing demographic questions and the four sport measures at the team's place of residence within 24 hours of the competitions beginning. The timing of this was approved by the teams' coach to ensure no interference with pre-competition training, and to ensure minimal effect on the performance of the teams during the competitions. The four measures were counterbalanced to eliminate order effects and took approximately 30 minutes to complete.

Data Analysis

Four analytical steps were used to examine the data. First, descriptive statistics such as means, standard deviations, and ranges were calculated for demographic questions and total and subscale scores were calculated for each of the measures. Second, factor analyses using maximum likelihood estimates with oblique rotations were used to analyze each of the four measures' hypothesized factor structure. Items that cross-loaded with several factors or did not factor into their hypothesized subscales were dropped so as to enhance scale interpretation. Reliability estimates were calculated for total and subscale scores for each measure. Third, one-way analysis of variance (ANOVA) were undertaken for each of the team level variables (e.g. mean GEQ, practice time, time spent on team building skills), to determine if variance was greater between groups rather than within groups (i.e. heterogeneity of responses between teams). This provided a justification of aggregation of individual responses to represent group characteristics (Moritz & Watson, 1998; Zhu, 1997). Significant F values provide evidence for greater between groups variability, which suggests that there is stronger agreement within teams (homogeneity of responses within groups). Intraclass correlations (ρ) were also calculated for the team level variables to examine the strength of the relationship between two peoples' responses or outcomes who were both in the same group (Kenny, Kashy, & Bolger, 1998). A statistically significant ICC implies homogeneity of responses within groups, and provides further evidence of a team level construct. Intraclass correlations were computed such that:

$$\frac{\text{MS between groups} - \text{MS within groups}}{\text{MS between groups} + [n-1]\,\text{MS with in groups}}, \qquad (1)$$

where n = the number of persons per group and MS = mean squares.

Finally, HLM models were constructed on the basis of theoretical research findings using the methods suggested Bryk and Raudenbush, (1992), with the following variables entered in to the models. Player level variables were:

1. Perceptions of Success Mastery orientation subscale score (POSMAST)
2. Perceptions of Success Competitive orientation subscale score (POSCOMP)
3. SSCQ Mastery subscale score (NSCMAST)
4. SSCQ Vicarious experiences subscale score (NSCVEXP)
5. SSCQ Coach's leadership subscale score (NSCLEAD)
6. SSCQ Social support subscale score (NSCSUPP)

At level two the following were modeled as team level predictors:

1. Mean ATG-Task subscale score (ATGTASK)
2. Mean ATG –Social subscale score (ATGSOC)
3. Mean GI-Social subscale score (GISOC)
4. Mean GI-Task subscale score (GITASK)
5. Mean time for team meetings

The Bryk and Raudenbush (1992), method involved a one-way analysis of variance (ANOVA) with random effects to provide preliminary information about the degree of variation in collective efficacy scores within and between teams. At the player level collective efficacy scores in each team were defined as the team mean of collective efficacy plus a random error at the player level. At the team level of analysis, each team's mean collective efficacy score was described as a function of the grand mean of collective efficacy score plus a random error at the team level.

Next, regressions were performed on player and team level variables. This produced a series of intercepts and slopes representing the collective efficacy score for a team, and the relationship between the predictor in question and collective efficacy in that team. This enabled identification of the amount of variation that was able to be explained by player-level variables and team-level variables.

If regression coefficients varied from team to team, and the player level variance component was small, then the intercepts and slopes-as-outcomes model was calculated. The results of this model furnished information regarding the variation in mean team collective efficacy, or the strength of association between the player level predictors and collective efficacy scores.

The modeling process involved entering only one team level predictor at a time, such that those retained were statistically significant ($p < 0.05$) in explaining coefficient variation on either intercepts or slopes and was similar to the approach used by (Zhu, 1997).

Results

Descriptive Statistics

The average age of the sample was 20.34 (SD= 4.29) years. Team members socialised with teammates for just under five hours per week, and spent 45 minutes (SD= 1.28) in team meetings other than practice meeting each week. Approximately 63 % of time during practice was spent on developing team skills, and 30 % was spent on developing individuals' skills. However, teams also stated that on average they spend approximately 43 % of time during practice on team building skills.

Table 2. Mean factor loadings and reliability estimates for each of the POS, GEQ, SSCQ and collective efficacy measures

Scale	Number of items	Subscale	Mean Factor Loading	α
POS	6	Competitiveness	0.69	0.86
	6	Mastery	0.76	0.90
	12	Total	0.73	0.90
GEQ	3	ATG-social	0.45	0.56
	4	ATG-task	0.57	0.69
	3	GI-social	0.57	0.62
	3	GI-task	0.68	0.73
	13	Total	0.56	0.77
SSCQ	5	Mastery	0.62	0.81
	6	Demonstration of ability	0.68	0.86
	3	Environmental comfort	0.82	0.87
	3	Physical self-presentation	0.77	0.83
	4	Vicarious experience	0.69	0.82
	5	Coach' s leadership	0.7	0.88
	5	Social support	0.48	0.69
	2	Unnamed Factor	0.29	0.55
	33	Total	0.66	0.92
Collective Efficacy	5	Attack	0.69	0.85
	5	Defence	0.73	0.89
	3	Motivation	0.44	0.85
	5	Obstacles	0.76	0.92
	4	Communication	0.59	0.90
	5	General	0.78	0.92
	27	Total scale	0.68	0.96

Factor Analysis

Table 2 shows the mean factor loadings for the POS, GEQ, SSCQ and the collective efficacy subscale and total scores. As suggested by Roberts et al. (1998), two factors were extracted for the POS (Perceptions of Success) scale and were interpreted as mastery and competitive orientations for success. The data from the present study supported the four factor structure of the GEQ (Group Environment Questionnaire), although only with the exclusion of several items. GEQ items that cross-loaded with other factors or did not factor into proposed subscales and were removed from further analyses (i.e. items 5, 9, 11, 14, and 18).

Overall, the nine factor structure of the SSCQ (Sources of Sport Confidence Questionnaire) as proposed by Vealey et al. (1998) was not supported. Ten items that cross-loaded with other factors or did not factor into proposed subscales were removed from the measure. Items 12 and 14 ("psych myself up" and "know I have support from others") cross-loaded with several other factors. However, if these two items were removed from the measure, the factor structure became more unclear. As a result, items 12 and 14 were retained in the measure as they loaded together in a separate factor. It should be noted that items 12 and 14 were not originally in the same proposed subscale, and although they loaded with one another, this unnamed subscale was not used in subsequent analyses.

Table 2 shows the mean factor loadings for the collective efficacy measure. From the original 72 items, 27 were retained for further analysis. The data supported a six factor structure. Some motivation items tended to cross-load with other factors, however the loadings still demonstrated a sixth factor, with all three motivation items loading greater than the minimum recommended loading of 0.30 (Giles, 2002).

Table 3. Analysis of variance and intraclass correlations for team level variables

Team level variables		*df*	MS	F	Intraclass Correlation α
Collective efficacy scale	Between groups	30	3515.41	5.64**	0.34
	Within groups	266	623.27		
GEQ	Between groups	30	459.87	3.38**	0.23
	Within groups	282	135.95		
Team Meetings	Between groups	30	11427.74	8.23**	0.42
	Within groups	279	1388.78		
ATG-Social	Between groups	30	18.56	1.52*	0.05
	Within groups	287	12.24		
ATG-Task	Between groups	30	59.82	2.43**	0.13
	Within groups	286	24.60		
GI-Social	Between groups	30	78.17	4.33**	0.25
	Within groups	283	18.05		
GI-Task	Between groups	30	53.31	2.39**	0.12
	Within groups	282	22.30		

Note. $^*p < .05$. $^{**}p < .001$.

Reliability estimates for the each of the four measures and their associated subscales were generally high ranging from α = 0.86 to 0.90 for the POS, α = 0.56 to 0.77 for the GEQ, α = 0.55 to 0.92 for the SSCQ, and α = 0.85 to 0.96 for the collective efficacy scale (see Table 2).

Table 7 presents the one-way ANOVA data for the team level variables. All team level variable *F* values were significant, which indicated that responses within each team were homogeneous and therefore players' responses could be aggregated to represent shared beliefs. ICC's were all statistically significant providing further evidence that team level variables were representing group level phenomena (see Table 3).

One-Way ANOVA with Random Effects

The one-way ANOVA with random effects provided necessary information to determine if there was a significant difference between teams in terms of the collective efficacy scores (Bryk & Raudenbush, 1992; Zhu, 1997). The grand mean (mean of all team collective efficacy means) of the collective efficacy scores was 199.74 with a standard error (*SE*) of 3.39 (see Table 4).

Table 4. Results of one-way ANOVA with random effects

Fixed effect	Coefficient		*SE*	
Average team mean	199.74		3.39	
Random effect	Variance component	*df*	Chi-square	*p* value
Team mean	299.45	30	158.33	0.001
Player level effect	617.53			

The variance component was 617.53 at the player level, and 299.45 at the team level suggesting that to some degree, players varied from each other within teams, however a substantial proportion of the difference was found between teams. The chi-square (χ^2 = 158.33, df = 30, p < 0.001, provides a test of whether the variance of the team means is significantly greater than zero, and the results of this model suggest that it was, therefore further team variables were needed to account for the variability in collective efficacy scores.

Random Coefficient Model

Fixed effects. Table 5 summarises the results of the random coefficients model that included POS and SSCQ subscale scores. In this model, the overall collective efficacy score (average of the intercepts) was 199.72 (*SE* = 3.39). The average of the Competitive and Mastery POS (Perceptions of Success) subscales slopes was 0.29 (*SE* = 0.39) and –0.05 (*SE* = 0.75) respectively. The averages of the SSCQ (Sources of Sport Confidence) subscale slopes were: average Mastery slopes was 1.83 (*SE* = 0.50); average Vicarious Experiences slopes was –0.15 (*SE* = 0.34); average Coach's Leadership slopes was 0.44 (*SE* = 0.40); and the average Social Support slope was 0.18 (*SE* = 0.54).

Only the SSCQ Mastery subscale was a significant factor in determining players' collective efficacy scores within teams. The ratio of the mastery slope was t = 3.66 (p < 0.001), which indicated that Mastery was positively related to players' collective efficacy scores. More specifically, controlling for all other level one predictors, for every standard deviation above the average Mastery score, the collective efficacy score for that team was 1.83 points higher.

Table 5. Results of the random coefficient model

Fixed effect	Coefficient	*SE*	*t* ratio	*p* value
Overall mean collective efficacy score	199.72	3.39	58.87	0.00
Mean POS Competitive slope	0.29	0.39	0.73	0.47
Mean POS Mastery slope	-0.05	0.75	-0.07	0.94
Mean SSCQ Mastery slope	1.83	0.50	3.66	0.00
Mean SSCQ Vicarious Experiences slope	-0.15	0.34	-0.45	0.65
Mean SSCQ Coach's Leadership slope	0.44	0.40	1.10	0.27
Mean SSCQ Social Support slope	0.18	0.54	0.33	0.74
Random effect	Variance component	*df*	Chi-square	*p* value
Team mean	326.40	30	257.90	0.00
POS Competitive slope	2.19	30	36.35	0.19
POS Mastery slope	10.76	30	65.10	0.00
SSCQ Mastery slope	1.78	30	43.21	0.056
SSCQ Vicarious Experience slope	0.79	30	31.89	0.37
SSCQ Coach's Leadership slope	1.61	30	45.18	0.03
SSCQ Social Support slope	5.35	30	37.99	0.15
Player level effect	379.12			

Random effects. Table 5 shows the regression coefficients' variability. The variance estimation of the intercepts (team means) was 326.40, and was statistically significant (χ^2 = 257.90, df = 30, p < 0.001). This confirmed the above results of the one-way ANOVA with random effects; Table 4). In other words, significant differences in collective efficacy scores were noted among teams. Similar results were found for the Mastery slopes of the POS, and Coach's Leadership slopes of the SSCQ. The Mastery slopes estimated variance components for the POS were statistically significant 10.76 ($\chi^2 = 65.10$, $df = 30$, $p < 0.001$), suggesting that the relationships between collective efficacy and mastery orientations did vary significantly among teams. The estimated variance of the Mastery slopes of the SSCQ were 1.78 and approached statistical significance ($\chi^2 = 43.21$, $df = 30$, $p = 0.056$). The Coach's Leadership slopes, however, were statistically significantly different with an estimated variance component of 1.61 ($\chi^2 = 45.18$, $df = 30$, $p < 0.05$). The results suggested that the relationship between collective efficacy scores and perceptions of mastery experiences and coach's leadership did vary significantly across teams. However, no significant differences were found among Competitive success orientations (POS), Vicarious Experiences, and Social Support slopes (SSCQ), which indicated that the relationships between collective efficacy scores and these subscales did not vary significantly among teams.

The variance in collective efficacy scores explained by player level predictors was:

$$\text{Variance Explained}_{\text{at player level}} = \frac{617.53 - 379.12}{617.53} = 0.386, \tag{2}$$

Therefore, the player level predictors (POS and SSCQ subscales) accounted for approximately 38.6 % of the player level variance of the players' collective efficacy scores.

Multilevel (Intercepts- and Slopes- as Outcomes) Model

Fixed effects: Intercepts. Table 6 reports the results of the intercepts- and slopes-as-outcomes model. For the intercepts, mean Team Meetings and mean GI-Task (Group Integration; subscale of the GEQ) were the only statistically significant predictors. Controlling for ATG-Social (Attractions to Group; subscale of the GEQ), ATG-Task, GI-Social, and GI-Task, for every standard deviation above average time spent in team meetings, average collective efficacy score was 0.20 points higher. Also, controlling for Team Meetings, ATG-Social, ATG-Task and GI-Social, for every one standard deviation above average Group Integration-Task score, average collective efficacy score was 4.44 points higher. The ratio for mean Team Meetings and mean GI-Task were $t = 5.80$ ($p < 0.001$) and $t = 4.00$ ($p < 0.001$) respectively. These ratios also indicated that mean Team Meetings and mean GI-Task scores were significantly positively related to collective efficacy scores.

Fixed effects: Slopes. The results of this model also suggest that the subscales of the GEQ also tend to predict the POS and SSCQ subscale slopes (see Table 6). More specifically, mean ATG-social, ATG-task and GI-social significantly moderated the relationship between of the POS mastery and collective efficacy with gamma coefficients for ATG-task (0.55) and GI-social (0.74) and ATG-social (–2.10).

Mean ATG-social and mean GI-task moderated the relationship between of SSCQ mastery and collective efficacy, with gamma coefficients of 1.48 and –0.51 respectively. Mean ATG-social was also shown to moderate the relationship between SSCQ coach's leadership slopes and collective efficacy ($\gamma = -1.00$).

Random effects. For the intercepts, the variance explained was:

$$\text{Variance Explained}_{\text{for intercepts}} = \frac{326.40 - 88.72}{326.40} = 0.728, \quad (3)$$

where the value 326.40 was the estimated variance of intercepts by the random coefficients model (see Table 5), and the value of 88.72 was the estimated variance by the intercepts- and slopes-as-outcomes model (see Table 6). Thus, the team level predictors in this model accounted for approximately 73 % of the intercept variation. In other words, 73% of the parameter variation in mean collective efficacy scores has been explained by mean time spent in team meetings and mean Group Integration-Task subscale score.

Table 6. Results for intercepts- and slopes-as-outcomes model

Fixed Effect	Gamma Coefficient	*SE*	*t* ratio	*p* value
For Intercepts at player level				
Intercept2	69.04	23.80	2.90	0.00
Meanmeet	0.20	0.03	5.80	0.00
Mean ATG-Soc	-0.17	1.14	-0.15	0.88
Mean ATG-Task	0.91	0.99	0.92	0.36
Mean GI –Soc	0.56	0.74	0.75	0.46
Mean GI-Task	4.44	1.11	4.00	0.00
For POS mastery slopes at player level				
Intercept2	11.14	10.22	1.09	0.28
Meanmeet	0.02	0.01	1.36	0.18
Mean ATG-Soc	-2.10	0.72	-2.93	0.00
Mean ATG-Task	0.55	0.19	2.84	0.00
Mean GI-Soc	0.74	0.28	2.62	0.01
Mean GI-Task	-0.41	0.29	-1.42	0.16
For SSCQ mastery slopes at player level				
Intercept2	-11.34	6.36	-1.78	0.08
Meanmeet	0.00	0.01	0.06	0.95
Mean ATG-Soc	1.48	0.44	3.33	0.00
Mean ATG-Task	0.14	0.14	1.03	0.31
Mean GI-Soc	-0.20	0.30	-0.67	0.51
Mean GI-Task	-0.51	0.19	-2.70	0.01
For SSCQ coach's leadership slopes at player level				
Intercept2	6.39	5.45	1.17	0.25
Meanmeet	0.01	0.01	1.53	0.13
Mean ATG -Soc	-1.00	0.32	-3.07	0.00
Mean ATG-Task	0.07	0.12	0.58	0.56
Mean GI-Soc	0.22	0.19	1.16	0.25
Mean-GI Task	0.11	0.19	0.58	0.57
Random Effect	Variance component	df	Chi-square $\chi 2$	p value
Intercepts at player level	88.72	25	66.20	0.00
POS mastery slopes at player level	7.39	25	56.20	0.00
SSCQ mastery slopes at player level	0.18	25	25.57	0.43
SSCQ coach's leadership at player level	1.95	25	40.62	0.02
Player level effect	480.59			

Discussion

Psychometric analyses of the four measures were generally mixed, but provided some support for the hypothesized factor structures within each of the measures. The two-factor structure of the POS, as suggested by Roberts et al. (1998) was evident in this sample of elite female athletes. However, the factor structure of the GEQ proposed by Widmeyer et al. (1985) was less apparent, as the present study only found 13 items that grouped into the four subscales. These results are similar to those noted by Schutz et al. (1994) (for a review of measurement issues in cohesion see Carron, Brawley, & Widmeyer, 1998). We acknowledge that the age range of sample used in this study was outside that used by Widmeyer et al. (1985), however, all athletes were experienced team members and thus the measure was appropriate to use in this study. As teams were formed approximately two months prior to the competition this may have impacted the structure of the GEQ. A further consideration regarding the factor structure is that the GEQ was developed in North America on mainly varsity athletes. Its use outside a North American context may have some bearing on the observed factor structure in this research. We agree with both Carron et al. (1998) and Schutz et al. (1994) that when using the GEQ one needs to establish its factor structure before using and interpreting any scores from it. Generally though validity is an ongoing process that requires evidence to support the theoretical rationale regarding the interpretation and use of test scores (Messick, 1989) and the result from this study highlight this point. This study did find some evidence of the factor structure proposed by Widmeyer et al. (1985) and, although weak, it suggested the teams in this study exhibited the facets suggested in the GEQ.

The nine factors of the SSCQ, as proposed by Vealey et al. (1998) were generally supported in the present study. However, two subscales were not evident (i.e., Situational Favourableness and Physical/Mental preparation), and several items from other subscales were not found to group into their proposed factors. The absence of two factors is concerning, and more empirical research on the SSCQ is needed to verify its factor structure. The factors that were present were strongly represented and could be used as the basis for future instrument refinement.

The theoretical basis for the collective efficacy measure as suggested by Paskevich et al. (1999) was supported, although more work needs to be done to enhance aspects of the measure, such as the motivation items. The results indicated a 27-item collective efficacy measure with six factors (Attack, Defence, Motivation, Overcoming Obstacles, Communication and General). The internal reliability estimates found in the present study provided strong support for the reliability of the POS, SSCQ and collective efficacy measures but generally were mixed for the GEQ and SSCQ.

All team level variables had significant F values, and significant moderate to high ICCs, which indicated that teams did in fact share beliefs in regards to the team level variables, and aggregation (via the use of team means) at the team level was appropriate, thus, allowing the level two model to be specified.

For the subscale scores at the player level, the results indicated that the mastery orientation of the POS was the only significant predictor of collective efficacy. That is, players who tended to derive success in sport from mastery related accomplishments (rather than beating opponents), also tended to have a higher level of collective efficacy beliefs. This result supported the suggestion by Spink (1990b) to some extent, who proposed that the individual focus of an athlete could affect collective efficacy. In this respect, the results of the study support the notion that players' success orientations have an effect on the collective efficacy of the team. In other words, players who perceived success in sport to come from accomplishing goals belong to teams that had a high sense of collective efficacy.

The player level model (see Table 5) indicated that POS Mastery slopes, SSCQ Mastery slopes and Coach's Leadership slopes were the only level one predictors to vary significantly across teams, and therefore be included in the team level model. Although the SSCQ subscales were not found to be significant predictors at Level 1 (within teams), they were found to vary significantly across teams, and so according to Bryk and Raudenbush (1992), should be included in the level two model.

The team level model indicated that length of time spent in team meetings (outside of normal practices) and GI-Task were the only significant predictors of collective efficacy. While it was not strictly specified what constituted a team meeting, it appeared that participants included pre- and post-game discussions as potential components of this variable. Therefore, it could be suggested that these meetings consisted of discussion with the coach about game specific skills (e.g. strategies to use during the game), as well as verbal feedback or encouragement about the game in general. If this was indeed the case, it makes sense then that this type of meeting would enhance a team's sense of efficacy.

The only GEQ subscale that had a significant positive relationship with collective efficacy was GI-Task. This subscale purports to measure an "individual team members' feelings about the similarity, closeness, and bonding within the team as a whole around the group's task" (Widmeyer et al., 1985, pp.17). Therefore, mean GI-Task represents a team's feelings about the similarity, closeness and bonding associated with the team's tasks and goals. Thus, the results indicated that the more cohesive a team was in relation to team tasks and goals, the higher the level of collective efficacy. This result did not support the finding of Spink (1990a), who found that both ATG-Task and GI-Social subscales of the GEQ differentiated between high and low efficacy groups. It should be noted however, that the relationships found by Spink (1990a) may have been affected by Type I error by discarding variance at one level of the data. It is also worth noting that different moderator variables were used in this study and that this also may explain the difference between the results other than Type-1 error. The results from this study partially supports the findings of Paskevich et al. (1999), who found that both task related aspects of team cohesion (i.e. ATG-Task and GI-Task) differentiated between high and low efficacy groups. This finding extends the previous research from a more robust statistical methodology given the increased statistical power due to the simultaneous analysis at both individual and team levels.

The team level model also showed significant relationships with the level one predictor slopes. These relationships were cross-level effects, or effects that occurred between the level one and level two variables. These cross-level effects were interesting findings as they indicated that team level variables (especially team cohesion variables) seem to impact on individuals within the team as well as on the team as a whole. Specifically ATG-Soc, ATG-Task, and GI-Soc moderated the relationship between POS mastery and collective efficacy. In other words, when personal acceptance and social interactions within teams were high, then the effect of mastery-based perceptions of success on collective efficacy was diminished. Teams where there was high attraction to group tasks, were more likely to enhance collective efficacy by drawing on the mastery-based perceptions of success. Teams where there was closeness and bonding around the groups social activities were also more likely to enhance collective efficacy using mastery-based perceptions of success.

There were also moderating effects on the SSCQ mastery slopes for ATG-Soc and GI-task. Where teams had a higher personal acceptance and social interaction, then sports self-confidence derived from mastery had more of a positive impact on collective efficacy. Also the higher the involvement in the group task suggested that collective efficacy was enhanced by drawing on mastery-based self-confidence.

The relationships between POS mastery slopes and TG-Soc and GI-Soc provide are interesting findings. One should remember, however, that the teams had only been formed two months prior to the competition, and therefore social bonding would likely be important in team development, whereas their personal acceptance and social interaction at this time point may have been low. This is not to say that the personal acceptance and social interactions would not have increased had the players been together for a longer period of time.

There was also a moderating effect on the SSCQ coach's leadership slope for ATG-Soc. Thus, where teams had less personal acceptance and social interaction, then coach's leadership was perceived to have a positive effect on collective efficacy. This finding provides some support for the above findings, in that the recent formation of the teams suggests that the coach may play an important part in developing positive collective efficacy in recently constructed teams. Thus to understand more about these team level relationships requires a season long investigation into social aspects of team development as well as the impact coach's have throughout the playing season. Overall the team level model suggested that 73% of the variance in collective efficacy was due to these team level predictors. The results indicate that team level variables account for a substantial proportion of the variance in collective efficacy, thus demonstrating that collective efficacy is primarily a function of team level characteristics.

Future Research

Future research should consider including prior performance as a predictor of collective efficacy. Performance data was collected in the current study, but its use was not appropriate as the teams were only formed approximately two months prior to the competition, and thus team members were not necessarily the same as the previous season. Therefore, previous seasons' results were not relevant to these teams' performance.

A second consideration for future research is collecting information on collective efficacy at more than one point in time. The inclusion of a single point in the current study meant that collective efficacy and the other information collected was probably situation (or competition) specific. However, this could also be seen as a strength, as the study therefore investigated context specific collective efficacy for two short (five day), but important national level competitions. In other words, as the competition was at one point in time, and not spread out over a couple of months, assessing context specific collective efficacy was appropriate.

Future studies would benefit from following or tracing teams across an entire season (i.e. spread over a couple of months) This would also allow for investigation of collective efficacy across an entire season to highlight any collective efficacy–performance spirals, which have recently been identified in group performance literature (c.f. Lindsley, Brass & Thomas, 1995).

The results of the present study suggest that the length of time spent in team meetings outside of regular practices is a significant predictor of collective efficacy. Therefore further investigation as to what happens in these meeting and their effect on a team's collective efficacy may be of benefit in future research in order to delineate these effects further. Based on the relationships team meetings had with collective efficacy, and goal orientations, it seems reasonable to suggest that this construct may be considered an important part of the development of the team and its beliefs. Future research should also consider the effect of team building and development techniques on collective efficacy. Although this was not investigated in much depth, the correlation between the total scores on the GEQ scores and team meetings was 0.20 ($p < 0.01$), indicating a small but significant relationship. It would be useful for future studies to include a more detailed investigation of this relationship to determine what it is about these team meetings that have an impact on other team level characteristics.

Although, the coach's leadership subscale did not contribute to the prediction of collective efficacy in these models, it was still found to be an important source of player's sport confidence. This supports Short and Feltz (2000) suggestion that the coach's efficacy and role as leader, as well as the team's perceptions of the coach should be included in future multilevel analyses of collective efficacy.

Conclusion

In conclusion, the results of the study suggest that players' tendency towards deriving sport success from accomplishing goals (i.e. mastery orientations), time spent in team meetings outside of normal practices, and team cohesiveness all have a significant impact on a team's collective efficacy beliefs. This study identified several factors that impact on collective efficacy. The fact that effects were analysed at both the player and team level gives more meaning to these results. Obtaining the fairly large number of teams (31) at the group level was a major highlight of the study, which also adds to the interpretation and statistical power of the analyses. This large number of teams also meant that the results of the study were representative of the larger population (with over half of the teams invited taking part).

The strength of this study is that it is one of the first to use HLM to analyse both individual and group levels, representing a new direction in group research. Results of the study provide substantial support for collective efficacy as a team level characteristic as team level predictors accounted for a substantial proportion of the variance in collective efficacy at the team level. It is clear that sport psychologists should be applying interventions, and aiming team development and team building strategies at the team level to enhance collective efficacy.

References

Arnold, C.L. (1992). Methods, plainly speaking: An introduction to hierarchical linear models. *Measurement and Evaluation in Counseling and Development, 25*, 58-90.

Bandura, A. (1986). *Social foundations of thought and action: A social cognitive theory.* Englewood Cliffs, NJ: Prentice Hall.

Bandura, A. (1990). Perceived self-efficacy in the exercise of personal agency. *Applied Sport Psychology, 2*, 128-163.

Bandura, A. (1997). *Self-efficacy: The exercise of control.* New York: W.H. Freeman and Company.

Bryk, A.S., & Raudenbush, S.W. (1992). *Hierarchical Linear Models: Applications and data analysis methods.* Newbury Park, CA: Sage Publications, Inc.

Carron, A.V., Widmeyer, W.N., & Brawley, L.R. (1985). The development of an instrument to assess cohesion in sport teams: The Group Cohesion Questionnaire. *Journal of Sport Psychology, 7,* 244-266.

Carron, A.V., Brawley, L. R., & Widmeyer, W. N. (1998).The measurement of Cohesiveness in sports groups. In Duda, J. (Ed). *Advances in sport and exercise psychology measurement.* (pp. 213-226). Morgantown, VA: Fitness Information Technology.

de Leeuw, J. (1992). Series editor's introduction to Hierarchical Linear Models. In A.S. Bryk and S.W. Raudenbush, *Hierarchical Linear Models: Applications and data analysis methods.* Newbury Park, CA: Sage Publications, Inc.

Feltz, D.L., & Chase, M.A. (1998). The measurement of self-efficacy and confidence in sport. In J.L. Duda (Ed.), *Advances in sport and exercise psychology measurement* (pp. 65-80). Morgantown, VW: Fitness Information Technology, Inc.

Feltz, D.L., & Lirgg, C.D. (1998). Perceived team and player efficacy in hockey. *Journal of Applied Psychology, 83* (4), 557-564.

Giles, D. C. (2002). *Advanced research methods in psychology.* New York: Routledge.

Greenlees, I.A., Graydon, J.K., & Maynard, I.W. (1999). The impact of collective efficacy beliefs on effort and persistence in a group task. *Journal of Sports Sciences, 17,* 151-158

Hodges, L., & Carron, A.V. (1992). Collective efficacy and group performance. *International Journal of Sport Psychology, 23,* 48-59.

Hox., J. J. & Maas., C. J. M. (2001). Sample sizes for multilevel modeling. In: J. Blasius, J.Hox , E. de Leeuw & P. Schmidt (eds.) *Social Science Methodology in the New Millennium.* Proceedings of the Fifth International Conference on Logic and Methodology. Second expanded edition. Opladen, RG: Leske & Budrich Verlag (CD-ROM).

Kenny, D.A., & LaVoie, L. (1985). Separating individual and group effects. *Journal of Personality and Social Psychology, 48* (2), 339-348.

Kenny, D.A., Kashy, D.A., & Bolger, N. (1998). Data analysis in social psychology. In D. Gilbert, S. Fiske, & G. Lindzey (Eds.), Handbook of Social Psychology (4th ed., Vol. 1, pp. 233-265). Boston, MA: McGraw-Hill.

Kozub, S.A., & McDonnell, J.F. (2000). Exploring the relationship between cohesion and collective efficacy in rugby teams. *Journal of Sport Behavior, 23* (2), 120-129.

Li, F., & Harmer, P. (1996). Confirmatory factor analysis of the Group Environment Questionnaire with an intercollegiate sample. *Journal of Sport and Exercise Psychology, 18,* 49-63.

Lindsley, D.H, Brass, D.J., & Thomas, J.B. (1995). Efficacy-performance spirals: A multilevel perspective. *Academy of Management Review, 20* (3), 645-678.

Messick, S. (1989). Validity. In R. L. Linn (Ed.) *Educational Measurement* (3rd ed, pp 13-103). New York, NY: American Council of Testing.

Moritz, S.E., & Watson, C.B. (1998). Level of analysis issues in group psychology: Using efficacy as an example of a multilevel model. *Group Dynamics: Theory, Research, and Practice, 2* (4), 285-298.

Novy, D.M., & Francis, D.J. (1989). An application of Hierarchical Linear Modeling to group research. Paper presented at the Annual Convention of the American Psychological Association, New Orleans, LA.

Paskevich, D.M., Brawley, L.R., Dorsch, K.D., & Widmeyer, W.N. (1999). Relationship between collective efficacy and team cohesion: Conceptual and measurement issues. *Group Dynamics: Theory, Research, and Practice, 3* (3), 210-222.

Paskevich, D. M., Estabrooks.,P. A., Brawley, L.R., & Carron, A.V. (2001). Group Cohesion and sport in exercise. In R. N. Singer, H. A. Hausenblas, & C. M. Janelle (Eds.), *Handbook of Sport Psychology* (2nd ed, pp 472-494). John Wiley & Sons Inc: New York.

Prussia, G.E., & Kinicki, A.J. (1996). A motivational investigation of group effectiveness using social-cognitive theory. *Journal of Applied Psychology, 81* (2), 187-198.

Roberts, G. C., & Balague, G. (1991). *The development and validation of the Perception of Success Questionnaire.* Paper presented at the FESPAC Congress, Cologne, Germany.

Roberts, G.C., Treasure, D.C., & Balague, G. (1998). Achievement goals in sport: The development and validation of the Perception of Success Questionnaire. *Journal of Sport Sciences, 16*, 337-347.

Schutz, R.W., Eom, H.J., Smoll, F.L., & Smith, R.E. (1994). Examination of the factorial validity of the Group Environment Questionnaire. *Research Quarterly for Exercise and Sport, 65,* 226-236.

Short, S.E., & Feltz, D.L. (2000). Collective efficacy and team performance in sport. Paper presented at the Annual Convention of the American Psychological Association, Washington, DC.

Spink, K.S. (1990a). Group cohesion and collective efficacy of volleyball teams. *Journal of Sport and Exercise Psychology, 12*, 301-311.

Spink, K.S. (1990b). Collective efficacy in the sport setting. *International Journal of Sport Psychology, 21*, 380-395.

Vealey, R.S. (1986). Conceptualization of sport-confidence and competitive orientation: Preliminary investigation and instrument development. *Journal of Sport Psychology, 8*, 221-246.

Vealey, R.S. (1988). Sport-confidence and competitive orientation: An addendum on scoring procedures and gender differences. *Journal of Sport and Exercise Psychology, 10*, 471-478.

Vealey, R.S., Hayashi, S.W., Garner-Holman, M., & Giacobbi, P. (1998). Sources of Sport-Confidence: Conceptualization and instrument development. *Journal of Sport and Exercise Psychology, 20,* 54-80.

Weldon, E., & Weingart, L.R. (1993). Group goals and group performance. *British Journal of Social Psychology, 32*, 307-334.

Widmeyer, W.N., Brawley, L.R., & Carron, A.V. (1985). *The measurement of cohesion in sport teams: The Group Environment Questionnaire.* London, Ontario: Sports Dynamics.

Zaccaro, S.J., Blair, V., Peterson, C., & Zazanis, M. (1995). Collective efficacy. In J.E. Maddux (Ed.), *Self-efficacy, adaptation, and adjustment: Theory, research and application* (pp. 305-328). New York: Plenum Press.

Zhu, W. (1997). A multilevel analysis of school factors associated with health-related fitness. *Research Quarterly for Exercise and Sport, 68* (2), 125-135.

In: Encyclopedia of Sports and Athletics
Editors: Jack L. Murray and Emily O. Watson

ISBN: 978-1-61209-959-0

Chapter XXVII

Is Positive Feedback Always Positive? In Women with High Social Physique Anxiety, Positive Physical Appearance Feedback Decreases Self-Presentational Efficacy

Heather A. Strong, Kathleen A. Martin Ginis and Steven R. Bray
McMaster University, Hamilton, Ontario, Canada

Abstract

Social physique anxiety (SPA) is the anxiety experienced in response to others' real or perceived evaluations of one's physique. In physical activity contexts, SPA can exacerbate performance anxiety concerns and diminish self-efficacy. In the present experiment, we examined the effects of positive and neutral performance feedback on self-presentational efficacy and whether SPA moderates those effects. Forty women (M_{age} = 20.93±2.77) were randomly assigned to receive either positive or neutral performance feedback after performing a strength and endurance task. They then completed a measure of self-presentational efficacy and the Social Physique Anxiety Scale. The performance feedback manipulation did not have a main effect on self-presentational efficacy. However, results of a hierarchical multiple regression analysis revealed that SPA did indeed moderate the effects of feedback on self-presentational efficacy. Women with higher SPA had lower self-presentational efficacy after receiving positive feedback than after receiving neutral feedback. Among women with lower SPA, there were no differential effects of feedback condition on self-presentational efficacy. These results are interpreted taken as indication that SPA can influence how women interpret feedback regarding their performance on physical tasks. In particular, for women with high SPA, it cannot be assumed that positive feedback will always have positive effects on self-presentational efficacy.

Introduction

Self-presentation is described as the processes by which people monitor and control how they are perceived and evaluated by others (Leary & Kowalski, 1990). When people try to manage their impressions, they usually have an expectation of the possibility of conveying a particular impression (Leary & Atherton, 1986). These expectations or self-beliefs are a form of self-efficacy known as "self-presentational efficacy" (SPE; Maddux, Norton & Leary, 1988) and they are situation and context-specific (Martin Ginis, Lindwall, & Prapavessis, 2007). In the specific context of the exercise environment, self-presentational efficacy is defined as the confidence people possess to present the image of a fit and competent exerciser (Gammage, Hall & Martin Ginis, 2004). However, in situations where people have low self-presentational efficacy, they may also experience social anxiety (Maddux et al., 1988). One specific form of social anxiety is social physique anxiety (SPA), which is defined as the anxiety people experience in response to others' real or imagined evaluations of their physique (Hart, Leary & Rejeski, 1989).

Consistent with the predictions of Social Cognitive Theory (Bandura, 1977) regarding self-efficacy's relationship with thoughts, feelings and behaviour, self-presentational efficacy has been shown to be related to physical activity-related cognitions, affect and behavior. For example, research has found that greater self-presentational efficacy is related to more frequent exercise (Gammage et al., 2004) and exercise intentions (Fleming & Martin Ginis, 2004), and negatively related to social physique anxiety (Gammage et al., 2004; Sinden, Martin Ginis & Angove, 2003), and the use of self-handicaps prior to a fitness test (Martin & Brawley, 2002). Given the potentially important role that self-presentational efficacy plays in terms of physical activity behaviors and cognitions, it is important to determine if it can be enhanced as a strategy to improve physical activity motivation, participation and psychological well-being.

Self-presentational efficacy is believed to be amenable to change through the sources of self-efficacy specified by Bandura's (1977) Social Cognitive Theory (Martin Ginis et al., 2007). Bandura posited that self-efficacy is generated from four sources: mastery experiences, vicarious experiences, physiological arousal and/or affect, and verbal or social persuasion. Verbal persuasion is described as the verbal judgments or evaluations that important others provide (Bandura). According to Social Cognitive Theory, when people have a limited understanding about a certain activity, their self-efficacy can be enhanced by receiving positive verbal feedback about their capabilities. In the present experiment, we manipulated the information that physically inactive women received regarding aspects of their physical self-presentation (e.g., how fit and strong they looked). Our purpose was to compare the effects of positive versus neutral feedback on self-presentational efficacy. We also examined the moderating effects of social physique anxiety. It was hypothesized that positive feedback would result in greater self-presentational efficacy, but especially in women with high social physique anxiety. Our reasoning was that women who were highly anxious about others' evaluations of their bodies would be more responsive to positive feedback which, in turn, would have a greater impact on their self-presentational efficacy. In contrast, women who had low anxiety about others' evaluations of their bodies would likely not be as influenced by others' feedback.

Method

Participants

Participants were 40 female undergraduate students (M_{age}=20.93 ±2.77 years) recruited from a larger unpublished experiment examining the effects of fatigue on performance of an isometric handgrip endurance task. All participants did less than three days per week of moderate to heavy exercise and had never been to the campus exercise facility, so as to control for their exercise experience and to maximize their susceptibility to the verbal feedback (cf. Bandura, 1997).

Measures

Self-presentational Efficacy for Exercise Scale (SPEES; Gammage et al., 2004). Self-presentational efficacy was measured using the SPEES which consists of five items that assess a person's confidence to present the image of a fit and competent exerciser. Participants indicated on a scale ranging from 0% to 100% how confident they were in their ability to perform behaviors and present images that would lead to specific self-presentational outcomes. Research has provided support for the factorial and construct validity of the SPEES (Strong & Martin Ginis, 2007) and in the present study, the internal consistency of the SPEES was adequate ($\alpha = .91$).

Social Physique Anxiety Scale (SPAS; Hart et al., 1989). The 9-item version (Martin, Rejeski, Leary, McAuley, & Bane, 1997) of the SPAS was employed in the present study. Each item was rated on a 5-point Likert-type scale ranging from 1 (*not at all characteristic of me*) to 5 (*extremely characteristic of me*). SPA scores were calculated by reverse scoring two items and then summing scores across the items, with higher scores reflecting more social physique anxiety. Research has provided support for the concurrent, discriminant, and factorial validity and test-retest reliability of the SPAS (for a review see Martin Ginis et al., 2007). In the present study, the internal consistency of the SPAS was adequate ($\alpha = .86$).

Procedure

Participants were recruited into the study if they exercised <3 times per week at a strenuous or moderate intensity and had never exercised in the campus exercise facility. As part of the larger experiment from which our participants were drawn, during the experimental session, participants completed two isometric handgrip endurance tests. They were then randomly assigned to the Positive or Neutral feedback condition and given written bogus feedback regarding their performance on the handgrip endurance tests. The written feedback was used to manipulate verbal persuasion and consisted of ratings on a series of items that paralleled items from the SPEES (Gammage et al., 2004). These items were: "appears to be physically fit", "appears to have good physical endurance", "appears to be in good shape", "appears to be generally healthy", "appears to look after their physical appearance", "appears to be strong", "appears to be muscular", "appears to be in good physical condition", "appears to live a healthy lifestyle", and "appears to enjoy the activity". Each item had three possible rating boxes: "above average", "average", and "below average." Participants were told that during the handgrip tests, the researcher had rated them on each dimension.

Participants in the Neutral condition received "average" ratings across all attributes as indicated by a check mark in the "average" box for each item. Participants in the Positive condition were rated "above average" on 6 of the 10 attributes (i.e., "appears to be physically fit", "appears to have good physical endurance", "appears to be generally healthy", "appears to look after their physical appearance", "appears to be strong", "appears to be in good physical condition") and "average" on the remaining 4 items. They did not receive "above average" ratings for all of the comments because we were concerned about the perceived credibility of such ubiquitous positive feedback. After participants read the feedback form, they completed the SPEES and SPAS.

Data Analysis

A simple linear regression analysis (general linear model) was computed to investigate the effect of the verbal feedback manipulation on self-presentational efficacy. Hierarchical multiple regression analysis was conducted to examine if social physique anxiety moderated the relationship between type of verbal feedback received and self-presentational efficacy. Given the difficulties associated with detecting statistically significant interactions (McClelland & Judd, 1993) and the limitations associated with significance testing (Cohen, 1994), effect sizes were also calculated and interpreted.

Results

Descriptive statistics were calculated for self-presentational efficacy and social physique anxiety and are shown in Table 1. The results of the hierarchical multiple regression analysis are presented in Table 2. Before conducting the regression analysis, the predictor variable (social physique anxiety) was zero-centered as recommended by Aiken and West (1991). The positive feedback condition was coded as 1, and the neutral feedback condition was coded as -1. The main effect for feedback condition was computed first, and was found to be non-significant ($B = -.24$, $p = .12$). In the second model, (model 2), the main effects for feedback condition and social physique anxiety were entered simultaneously. In the final model (model 3), the main effects for feedback condition and social physique anxiety were entered simultaneously, followed by the interaction term. Together, feedback condition and social physique anxiety explained a significant 22% of the variance in self-presentational efficacy (model 2). In model 3, the interaction term explained an additional 6% of the variance. Although not statistically significant (p=.09), according to Cohen's (1988) guidelines, 6% of variance explained constitutes a large effect. Thus, the interaction term was decomposed for further analyses by plotting the interaction (Aiken & West, 1991).

Table 1. Means and Standard Deviations for Social Physique Anxiety and Self-Presentational Efficacy as a Function of Feedback Condition

	Positive Feedback ($n = 21$) *M (SD)*	Neutral Feedback ($n = 20$) *M (SD)*
Social Physique Anxiety	27.33 (7.94)	25.20 (7.68)
Self-Presentational Efficacy	48.47 (22.99)	57.78 (13.53)

Table 2. Hierarchical Multiple Regression Analysis Predicting Self-presentational Efficacy

Predictor	R^2	Adj R^2	B	*p*
Model One	.06	.03		
Feedback Condition			-.24	.12
Model Two	.22	.19**		
Feedback Condition			-.18	.20
Social Physique Anxiety			-.41	<.01
Model Three	.28	.24**		
Feedback Condition			-.19	.18
Social Physique Anxiety			-.15	.46
Social Physique Anxiety x Feedback Condition			-.35	.09

Note. $^{**}p < .01$

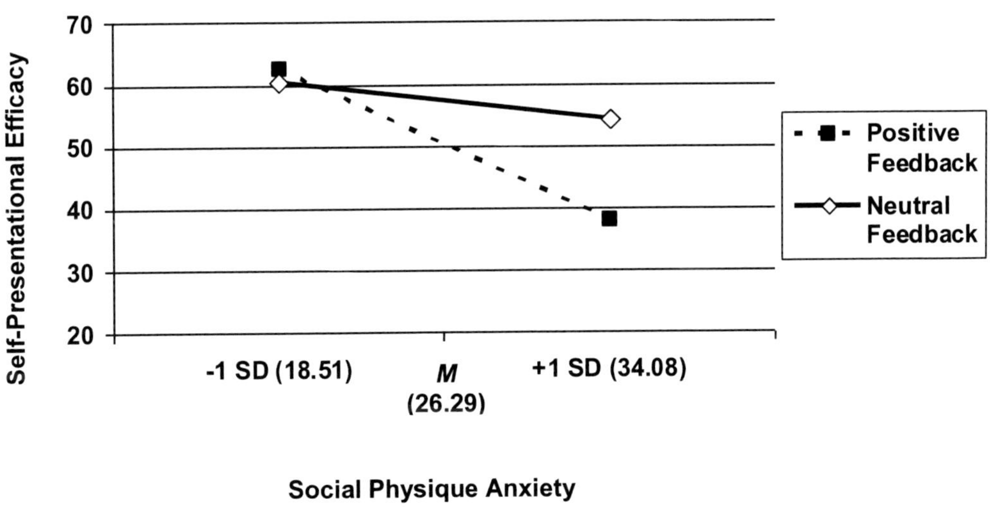

Figure 1. Plot of the interaction between feedback condition and social physique anxiety.

Two regression equations were calculated (one for each feedback condition), whereby self-presentational efficacy was regressed on social physique anxiety. Next, self-presentational efficacy scores were calculated for each regression equation using the mean social physique anxiety score and 1 *SD* above and below the mean. The predicted values were then plotted for each condition. As shown in Figure 1, for women with low social physique anxiety, there was no difference in self-presentational efficacy between those who received positive feedback and those who received neutral feedback. However, among women with higher social physique anxiety, those who received positive feedback had lower self-presentational efficacy than those who received neutral feedback.

Discussion

The purpose of the present study was to compare the effects of positive versus neutral feedback on self-presentational efficacy, and determine whether social physique anxiety moderates the effects. Our results partially supported our hypotheses. Contrary to the first hypothesis, exposing participants to verbal feedback consisting of positive comments regarding their physical characteristics and capabilities did not result in higher self-presentational efficacy scores compared to a condition that received neutral comments. However, as predicted, the difference in self-presentational efficacy between the neutral and positive feedback conditions was greater for women with higher social physique anxiety than those with lower social physique anxiety. It is important to note, however, that these results were in an unexpected direction. That is, among women with high social physique anxiety, those who received positive feedback had lower self-presentational efficacy than those who received neutral feedback.

One possible explanation for these seemingly counterintuitive findings may be that for women with high social physique anxiety, the positive feedback embarrassed them and drew attention to the discrepancy between how they were perceived by the researcher and how they perceived themselves. According to Leary and Kowalski (1995), people become more aware of the way they present themselves when others comment on, or observe, their physical features or behavior. The positive feedback may have heightened self-awareness in participants, thus eliciting self-presentational concerns and doubts, and decreasing their self-presentational efficacy. In support of this explanation, one study found that when a fitness instructor drew attention to new exercisers in a fitness class by praising their abilities and effort, they experienced greater social anxiety than exercisers who did not receive praise (Martin & Fox, 2001).

From a theoretical perspective, our results demonstrate that self-presentational efficacy is amenable to change through at least one of the four sources of efficacy beliefs (cf. Bandura, 1997). This is an important finding that speaks to the conceptualization of self-presentational efficacy within the broader framework of Social Cognitive Theory. As most of the self-presentational literature in physical activity contexts has been atheoretical (Martin Ginis et al., 2007), our findings demonstrate that Social Cognitive Theory is at least one viable framework that researchers can use to study and understand self-presentational phenomena.

From a practical perspective, our results suggest that when women with high social physique anxiety engage in physical activity, instructors and observers should avoid giving feedback and comments that draw attention to the women's appearance. It may be more appropriate to give feedback regarding how a task was performed or how much effort was expended (e.g. "You looked like you put all your effort into that bike ride, great job!"). Providing task-and effort-related verbal feedback should minimize further appearance-related anxiety and may enhance confidence in a woman's ability to present the image of an exerciser. This recommendation may be particularly important for women who are not regular exercisers (such as those included in our study), because they are most likely to be responsive to verbal feedback regarding their physical abilities (cf. Bandura, 1997).

Despite our study's theoretical and practical contributions, a few limitations need to be addressed. First, had we included only women with extreme social physique anxiety scores (i.e., very high and very low) in this study, we would have had greater power to detect a statistically significant interaction (McClelland & Judd, 1993). Nevertheless, explaining 6% of the variance in self-presentational efficacy is impressive considering the difficulty of detecting significant interaction effects in samples that are not comprised of people with extreme scores on the moderator variable (McClelland & Judd). Second, self-presentational efficacy was not measured before and after the manipulation. A post-test only design was used because we were concerned that the women would be suspicious about the authenticity of the feedback if we measured self-presentational efficacy before and after the manipulation. When feasible, future research that involves manipulating self-presentational efficacy should utilize a pre-test post-test study design, to test whether verbal feedback can change self-presentational efficacy. Finally, only one of the four sources of self-efficacy was manipulated (i.e., verbal persuasion) because we were interested in isolating the impact of verbal persuasion. We suspect that if all four sources of self-efficacy were manipulated in a single experiment, there would be an even greater difference in self-presentational efficacy between experimental and control conditions.

Conclusion

Despite these limitations, our study findings suggest that for women who are not habitually physically active, instructors, coaches and others may need to be cautious about the type of verbal feedback that they provide. Specifically, women with high social physique anxiety may respond to positive feedback regarding their appearance with a decrease in self-presentational efficacy. Clearly, it cannot be assumed that positive verbal feedback always has positive effects on women's self-perceptions.

References

Aiken, L. S., & West, S. G. (1991). *Multiple regression: Testing and interpreting interactions.* Newbury Park, CA: Sage Publications.

Bandura, A. (1977). Self-efficacy: Toward a unifying theory of behavior change. *Psychological Review, 84,* 191-215.

Bandura, A. (1997). *Self-Efficacy: The Exercise of Control.* New York: Freeman.

Cohen, J. (1988). *Statistical power analysis for the behavioral sciences (2nd ed.).* Hillsdale, NJ: Erlbaum.

Cohen J (1994). The world is round (p < .05). *American Psychologist, 49,* 997–1003.

Fleming, J. C., & Martin Ginis, K. A. (2004) The effects of commercial exercise video models on women's self-presentational efficacy and exercise task self-efficacy. *Journal of Applied Sport Psychology, 16,* 92-102.

Gammage, K. L., Hall, C. R., & Martin Ginis, K. A. (2004). Self-presentation in exercise contexts: Differences between high and low frequency exercisers. *Journal of Applied Social Psychology,34,* 1638-1652.

Hart, E. A., Leary, M. R., & Rejeski, W. J. (1989). The measurement of social physique anxiety. *Journal of Sport & Exercise Psychology*, *11*, 94-104.

Leary, M. R. & Atherton, S. C. (1986). Self-efficacy, social anxiety, and inhibition in interpersonal encounters. *Journal of Social and Clinical Psychology, 4,* 256-267.

Leary, M. R., & Kowalski, R. M. (1990). Impression management: A literature review and two -component model. *Psychological Bulletin, 107*, 34-47.

Leary, M. R. & Kowalski, R. M. (1995). *Social anxiety.* New York, NY: Guilford.

Maddux, J. E., Norton, L. W., & Leary, M. R. (1988). Cognitive components of social anxiety: An investigation of the integration of self-presentation theory and self-efficacy theory. *Journal of Social and Clinical Psychology, 6,*180-190.

Martin, K. A., & Brawley, L. R. (2002). Self-handicapping in physical achievement settings: The contributions of self-esteem and self-efficacy *Self and Identity, 1,* 337-351.

Martin, K. A. & Fox, L. D. (2001). Group and leadership effects on social anxiety experienced during and exercise class. *Journal of Applied Social Psychology, 31*, 1000-1016.

Martin, K. A., Rejeski, W. J., Leary, M. R., McAuley, E., & Bane, S. (1997). Is the Social Physique Anxiety Scale really multidimensional? Conceptual and statistical arguments for a unidimensional model. *Journal of Sport & Exercise Psychology, 19*, 359-367.

Martin Ginis, K. A., Lindwall, M., & Prapavessis, H. (2007). Who cares what other people think? Self-presentation in sport and exercise. In G. Tenenbaum & R. Eklund, (Eds.) *Handbook of Sport Psychology, 3rd ed.* (pp.136-157). Hoboken, NJ: Wiley.

McClelland, G. H. & Judd, C. M. (1993). Statistical difficulties of detecting interactions and moderator effects. *Psychological Bulletin, 114,* 376-390.

Sinden, A. R., Martin Ginis, K. A., & Angove, J. (2003). Older women's reactions to revealing and non-revealing exercise attire. *Journal of Aging and Physical Activity, 11,* 387-400.

Strong, H. A. & Martin Ginis, K. A. (2007). Factorial and construct validity of the self - presentational efficacy in exercise scale. *Journal of Sport and Exercise Psychology, 29,* S206.

In: Encyclopedia of Sports and Athletics
Editors: Jack L. Murray and Emily O. Watson
ISBN: 978-1-61209-959-0

Chapter XXVIII

The Role of Physical Activity in the Treatment and Prevention of Anxiety and Depression in Children: An Overview

Patrick W.C. Lau and Erica Y.Y. Lau
Department of Physical Education, Hong Kong Baptist University,
Kowloon Tong, Hong Kong

Abstract

Anxiety and depression were the major mental health disease in worldwide (Zoeller, 2007). The prevalence of anxiety and depression in children and adolescents were accelerating at an alarming rate. Previous studies reported that 5.7% to 17.7% children were suffering form anxiety and 2% to 5% of them with diagnosed depression. Anxiety might lead to serious impairment to individual daily lives and depressed individuals were more likely to suffer from other chronic disease (i.e. diabetes, cardiovascular disease), health risk behaviors (i.e. drug abuse and alcoholism) and committed suicide.

Growing body of research indicated that physical activity (PA) was a protective factor of anxiety and depression and adopted it as a non-pharmaceutical for treating anxiety and depression in adults. However, issue in respect to the effectiveness, mechanism and the application of PA in the treatment and prevention of childhood anxiety and depression is still equivocal. Therefore, this chapter provided an overview on 1) the effect of PA in the treatment and prevention of anxiety and depression in children; 2) the mechanism of PA on anxiety and depression, and 3) PA recommendation for treating and preventing anxiety and depression treatment and prevention in children.

Introduction

Physical activity (PA) has positive impacts on children's mental health. Regular PA was associated with improved mood and self-perception and reduced risk of two major mental disorders in children and adolescent: Anxiety and depression (Fox, 1999). Anxiety and depression are the major mental health diseases in worldwide (Zoeller, 2007). The prevalence of anxiety and depression in children and adolescents are also accelerating at an alarming rate. Previous studies reported that 5.7-17.7% and 2-5% of the children were suffering form anxiety and depression respectively.

Anxiety disorder could be categorized into panic disorder, obsessive-compulsive disorder, post-traumatic disorder, social phobia disorder, specific phobias disorder and generalized anxiety disorder. Although each disorder has its unique symptom but they all share the feelings of excessive apprehension, worry and fear (Barlow, 2004). Untreated anxiety may lead to serious impairment to individual's daily lives and interference their ability to establish and maintain relationship with others (World Health Organization, 2006). Moreover, it was associated with increased risk cardiovascular disease depression and suicide (Barlow, 2004).

Depression is a mood disorder which could be classified as depressive disorder (major depressive disorder (MDD) and dysthymic disorder) and bipolar disorder (bipolar I and bipolar II) (American Psychiatric Association (APA), 2002). Depressed individuals may have the following symptoms: depressed mood, loss of interest or pleasure, feelings of guilt or low self-worth, disturbed sleep or appetite, low energy, and poor concentration. These symptoms could be chronic or recurrent. Without appropriate treatment, depression might affect individual's ability to take care of his or her everyday responsibilities substantially (World Health Organization, 2006). Depression was associated with cardiovascular disease and diabetes (Mykletun *et al.*, 2007; Thakore, 2001), and other health risk behavior (i.e. drugs abuse, alcoholism, cigarette smoking and teen pregnancy) (Dunn & Weintraub, 2008). It was also the most frequent mental problem for people who committed suicide (Chan & Hung, 2006). These urged the needs for effective treatment.

In addition to treatment, prevention prior to the initial onset of the disorder is also important. Previous studies showed that children with a history of these disorders was at least 3 times more likely than those with no previous history to suffer from the disorders in their later life (Costello et al., 2003; Fergusson & Woodward, 2002). Moreover, prevention also plays an imperative role in reducing the prevalence if developing significant anxiety and depression. The reasons are that the symptoms of anxiety and depression are not easy to be recognized in children (Tomb & GHunter, 2004). Researchers believed that there may be a large proportion of children with undiagnosed anxiety and depression just because the extent did not reach to the diagnostic criteria. However, most of them were not receiving any treatment (Barrett & Turner, 2004). These evidences indicated the importance of early prevention or intervention.

Current Treatment of Childhood Anxiety and Depression

Currently, medication (i.e. Tricyclic antidepressants) and psychosocial treatments (i.e. Cognitive Behavior Therapy (CBT)) are the standard approaches in the treatment of anxiety and depression. However, medication showed little effect in children (Michael & Crowley, 2002). Importantly, it may lead to adverse effects to children's health such as weight gain, hyperlipidemia, elevated blood pressure and increased risk of suicidal behavior (Wipfli *et al.*, 2008). Although psychosocial treatment appeared to be an effective treatment (Cartwright-Hatton *et al.*, 2004), it requires certain level of cognitive ability which may not be well developed in young children. Therefore, its effectiveness was limited in older children. Moreover, psychosocial treatment may not be available in most communities (Cheung *et al.*, 2006). These evidences indicated that children with anxiety and depression were not treated effectively in the current state.

Current Prevention of Childhood Anxiety and Depression

Psychosocial therapy (i.e. cognitive reconstruction therapy) and education program were the approaches commonly used in the prevention of anxiety and depression in children (Clark, 1999; Garber, 2006; Merry et al., 2004). Previous studies showed that the effectiveness of these programs was modest (Barrett & Turner, 2004; Clark, 1999; Merry et al., 2004). In fact, majority of the prevention programs were secondary prevention that targeted to participants who were already experiencing the symptoms rather than before the onset of the disorders (Horowitz & Garber, 2006). That means the effectiveness of these approaches on preventing childhood anxiety and depression was remained unknown. Therefore, an effective, absence of unwanted adverse effects, and widely accessible and acceptable approach for treating and preventing anxiety and depression in children is warranted, and PA has considerable potential (Cartwright-Hatton et al., 2006; Dimeo et al., 2001; Dunn & Weintraub, 2008).

Several reviews studies (Dunn & Weintraub, 2008; Larun et al., 2008; Martinsen, 2007; Martinsen, 2008; Wipfli et al., 2008) provided evidences for adopting PA in the treatment and prevention of depression and some forms of anxiety disorder. These also concluded that PA may be a preventive factor of anxiety and depression in adults. However, issue in respect to the effectiveness, mechanism and the application of PA in the treatment and prevention of childhood anxiety and depression is still equivocal. Therefore, this chapter would discuss the role of PA in the treatment and prevention of anxiety and depression in children. As these reviews were all recent publication and have included most of the updated and relevant studies, this chapter would provide an overview in the following issues based on their findings:

1) the effect of PA in the treatment and prevention of anxiety and depression in children
2) the mechanism of PA on anxiety and depression
3) to provide PA recommendations for treating and preventing anxiety and depression in children

PA in the Treatment of Anxiety and Depression

Anxiety

Few studies have been examined the treatment effect of PA on anxiety. Larun and colleague (2008) found that no randomized controlled trial (RCT) was conducted to investigate the effect of PA in the treatment of childhood anxiety in the last 20 years. Though, there was positive effect reported in recent non randomized controlled trial in clinical pediatric population. Kiluk and colleague (2009) found that children with Attention-deficit hyperactivity disorder (ADHD) who participated in three or more sports displayed significantly fewer anxiety or depression symptoms than those who participated in fewer than three sports. However, Strohle (2008) noted that the effect of PA in the treatment of childhood anxiety was difficult to justify because a specific type of disorder could not be generalized in other disorders as they are diverse in nature.

Depression

Comparatively, more studies have investigated the effect of PA on treating childhood depression (Dunn & Weintraub, 2008; Ströhle, 2008). Larun and colleague (2008) claimed that the treatment effect of PA on childhood depression was not confirmed by small number of study, although existing evidences showed that PA had a significant and positive effect in treating depressed children compared with no intervention control group. However, Dunn and colleague (2008) provoked that the positive finding in adults and animals model were strong enough to support the potential benefits of PA in the treatment of depression in children. This notion was supported by recent non randomized controlled trial. Stella and colleague (2005) conducted a 12-week PA intervention to reduce depression in 40 obese female adolescents. The result demonstrated that aerobic exercise produced significant reduction in the depression score. Similarly, Nabkasorn and colleague (2006) examined the effectiveness of an 8-week jogging exercise in 49 adolescent girls with mild-to-moderate depressive symptoms. The result indicated a significant decrease in depression scores and 24 hour excretions of urinary cortical and epinephrine level. In general, majority of the studies tended to illustrate positive impact of PA in the treatment of childhood depression.

PA in the Prevention of Anxiety and Depression

Anxiety

Martinsen (2008) found that there was lack of longitudinal studies to support the prevention effect of PA on anxiety. Larun and colleague (2008) concluded that PA intervention has significant and positive effect on preventing anxiety compared to no intervention control group. Strohle (2008) studied 2548 adolescents found that people with regular PA had substantially lower incidence of any and comorbid mental disorder after 4 years and a lower incidence of somatoform- dynamic- and some anxiety disorder. Lindwall and Lindgren (2004) conducted a 6-month PA intervention program on physical self-perception and social physique anxiety in inactive adolescent girl. The result showed that the intervention significantly reduced the anxiety score after 6 months. The evidences regarding the positive effect of PA in the prevention of anxiety was relatively consistent.

Depression

In the study of Larun et al (2008), the result indicated that PA has a significant effect on preventing depression compared with no intervention or placebo control group. However, the prevention effect of PA on childhood depression is reserved. First, only small number of studies (n=16) were included. In addition, most of the include studies were targeted to older children aged above 12 years while the prevention effect of PA in young children was still equivocal. A longitudinal study (Harris *et al.*, 2006) in adults suggested that PA may have an indirect prevention effect on depression. It counteracted with medical conditions and negative life events.

Moreover, some studies (Dunn & Weintraub, 2008; Ströhle, 2008; Wipfli et al., 2008) argued that there was actually no study examined the preventive effect of PA on depression in healthy population. It is because majority of the participants in the previous studies were those who have previous episode of MDD. Therefore, these studies were in fact exploring the effect of PA on preventing the reoccurrence rather than the development of depression. The effect of PA in the prevention of depression was inconclusive.

In summary, existing evidences supported that PA appears to have significant and positive effect in the treatment of depression but inconclusive in anxiety. This only indicated that there was lack of consistent findings with respect to the treatment effect of PA on childhood anxiety. It is because the anxiety disorders are diverse in nature which limits the generalization of a significant result from a specific anxiety disorder to others. In contrast, PA seems to show consistent positive effect in the prevention of anxiety. However, no consensus exited in depression due to lack of pure prevention program (program intervene prior the initial onset t of the depressive symptom). Dunn and colleague (2008) suggested that this finding may be confounded by the floor effect. That is the intervention would not be able to produce further reduction in the depression level when participant's baseline level was very low.

Mechanism of PA on Anxiety and Depression

Although none of the mechanism of PA on anxiety and depression was proven, a number of explanations were commonly accepted. From the biochemical perspective, PA increased the concentration of endorphin and serotonin that have been reported to affect mood (Dimeo et al., 2001; Nabkasorn et al., 2006; Sjoten & Kivel, 2006). Endorphin is a neuro-chemical substance that provides the euphoria sensation (Petruzzello et al., 1991). Serotonin is a neurotransmitter which is responsible for mood enhancement (Graeff et al., 1996). A deficit of endorphin and serotonin was found to be associated with anxiety and depression. These hypotheses were supported by the study in animal model (Russo-Neustadt et al., 2001).

Physiologically, increased in core body temperature, cerebral blood flow and muscle relaxation during and after exercising may also attributed to stress relaxation and mood improvement (Fox, 1999). Stathopoulou and colleague (2006) suggested that improved quality of sleep after performing PA may produce positive effect on ameliorating anxiety and depression, which is similar to certain types of antidepressant. To date, the findings were mixing. More studies are needed to investigate the impact of sleeping quality on anxiety and depression.

Furthermore, PA was associated with improved psychological outcome which may also reduce anxiety and depression. Self-esteem was closely related to anxiety and depression (Bragado et al., 2008). Self-esteem is the belief on how a person feels and thinks about themselves physically (i.e. body appearance), psychologically (i.e. self-efficacy) and socially (i.e. social skills) (Murk, 2006). PA offers a mean for improving and maintaining body appearance (i.e. fat loss and body shaping), enhancing one's self-efficacy (i.e. providing positive experience of mastering new tasks), and improving social skills (i.e. communication and cooperation with others). These may increase one's confidence on coping with anxiety and depression (Bandura, 2004; Fox, 1999; Stathopoulou et al., 2006)..

Operationally, PA was used as a medium to help distracting individual from negative and stressful aspects (Biddle et al., 2000; Stathopoulou et al., 2006). It was also adopted in the treatment to produce similar bodily sensation with anxiety like increases in heart rate, body temperature, respiration and perspiration. Anxious individual would expose to those anxiety reactions *repetitively* while engaging in PA. Individuals may be able to recognize and positively interpret those anxiety reactions as a normal sign of stress under the supervision of psychiatric and PA professionals (Borman-Fulk et al., 2003; Martinsen, 2008)

PA Recommendation in the Treatment and Prevention of Childhood Anxiety and Depression

The design of PA intervention should be varied in respect to different purposes (i.e. treatment and prevention) and several factors like severity of the illness, type, frequency, duration and intensity of PA should be considered.

For treatment purpose, PA intervention may produce greater effect in the treatment of childhood anxiety and depression in several population: 1) Inpatient with mild to moderate depression as they are not suffering from severe physical impairment (Martinsen, 2000; Sjoten & Kivel, 2006). 2) Children whom are conventional psychological intervention are less acceptable (Salmon, 2000). For instance, children who aged below 12 years-old may not possess sufficient cognitive ability to receive CBT. 3) Parents with children suffering in anxiety and depression disorders. Previous studies showed that parental involvement was positively associated with the success of anxiety and depression treatment (Beardslee et al., 2003), as well as PA intervention (Sharma, 2006).

Settings

Previous study in adult but not in children showed that supervised program was more effective than home-based self-help program (Ströhle, 2008). Therefore, a clinical-based treatment is suggested. For the prevention, school was suggested as the ideal setting for disseminating health promotion program because most of the children spend their day in schools (Sharma, 2006; van Sluijs et al., 2007). Compulsory basis was found to be an important determinant to the success of children's PA intervention (Lee, 2003; Palmer et al., 2005; Prochaska & Sallis, 2004; Winett et al., 1999).

Frequency and Intensity

Based on the experience from previous studies, at least 3 times per week with at least 20 minutes per session (Dunn & Weintraub, 2008; Larun et al., 2008). In respect to the intensity, some evidences indicated that mood improvement was associated with medium and long term moderate-intensity PA, while worsened mood was related with high-intensity which lasted for 10 days to a few weeks (Peluso & de Andrade, 2005). Considering anxious and depressed children may have lower physical fitness level than the general population (Martinsen, 2008), the exercise frequency should start at elementary level and progress gradually so as to minimize the risk of injury (Centers for Disease Control and Prevention, 2008). For instance, children with depressive and anxiety symptoms may start engaging in PA from the light-to-moderate PA from 2-3 times per week with 15-20 per day, then increase gradually according to individual condition.

Time

Previous studies demonstrated that an acute effect could be occurred even in one single session (Peluso & de Andrade, 2005). In general, the normal range of the intervention duration was 6- week to 20-week (Dunn & Weintraub, 2008; Larun et al., 2008). However, no study has been conducted to examine the optimal duration for reducing anxiety and depressive symptom in children. Indeed, there were strong evidences supporting the beneficial effect of PA to children's health (US Department of Health & Human Services, 2008). It seems harmless to adopt PA as a lifelong habit if no clinical condition was reported.

Types

In general, rhythmic aerobic exercise was agreed to be an appropriate types of exercise for alleviating anxiety and depression (Petruzzello et al., 1991). However, no significant difference was found between different aerobic (i.e. walking) and anaerobic exercise (i.e. weight training) in the treatment of depression (Larun et al., 2008). However, mixed results were found with respect to the treatment of anxiety (Peluso & de Andrade, 2005). From the exercise science perspective, positive experience was an important factor for repeated PA participation (Bandura, 2004). Therefore, activity like fun game rather than of harsh discipline and skill-dependent games are suggested. Also, exercise on individual and small group basis may be more appropriate than large collective activities to create enjoyable PA experience (Lagerberg, 2005).

In comparison, the PA recommendation for prevention program is much simpler. The Centers for Disease Control and Prevention (2008) recommended children to engage in at least 60 minutes PA per day. Three types of exercises are suggested: 1) moderate-to-vigorous-intensity aerobic exercise (i.e. brisk walking and running); 2) muscle strengthening (i.e.

gymnastics and push up) and 3) Bone strengthening (i.e. jumping rope or running). As children's PA pattern is spontaneous, activities could be divided into several 10- to 15-minute bouts. This guideline is certainly appropriate for all children in the general population to prevent and enhance both physical and mental health.

Conclusion

This chapter provided an overview in respect to the effect, mechanism and application of PA in the treatment and prevention of childhood anxiety and depression. PA appears to demonstrate certain extent of positive impact and no negative effect in treatment and prevention of childhood anxiety and depression. In addition, PA was associated with other health benefits to children's health physically (i.e. increase in fitness level, bone health, weight reduction and maintenance and stimulate brain development) (Warburton et al., 2006) and psychologically (i.e. increase in self-efficacy and self-esteem) (Biddle et al., 2000; Fox, 1999). Regarding to the implementation, PA seems to be more accessible than traditional approaches where psychiatric professionals may not presence. These evidences provide support for incorporating PA as a mean in the treatment and prevention of childhood anxiety and depression. However, the effect of PA in the treatment and prevention of childhood anxiety and depression should not be overstated. PA plays an imperative role in the prevention, but it only acts as an assistant in the pharmaceutical treatment, especially for those with severe anxiety and depression. Moreover, professional consultation should be conducted before starting any exercise treatment.

Research on the treatment and prevention effect of PA on childhood anxiety and depression is still on an early stage. More studies regarding the dose response and its effectiveness are needed to robust the evidences.

References

American Psychiatric Association (APA). (2002). *Diagnostic and statistical manual of mental disorders* (4 ed.). Washington, D.C.: Author.

Bandura, A. (2004). Health promotion by social cognitive means. *Health Education & Behavior, 31*, 143-164.

Barlow, D. H. (2004). *Anxiety and its disorder: The nature and treatment and anxiety and panic* (2 ed.): Guilford Press.

Barrett, P. M., & Turner, C. M. (2004). Prevention strategies. In T. L. Morris & J. S. March (Eds.), *Anxiety disorder in children and adolescents* (2 ed.). New York,

London: The Gulford Press.

Beardslee, W. R., Gladstone, T. R. G., Wright, E. J., & Cooper, A. B. (2003). A family-based approach to the prevention of depressive symptoms in children at risk: Evidence of parental and child change. *Pediatrics, 112*(2), e119-131.

Biddle, S., Fox, K. R., & Boutcher, S. H. (2000). *Physical activity and psychological well-being: An evidence based approach*: Routledge.

Borman-Fulk, J. J., Berman, M. E., & Rabian, B. A. (2003). Effects of aerobic exercise on anxiety sensitivity. *Behaviour Research and Therapy, 42*(2), 125-136.

Bragado, C., Hernández-Lloreda, M. J., Sánchez-Bernardos, M. L., & Urbano, S. (2008). Physcial self-concept, anxiety, depression, and self-esteem in children with cancer and healthy children without cancer history. *Psicothema, 20*(3), 413-419.

Cartwright-Hatton, S., McNicol, K., & Doubleday, E. (2006). Anxiety in a neglected population: Prevalence of anxiety disorders in pre-adolescent children. *Clinical Psychology Review, 26*(7), 817.

Cartwright-Hatton, S., Roberts, C., Chitsabesan, P., Fothergill, C., & Harrington, R. (2004). Systematic review of the efficacy of cognitive behaviour therapies for childhood and adolescent anxiety disorders. *British Journal of Clinical Psychology, 43*(4), 421.

Centers for Disease Control and Prevention. (2008). How much physical activity do children need? Centers for Disease Control and Prevention.

Chan, P. M., & Hung, S. F. (2006). Depression in children and adolescents. *The Hong Kong Particitioner, 28*.

Cheung, A. H., Emslie, G. J., & Mayes, T. L. (2006). The use of antidepressants to treat depression in children and adolescents. *CMAJ, 174*(2), 193-200.

Clark, G. N. (1999). Prevention of depression in at-risk samples of adolescents. In C. A. Essau & E. Petermann (Eds.), *Depressive disorders in children and adolescents. Epidemiogy, risk factors, and treatment*: Jason Aronsaon Inc.

Costello, E. J., Mustillo, S., Erkanli, A., Keeler, G., & Angold, A. (2003). Prevalence and development of psychiatric disorders in childhood and adolescence. *Arch Gen Psychiatry, 60*(8), 837-844.

Dimeo, F., Bauer, M., Varahram, I., Proest, G., & Halter, U. (2001). Benefits from aerobic exercise in patients with major depression: A pilot study. *British Journal of Sports and Medicine, 35*, 114-117.

Dunn, A. L., & Weintraub, P. (2008). Exercise in the prevention and treatment of adolescent depression: A promising but little researched intervention. *American Journal of Lifestyle Medicine, 2*(6), 507-518.

Fergusson, D. M., & Woodward, L. J. (2002). Mental health, educational, and social role outcomes of adolescents with depression. *Arch Gen Psychiatry, 59*(3), 225-231.

Fox, K. R. (1999). The influence of physical activity on mental well-being. *Public Health Nutrition, 2*(3a), 411-418.

Garber, J. (2006). Depression in children and adolescents:Linking risk research and prevention. *American Journal of Preventive Medicine, 31*(6), 104-125.

Graeff, F. G., Guimarães, F. S., De Andrade, T. G. C. S., & Deakin, J. F. W. (1996). Role of 5-ht in stress, anxiety, and depression. *Pharmacology Biochemistry and Behavior, 54*(1), 129-141.

Harris, A., H.S., Cronkite, R., & Moos, R. (2006). Physical activity, exercise coping and depression in a 10-year cohort study of depression patients. *Journal of Affective Disorder, 93*, 79-85.

Horowitz, J. L., & Garber, J. (2006). The prevention of depressive symptoms in children and adolescents: A meta-analytic review. *Journal of Consulting and Clinical Psychology, 74*(3), 401-415.

Kiluk, B. D., Weden, S., & Culotta, V. P. (2009). Sport participation and anxiety in children with adhd. *J Atten Disord, 12*(6), 499-506.

Lagerberg, D. (2005). Physical activity and mental health in schoolchildren: A complicated relationship. *Acta Pædiatrica, 94*, 1699-1705.

Larun, L., Nordheim, L. V., Ekeland, E., Hagen, K. B., & Heian, F. (2008). Exericse in prevention and treatment of anxiety and depression among children and young people (review). *The Cochrance Library*(4).

Lee, W. (2003). Fighting fat: With taf in singapore. *Diabetes Voice, 48*(May), 49-50.

Lindwall, M., & Lindgren, E.-C. (2004). The effects of a 6-month exercise intervention program on physical self-perceptions and social physique anxiety in non physically active adolescent swedish girls. *Psychology of Sport and Exercise, 6*(6), 643-658.

Martinsen, E. W. (2000). Physical activity for menatl health. *Tidsskrift for den Norske lægeforening, 230*(25), 3054-3056.

Martinsen, E. W. (2007). Themed review: Anxiety/depression. *American Journal of Lifestyle Medicine, 1*(3), 159-166.

Martinsen, E. W. (2008). Physical activity in the prevention and treatment of anxiety and depression. *Nordic Journal of Psychiatry, 62*, 25.

Merry, S., McDowell, H., Hetrick, S., Bir, J., & Muller, N. (2004). Psychological and/or educational interventions for the prevention of depression in children and adolescents. *Cochrane Database of Systematic Reviews*(1), CD003380.

Michael, K. D., & Crowley, S. L. (2002). How effective are treatments for children and adolescents depression? A meta-analytic review. *Clinical Psychology Review, 22*(3), 247-269.

Murk, C. J. (2006). *Self-esteem research, theory, and practice: Toward a positive psychology of self-esteem* (3 ed.): Springer Publishing Company.

Mykletun, A., Bjerkeset, O., Dewey, M., Prince, M., Overland, S., & Stewart, R. (2007). Anxiety, depression, and cause-specific mortality: The hunt study. *Psychosom Med, 69*(4), 323-331.

Nabkasorn, C., Miyai, N., Sootmongkol, A., Junprasert, S., Yamamoto, H., Arita, M., et al. (2006). Effects of physical exercise on depression, neuroendocrine stress hromones and physiological fitness in adolescent females with depressive symptoms. *European Journal of Public Health, 16*(2), 179-184.

Palmer, S., Graham, G., & Elliott, E. (2005). Effects of a web-based health program on fifth grade children's physical activity knowledge, attitudes and behavior. *American Journal of Health Education, 36*(2), 86-93.

Peluso, M. A. M., & de Andrade, L. H. S. G. (2005). Physical activity and mental health: The association between exercise and mood. *Clinics, 60*(1).

Petruzzello, S. J., Landers, D. M., Hatfield, B. D., Kubitz, K. A., & Salazar, W. (1991). A meta analysis on the anxiety-reducing effects of acute and chronic exercise: Outcome and mechanism. *Sports Medicine, 11*(3), 143-182.

Prochaska, J. J., & Sallis, J. F. (2004). A randomized controlled trial of single versus multiple health behavior change: Promoting physical activity and nutrition among adolescents. *Health Psychology, 23*(3), 314-318.

Russo-Neustadt, A., Ha, T., Ramirez, R., & Kesslak, J. P. (2001). Physical activity-antidepressant treatment combination: Impact on brain-derived neurotrophic factor and beahvior in an animal model. *Behavior Brian Research, 11*, 1495-1510.

Salmon, P. (2000). Effects of physical exercise on anxiety, depression, and sensitivity to stress: A unifying theory. *Clinical Psychology Review, 21*(1), 33-61.

Sharma, M. (2006). International school-based intervention for preventing obesity in children. *Obesity Reviews, 8*, 155-167.

Sjoten, N., & Kivel, S.-L. (2006). The effects of physical exercise on depressive symptoms among the aged: A systematic review. *International Journal of Geriatric Psychiatry, 21*(5), 410-418.

Stathopoulou, G., Power, M. B., Berry, A. C., Smits, J. A., & Otto, M. W. (2006). Exercise interventions for mental health: A quantitative and qualitative review. *Clinical Psychology: Science & Practice, 13*, 179-193.

Stella, S. G., Vilar, A. P., Lacroix, C., Fisberg, M., Santos, R. F., Mello, M. T., et al. (2005). Effects of type of physical exercise and leisure activities on the depression scores of obese brazilian adolescents girls. *Brazilian Journal of Medical and Biological Research, 38*(11), 1683-1689.

Ströhle, A. (2008). Physical activity, exercise, depression and anxiety disorders. *J Neural Transm.*

Thakore, J. H. (2001). *Physical consequences of depression.* Peterfield, United Kingdom: Wrightson Biomedical.

Tomb, M., & GHunter, L. (2004). Prevention of anxiety in children and adolescents in a school setting: The role of school-based practitioners. *Children & Schools, 26*(2), 87-101.

US Department of Health & Human Services. (2008). 2008 physical activity guidelines for americans. Retrieved 18-05, 2009, from *www.health.gov/paguidelines*

van Sluijs, E. M. F., McMinn, A. M., & Griffin, S. J. (2007). Effectiveness of interventions to promote physical activity in children and adolescents: Systematic review of controlled trials. *British Medical Journal, 335*(7622), 703-.

Warburton, D. E. R., Nicol, C. W., & Bredin, S. S. D. (2006). Health benefits of physical activity: The evidence. *CMAJ, 174*(6), 801-809.

Winett, R. A., Roodman, A. A., Winett, S. G., WBajzek, W., Rovniak, L. S., & Whiteley, J. A. (1999). The effect of the eat4 life internet-based health behavior program in the nutrition and activity practice of high school girls. *Journal of Gender, Culture, and Health, 4*(3), 239-254.

Wipfli, B. M., Rethorst, C. D., & Landers, D. M. (2008). The anxiolytic effects of exercise: A meta-analysis of randomized trials and dose-response analysis. *Journal of Sport & Exercise Psychology, 30*(4), 392.

World Health Organization. (2006, 18-04-2006). Diagnosing depression. *Mental health and substance abuse.Facts and figures: conquering depression* Retrieved 15-04, 2008, from *http://www.searo.who.int/en/Section1174/Section1199/Section1567/Section1826_8100.htm*

Zoeller, R. F. J. R. (2007). Physical activity: Depression, anxiety, physical activity, and cardiovascular disease: What's the connection? *American Journal of Lifestyle Medicine, 1*(3), 175-180.

In: Encyclopedia of Sports and Athletics
Editors: Jack L. Murray and Emily O. Watson
ISBN: 978-1-61209-959-0

Chapter XXIX

Contemporary Themes in Group Cohesion

Sara LeBlanc and Changiz Mohiyeddini
Roehampton University, London, UK

Group cohesion is a ubiquitous, multi-dimensional construct investigated within the military, organizational and industrial settings, sports teams and exercise classes (Seibold, 2007; Burke, Carron & Shapcott 2008; Gill & Williams 2008). According to Carron, Brawley and Widmeyer (1998), cohesion is "a dynamic process that is reflected in the tendency for a group to stick together and remain united in the pursuit of its instrumental objectives and/or for the satisfaction of member affective needs" (p. 213). This theory- driven definition was posited by Carron, Widmeyer & Brawley (1985) and has become the universally accepted definition within the field of sport psychology (Horn, 2008). Cohesion has been cited as the most important small group variable (Lott & Lott, 1965, Cartwright, 1968; Golembiewski, 1962; Paskevich, Estabrooks, Brawley, & Carron, 2001; Carron & Brawley 2000; Carron Widmeyer & Brawley, 1988; Prapavessis & Carron, 1996) and has been shown to have a profound impact on group processes, with links to various factors such as collective efficacy (Heuzé, Sarrazin, Masiero, Raimbault & Thomas, 2006), mood (Lane & Lowther, 2002), performance (Carron, Colman, Wheeler & Stevens, 2002; Patterson Carron & Loughead 2005) and adherence (Spink, Wilson & Odnokon, 2010). In addition, intervention studies have demonstrated efficacy, enhancing cohesion through goal-setting (Senécal, Loughead & Bloom, 2008) and physical exercise programs developed for cancer patients which concurrently improved mental health, performance levels, as well as emotional and social functioning (Midtgaard, Rorth, Stelter & Adamsen, 2006).

Due to its profound impact on group dynamics, cohesion will continue to be a salient research topic investigated well into the 21st century across both the social and psychological sciences; yet important challenges persist, as key questions remain unanswered (Dion, 2000). Hence, the current paper aims to critically review recent findings, address limitations and provide suggestions for future research.

Dimensions of Group Cohesion

The evolution of cohesion research shifted drastically as Carron and colleagues advanced a theory-driven, hierarchical definition of cohesion measured via the Group Environment Questionnaire (Carron et al., 2002; GEQ; Carron et al., 1985). In his influential review of cohesion Dion (2000) highlighted the utility of the GEQ citing it as one of the most useful contemporary measurement tools available to investigate the myriad of research questions associated with groups and teams within the domain of athletics and exercise classes (Gill & Williams 2008; see also Eys, Carron, Bray & Brawley, 2007 for the GEQ's limitations when used in different settings and with different groups). The GEQ differentiates between both the task and social aspects of cohesion (Carron et al., 1985). It breaks cohesion into four dimensions which are attraction to the group-task (ATG-T), attraction to the group-social (ATG-S), group integration-task (GI-T) and group integration-social (GI-S). Group integration task (GI-T) refers to members' beliefs regarding the teams' unity towards group objectives (Eys et al., 2007). The ATG-T dimension delineates personal perceptions regarding one's individual contribution to the achievement of group goals (Carron & Brawley, 2000). The GI-S sub-unit refers to individual perceptions of social unity among the group (Carron & Brawley 2000), while the ATG-S sub-unit refers to individual's perception of their social interactions with respective group members (Carron & Brawley, 2000). This dynamic, multifaceted definition of cohesion recognizes and distinguishes between individual and group differences in order to gain a deeper understanding of the driving forces that fuel team processes.

Although the GEQ has become the predominant measurement tool within athletics, internal consistency values of each dimension have been variable, with ATG-S often demonstrating inadequate Cronbach's alpha values (Eys et al., 2007). A plausible explanation for this instability is the employment of mixed format scales which were initially included to combat response acquiescence (Eys et al., 2007). However, Carron and colleagues (1998) offered an alternative explanation noting the dynamic nature of cohesion which implies different dimensions of cohesion will be present in varying degrees at different times within a group. Therefore, when studying elite sport or business teams which both have a high task involvement, aspects of social cohesion may be secondary or non-existent which would explain the low consistency of the ATG-S dimension in certain environments. A study by Eys and colleagues (2007) addressed this issue by developing a revised version of the GEQ that exclusively utilized positive format scales; both the original and revised version of the GEQ were given to a sample of 276 athletes on two separate occasions. Results indicated the revised version demonstrated significantly higher internal consistency for three of the four GEQ dimensions (i.e. GI-T = .84, ATG-S = .74, GI-S = .86). Expanding on this line of research Eys Loughead and Brawley (2009) developed the Youth Sport Environment Questionnaire (YSEQ) which consists of two negatively worded items and 14 positively worded items. Currently there is a lack of cohesion research within youth athletics, nevertheless the development and subsequent validation of a viable measure will encourage researchers to investigate the impact cohesion has on this population. As stated by Carron, Eys & Burke (2007), "if cohesion is the most important group variable—as many authors have suggested—some measure of the degree to which it is present in youth sport is necessary" (p. 100).

Cohesion and Collective Efficacy

Recent research in athletics has recognized the important influence cohesion and collective efficacy have on performance outcomes (Heuzé et al., 2006; Myers, Feltz, & Short, 2004). Although previous studies have demonstrated a link between cohesion and collective efficacy, the relationship between these constructs remains unclear, as the majority of research has been cross-sectional and correlational in nature so causality could not be inferred (Heuzé, Bosselut & Thomas, 2007). Gaining deeper incite into this relationship has significant implications in both an applied and research setting as both exert a strong influence on performance outcomes.

A recent study by Heuzé and colleagues (2006) examined the interactions between cohesion, collective efficacy and motivational climate in elite female athletes participating in interactive sports. The results determined that changes in both collective efficacy and GI-T were positively associated with a task-involving motivational climate. This was sharply contrasted in an ego-involving motivational climate which was negatively related to changes in the cohesion dimensions GI-S, GI-T and ATG-S. These findings provide empirical support for a link between the perception of group related factors and situational perspectives by demonstrating that athletes base their perceptions of team characteristics on the perceived motivational climate that exists within their athletic microcosm (Heuzé et al., 2006). In the Heuzé and colleagues (2006) study, data was analyzed at the individual level due to the limited number of elite teams available for sampling. Future research should investigate the interrelationship between collective efficacy, group cohesion and perceived motivational climate with a larger more divergent sample that consists of both male and female athletes who compete across a variety of different sports so that group level analysis can occur.

Heuzé and colleagues (2007) continued this line of research, examining the cohesion-collective efficacy relationship in greater depth in order to determine the direction of effect between these two constructs in elite female handball players. Controlling for variables such as group level, influence of past performance and ATG-T scores early in the season, collective efficacy alone early in the season, explained 6-8 % of the variance observed in ATG-T at mid-season (ATG-T was the only dimension of cohesion explained by collective efficacy). Thus, athletes' perceptions of group competency regarding task goals enhanced their feelings regarding personal engagement with their teams' task objectives. Although this study adds depth to the interaction between cohesion and collective efficacy, certain limitations persist. Firstly, due to the difficulty of gathering data at the end of the season when teams are in pursuit of a playoff position, data was gathered at the beginning and the middle of the season only. Due to the dynamic nature of cohesion and collective efficacy this relationship may be substantially different at the end of the season, as task aspects of cohesion have been shown to develop earlier than social dimensions (Carron & Brawley, 2000). Future research should investigate the collective efficacy-cohesion relationship over the span of an entire season to determine what changes occur and when they are manifested. A second limitation was the level of analysis utilized. Due to the fact that these relationships were examined at the individual level, it is logical that individual conceptions of collective efficacy were linked to individual dimensions of cohesion rather than group aspects. Thus, these findings cannot explain group level dynamics and minimize the cross-level impact of group factors (Heuzé et al., 2007). Future research should utilize larger, more diverse samples, gathering data from a larger number of teams so that group-level analysis is possible (Castro, 2002). In addition, a few troubling trends emerged in the data set as teams with stronger levels of cohesion at the beginning of the season were more likely to participate in the second data collection as were teams that were more successful according to rank which limits the generalizability of these findings. A final limitation in this study was the measurement of these constructs. Although cohesion was measured via the GEQ which is widely used and has demonstrated adequate internal reliability in an athletic setting (Li & Harmer, 1996), the collective efficacy measure was created exclusively for this study and the psychometric integrity of this measure was not investigated exhaustively. Future studies should investigate the internal validity of this measure within an athletic context.

Cohesion and Performance

In the past, results have been inconclusive regarding the impact that cohesion has on performance outcomes, a fact illustrated by Gill (1986) who said "we can answer the question 'Do cohesive teams win more games?' with 'Yes,' 'No,' and 'Maybe'" (p. 226). Consequently, Carron and colleagues (2002) conducted a comprehensive meta-analysis that investigated this compelling question within an athletic setting with a robust sample of 9,988 athletes from 1,044 teams. They determined a reciprocal cohesion-performance relationship exists as high cohesion increases performance, while increased performance in turn enhances cohesion. The results from this meta-analysis revealed a significant, moderate to large cohesion-performance relationship exists (ES = .66) while studies utilizing the GEQ specifically determined a moderate relationship that did not vary between published and non-published articles. Overall this meta-analysis demonstrated a greater cohesion-performance relationship was evident in published sources and in studies that utilized a female sample (trends that were not evident in studies utilizing the GEQ). In addition, both social and task aspects of cohesion were found to influence performance in both coactive (ex. golf) and interactive sports (ex. football). In performance research the validity of self-reported measures has often been questioned, yet the relationship remained the same whether actual performance was measured (ES = .686) or self-reported data was utilized (ES = .577). Furthermore, the experience or skill level of the athlete did not moderate the cohesion-performance relationship and the results supported the contention that there is a degree of generalizability in this relationship from high school to elite sport. However this finding should be considered with caution as the magnitude of the cohesion-performance effect varied substantially among athletes competing at varying levels of competition, as ES for professional teams was .192 while ES for high school teams was .769 (Carron et al., 2002). Thus the impact of skill level on the cohesion-performance relationship still warrants further investigation. Now that the cohesion-performance relationship has been proven definitively, future research should begin to investigate why this relationship exists and what potential variables mediate or moderate this relationship (Patterson et al., 2005).

The meta-analysis by Carron and colleagues (2002) encouraged researchers to investigate mediating factors such as collective efficacy, role clarity and team norms to help explain the nature of cohesion-performance relationship. This line of research was pursued by Patterson and colleagues (2005) who investigated the impact of team norms on the cohesion–

performance relationship in a sample of 298 athletes from 24 different teams who participated in both coactive and interactive sports. This study determined players on teams with higher social cohesion (GI-S) and with greater social interaction norms reported higher performance levels. However, athletes who reported the lowest performance levels played on teams that were low in social cohesion but high in social interaction norms which was contrary to the hypothesis put forth by the researchers. This led them to conclude that the relationship between group cohesion, performance and team norms is convoluted and requires further investigation. Future research should investigate the impact of further moderating variables such as starting status, skill level and task type in addition to team norms utilizing a larger sample size where data is gathered at different points over the course of the competitive season (Patterson et al., 2005).

The general findings in the literature have determined high levels of cohesion increase performance levels, making cohesiveness a sought after goal for sports teams (Carron et al., 2002). However a recent study by Rovio, Eskola, Kozub, Duda & Lintunen (2009) which followed a junior ice hockey team over the course of a season determined high levels of cohesion had a deleterious impact on performance. Furthermore, the desire to evaluate performance declined as pressure to conform to group norms increased. Little research has been done on the harmful effects of cohesion, however a study by Paskevich and coleagues (2001) linked cohesion to deindividuation, groupthink and the need to conform. Paskevich and colleagues (2001) emphasized that one of the reasons the negative impact of cohesion is not investigated is because athletes, coaches and researchers take it as fact that cohesion is advantageous to performance leading them to enhance and promote its existence. In a related vein, a study by Hoigaard, Säfvenbom, & Tonnessen (2006) found that when high social cohesion exists in conjunction with low task cohesion the degree of social loafing is at it's highest level and group performance norms are low. In the Rovio and colleagues (2009) study the researchers posited that group think, conformism and group polarization led to a misconception of reality among the team which led them to overestimate their performance achievements and training deficiencies, thus no actions were taken to improve. In this case study a high level of social cohesion was associated with a myriad of detrimental group processes as well as the unwillingness to provide constructive criticism to teammates which led to an elevated and unrealistic perception of the teams' performance. The findings of this study illuminate the complex nature of cohesion and the need for critical analysis of its influence on performance in different settings. This longitudinal, mixed method study raises serious doubt on the *prima facie* acceptance of the beneficial influence of cohesion. However, these results needs further exploration in different sports and with larger sample sizes that utilize both male and female athletes considering that significant gender differences exist in the cohesion-performance relationship (Carron et al., 2002).

Cohesion and Intention to Return

Cohesion has been shown to exert a powerful influence on group dynamics impacting adherence rates in a variety of settings from recreational exercise classes to elite sports teams (Carron, 2006). The cohesion-attendance relationship is significant as both the physical and mental benefits of physical activity are numerous (see Carron, Hausenblas, & Estabrooks,

2003 for a summary). Empirical research in the early 80's linked drop out rates to low levels of cohesion, more specifically dropouts perceived the team to be a close-knit group that they failed to identify with (Robinson & Carron, 1982). This is a significant finding as attrition rates for fitness related programs exceed 50 percent six months after program initiation which demonstrates a discrepancy between intention and adherence behaviours (Robison and Rogers, 1994). In the Robertson & Carron (1982) study, adherence behaviour was operationalized within an intact group over the course of a season. Spink and colleagues (2010) extended this research by investigating the link between cohesion and intention to return the following season in sample of 122 elite male ice hockey players who played for eight different teams. In this study, players who exhibited significantly higher levels of task cohesion where more likely to return to their respective team the following season. These findings are significant but limitations and recommendations for future research should be noted. A weakness of this study was the fact that it was correlational in nature therefore causality could not be inferred. Furthermore, the adherence behaviour was only measured at the start of the season when adherence rates have been shown to be substantially higher (Robison and Rogers, 1994). Future research should utilize a longitudinal research design so that changes in cohesion and adherence can be explored and the directionality of the relationship can be determined. In addition, significant differences have been found between the motivating aspects of cohesion in an elite setting when compared with a recreational setting, with social aspects being the discriminating factor in the latter while task aspects are a more salient concern in the former (Heuzé et al., 2006). Future research should investigate the relationship between cohesion, intention to return and actual return rates in a more diverse sample of athletes and recreational exercisers with a range of experience, skill level and ability to promote the generalizability of these findings.

Cohesion Interventions

It is generally believed within the athletic community that increased group cohesion leads to enhanced performance levels (Loughead & Hardy, 2006). A contention supported by the seminal meta-analysis by Carron and colleagues (2002) discussed earlier, which determined a moderate to strong relationship exists between performance and cohesion. Thus, many attempts have been made to enhance cohesion amongst teams and exercise classes. A recent study by Mitgaard and colleagues (2006) investigated the influence of group cohesion and the quality of life changes that occurred during an intensive, six-week exercise intervention program developed for 55 cancer patients (55% of the participants had advanced forms of malignant cancer) currently undergoing treatment. This study utilized a mixed method design that involved both qualitative and quantitative methods. Through group interviews, this study determined that forming a cohesive unit became an interim goal of the participants, which helped maximize performance levels promoting, an '*esprit de corps*' among the participants which inspired them, making them feel like they were part of a sports team (Mitgaard et al., 2006, pg. 30). In this study, training occurred in a supportive yet competitive environment that involved upward social comparisons that were reciprocated between members, motivating them to tap unused resources in order to push the boundaries of their physical capabilities. The formation of a tight-knit group empowered participants uniting them around a common goal (to increase their physical fitness levels) while their illness took a back seat. In addition to the qualitative data gathered in this study, quantitative data revealed significant improvements in emotional and social functioning as well as enhanced mental well-being. Although the findings of this exploratory study are auspicious, certain limitations should be highlighted. Firstly, the fact that the qualitative data was gathered through group interviews which can promote homogenization and groupthink as all group members may not have expressed their genuine opinions if they deviated from the group norm (Rovio et al., 2009). Secondly, the fact that participants where a highly motivated, specialized group of cancer patients who joined the exercise group of their own volition a fact that may limit the generalizability of these findings. Furthermore, the fact that no placebo or control group was utilized in this study prevents the efficacy of the intervention program from being tested empirically. Future research should replicate this study with a placebo, control and experimental group to see if the health benefits conferred can in fact be attributed to the intervention.

Cohesion interventions have also been utilized in an athletic setting; Senécal and colleagues (2008) conducted a season-long goal setting intervention examining the impact goal setting exerts on team cohesion. At season's end the goal-setting condition had higher levels of perceived cohesion when compared with an experimental control. These results suggest that a goal-setting intervention is an effective way of maintaining cohesion levels over the course of a competitive season. During the year, no significant changes of cohesion were observed in the experimental group which may be attributed to a ceiling effect, as high levels of cohesion were already present at the beginning of the season. It should be noted however that the control group experienced a significant decline in cohesion as the season progressed, which illustrates the utility of the goal-setting intervention as the experimental group had significantly higher levels of cohesion when compared with the experimental control. The research design of this study was strong as it involved a longitudinal intervention that charted changes in cohesion over an entire season which is important due to the dynamic nature of the construct. In addition, this study utilized a control group which allowed inter-group comparisons to be made. A potential weakness in this study however was the lack of a placebo group which makes it unclear whether the intervention had a significant impact on cohesion or whether the act of intervening itself was enough to impact cohesion rates among team members.

Future Directions

Cohesion research has forged ahead in the last ten years definitively proving a strong cohesion-performance relationship exists, perhaps validating Lott & Lott's (1965) bold assertion that cohesion is in fact the most important small group variable. However the Rovio (2009) study casts a shadow of doubt on this finding as it determined social cohesion can have a deleterious impact on performance levels. The disadvantages of cohesion need to be investigated in greater detail to determine if the Rovio (2009) finding was an anomaly or if there is specificity (i.e. task vs. social) within the cohesion-performance relationship.

Researchers should expand on these findings, determining which variables mediate and moderate the cohesion-performance relationship so it can be understood in greater depth and interventions can be created accordingly.

The GEQ has been identified as a sound psychometric tool within athletics, researchers are encouraged to test the boundary of it's utility and when appropriate put to use alternative variations such as the adolescent GEQ so that specialized populations can be investigated in greater depth.

As a whole, cohesion research needs to produce more longitudinal studies with larger, more diverse samples so that specific findings can be generalized to the greater athletic population and group-level analysis can occur. Cohesion is a dynamic construct that is malleable within a group, thus intervention studies need to employ sound research designs which include appropriate control and placebo groups so that we can begin to mould cohesion to produce greater team satisfaction and performance outcomes and bridge the gap between research and application.

References

Burke S.M., Carron A.V., Shapcott K.M. (2008). Cohesion in Exercise Groups: An Overview. *Review of Sport and Exercise Psychology*, 1, 107-123.

Carron, A.V. Brawley, L.R., & Widmeyer, W.N. (1985). The Development of an Instrument to Measure Cohesion in Sport Teams: The Group Environment Questionnaire. *Journal of Sport Psychology*, 7, 244-266.

Carron, A.V., Widmeyer, W.N., & Brawley, L.R. (1988). Group Cohesion and Individual Adherence to Physical Activity. *Journal of Sport & Exercise Psychology*, 10, 127-138.

Carron, A.V., Brawley, L.R., & Widmeyer, W.N. (1998), The Measurement of Cohesiveness in Sports Groups. In J. L. Duda (ed.), *Advances in Sport and Exercise Psychology Measurement* (213-226). Morgantown, WV: Fitness Information Technology.

Carron, A.V. & Brawley, L.R. (2000). Cohesion: Conceptual and Measurement Issues. *Small Group Research*, 31, 89-108.

Carron, A.V., Colman, M.M., Wheeler, J., & Stevens, D. (2002). Cohesion and Performance in Sport: A Meta-Analysis. *Journal of Sport and Exercise Psychology*, 24, 168-188.

Carron, A.V., Hausenblas, H.A., & Estabrooks, P.E. (2003). *The Psychology of Physical Activity.* Dubuque, IA: McGraw-Hill.

Carron, A.V. (2006). Cohesion: Conceptual and Measurement Issues. *Small Group Research*, 37, 701-720.

Carron, A.V., Eys, M.A., & Burke, S.M. (2007). Team Cohesion. In S. Jowett & D. Lavallee (Eds.), *Social psychology in sport* (91-102). Champaign, IL: Human Kinetics.

Cartwright, D. (1968). *The Nature of Group Cohesiveness*. In D. Cartwright & A. Zander (Eds.), Group dynamics: Research and theory (3rd ed., pp. 91-109). New York: Harper & Row.

Castro, S.L. (2002). Data Analytic Methods for the Analysis of Multi Level Questions: A Comparison of Intraclass Correlation Coefficients, $r_{WG(j)}$, Hierarchical Linear Modeling, Within- and Between-Analysis, and Random Group Resampling. *The Leadership Quarterly*, 13, 69-93.

Dion, K. L. (2000). Group Cohesion: From "Field of Forces" to Multidimensional Construct. *Group Dynamics: Theory, Research, and Practice*, 4, 7-26.

Eys, M.A., Carron, A.V., Bray, S.R., Brawley, L.R. (2007). Item Wording and Internal Consistency of a Measure of Cohesion: The Group Environment Questionnaire. *The Journal of Sport and Exercise Psychology*, 29, 395-403.

Eys, M.A., Loughead, T.M. Brawley, L.R. (2009). Development of a Cohesion Questionnaire for Youth: The Youth Sport Environment Questionnaire. *Journal of Sport and Exercise Psychology*, 31, 390-408.

Gill, D.L. (1986). *Psychological Dynamics of Sport*. Champaign, IL: Human Kinetics.

Gill D.L. & Williams L. (2008). *Psychological Dynamics of Sport and Exercise*. Human Kinetics.

Golembiewski, R. (1962). *The Small Group*. Chicago: University of Chicago Press.

Heuzé, J.P., Sarrazin, P., Masiero, M., Raimbault, N., & Thomas, J.P. (2006). The Relationships of Perceived Motivational Climate to Cohesion and Collective Efficacy in Elite Female Teams. *Journal of Applied Sport Psychology*, 18, 201-218.

Heuzé, J.P., Bosselut G. & Thomas J.P. (2007). Should the Coaches of Elite Female Handball Teams Focus on Collective Efficacy or Group Cohesion? *The Sport Psychologist*, 21, 383-399.

Hoigaard, R., Safvenbom, R., Tonnessen, F.E. (2006). The Relationship Between Group Cohesion, Group Norms, and Perceived Social Loafing in Soccer Teams. *Small Group Research*, 37, 217-32.

Horn T. (2008). *Advances in Sport Psychology* (223-229). Champaign, IL: Human Kinetics.

Lowther, J. & Lane, A.M. (2002). Relationships Between Mood, Cohesion and Performance Among Soccer Players. *Athletic Insight*, 4, Available from URL: http://www.athleticinsight.com/Vol4Iss3/Moodand Performance.htm

Li, F., & Harmer, P. (1996). Confirmatory Factor Analysis of the Group Environment Questionnaire with an Intercollegiate Sample. *Journal of Sport & Exercise Psychology*, 18, 49-63.

Lott, A.J. & Lott, B.E. (1965). Group Cohesiveness as Interpersonal Attraction: A Review of Relationships with Antecedent and Consequent Variables. *Psychological Bulletin*, 64, 259-309.

Loughead, T.M., & Hardy, J. (2006). Team cohesion: From Theory to Research to Team Building. In S. Hanton, & S. Mellalieu (Eds.), *Literature reviews in sport psychology*, (257-287). Hauppauge, NY: Nova Science Publishers.

Myers, N.D., Payment, C.A., & Feltz, D.L. (2004). Reciprocal Relationships Between Collective Efficacy and Team Performance in Women's Ice Hockey. *Group Dynamics: Theory, Research, and Practice*, 8, 182-195.

Midtgaard, J. Rorth, M. Stelter R. & Adamsen, L. (2006). The Group Matters: An Explorative Study of Group Cohesion and Quality of Life in Cancer Patients Participating in Physical Exercise Intervention During Treatment. *European Journal of Cancer Care*, 15, 25-33.

Carron, A.V., Prapavessis, H. (1996). The Effect of Group Cohesion on Competitive Anxiety. *Journal of Sport & Exercise Psychology*, 18, 64-74.

Paskevich, D.M., Estabrooks, P.A., Brawley, L.R., & Carron, A.V. (2001). Group Cohesion in Sport and Exercise. In R. N. Singer, H.A. Hausenblas, & C.M. Janelle (Eds.), *Handbook of sport psychology* (2nd Edition, 472-494). New York: Wiley.

Patterson M.M. Carron A.V. Loughead T.M. (2005). The Influence of Team Norms on the Cohesion–Self-Reported Performance Relationship: A Multi-Level Analysis. *Psychology of Sport and Exercise*, 6, 479-493.

Robinson, T. T., & Carron, A. V. (1982). Personal and Situation Factors Associated with Dropping Out Versus Maintaining Participation in Competitive Sport. *Journal of Sport Psychology*, 4, 354-378.

Robison, J.I. & Rogers, M.A. (1994). Adherence to Exercise Programmes: Recommendations. *Sports Medicine*, 17, 39-52.

Rovio, E. Eskola, J. Kozub, S. Duda J. & Lintunen T. (2009). Can High Group Cohesion Be Harmful? *Small Group Research*, 40, 421-435.

Senécal, J. Loughead T.M. & Bloom, G.A. (2008). A Season-Long Team-Building Intervention: Examining the Effect of Team Goal Setting on Cohesion. *Journal of Sport & Exercise Psychology*, 30, 186-199.

Siebold G.L. (2007). The Essence of Military Group Cohesion. *Armed Forces & Society*, 33, 286-295.

Spink K.S., Wilson K.S. & Odnokon P. (2010). Examining the Relationship Between Cohesion and Return to Team in Elite Athletes. *Psychology of Sport and Exercise*, 11, 6-11.

In: Encyclopedia of Sports and Athletics
Editors: Jack L. Murray and Emily O. Watson

ISBN: 978-1-61209-959-0

Chapter XXX

Flow Impairs Risk Perception in Kayakers

Julia Schüler[1] and Mirjam Pfenninger[2]
University of Zürich, Switzerland

Abstract

Previous research has focused on the positive effects of the experience of flow in sports, such as peak performance and well-being. In the present research we assumed that, due to some flow characteristics, the consequences of flow are not always beneficial. For example, the dissociative nature of flow and its association with a loss of self-reflection should lead to an underestimation of one's personnel risk. We tested our hypothesis in a field study with 63 male and female kayakers. Right after kayaking (one easy and one demanding route) they rated their flow experience and their perceived risk. Underestimation of risk was operationalized as the difference between participants' subjective rating of risks (e.g. risk of capsizing) and an objective expert's rating of those risks. As expected, the experience of flow was associated with an underestimation of risks in kayaking. This result remained stable even when controlled for fear, which was highly negatively associated with risk perception, and even when controlled for the conceptually related concept of sensation seeking. The positive and negative consequences of flow in sports are discussed critically in terms of practical implications.

[1] Corresponding Author: Julia Schüler, PhD
University of Zürich Binzmühlestrasse 14/6 8050 Zürich, Switzerland E-mail: j.schueler@psychology.uzh.ch
Phone:+ 41 44 635 75 08
[2] Mirjam Pfenninger. University of Zürich
Binzmühlestrasse 14/6 8050 Zürich, Switzerland E-mail: mirjam78@hotmail.com

Introduction

Flow experience is defined as a state "in which people are so involved in an activity that nothing else seems to matter; the experience itself is so enjoyable that people will do it even at great cost, for the sheer sake of doing it" (Csikszentmihalyi, 1990, p. 4). At first sight this state of optimal experience seems highly desirable and previous research has confirmed this view by showing positive consequences of flow experience such as positive affect and high performance (Jackson & Wrigley, 2004). However, on closer inspection the above definition of flow also suggests a potential disadvantage of flow in that individuals are prepared to accept great costs. These costs can be time costs, for example spending night after night writing computer programs, or financial costs, performing an expensive hobby (diving in the South Seas; restoring vintage cars), or costs that result through neglecting other domains of one's life (e.g., neglecting one's family and friends). At worst, the cost may be to one's physical integrity, for example when endangering one's health or even one's life in risky sports. In the present paper we will compile theoretical considerations and facts about how flow is associated with risk behavior and we will present a study involving kayakers showing that flow does indeed lead to an underestimation of risk. However, first the phenomenon of flow will be described in detail.

Conditions and Characteristics of Flow

The flow experience is conceptualized as a multifaceted phenomenon that is mainly characterized by a deep involvement in the activity concerned, which makes it feels as if action and awareness were merged (Csikszentmihalyi, 1990; Csikszentmihalyi, Abuhamdeh, & Nakamura, 2005). This feeling of immersion in the task is accompanied by a "[...] sense of effortless ease and fluency in our movements" (Jackson & Wrigley, 2004, p. 430), which is the reason for calling the phenomenon "flow". Additionally, individuals experiencing flow concentrate strongly on the task at hand, leaving no room for other thoughts and self-reflective processes. Csikszentmihalyi and colleagues (Csikszentmihalyi et al., 2005) describe it as a "loss of self-consciousness" that is also often accompanied by losing one's sense of the ordinary passage of time. Often time seems to pass more quickly. During flow, individuals feel a high sense of control and trust their skills fully. No worries about one's competence disturb the action or the positive state of mind. The most important condition for experiencing flow is the perceived balance of the challenge of a task and one's own skills (Csikszentmihalyi et al., 2005). Further conditions are a clear set of goals that, combined with an unambiguous feedback about how well one is doing, direct the activity towards a positive goal state and continuously provide information about what exactly has to be done next.

Consequences of Flow

Previous research has focused on analyzing the positive consequences of the flow experience. The definition of flow as "[...] a psychological state in which the person feels simultaneously cognitively efficient, motivated and happy" (Moneta & Csikzentmihalyi,

1996, p. 277) already shows that flow is assumed to be related to peak performance as well as to peak experience (Jackson & Wrigley, 2004; Privette, 1981).

The positive quality of the experience accompanied by flow in sport is described by Jackson and Wrigley (2004, p. 428) as a state in which "our mind and body are working together effortlessly so that there is an intrinsic experience of harmonious enjoyment and pleasure". Flow is also related to positive post-exercise feelings such as revitalization and positive engagement (Karageorghis, Vlachopoulos, & Terry, 2000). Thus, the optimal experience of flow encourages sports activities by providing positive affective states during and after exercising.

Flow is associated with a high level of performance in different life domains (e.g., Jackson & Roberts, 1992; Jackson, Thomas, Marsh & Smethurst, 2001; Martin & Cutler, 2002; Moneta & Csikszentmihalyi, 1996) including sports (Jackson, 1992; Jackson & Roberts, 1992; McInman & Grove, 1991; Jackson, Kimiecik, Ford, & Marsh, 1998; Jackson et al., 2001; Jackson & Wrigley, 2004), learning settings (Engeser & Rheinberg, 2008; Schüler, 2007), and artistic and scientific creativity (e.g., Perry, 1999; Sawyer, 1992). Additionally, flow in sports is associated with duration of sport involvement, positive self-concepts and psychological skills (for an overview see Jackson & Wrigley, 2004).

However, while focusing on the positive consequences of flow, it has so far been neglected that the mechanism that links flow with its positive effect also implies certain disadvantages. For example, the mechanism that links flow to performance is a rewarding effect. The positive experience that accompanies the deep involvement during flow functions as a reward which enhances the probability that the activity will be performed again (e.g., Csikszentmihalyi et al., 2005). In order to maintain the positive experience of flow, individuals have to find greater challenges which enhance their skills and competence over time. Thus, experiencing flow is a powerful motivating force associated with a positive quality of the experience and an enhancement of performance in the long run. However, the rewarding quality of flow is also a source of danger in that it can become addictive. According to Csikszentmihalyi, enjoyable activities can become addictive, "[…] in the sense that instead of being a conscious choice, it becomes a necessity that interferes with other activities. […] When a person becomes so dependent on the ability to control an enjoyable activity that he cannot pay attention to anything else, then he loses the ultimate control: the freedom to determine the contents of consciousness. Thus, enjoyable activities that produce flow have a potentially negative aspect" (Csikszentmihalyi, 1990, p. 62).

Recent studies have confirmed the addictive character of flow, for example when using the Internet (Thatcher, Wretschko, Fridjhon, 2008) or during cyber-gaming (Chou & Ting, 2003) and sports. In sports, Partington, Partington and Olivier (2009) interviewed passionate big wave surfers and found flow to be associated with positive consequences such as improved mood states, performance and fulfillment. However they also found characteristics of dependence on surfing that match diagnostic criteria for exercise dependence. The description given by one of their participants of the feeling produced while big wave surfing illustrates this: "[…]. The best drugs cannot get you the same level of ecstasy, feeling of really good adrenaline. Once you get familiar with that feeling it's an addiction" (Partington et al., 2009, p. 176). Next to the danger of becoming addictive, Csikszentmihalyi and Rathunde (1992, p. 91) mention another negative consequence of flow. "There are two dangers inherent in flow: one is that the enjoyment can become addictive, the other that it can be experienced in antisocial contexts." The authors explain that when people lack other opportunities they will seek flow in destructive activities such as violence, crime and gambling.

The Present Research

With the present research we would like to add a third negative consequence of the flow experience, namely risk taking. The loss of self-reflection, the lost control of time, the absence of anxiety, the restricted perception to a limited field of activity combined with the feeling of having everything under control are important flow features that can be problematic when performing high-risk sports such as rock-climbing or kayaking. We assume that these features result in an underestimation of personal risks, which in turn leads to risk-taking behavior.

First evidence for the relationship between flow and risk-taking behavior was reported by Rheinberg (1991). He asked motorcyclists to describe their experiences when riding and found that they mentioned flow components such as the loss of self-reflection ("I am so gone that I feel that I don't exist", p. 357) and a feeling of control ("In this condition I feel absolutely safe", p. 358). Interestingly, the more intense the experience of flow described by the motorcyclists, the less afraid they were when riding a motorcycle. The motorcyclist's self-assessments of their driving style support our assumption that flow is related to risk taking. The higher the experience of flow the more the motorcyclists agreed with items like "preferred speed on highways", "preferred speed in city limits" and "number of crashes/accidents" and the less they agreed with the item "always ride cautiously". Rheinberg's (1991) interviews also showed that most motorcyclists mentioned the positive aspects of flow when asked to describe what makes motorcycling so enjoyable. However, scarcely anybody realized that the joyful merging with the activity can be dangerous. Consequently, participants "act at times completely contrary to their commendable safety standards" (Rheinberg, 1991, p. 361).

In the present research, we hypothesized that the experience of flow leads to an underestimation of risk in kayaking. We chose kayaking as a context to explore the relationship between flow and risk because it is a risky sport that involves the danger of being seriously hurt or even losing one's life by drowning. Thus, an analysis of antecedents of risk behavior seems particularly valuable. We operationalized the underestimation of risk by comparing an objective risk rating by experts with the participant's perceived subjective risk when kayaking two river routes. We analyzed one easy and one demanding river route in order to determine whether the difficulty of the river route makes any difference to the intensity of flow experience. In accordance with Csikszentmihalyi's (Csikszentmihalyi & Rathunde, 1992) assumption that flow is facilitated by demanding activities that offer the expression of one's potential, we assumed that participants would experience more flow on the demanding than on the easy river route. Because there is no theoretical reason why the effects of flow on risk perception should be different in easy and demanding routes, we assume the same effects for both kinds of routes.

Since risk-taking behavior in various domains of human life is related to Zuckerman's (1994) concept of sensation seeking (Zuckerman, 2006) and since flow shares some characteristics with sensation seeking, such as the quest for exceptional experiences, we also measured sensation seeking to disentangle the effects of these two variables on risk perception. Another (negative) predictor of risk taking that is also discussed as an antithesis of flow is fear (Csikszentmihalyi, 1990; Jackson, 1995). In order to examine the pure effect of flow on risk perception in our analyses, we also controlled for fear.

Study: Flow and Risk Perception in Kayakers

Participants and Procedure

Forty-two male and 21 female students of sports with a mean age 21.8 (*SD* = 2.16) took part in a study on "experiences in kayaking". They were participating in a kayaking education program and had similar levels of kayaking experience. Beforehand, participants filled in a questionnaire that asked them about their age and experience in kayaking, and contained the sensation seeking measure. Before boarding their kayaks, the procedure for data collection was explained and participants were informed that they would go kayaking on an easy and on a demanding route with breaks in between during which they would be asked to fill in a questionnaire. Right after the participants had performed the easy route (still sitting in their kayaks) they filled in the flow and fear measures that referred temporally to the experiences they had had on the river a few seconds earlier. Then they rated the risk (e.g. risk of capsizing) they perceived on the river route. The same procedure was repeated for the demanding route which they performed subsequently.

Measures

Sensation Seeking

Sensation seeking was measured using the Thrill and Adventure Seeking scale which is a subscale of a German version of the Sensation Seeking Scale Form F (Zuckerman, 1996; German version by Beauducel, Strobel & Brocke, 2003). Two alternative statements were presented at a time and the participant had to tick the statement that fit best (e.g., "A sensible person will avoid activities that are dangerous" versus "I sometimes enjoy doing things that are a bit scary"). Ten item pairs were rated overall. The items representing sensation seeking were summed.

Flow Experience

Flow experience was assessed using the 10-item Flow Short-Scale (Rheinberg, Vollmeyer, & Engeser, 2003). Participants were asked to rate whether they agreed with the items (e.g., "I do not recognize that time is going by", "I feel that everything is under control"), each item concerning the previous river route using a 7-point scale from 1 (no agreement) to 7 (agreement). A mean score of all items was computed.

Fear

Fear was measured using three items that have often been administered together with the flow items of the Flow Short-Scale (Rheinberg et al., 2003). Participants rated their agreement with the items "Something important to me is at stake here", "I won't make any mistakes here" and "I am worried about failing" on a 7-point scale (1: no agreement to 7: agreement).

Underestimation of Risk

To assess participant's *underestimation of risk*, in a first step experts (experienced kayaking athletes and trainers) objectively rated the main risk factors of kayaking, which are the risk of capsizing, the risk of hurting oneself and the general risk (e.g., "How high is the risk of capsizing on this river route?") of the two river routes on a scale ranging from 1 (very low) to 7 (very high). Then the items were rephrased in such a way that they could be rated by the participants regarding their experience during kayaking (e.g., "How high did you experience the risk of capsizing on the river route during kayaking?"). An index of underestimation of risk was computed by subtracting the objectively measured risk ratings from the participant's ratings.

Results

Descriptive Statistics and Correlations

Table 1 shows that the means, standard deviations and reliability coefficients measured for the easy and at the difficult route (T1 and T2) are very similar. The reliability coefficients for flow and fear were sufficiently high, whereas the Cronbach Alpha for sensation seeking was rather low. Also, the correlation coefficients were highly comparable for both routes. As expected, the higher the participants flow experience, the more they underestimated their personal risk in kayaking (T1: $r = .30$, T2: $r = .24$). The assumed alternative predictors were only partly related to risk perception. Fear was negatively related to the underestimation of risk (T1: $r = -.39$, T2: $r = -.38$), whereas sensation seeking was only marginally related to risk perception during the easy route (T1: $r = .22$, T2: $r = .06$). Flow was unrelated to sensation seeking, whereas the latter negatively correlated with fear.

Testing the Hypothesis

In order to test the hypothesis that flow predicted an unrealistic risk perception even when controlled for further variables that are related to the dependent variable (sensation seeking and fear), we conducted hierarchical regression analyses for each river route. We entered sensation seeking and fear into the regression equation as Step 1, followed by flow experience as a second step. Table 2 illustrates the results of the regression analyses for the easy (T1) and difficult route (T2, in brackets). Flow still predicted the underestimation of risk in the hypothesized direction. Also, fear remained a significant risk perception predictor, whereas sensation seeking was unrelated.

Table 1. Means, standard deviations, reliabilities (Cronbach Alpha) and correlations of variables at T1 and T2

T1 :	1	2	3	4	*M*	*SD*	Alpha
1 Flow	-	.14	.01	.30*	5.19	.77	.85
2 Sensation Seeking		-	-.32*	.22+	8.57	1.49	.53
3 Fear			-	-.39**	3.09	1.69	.81
4 Risk underestimation				-	-1.27	1.00	-
T2 :	1	2	3	4	*M*	*SD*	Alpha
1 Flow	-	.20	.05	.24*	5.73	.72	.85
2 Sensation Seeking		-	-.30*	.06	8.57	1.49	.53
3 Fear			-	-.38**	3.03	1.57	.84
4 Risk underestimation				-	-1.32	1.02	-

+$p < .10$ *$p < .05$ **$p < .01$

Table 2. Hierarchical regressions of underestimation of risk on easy route (T1) and demanding kayaking route (T2, scores in brackets) on flow controlled for fear and sensation seeking

Step	Variable	ΔR^2	*df*	ΔF	b^a
1	Control Variables	.17 (.15)	2, 60	5.99** (5.20**)	
	Fear				-.38** (-.43**)
	Sensation Seeking				.06 (.12)
2	Flow experience	.09 (.08)	1,59	6.94* (6.00*)	.30* (.29*)
	Cumulative R^2	.25 (.23)	2,59	6.70** (5.75**)	

Note. [a] *b* is the standardized regression coefficient in the regression equation.
*$p < .05$. **$p < .01$.

A GLM repeated measure analysis confirmed our supplemental hypothesis that participants experienced more flow on the demanding route ($M = 5.73$, $SD = .72$) than on the easy river route ($M = 5.19$, $SD = .77$), $F(1,62) = 47.07$, $p < .001$.

Brief Discussion of the Study

In the present study we argued that, due to its characteristics loss of self-reflection and a feeling of control over the activity, flow experience influences risk perception. Our results confirmed the hypothesized effect showing that the experience of flow while kayaking predicts an underestimation of one's personal risk in kayaking. This is also true when controlling for sensation seeking. As a limitation it has to be mentioned that the German Sensation Seeking Scale (Beauducel et al., 2003) lacks sufficient reliability in this study. As predicted, fear emerged as a strong predictor of overestimating risk, but did not influence the effects of flow on risk perception.

Our results also confirmed our hypothesis that the intensity of flow experience is significantly higher on the demanding route than on the easy route. However, the mean flow scores of 5.73 (demanding route) and 5.19 (easy route) on a 7-point rating scale suggest that kayaking per se is a sport that easily provokes the experience of flow.

In order not to endanger the health of our participants we measured risk perception but not risk-taking behavior directly. Although risk perception is strongly associated with risk taking, the current state of research could be extended by assessing real risk behavior in future research.

Discussion and Conclusion

Previous research has focused on the positive consequences of flow such as the positive quality of its experience and its association with high performance (Jackson & Wrigley, 2004). However, we have summed up some theoretical considerations and showed in a study with kayakers that flow might also have severe negative consequences. The underestimation of one's risk, not being aware of or even denying one's physical vulnerability while simultaneously overestimating one's competences in risky sports may have serious negative consequences for one's health.

Interestingly, the same features that define the positive quality of the experience of flow (loss of self-reflection, feeling of having everything under control) are also the reasons for its negative consequences. Thus, "feeling simultaneously cognitively efficient, motivated, and happy" (Moneta & Csikszentmihalyi, 1996, p. 277) and endangering one's health are two sides of the same coin which is flow experience. This puts practitioners in a real dilemma. On the one hand, interventions that aim to enhance flow in sport, for example by providing important flow conditions (e.g., confidence, optimal arousal, motivational state; Catley & Duda, 1997; Jackson, 1995; Jackson, et al., 2001) are desirable because the positive quality of the experience associated with flow enhances persistence in sports and thereby promotes the positive health effects of regular exercising, for example. On the other hand the experience of flow facilitates addiction and an unrealistic risk perception and therefore interventions that disturb the experience of flow, for example by initiating self-reflection processes, would be the better way to promote healthy sports activities. However, the dilemma can be resolved by matching the intervention strategies to the problems of specific populations. An expert in a certain kind of sport, such as an experienced and passionate rock climber, big wave surfer or kayaker, does not need a flow-enhancing strategy but might benefit from the knowledge of strategies to control his flow experience and the risks associated with it. In contrast, a person who is beginning a sport needs flow-enhancing strategies so that the sport activities become rewarding quickly. This again leads to long-term adherence to the sport. Thus, flow-enhancing strategies might tackle the problems of the high drop-out rate in leisure- and health-oriented sports programs.

To sum up the present paper using Csikszentmihalyi's words, "The flow experience, like everything else, is not "good" in an absolute sense. It is good only in that it has the potential to make life more rich, intense and meaningful" (Csikszentmihalyi, 1990, p. 70). However, as we have aimed to show in the present paper, flow also has the potential to make life dangerous and thus "learning to distinguish the useful and harmful forms of flow, and then making the most from the former while placing limits on the latter" (Csikzsentmihalyi, 1990, p. 70) is an important aim of future research.

References

Beauducel, A., Strobel, A., & Brocke, B. (2003). Psychometrische Eigenschaften und Normen einer deutschsprachigen Fassung der Sensation Seeking-Skalen, Form V [Psychometric characteristics of a German version of the Sensation Seeking-Scales, Form V]. *Diagnostica, 49, 2,* 61-72. Göttingen: Hogrefe.

Catley, D., & Duda, J. L. (1997). Psychological antecedents of the frequency and intensity of flow in golfers. *International Journal of Sport Psychology, 28*(4), 309 – 323.

Chou, T. J., & Ting, C. C. (2003). The role of flow experience in cyber-game addiction. *Cyberpsychology and Behavior, 6*(6), 663 – 675.

Csikszentmihalyi, M. (1990). *Flow: The psychology of optimal experience.* New York: Harper & Row.

Csikszentmihalyi, M., Abuhamdeh, S., & Nakamura, J. (2005). Flow. In A. J. Elliot & C. S. Dweck (Eds), *Handbook of competence and motivation* (pp. 598-608). New York: Guilford Publications, Inc.

Csikszentmihalyi, M., & Rathunde, K. (1992). The measurement of flow in everyday life: Toward a theory of emergent motivation. In R. Dienstbier & J.E. Jacobs (Eds.), *Nebraska Symposium on motivation, 1992, 40, Developmental Perspectives on motivation* (pp. 57-97). Lincoln and London: University of Nebraska Press.

Engeser, S., & Rheinberg, F. (2008). Flow, performance and moderators of challenge-skill-balance. *Motivation and Emotion,32*, 158–172.

Jackson, S. A. (1992). Athletes in flow: A qualitative investigation of flow states in elite figure skaters. *Journal of Applied Sport Psychology, 4*(2), 161-180.

Jackson, S. A. (1995). Factors influencing the occurence of flow in elithe athletes. *Journal of Applied Sport Psychology, 7*(2), 135 -163.

Jackson, S. A., Kimiecik, J., Ford, S., & Marsh, H.W. (1998). Psychological correlates of flow in sport. *Journal of Sport & Exercise Psychology, 20*, 358–378.

Jackson, S. A., & Roberts, G. C. (1992). Positive performance states of athletes: Toward a conceptual understanding of peak performance. *The Sport Psychologist, 6,* 156 -171.

Jackson, S. A., Thomas, P. R., Marsh, H. W., & Smethurst, C. J. (2001). Relationship between flow, self-concept, psychological skill, and performance. *Journal of Applied Sport Psychology, 13,* 129 -153.

Jackson, S. A., & Wrigley, W. J. (2004). Optimal experience in sport: current issues and future directions. In T. Morris, & J. Summers (2004), *Sport Psychology: theory, applications and issues.* Milton : John Wiley & Sons Australia, Ltd.

Karageorghis, C. I., Vlachopoulos, S. P., & Terry, P. C. (2000). Latent variable modeling of the relationship between flow and exercise-induced feelings: an intuitive appraisal perspective. *European Physical Education, 6*(3), 230 – 248.

Martin, J. J., & Cutler, K. (2002). An exploratory study of flow and motivation in theatre actors. *Journal of Applied Sport Psychology, 14*, 344 - 352.

Moneta, G. B., & Csikszentmihalyi, M. (1996). The effect of perceived challenges and skills on the quality of subjective experience. *Journal of Personality, 64,* 274-310.

McInman, A. D., & Grove, J. R. (1991). Peak moments in sport: a literature review. *Quest, 43*, 333 - 351.

Partington, S., Partington, E., & Olivier, S. (2009). The dark side of flow : a qualitative study of dependence in big wave surfing. *The Sport Psychologist, 23*, 170 - 186.

Perry, S. K. (1999). *Writing in flow*. Cincinnati: Writer's Digest Books.

Privette, G. (1981). Dynamics of peak performance. *Journal of Humanistic Psychology, 21*(1), 57-67.

Rheinberg, F., Vollmeyer, R., & Engeser, S. (2003). Die Erfassung des Flow Erlebens [Measuring flow experience]. In J. Stiensmeier-Pelster & F. Rheinberg (Hrsg.), *Diagnostik von Motivation und Selbstkonzept* (pp. 261-279). Göttingen: Hogrefe.

Rheinberg, F. (1991). Flow-Experience when motorcycling: A study of a special human condition. In R. Brendicke (Ed.), *Safety, environment, future*. (pp. 349-362). Bochum, Germany: Institut für Zweiradsicherheit (ifZ).

Sawyer, K. (1992). Improvisational creativity: an analysis of jazz performance. *Creativity Research Journal, 5*, 253–263.

Schüler, J. (2007). Arousal of flow-experience in a learning setting and its effects on exam-performance and affect. *Zeitschrift für Pädagogische Psychologie, 21*, 217 - 227.

Thatcher, A., Wretschko, G., & Fridjohn, P. (2008). Online flow experiences, problematic internet use and internet procrastination. *Computers in Human Behavior, 24*, 2236 -2254.

Zuckerman, M. (1994). *Behavioral Expressions and Biosocial Bases of Sensation Seeking*. Cambridge, England: Cambridge University Press

Zuckerman, M. (1996). Item revisions in the Sensation Seeking Scale Form V(SSS-V). *Personality and Individual Difference, 20,* 515

Zuckerman, M. (2006). *Sensation seeking and risky behavior*. American Psychological Association.

Index

B

C

D

E

F

G

H

I

J

K

L

M

N

O

P

Q

R

S

T

W

X

Y

Z

8